A Color Handbook

Small Animal Anesthesia and Pain Management

SECOND EDITION

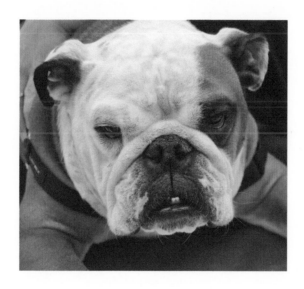

A Color Handbook

Small Animal Anesthesia and Pain Management

SECOND EDITION

A Color Handbook

Small Animal Anesthesia and Pain Management

SECOND EDITION

Edited by Jeff C Ko
DVM, MS, Dip ACVAA

Professor of Anesthesiology
Department of Veterinary Clinical Sciences
College of Veterinary Medicine, Purdue University
West Lafayette, Indiana, USA

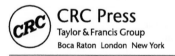

CRC Press
Taylor & Francis Group
Boca Raton London New York

CRC Press is an imprint of the
Taylor & Francis Group, an **informa** business

CRC Press
Taylor & Francis Group
6000 Broken Sound Parkway NW, Suite 300
Boca Raton, FL 33487-2742

Printed on acid-free paper

International Standard Book Number-13: 978-1-138-03568-3 (Paperback)
978-1-138-34563-8 (Hardback)

Library of Congress Cataloging-in-Publication Data

Names: Ko, Jeff C., editor. | Ko, Jeff C. Anesthesia and pain management in dogs and cats.
Title: Small animal anesthesia and pain management : a color handbook / editor, Jeff Ko.
Other titles: Anesthesia and pain management in dogs and cats
Description: Second edition. | Boca Raton : CRC Press/Taylor & Francis, 2019. | Preceded by Anesthesia and pain management in dogs and cats / Jeff C. Ko. c2013. | Includes bibliographical references and index.
Identifiers: LCCN 2018024366| ISBN 9781138035683 (pbk. : alk. paper) | ISBN 9781138345638 (hardback : alk. paper)
Subjects: LCSH: Veterinary anesthesia--Handbooks, manuals, etc. | MESH: Anesthesia--veterinary | Analgesia--veterinary | Pain Management--veterinary | Pets
Classification: LCC SF914 .S634 2018 | NLM SF 914 | DDC 636.089/796--dc23
LC record available at https://lccn.loc.gov/2018024366

Visit the Taylor & Francis Web site at
http://www.taylorandfrancis.com

and the CRC Press Web site at
http://www.crcpress.com

Contents

CHAPTER 3
Preanesthetic medication: drugs and dosages.................... 51
Jeff C Ko

CHAPTER 11
Airway management and
ventilation 211
Ann B Weil and Jeff C Ko

CHAPTER 12
Anesthetic considerations
for patients requiring upper
airway surgery and patients
requiring thoracic surgery.......219
Jennifer C Hess

CHAPTER 17
Anesthesia and sedation for radiography, ultrasound, CT, and MRI patients................259
Jeff C Ko

CHAPTER 18
Anesthetic considerations for orthopedic surgical patients ...265
Bonnie L Hay Kraus

CHAPTER 19
Anesthetic considerations for dental and oral–facial surgeries 279
Jeff C Ko

CHAPTER 20
Analgesia and sedation of emergency/intensive care unit patients.............................287
Elizabeth J Thomovsky and
Aimee C Brooks

CHAPTER 24
Acute pain management........353
Jeff C Ko

Preface

The first edition of this *Small Animal Anesthesia and Pain Management – A Color Handbook* was published in October 2012. The book has been a popular anesthesia textbook among veterinary practitioners, veterinary nurses/technicians, and students alike, simply because it contains high-quality photographs on various anesthesia techniques and related subjects.

In this second edition, we not only include the content of the first edition in essence, but also greatly expand on the anesthetic techniques used in dealing with patients with various diseases subjected to diagnostic or surgical procedures. In addition, we have included new drugs, monitors, anesthetic/analgesic techniques, and information made available since the first edition was published.

The goals of this handbook, similar to those of the first edition, are to provide the anesthetist with (1) a quick information source about anesthetic equipment, monitors, drug dosages, and anesthetic techniques via high-quality photographs, flow charts, tables, and illustrations; (2) a resource for making anesthetic/analgesic decisions for both healthy and various organ-dysfunctional animals. Each chapter from the first edition has been updated, and the number of authors increased from the initial 6 to 17 specialists, to reflect the wide range of experience and expertise of practitioners in this field.

Because this book is not intended to be a comprehensive or theory-based textbook, it allows the authors to be able to provide complex anesthetic information and techniques in a very precise and practical way. As the key author of this book, I hope that the reader continues to find this color handbook a useful tool when practicing anesthesia and pain management.

Jeff C Ko

Acknowledgments

This book is dedicated to my parents and family, especially my father who passed away in 2017. He was unable to read and write English but worked as hard as he could as an immigrant citizen to the United States for 40 years. This book is also dedicated to my wife and two sons, who provided encouragement and support during the writing of this book. Special thanks also go to all the contributing authors for unselfishly sharing their wealth of veterinary experience with the reader. I would also like to thank Kim Sederquist, BS, RVT, VTS (Cardiology), who kindly provided ECG strips for Chapter 22.

My thanks also to all the readers who bought the first edition of this book and continue to provide their support and encouragement. Special gratitude goes to Alice Oven, Paul Bennett, and Ruth Maxwell of the Taylor & Francis Group, who worked tirelessly in editing and proofreading the manuscript with great care. Warm acknowledgment also goes to my DVM students, veterinary technology students, graduate students, residents, and veterinary technicians/nurses who challenged my thoughts and ideas throughout the writing of both first and second editions of the book.

Contributors

Tokiko Kushiro-Banker BVM, MS, PhD, Dip ACVAA
Clinical Assistant Professor, Veterinary Anesthesiology
Department of Veterinary Clinical Sciences
College of Veterinary Medicine, Purdue University
West Lafayette, Indiana, USA

Aimee C Brooks DVM, MS, Dip ACVECC
Clinical Assistant Professor, Emergency and Critical Care
Department of Veterinary Clinical Sciences
College of Veterinary Medicine, Purdue University
West Lafayette, Indiana, USA

Lauren R Frank DVM, MS, CVA, CVCH, CCRT, Dip ACVSMR
Physical Rehabilitation and Acupuncture Service
Long Island Veterinary Specialists
Plainview, New York, USA

Stefania C Grasso DVM, MS, Dip ACVAA
Faculté de Médecine Vétérinaire
Université de Montréal
Montréal, Quebec, Canada

Tamara L Grubb DVM, PhD, Dip ACVAA
Assistant Clinical Professor, Anesthesia and Analgesia
Department of Veterinary Clinical Sciences
College of Veterinary Medicine, Washington State University
Pullman, Washington, USA

Jennifer C Hess DVM, MS, Dip ACVAA
Department of Veterinary Clinical Sciences
College of Veterinary Medicine, Purdue University
West Lafayette, Indiana, USA

Tomohito Inoue DVM
Department of Veterinary Clinical Sciences
College of Veterinary Medicine, Purdue University
West Lafayette, Indiana, USA

Paula A Johnson DVM
Clinical Assistant Professor, Emergency and Critical Care
Department of Veterinary Clinical Sciences
College of Veterinary Medicine, Purdue University
West Lafayette, Indiana, USA

Jeff C Ko DVM, MS, Dip ACVAA
Professor of Anesthesiology
Department of Veterinary Clinical Sciences
College of Veterinary Medicine, Purdue University
West Lafayette, Indiana, USA

Rebecca A Krimins DVM, MS
Assistant Professor of Radiology and Radiological Science
School of Medicine, John Hopkins University
Baltimore, Maryland, USA

Bonnie L Hay Kraus DVM, Dip ACVAA, Dip ACV
Assistant Professor
Iowa State University College of Veterinary Medicine
Ames, Iowa, USA

Andrea L Looney DVM, Dip ACVAA, CCRP, Dip ACVSMR
Anesthesiologist, Learning & Development Team, Specialists
Ethos Veterinary Health
Woburn, Massachusetts, USA

Talisha M Moore DVM, Dip ACVIM (Neurology)
Assistant Clinical Professor, Neurology/Neurosurgery
Mississippi State University, College of Veterinary Medicine
Mississippi, USA

Nicholas J Rancilio DVM, MS, Dip ACVR (Radiation Oncology)
Assistant Professor, Radiation Oncology
Department of Clinical Sciences
College of Veterinary Medicine, Auburn University
Auburn, Alabama, USA

Patrick Roynard DVM, Dip ACVIM (Neurology)
Neurology/Neurosurgery Department
Long Island Veterinary Specialists
Plainview, New York, USA
and
Fipapharm
Mont-Saint-Aignan, France

J Catharine Scott-Moncrieff VetMB, MA, MS,
DECVIM (Companion Animal), DSAM,
Dip ACVIM (Small Animal Internal Medicine)
Department Head, Professor, Small Animal
Internal Medicine
Department of Veterinary Clinical Sciences
College of Veterinary Medicine, Purdue
University
West Lafayette, Indiana, USA

Elizabeth J Thomovsky DVM, MS, Dip ACVECC
Clinical Assistant Professor, Small Animal
Emergency and Critical Care
Department of Veterinary Clinical Sciences
College of Veterinary Medicine, Purdue
University
West Lafayette, Indiana, USA

Stephanie A Thomovsky DVM, MS, Dip ACVIM
(Neurology), CCRP
Clinical Assistant Professor, Veterinary
Neurology
Department of Veterinary Clinical Sciences
College of Veterinary Medicine, Purdue
University
West Lafayette, Indiana, USA

Ann B Weil MS, DVM, Dip ACVAA
Clinical Professor
Department of Veterinary Clinical Sciences
College of Veterinary Medicine, Purdue
University
West Lafayette, Indiana, USA

Huisheng Xie DVM, PhD
Clinical Professor – Integrative Medicine
Department of Comparative, Diagnostic and
Population Medicine
University of Florida
Gainesville, Florida, USA

Abbreviations

ABG	arterial blood gas
ACD	anticoagulant citrate dextrose
ACh	acetylcholine
ACVAA	American College of Veterinary Anesthesia and Analgesia
AKI	acute kidney injury
ALP	alkaline phosphatase
ALT	alanine aminotransferase
APL	adjustable pressure limiting (valve)
aPTT	activated partial thromboplastin time
ASA	American Society of Anesthesiologists
AST	aspartate aminotransferase
ASTM	American Society for Testing and Materials
ATP	adenosine triphosphate
AV	atrioventricular
AVMA	American Veterinary Medical Association
BBB	bundle branch block
BCS	body condition score
BG	blood glucose
BIS	bispectral index (monitor)
BLK	butorphanol–lidocaine–ketamine
BMBT	buccal mucosal bleeding time
BNZ	benzodiazepines
bpm	beats per minute
BP	blood pressure
BUN	blood urea nitrogen
BW	body weight
cAMP	cyclic adenosine monophosphate
CBC	complete blood count
CBF	cerebral blood flow
$CMRO_2$	cerebral metabolic rate
CNS	central nervous system
CO	cardiac output
CO_2	carbon dioxide
COX	cylcooxygenase
CPDA	citrate-phosphate-dextrose-adenine
CPP	cerebral perfusion pressure
CPR	cardiopulmonary resuscitation
CRI	constant rate infusion
CRT	capillary refill time
CSF	cerebrospinal fluid
CT	computed tomography

Cytoco	cytochrome c oxidase
DBK	dexmedetomidine–butorphanol–ketamine
DCM	dilated cardiomyopathy
DEA	dog erythrocyte antigen
DIC	disseminated intravascular coagulation
DISS	diameter index safety system
DKA	diabetic ketoacidosis
EBRT	external beam radiation therapy
DRT	definitive radiation therapy
ECG	electrocardiogram/electrocardiography
EDTA	ethylenediaminetetraacetic acid
EEG	electroencephalogram/electroencephalography
ERG	electroretinography
$ETCO_2$	end-tidal carbon dioxide
ETT	endotracheal tube
FDA	Food and Drug Administration
FiO_2	inspiratory fraction of oxygen
FLK	fentanyl–lidocaine–ketamine
FFP	fresh frozen plasma
FLK	fentanyl–lidocaine–ketamine
FP	frozen plasma
FROGS	Flowmeter, Regulator, vapOrizer, Gas supply, Scavenger
FSNB	femoral/sciatic nerve block
GABA	gamma-aminobutyric acid
GDV	gastric dilatation/volvulus
GER	gastroesophageal reflux
GFR	glomerular filtration rate
GGT	gamma glutamyltransferase
GI	gastrointestinal
Gy	Gray
H_2O	water
HCM	hypertrophic cardiomyopathy
Hct	hematocrit
HFV	high-frequency ventilation
HLK	hydromorphone–lidocaine–ketamine
HPBCD	2-alpha-hydroxypropyl beta cyclodextrin
HR	heart rate
IAP	intra-abdominal pressure
IC	intercostal
ICP	intracranial pressure
ICU	intensive care unit

ID	internal diameter	PG	propylene glycol
I:E	inspiratory to expiratory (time ratio)	PI	perfusion index
		PIP	peak inspiratory pressure
IM	intramuscular/intramuscularly	PISS	pin index safety system
IOP	intraocular pressure	PK/PD	pharmacokinetic/dynamic
IPPV	intermittent positive-pressure ventilation	PNST	peripheral nerve sheath tumor
		PO	per os/orally
IT	intratracheal/intratracheally	pRBC	packed red blood cell
IV	intravenous/intravenously	PRT	palliative radiation therapy
IVDD	intervertebral disc disease	PSGAG	polysulfated glycosaminoglycan
KCl	potassium chloride	psi	pounds per square inch
kPa	kilopascals	PT	prothrombin time
LA	local anesthetic	PTT	partial thromboplastin time
LASER	low-level impulse light amplification by stimulated emission of radiation	PVC	polyvinyl chloride
		PVI	plethysmographic variability index
LED	light-emitting diode	RBC	red blood cell
LLLT	low-level laser therapy	RNA	renal nerve activity
LRS	lactated Ringer's solution	ROS	reactive oxygen species
LS	lumbosacral (epidural)	RPE	re-expansion pulmonary edema
MAC	minimum alveolar concentration	RR	respiratory rate
MAP	mean arterial blood pressure	RUMM	radius/ulna/median/musculocutaneous (block)
MCH	mean corpuscular hemoglobin		
MCHC	mean corpuscular hemoglobin concentration	SA	sinoatrial
		SaO_2	hemoglobin oxygen saturation measured by arterial blood gas analysis
MCV	mean corpuscular volume		
MLK	morphine–lidocaine–ketamine		
MOA	mu opioid agonist	SC	subcutaneous/subcutaneously
MRI	magnetic resonance imaging	SG	specific gravity
MV	minute volume	SNS	sympathetic nervous system
NAALT	North American Association of Photobiomodulation	SpO_2	hemoglobin oxygen saturation measured by pulse oximeter
NaCl	sodium chloride	SSI	surgical site infection
NIOSH	National Institute of Occupational Safety and Health	SV	stroke volume
		SVR	systemic vascular resistance
NMBA	neuromuscular blocking agent	SVT	supraventricular tachycardia
NMDA	N-methyl D-aspartate	TCM	Traditional Chinese Medicine
NO	nitric oxide	TCVM	Traditional Chinese Veterinary Medicine
NRS	numerical rating scale		
NSAID	non-steroidal anti-inflammatory drug	TENS	transcutaneous electrical nerve stimulation
OA	osteoarthritis	THDex	Telazol–hydromorphone–Dexdomitor
OSHA	Occupational Safety and Health Administration		
		TIVA	total intravenous anesthesia
OTM	oral transmucosal/transmucosally	TKX	Telazol–ketamine–xylazine
		TMDex	Telazol–morphine–Dexdomitor
$PaCO_2$	partial pressure of arterial carbon dioxide	TNDex	Telazol–nalbuphine–Dexdomitor
		TOF	train-of-four
PaO_2	partial pressure of arterial oxygen	TP	total protein
PBM	photobiomodulation	TPLO	tibial plateau leveling osteotomy
PCV	packed cell volume	TS	total solids
PDA	patent ductus arteriosus	TSDex	Telazol–Simbadol–dexmedetomidine
PEEP	positive end expiratory pressure		

TTA	tibial tuberosity advancement	VOC	vaporizer-out-of-the-circuit
TTD	Telazol–Torbugesic–Domitor	VPC	ventricular premature
TTDex	Telazol–Torbugesic–Dexdomitor		contraction
TV	tidal volume	V/Q	ventilation–perfusion
VAS	visual analog scale		(mismatch)
VIC	vaporizer-in-the-circuit	WBC	white blood cell

CHAPTER 1

Equipment for inhalant anesthesia

Jeff C Ko

Introduction

Inhalant anesthetic equipment includes an anesthesia machine and a breathing circuit (**Figs. 1.1, 1.2**). Other important equipment for inhalant anesthesia includes a reservoir bag, endotracheal tube, laryngoscope, and blade, as well as oxygen and other medical gases. The purpose of the inhalant anesthesia machine, together with the breathing circuit, is to deliver oxygen and inhalant anesthetic effectively to the animal and to remove carbon dioxide (CO_2) from the animal's respiratory system. This chapter describes the primary components of inhalant anesthetic equipment and their functions.

Components of the anesthesia machine

No matter how simple or complicated an anesthesia machine looks, it has five basic components (Flowmeter, Regulator, vapOrizer, Gas supply, Scavenger), which can be remembered using the acronym **FROGS**.

FLOWMETERS (FIGS. 1.3, 1.4)

Key points about flowmeters:

- The flowmeter is used to control precisely the delivery of a specific amount of medical gas through the vaporizer to the patient.
- A flowmeter is required for each medical gas.
- There are two types of flowmeter: pediatric and adult (**Fig. 1.4**). A pediatric flowmeter provides more precise control of the flow rate and allows the anesthesia machine to run with a precise, low flow rate. It is therefore preferred for running a low-oxygen flow rate.
- The flow rate is determined by observing the position of the bobbin or float in the flowmeter. The bobbin or float comes in various shapes and sizes. Ball-shaped bobbins are read at the center or widest diameter of the float (**Fig. 1.5**). Bobbins with other shapes are read at the top of the float (**Fig. 1.6**).
- Flowmeters are agent specific and color coded (**Fig. 1.3**). For example, in the USA, flowmeters for oxygen are coded green, while flowmeters for nitrous oxide are coded blue and medical room air flowmeters are coded yellow. This may not be the same in other parts of the world.

REGULATORS (PRESSURE REDUCING VALVES)

Key points about regulators:

- The pressure regulator, also called a pressure reducing valve, is designed to reduce the high pressure from the medical gas, which is supplied from a portable or storage tank (up to 2,200 psi [15,168.4 kPa] in a size E portable oxygen tank, **Fig. 1.7**), to a working pressure (15–30 psi [103.4–206.8 kPa]) that does not damage the anesthesia machine or the patient's airway.

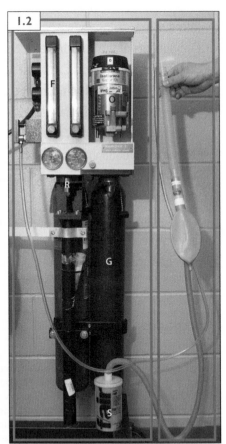

Fig. 1.2 An anesthesia machine (portion outlined with the green color box) with a non-rebreathing circuit (portion outlined with the red color box). The acronym for the five basic components (FROGS) is marked. Note the simple structure of a non-breathing circuit, which is built to have minimal resistance to breathing.

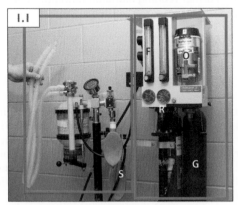

Fig. 1.1 An anesthesia machine (portion outlined with the green color box) with a rebreathing circuit (portion outlined with the red color box) and an isoflurane vaporizer-out-of-the-circuit. The acronym for the five basic components (FROGS) is marked on the image. The rebreathing circuit has a pair of breathing hoses and a CO_2 absorbent.

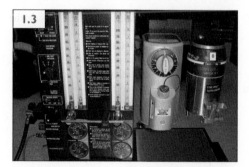

Figs. 1.3, 1.4 Two sets of flowmeters each with a rotameter and a needle valve at the bottom (**Fig. 1.3**); note the nitrous oxide (blue color) and oxygen (green color) each has their own set of flowmeters. Note the metal bar in front of the rotameters to prevent accidental adjustment of the flowmeters. Pediatric flowmeters (on the left side, **1.4**) are graduated in milliliters from zero to 1,000 ml, while adult flowmeters (on the right side, **1.4**) are graduated in liters.

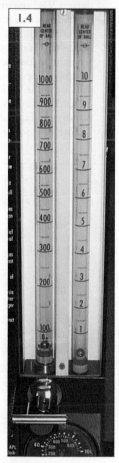

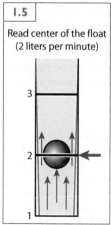

1.5 Read center of the float (2 liters per minute)

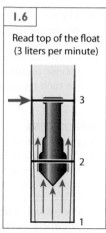

1.6 Read top of the float (3 liters per minute)

Figs. 1.5, 1.6 Oxygen enters the rotameter and passes through a bobbin (float), exiting at the top of the flowmeter to enter the machine and vaporizer. Ball-shaped bobbins are read at the center or widest diameter of the bobbin (**1.5**). Other shapes of bobbins are read at the top of the bobbin (**1.6**). Note that the flowmeter is tapered in shape. The clearance between the bobbin and the wall of the flowmeter increases from bottom (narrow) to top (wide).

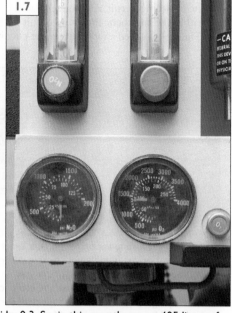

Fig. 1.7 This pressure gauge indicates a partially full size E oxygen tank of approximately 1,350 psi (9308 kPa). A full size E oxygen tank has a pressure of approximately 2,200 psi (15,168.4 kPa). A quick way to calculate the amount of oxygen (in liters) left in the size E tank is to multiply the pressure in psi by 0.3. So, in this case there are 405 liters of oxygen left in the tank. Note the regulator (brass color) located directly below the pressure gauge. Regulators (and flowmeters) are marked with the corresponding medical gas color.

- The regulator provides a constant flow of gas irrespective of measured changes at the source.
- Given that each medical gas requires a specific regulator, there is one regulator for each medical gas within the anesthesia machine.

VAPORIZERS

Key points about vaporizers:

- A vaporizer (**Fig. 1.8**) is used to add a specific amount of inhalant anesthetic agent to the oxygen/gas (nitrous oxide) mixture in order to anesthetize the patient. The amount of inhalant anesthetic is expressed either as a percentage of the saturate vapor added to the oxygen/gas flow or as a volume percentage of the vapor output.
- Because anesthetic gas (isoflurane or sevoflurane) can vaporize to dangerously high concentrations (isoflurane to 32% and sevoflurane to 22% at sea level in room temperature), a precision vaporizer is required to control precisely the volume of inhalant anesthetic delivered to the patient.
- Vaporizers are largely divided into two types based on their location in relation to the breathing circuit. A vaporizer placed within the anesthetic breathing circuit (**Fig. 1.9**) is called a vaporizer-in-the-circuit (VIC), while a vaporizer placed outside the breathing circuit is called a vaporizer-out-of-the-circuit (VOC).

Vaporizers-in-the-circuit

Specific points related to VICs:

- VICs are non-precision vaporizers of simple construction designed to minimize resistance to breathing. The VIC is less commonly used in current anesthesia practice. However, some practices still have a VIC system. The advantage of the VIC is that it can be used with many different types of anesthetic inhalants, given that it is not calibrated for a specific anesthetic gas (hence the term non-precision vaporizer). The most common VICs are the Ohio #8 bottle vaporizer (**Fig. 1.10**) and Stephen's Universal vaporizer (**Fig. 1.9**); both can be used for halothane, isoflurane, or sevoflurane.

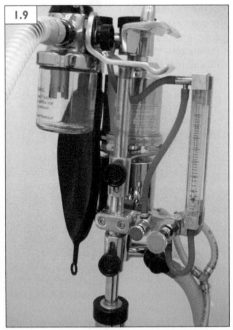

Fig. 1.9 A vaporizer-in-the-circuit is usually a non-precision vaporizer constructed of glass and without flow or temperature compensation. A Stephen glass vaporizer with a Stephen machine is shown. (Image courtesy M. Iqbal Javaid.)

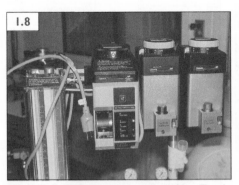

Fig. 1.8 A desflurane vaporizer (left), a Tec 4 isoflurane vaporizer (middle with purple color label), and a Tec 4 halothane vaporizer (on the right with the red label). Note the electric cable and plug on the desflurane vaporizer for the external heat supply required for proper vaporization.

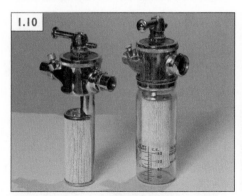

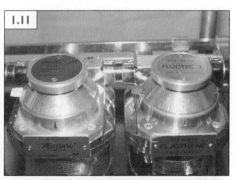

Fig. 1.11 A Tec 3 isoflurane vaporizer (left) and a Tec 3 halothane vaporizer (right).

Fig. 1.10 Ohio #8 bottle vaporizers with a wick in the center of the bottle. The vaporizer on the left is pictured with the glass jar removed to show the wick. When operating with a highly volatile inhalant, such as halothane, isoflurane, or sevoflurane, the wick is removed to reduce the area of vaporization.

- As VICs are not calibrated for a specific anesthetic agent, the calibrators on the vaporizer dial do not indicate the percentage of inhalant delivered to the patient, but rather indicate that the vaporizer is closed, approximately half-way closed, or fully open.
- The anesthetic is vaporized while the patient breathes through the vaporizer. As a result, a VIC must be low resistance in order to minimize the effort required for a patient to breathe through it.

Vaporizer-out-of-the-circuit

Specific points related to VOCs:

- VOCs are precision vaporizers. They are specifically designed for a particular inhalant anesthetic agent, as the vapor pressure differs between agents. These vaporizers are usually complex in design and have a relatively high resistance to breathing. Each precision vaporizer is identified by color and clearly labeled to indicate the associated anesthetic agent (**Fig. 1.11**).
- Most modern vaporizers are designed specifically for isoflurane, sevoflurane, or desflurane and are calibrated precision vaporizers. The advantages of these agent-specific vaporizers are flow rate and temperature compensations. That is, they

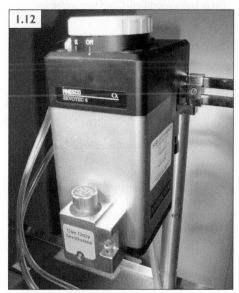

Fig. 1.12 A Tec 4 sevoflurane vaporizer. Note the square shape.

have a stabilized anesthetic concentration output over a wide range of environment temperatures and oxygen flow rates (200 ml to 15 liters per minute).
- Due to the complex internal structure of precision vaporizers, they are high resistance vaporizers and cannot be placed within the breathing circuit.
- There are many different types of modern vaporizers for use with inhalant anesthetic agents (e.g. isoflurane or sevoflurane) including the Tec 3 (**Fig. 1.11**), Tec 4 (**Fig. 1.12**), Tec 5 modified-Ohio (**Fig. 1.13**), Vapor 19.1, and Penlon (**Fig. 1.14**).

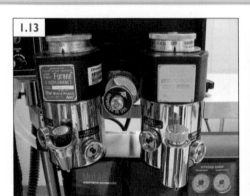

Fig. 1.13 An Ohio vaporizer for isoflurane (left) and a modified-Ohio vaporizer for sevoflurane (right).

Differences between a VIC and a VOC
(See *Table 1.1*)

GAS SUPPLY
- Gas supply refers to the medical gas supply to the anesthesia machine and it may come from a local (portable) source or from a central pipeline source (**Fig. 1.15**).

Carrier gas supply
- The inhalant anesthetic is carried by a carrier gas supply from the machine through the breathing circuit to the patient.

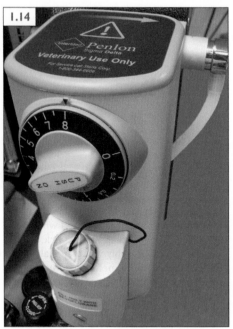

Fig. 1.14 A Penlon sevoflurane vaporizer.

- While oxygen is the most common carrier gas, nitrous oxide is sometimes used as a second carrier gas for isoflurane or sevoflurane. Medical air is sometimes used as well.

Table 1.1 Differences between a VIC and a VOC	
VIC	VOC
Simple construction	Complex construction
Low resistance to breathing	Relatively high resistance to breathing
Non-precision (meaningless for calibration)	Precision (requires calibration)
No compensation for changes in temperature or oxygen flow rate	Compensation for changes in temperature and oxygen flow rate
Can be used for multiple inhalant anesthetic agents	Inhalant anesthetic agent specific

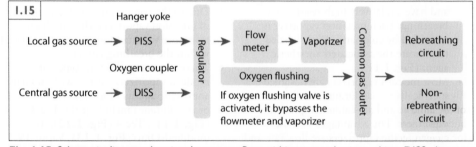

Fig. 1.15 Schematic diagram showing the oxygen flow within an anesthesia machine. DISS, diameter index safety system; PISS, pin index safety system.

Central gas supply (piped gas system)
- An anesthesia machine connected to a central gas supply has a separate connector (**Fig. 1.16**) from the local (portable) gas supply.

Hanger yoke (cylinder yoke)
- The hanger yoke is a device that allows the portable gas tank to be connected to the anesthesia machine (**Fig. 1.17**).
- A pin index safety system (PISS) within the hanger yoke (**Fig. 1.18**) is designed to prevent accidental connection of another medical gas to the oxygen connector and vice versa (**Fig. 1.19**). A similar safety system called the diameter index safety system (DISS) is designed to prevent accidental connection of another medical gas to the oxygen connector from the central gas supply (**Fig. 1.20**).

Common gas outlet
- The common gas outlet (**Fig. 1.21**) is an outlet on the body of the anesthesia machine that allows the carrier gas with the inhalant anesthetic agent to flow out of the machine and into the rebreathing or non-rebreathing circuit.

Oxygen flushing valve
- The oxygen flushing valve is a button on the body of the anesthesia machine. When activated, this valve directs a high volume of oxygen (35–75 liters per minute) at a

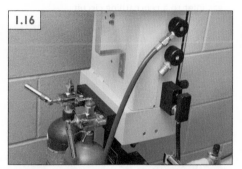

Fig. 1.16 This anesthesia machine, connected to a central pipeline gas supply, has a separate connector (green pipe on the upper right). Oxygen and nitrous oxide size E portable tanks (oxygen, green color tank; nitrous oxide, blue color tank) are mounted on the hanger yoke.

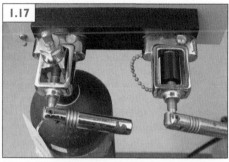

Fig. 1.17 Hanger (or cylinder) yokes are also color coded and designed with a pin index system to prevent accidental placement of the incorrect gas tank. A yoke block has been placed on the nitrous oxide hanger (on the right) as the tank is not being used.

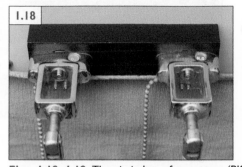

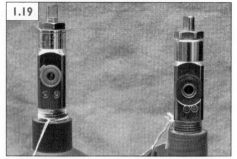

Figs. 1.18, 1.19 The pin index safety system (PISS) is designed to match the different positions of the pin on the hanger yoke and the compressed medical gas tank stem. Note the distance between the two pins (**1.18**) on the hanger yoke and the stems of the compressed gas tanks for oxygen (green code) and nitrous oxide (blue code). Also note that the oxygen tank (**1.19**) has a washer (red color). The washer on the nitrous oxide tank has been removed to show the structure. Without the washer in place the tank will leak when mounting onto the hanger yoke.

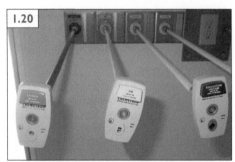

Fig. 1.20 The diameter index safety system (DISS) is another safety feature to prevent accidental connection of medical gas to the unintentional gas supply from the central medical gas bank. Note the color codes and clear labels as well as the different diameter/shapes of the connecters in this picture.

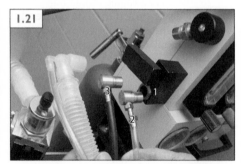

Fig. 1.21 A common gas outlet (1), which is also called a fresh gas outlet, is shown. The metal adapter connected to the transparent hose (2) is a fresh gas inlet to a non-rebreathing circuit (see part of the non-rebreathing circuit on the left). The second metal adapter (3), which is connected to the black hose, is a fresh gas inlet to a rebreathing circuit.

pressure of approximately 58 psi (400 kPa) to bypass the vaporizer and flow directly through the common gas outlet into the breathing circuit.

- The purpose of the oxygen flushing valve is to allow large amounts of oxygen to enter the machine and breathing circuit in a short time to dilute the anesthetic agent concentration during an anesthetic emergency and rapidly decrease the concentration of anesthesia, or, during recovery, to eliminate waste gas.
- Excessive airway pressure will build up with high oxygen flow when using an oxygen flushing valve with a non-breathing circuit. Extreme caution should be taken to avoid using an oxygen flushing valve when a patient is connected to a non-breathing circuit. In contrast, using an oxygen flushing valve with a rebreathing circuit is safe; its complex structures prevent excessive pressure building up in the airway of the patient within a short time.

Portable medical gas source and supply systems

- Portable medical gas source and supply systems are usually in the form of a compressed gas tank or cylinder attached to the anesthesia machine via the hanger yoke (**Fig. 1.16**).

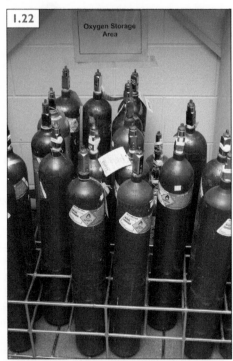

Fig. 1.22 Compressed gas tanks (size E tank in this case) should be stored securely in a designated place.

- Compressed gas tanks are classified by size (e.g. E or H). Size E (**Fig. 1.22**) and size H tanks are most commonly used in the USA.

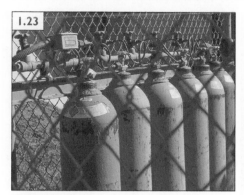

Fig. 1.23 A series of size H tanks can be connected to form a cylinder bank for a pipeline oxygen supply.

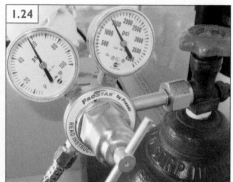

Fig. 1.24 A size H tank is connected to a two-stage regulator. Note that both pressure gauge units register as pounds per square inch (psi).

- A full size E oxygen tank registers a pressure of 2,200 psi (15,168.4 kPa) and contains 660 liters, a 0.3 factor relationship. This can be used to estimate how much oxygen remains in the tank. The oxygen tank pressure reading on the pressure gauge (**Fig. 1.7**) in psi multiplied by 0.3 yields the number of liters of oxygen remaining. Compressed gas tanks should be secured to prevent them falling during storage or transportation (**Fig. 1.22**). The size H tank contains approximately 10 times more oxygen (6,600 liters) than the size E tank and is therefore more economical.
- A series of size H tanks can be connected to form a cylinder-bank system (cylinder manifold system) (**Fig. 1.23**) for a central pipeline gas supply. The size H tanks are usually attached to a two-stage (or dual-stage) regulator (**Fig. 1.24**).

Single-stage and two-stage pressure regulators

Practical questions related to pressure regulators:

- What are the main differences between a single-stage and a two-stage regulator? One distinct difference is the units on the gauges. Both gauges on the two-stage regulator use psi units (pounds per square inch). The single-stage regulator reflects pressure psi, while the flow control valve reflects liters per minute. The advantage of the two-stage regulator is that the pressure flow remains constant until the gas tank is nearly empty. The two-stage regulator, however, should not be confused with a single-stage regulator with a flow control valve or flow gauge. With single-stage regulators the flow control valve does not control the pressure from the tank, only the amount of gas flowing from the tank. It acts as a flowmeter, but registers the flow rate (in liters per minute) on the flow gauge. While the two-stage regulator and the single-stage regulator with a flow control valve and flow gauge look alike, they function very differently.

- Why does the oxygen rate shown on the flowmeter go down to zero when the oxygen flushing valve on the anesthesia machine is pressed? If an anesthesia machine is inadvertently connected to the outlet of the flow control valve of a single-stage regulator on the oxygen bank, the oxygen pressure in the pipeline is inadequate to operate the machine. As a result, the flowmeter on the machine will fluctuate dramatically or fall to a very low flow rate. If the oxygen flush valve on the anesthesia machine is activated, it completely depletes the oxygen supply from the pipeline and the flow of oxygen decreases to zero on the flowmeter.

Central pipeline oxygen supply and source
Liquid oxygen storage tanks
- Liquid oxygen storage tanks (**Fig. 1.25**) are large vacuum-insulated evaporators used to store and supply oxygen.

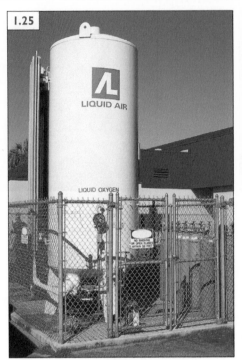

Fig. 1.25 Liquid oxygen storage tanks are usually located outside the hospital building, as shown here.

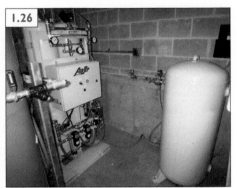

Fig. 1.26 An air compressor collects and compresses room air into a storage tank. The room air is then filtered and concentrated to 90% or greater medical oxygen, which is stored in the oxygen tank for hospital use.

- They are thermally insulated double-walled steel tanks with a pressure regulator that allows oxygen gas to enter the pipelines and maintains the pipeline pressure at about 58 psi (400 kPa).
- Liquid oxygen is stored at –150° to –170° C (–238° to –274°F). As it warms, it becomes gaseous and can be used for central oxygen supply. Bulk liquid oxygen is usually stored in a storage tank located outside the hospital building and the gas is delivered by means of a hospital pipeline system.

Oxygen concentrator
- An oxygen concentrator (also called condenser or compressor, **Fig. 1.26**) is a medical device that concentrates 21% room air oxygen to medical grade oxygen (at 90% or greater) by extracting oxygen through zeolite filters and removing nitrogen as well as other unwanted components of air. Zeolites are hydrated aluminum silicate granules.

- Oxygen concentrators consist of an air intake, compressor, storage tank, zeolite sieve columns, moisture remover, coolers, filters to remove oil, water, and dust, and a pipeline for oxygen delivery. Some oxygen concentrators are small and portable; they have been recently combined with anesthetic machines and serve as an oxygen source.
- Most hospital oxygen concentrators have a large capacity, are stationary and have a large storage tank that allows converted high-percentage oxygen to be dispensed at multiple sites simultaneously.

Pressure regulation
- The pressure of a medical gas delivered from a central pipeline supply is typically regulated down to 50–52 psi (344.7–358.5 kPa) at the wall outlet by the manifold pressure regulator.
- Similarly, the pressure of the size E oxygen cylinder is regulated from 2,200 psi (15,168.4 kPa) down to 48 psi (331 kPa) by the pressure regulator of the anesthesia machine. A result of this final delivered pressure gradient differentiation (i.e. 52 versus 48 psi) is that the anesthesia machine preferentially uses the higher pressure source (52 psi). In other words, the central oxygen pipeline supply is preferred over the portable oxygen tanks (cylinders, 48 psi) when the anesthesia machine is supplied from both

sources (i.e. the oxygen tank is opened and the anesthesia machine is attached to the central pipeline oxygen supply simultaneously).

- There is a one-way check valve in the hanger yoke that prevents the higher pressure central supply from filling the lower pressure tank.

SCAVENGERS

- The waste gas scavenging system is the most effective way of minimizing pollution of the working environment. There are passive and active methods of scavenging waste gas.

Passive scavenging systems

- A simple passive scavenging system is a waste gas hose connecting the anesthesia machine pop-off valve to the wall connector and allowing waste gas to vent outside the building and into the atmosphere. The exhaled gases are directed by the upstream flow of oxygen and passively force the waste gases downstream into the scavenging hose. It must be remembered, however, that if the connector or outlet to the outside environment is physically higher than the vaporizer of the anesthesia machine (e.g. the exit is located in the ceiling), the waste gas cannot rise and be eliminated passively. Waste gas is heavier than ambient air and will not flow upwards passively, unless an active pump is used for evacuation.
- Another passive method of waste gas elimination is to connect the scavenging hose from the pop-off valve in such a way that the waste gas exits to an active

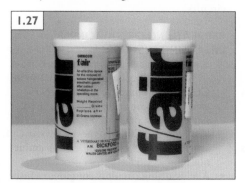

Fig. 1.27 Active charcoal canisters.

charcoal canister (**Fig. 1.27**). If the waste gas flow rate is too high, it can exceed the capacity of the active charcoal to absorb the waste gas, resulting in pollution. If the flow rate of the waste gas is too high, the active charcoal absorbent canister will rattle because of the high resistance of the canister obstructing the gas flow.

- The advantages of an active charcoal canister are that it is effective in absorbing halogenated hydrocarbon anesthetic agents, it has a simple construction, and it can be moved around with the anesthesia machine. The disadvantages of an active charcoal canister system are its high resistance to waste gas flow, its ineffectiveness at eliminating nitrous oxide, and the limited time of use before the canister must be changed. To monitor this, the charcoal absorbent should be weighed before use and frequently during use. When the charcoal canister weighs 50 g more than its initial weight, it should be changed.

Active scavenging system

- An active scavenging system has a similar collecting and transfer system to that of the passive scavenging system, but it has a vacuum pump and an interface that allows negative pressure to vacuum the waste gas from the collecting system as it exits the breathing circuit. An ideal active scavenging system should not actively compete with the fresh oxygen flow within the breathing circuit, or affect the patient's ventilation and oxygenation, if it is correctly set up.
- The advantage of the active scavenging system is its effectiveness at removing waste gas.
- The disadvantages are that, if the system is not connected properly or is not functioning properly, it can competitively vacuum the fresh gas supply and affect the patient's ventilation and oxygenation (as evidenced by a constantly empty reservoir bag) into the scavenging system, resulting in an inadequate supply of fresh gas to the patient.
- An active scavenging system is also more expensive and more complicated to set up.

Health and safety considerations

- In the USA, the Occupational Safety and Health Administration (OSHA) requires veterinary clinics and hospitals to maintain a proper waste gas scavenging system to prevent pollution of the work environment. Other countries also enforce this requirement to ensure safety of the work place through similar legislative bodies (e.g. the National Safety Executive in the UK).
- The OSHA recommends that the maximum accepted concentrations of any volatile halogenated anesthetic agent (isoflurane, halothane, sevoflurane, and desflurane) should not exceed 2 ppm when used alone or 0.5 ppm when used with nitrous oxide. The maximum, time-weighted (8-hour) average concentration of nitrous oxide should not exceed 25 ppm. These requirements vary from country to country and all practitioners must ensure that the safety standards in their region are met.

Breathing circuits and components

An anesthetic breathing circuit (or system) is a conduction system that allows fresh gas and the inhalant anesthetic agent to be delivered from the anesthesia machine to the patient

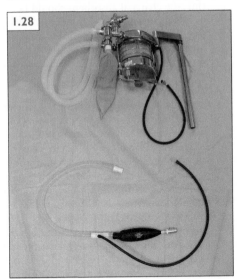

Fig. 1.28 A rebreathing circuit (top) and a Bain's non-rebreathing circuit (bottom). A rebreathing circuit usually is attached to the anesthesia machine (see **Fig. 1.1**) and is supplied with the machine because of its complex structure. The rebreathing circuit shown has been detached from the machine so that it can be contrasted with the non-rebreathing circuit. Note the fresh gas inlet hose (black) in both the rebreathing and the non-rebreathing circuits. This fresh gas inlet hose is connected to the fresh gas outlet (see **Fig. 1.21**) of the anesthesia machine and serves as a conduit to bridge the breathing circuit and the machine.

while eliminating expired CO_2 and other trace gases from the patient to the machine's scavenging system (see **Figs. 1.1** and **1.2** for the location of the breathing circuits). Anesthetic breathing circuits can be largely divided into rebreathing or non-rebreathing circuits (**Fig. 1.28**).

Regardless of the type, breathing circuits all have the following characteristics:
- They allow either spontaneous breathing, manually controlled breathing, or controlled ventilation with positive pressure.
- An ideal breathing circuit allows the patient to breathe easily with minimal resistance and minimal dead space.
- Most breathing circuits consist of a breathing hose (tubing), a reservoir bag, and a pressure relief valve.

The classification of breathing circuits is complicated and at times confusing. *Table 1.2* lists the similarities and differences of rebreathing and non-rebreathing circuits.

REBREATHING CIRCUIT (CIRCLE BREATHING SYSTEM)

- A rebreathing circuit enables part of the expired alveolar gas, which contains CO_2, unused oxygen, and anesthetic gases, to be circled back and inspired as part of the next fresh gas input; however, the CO_2 is removed by the CO_2 absorbent via chemical reactions and is not rebreathed.
- A rebreathing circuit is composed of two one-way valves (one on the inspiratory

Table 1.2 Similarities and differences between rebreathing and non-rebreathing circuits

Differences	Rebreathing	Non-rebreathing
Reuse of oxygen and inhalant	Yes	No
Construction of the circuit	Complex	Simple
Structure contains carbon dioxide absorbent	Yes	No
Structure has one-way (unidirectional) valve	Yes	No
Work of breathing (resistance to breathing)	High	Low
Required fresh gas (oxygen) flow rate	Low	High
Selection for use in body weight	≥7–7.5 kg	≤7–7.5 kg
Terminology used	Semi-closed, closed circuit	Mapleson A–F circuit, semi-opened

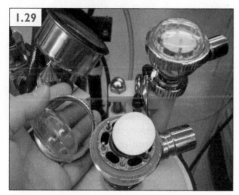

Fig. 1.29 The one-way valve has been removed from the dome of an expiratory limb. Note that the inspiratory one-way valve is located in the dome of the inspiratory limb. Also, this modern one-way valve is constructed of plastic instead of metal to minimize resistance. One-way valves should be removed for cleaning and air dried to prevent a build-up of moisture.

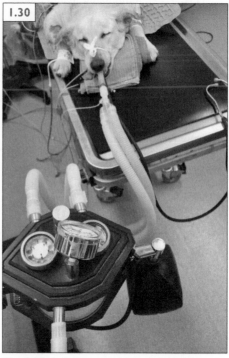

Fig. 1.30 A dog connected to a rebreathing circuit. Because of the complex structures in the air passage, a rebreathing circuit provides relatively high resistance to breathing compared with a non-rebreathing circuit. Note the pressure manometer and the pop-off valve are located between the two one-way valves (round shape), which sit on the top of the soda lime canister.

limb and one on the expiratory limb) (**Fig. 1.29**), a reservoir bag, a fresh gas inlet, a canister for holding a CO_2 absorbent, and a pop-off valve (sometimes called an overflow valve or an airway pressure limiting valve). Because of these structures, breathing resistance is higher with a rebreathing circuit than with a non-rebreathing circuit (**Fig. 1.30**). Since some of the exhaled alveolar gases are reused in the rebreathing circuit, and the elimination of CO_2 is accomplished by CO_2 absorbents, a lower oxygen or fresh gas flow rate can be used (approximately 10–20 ml/kg body weight/min) than the oxygen or fresh gas flow rate on a non-rebreathing circuit.

- The key components of a rebreathing circuit are described below.

Inspiratory and expiratory valves (one-way valves)

- One-way valves allow the anesthetic agent and exhaled gases to flow in one direction only (**Fig. 1.29**). They are seated in the domes of the inspiratory and expiratory limbs of the rebreathing circuit and direct inspired gases toward the animal on inspiration and expired gases away from the animal on expiration.
- One-way valves used to be constructed of metal and contributed to most of the breathing resistance in a rebreathing circuit. Newer one-way valves are plastic (**Fig. 1.29**), minimizing weight-induced resistance to breathing.
- Dust and moisture from the airway tend to cause these one-way valves to stick open. As a result, the valves should be cleaned regularly.
- An open expiratory one-way valve generates mechanical dead space from the entire expiratory limb and CO_2 is rebreathed. If an inspiratory one-way-valve remains open, it also contributes to CO_2 accumulation in the rebreathing tubing and CO_2 is rebreathed.

Pressure manometer

- A pressure manometer is a pressure gauge connected to the rebreathing circuit (**Fig. 1.31**). Non-rebreathing circuits usually do not have a pressure manometer in order to avoid additional resistance to the airway. Furthermore, the manometer is heavy and tends to drag on the endotracheal tube when attached to a non-rebreathing circuit, and this could lead to accidental extubation.
- The manometer is used to monitor the pressure within the breathing circuit during spontaneous, assisted, or controlled ventilation and to check for leaks in the breathing circuit.
- During assisted or controlled ventilation, the peak inspiratory pressure should not exceed 15–20 cmH$_2$O in small patients. To monitor the peak inspiratory pressure it is necessary to use a pressure manometer.
- A pressure manometer can also be used to check for leaks around the endotracheal cuff when connected to a breathing circuit. Immediately following endotracheal intubation and inflation of the endotracheal tube cuff, the pop-off valve should be

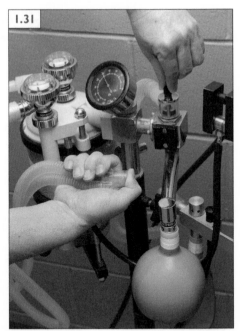

Fig. 1.31 A pressure manometer is useful for monitoring positive pressure within the breathing circuit and ensuring that safety pressure is applied to the airway. It is also useful for checking for leaks in the anesthesia machine and breathing circuit. During leak checking, the breathing bag distends when the pop-off valve is closed and the Y-piece is occluded. The pressure manometer registers 30 cmH$_2$O. The pop-off valve (being turned by the fingers) is part of the rebreathing circuit and allows excess gas to escape from the machine and breathing circuit.

closed and the reservoir bag squeezed to build an airway pressure of 15–20 cmH$_2$O, while at the same time listening for leaks around the endotracheal tube (**Fig. 1.32**).
- Pressure manometers use a scale of cmH$_2$O and/or mmHg.

Pop-off valve

- A pop-off valve (also called an adjustable pressure limiting [APL] valve, **Fig. 1.31**) is an adjustable, spring-loaded one-way valve. When the valve is in an open position it allows exhaled gases, waste gas, and unused fresh gas to exit the breathing circuit. During the expiration phase of spontaneous breathing, a positive pressure within the breathing circuit is generated, which causes the spring-loaded valve to

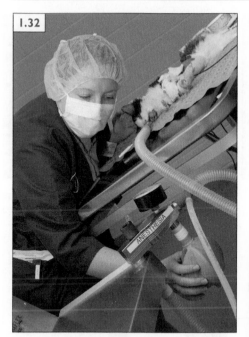

Fig. 1.32 Proper inflation of the endotracheal tube cuff can be checked by squeezing the reservoir bag of the breathing circuit to a peak airway pressure of 15–20 cmH$_2$O while at the same time listening for leaking gas from the endotracheal tube.

open and allows the exhaled gases to exit. It only takes 1–2 cmH$_2$O (0.1–0.2 kPa) of pressure to open the valve when the pop-off valve is in the open position.
- If a pop-off valve is malfunctioning, the valve is open at all time while it is in its open position. This allows the exhaled gases to exit without there being a 1–2 cmH$_2$O pressure build up within the breathing circuit. As a result, the anesthetic gas and oxygen within the reservoir bag and breathing circuits are vacuumed by the active scavenging system, resulting in a deflated reservoir bag.
- All the gases in the pop-off valve are passed to the waste gas scavenger collection system.
- The spring adjustment allows the pop-off valve to be opened in various positions to alter the amount of gas that exits the breathing circuit.
- If the pop-off valve is completely closed, no gas exits and pressure builds within the breathing circuit. Since fresh gas continues

to enter the breathing circuit and the animal continues to expire waste gas, the pressure increases in the animal's airway and lungs, eventually resulting in barotrauma. It is therefore important to watch for an inadvertently closed pop-off valve.

Y-piece of breathing hose
- The Y-piece of a rebreathing circuit (**Fig. 1.33**) connects the endotracheal tube adapter to the inspiratory and expiratory limbs of the breathing circuit (**Fig. 1.34**). This is usually called a "Y-breathing circuit".

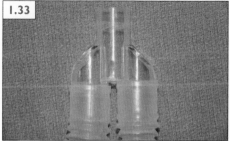

Fig. 1.33 The Y-piece of a breathing hose.

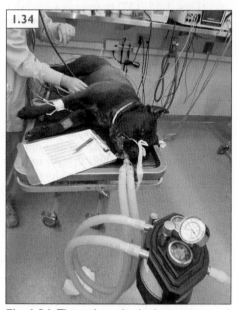

Fig. 1.34 The endotracheal tube is connected to the patient end of the Y-piece and the breathing hoses are attached to the inspiratory and expiratory limbs of the breathing circuit. The Y-piece serves to connect the endotracheal tube to the breathing hoses.

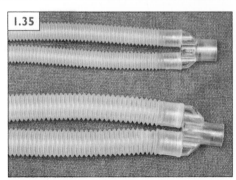

Fig. 1.35 Human pediatric (top) and adult (bottom) breathing hoses.

- The Y-piece contributes to the mechanical dead space and contains some of the exhaled air respired during each breath.
- The Y-piece usually has a 22 mm internal diameter (ID) to accept the 15 mm ID endotracheal tube adapter.

Breathing hoses (or tubings)

- Rebreathing circuits usually have two breathing tubes in parallel (**Figs. 1.35, 137**) to serve as a conduit for anesthetic gas and oxygen. One breathing tube connects to the inspiratory limb of the rebreathing circuit and the other connects to the expiratory limb of the rebreathing circuit.
- Breathing hoses are constructed of either rubber or clear plastic materials. The plastic hoses are easy to inspect, are light weight, and are usually disposable, although they can sustain a medium duration of use. Rubber (usually in black color) breathing hoses are no longer popular because they are heavy, difficult to inspect, and less durable for use over time.
- Breathing hoses are corrugated to resist kinking, increase flexibility, and minimize obstruction within the tubing from airway secretions. However, the corrugation increases resistance to breathing. For animals >7.5 kg (16.5 lb) but <15 kg (33 lb), a human pediatric breathing tubing (9.52 mm ID with a shorter length, **Fig. 1.35**) can be used to minimize breathing resistance.

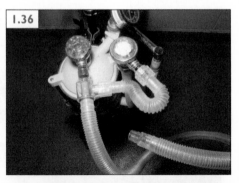

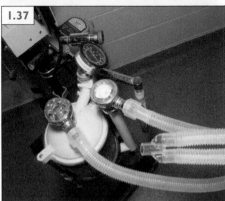

Figs. 1.36, 1.37 A new rebreathing hose design, called a 'unilimb' or 'universal F' breathing circuit (**1.36**), is shown. While the hose is called 'university F breathing circuit', it has in fact dual hoses, one connected to the inspiratory limb and one to the expiratory limb. When these hoses are connected backward with the inspiratory and expiratory limb, respectively, all the advantages of thermal efficiency and humidification are lost. The universal F breathing circuit should not be confused with a Bain's non-rebreathing circuit, even though they look very similar because both are of coaxial design (with a green colored house inside the white colored hose). A traditional bi-lateral breathing hose is shown (**1.37**).

- The 'unilimb' or 'universal F' breathing circuit (**Fig. 1.36**) is a different design of rebreathing hose that is commonly used in the USA and is available in other countries around the world. The advantages of the universal F breathing circuit include the single-limbed design that eliminates the bulkiness of the conventional parallel limbed breathing tubes. The coaxial design is thermally efficient with humidification, so inspired gases are spontaneously warmed and humidified by the exhaled gases exiting the outer tubing. The universal F breathing circuit is available in adult and pediatric sets with different diameters (and frequently with different color coded) to minimize the resistance to breathing. One disadvantage of the universal breathing circuit is that it has a slightly higher resistance to breathing than the regular Y-breathing circuit. The other disadvantage is that when the inspiratory and expiratory hoses are connected backward with the inspiratory and expiratory limb, respectively, of the rebreathing circuit, it loses all the thermal efficiency and humidification advantages.

Fresh gas inlet (Fig. 1.21)

- A fresh gas inlet allows oxygen and anesthetic gas to enter the rebreathing circuit or the non-rebreathing circuit from the common gas outlet of the anesthesia machine.
- The fresh gas inlet is an important connection between the anesthesia machine and the breathing circuit.

Reservoir bag

- Reservoir bags are also called rebreathing bags when they are used in a rebreathing circuit (**Fig. 1.38**).
- The bag accommodates the peak inspiratory flow rate during inspiration and provides adequate fresh gas volume to the patient. Without a bag in place, a peak inspiratory

flow rate that exceeds the amount of gas in the breathing circuit will result in the animal inspiring ambient air and the anesthetic concentration and oxygen will be diluted by the entrapped room air.

- A reservoir bag can be used to assist or control ventilation by squeezing the bag manually. It also allows anesthetists to monitor the patient's breathing pattern during spontaneous ventilation.
- Selecting the size of reservoir bag to be used is based on the tidal volume of the animal. The bag should be 3–5 times the anesthetized animal's tidal volume (10 ml/kg). A quick way of selecting a reservoir bag is to use 1 liter for every 13.5–16.0 kg (30–35 lb) body weight or 0.5 liter for every 6.8 kg (15 lb) body weight (*Table 1.3*).
- Reservoir bags are commercially available for small animals in 0.5, 1, 2, 3, and 5 liter sizes.
- A reservoir bag that is too large slows the change in anesthetic concentration during induction and recovery because the breathing circuit volume barrier is increased. In addition, a large bag makes observation of respiration difficult because the movement is so small. A large size bag is also difficult to squeeze during positive ventilation.
- A reservoir bag that is too small results in an inadequate gas supply to meet the peak inspiratory volume of the animal; the reservoir bag will completely collapse during inspiration and overinflate during expiration.
- During expiration, a bag that is too small is unable to provide a safety margin against pressure build up within the breathing circuit.

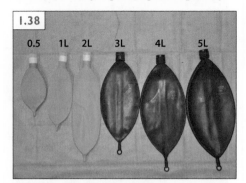

1.38

| 0.5 | 1L | 2L | 3L | 4L | 5L |

Fig. 1.38 Various sizes and shapes of reservoir bags are shown. A reservoir bag is also called a rebreathing bag when the bag is used in a rebreathing circuit.

Table 1.3 Size of reservoir bag related to the weight of the animal

Reservoir size (liters)	Animal's body weight
0.5	≤7 kg (≤15 lb)
1	8–13 kg (16–30 lb)
2	14–27 kg (31–60 lb)
3	28–41 kg (61–90 lb)
5	42–68 kg (91–150 lb)

CO₂ absorbents

- There are two kinds of CO_2 absorbents: soda lime (**Fig. 1.39**) and barium hydroxide lime. Both are produced in granule form.
- Calcium hydroxide is the main component of both CO_2 absorbents.
- Soda lime consists of 94% calcium hydroxide, 5% sodium hydroxide, and 1% potassium hydroxide. When CO_2 passes through soda lime, the reaction forms calcium carbonate. Soda lime also contains small amounts of silica to prevent the granules from disintegrating into a powder.
- Barium hydroxide lime consists of 80% calcium hydroxide and approximately 20% of barium hydroxide lime. Barium hydroxide lime does not contain silica since it is inherently hard and will not disintegrate into a powder.
- Chemical dye is incorporated into CO_2 absorbents and the color changes according to the pH of the CO_2 absorbent. Soda lime has a pH of 13.5. As more CO_2 is absorbed, the pH decreases to <10 and the color changes from white to purple (with ethyl violet dye) (**Fig. 1.40**) or pink to yellow/white (titan yellow dye), depending on the type of chemical dye used.
- When approximately 75% of the soda lime or barium hydroxide lime has changed color, all of the CO_2 absorbent should be replaced.
- CO_2 absorbents are housed in the CO_2 absorbent canister of the rebreathing circuit (**Figs. 1.40, 1.41**).
- One kg of CO_2 absorbent has a volume of 1.5 liters. One kg of soda lime can absorb 120 liters of CO_2. The reaction between CO_2 and sodium hydroxide (if soda lime is used)/barium hydroxide (if barium hydroxide lime is used) produces heat, which can be felt through the wall of the CO_2 absorbent canister.

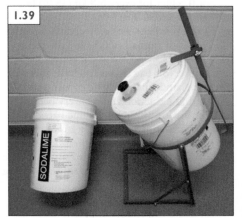

1.39

Fig. 1.39 Soda lime in a 5-gallon bucket is mounted in a stand for easy filling.

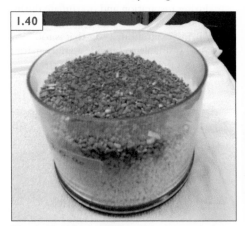

1.40

Fig. 1.40 When soda lime is exhausted, the color changes from white to blue-purple.

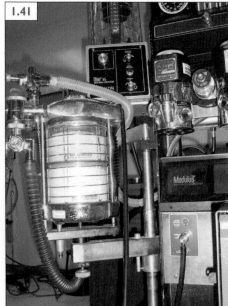

1.41

Fig. 1.41 A dual CO_2 absorbent canister staggered with one canister on top of the other.

- Some rebreathing circuits have dual canisters, with one canister staggered on top of the other (**Fig. 1.41**). The advantage of the dual canister system is that it does not require frequent changes of the CO_2 absorbent. The disadvantages are increased resistance to breathing and slow changes in inhalant anesthetic concentrations during induction and recovery.
- Soda lime or barium hydroxide lime should be packed loosely in the CO_2 absorbent canister to maintain adequate intergranule space and to prevent cake formation. The intergranular space should be approximately the minute volume of the anesthetized animal. The CO_2 absorbent should be filled to approximately 2/3 full of the canister.
- A tightly packed CO_2 absorbent canister causes exhaled CO_2 to form gas channels through the absorbent, exhausting the capacity of the channels while underutilizing the other areas. This results in ineffective CO_2 absorption.
- The duration of CO_2 absorbents depends on the size of the CO_2 canister, total hours of use, the size of the animal, and the fresh gas flow rate used. In general, the CO_2 absorbent should be changed after 8–12 hours of continuous use or when 50–75% of the CO_2 absorbent granules have changed color.
- In addition, fresh CO_2 absorbent granules crumble easily.
- Regeneration occurs when CO_2 absorbents are stored after use, so expired absorbent that had previously changed color may return to normal color and can be mistakenly identified as fresh absorbent.

NON-REBREATHING CIRCUITS
- A non-rebreathing circuit does not allow reutilization of the exhaled alveolar gas; all exhaled alveolar gases are eliminated through the scavenging system. Unlike a rebreathing circuit, a non-rebreathing circuit contains few if any valves and parts, and it therefore provides minimal resistance to breathing by the anesthetized animal. Rebreathing circuits are used in dogs and cats weighing <7.0–7.5 kg (15.4–16.5 lb). Some anesthestists use a lower body weight (as small as 3 kg [6.6 lb]) as the cut-off point between using a rebreathing circuit or a non-rebreathing circuit. However, there is no universal agreement on the cut-off body weight for such use.
- A non-rebreathing circuit does not utilize a CO_2 absorbent (**Fig. 1.28**) to remove exhaled CO_2 from the circuit. All non-rebreathing circuits use high fresh gas flow in lieu of a CO_2 absorbent to eliminate exhaled CO_2. An average oxygen flow rate of 200–300 ml/kg (approximately 100–200 ml/lb) body weight/minute is used with a non-rebreathing circuit.
- Non-rebreathing circuits are usually classified as Mapleson systems and are used frequently in veterinary clinics. They include Ayre's T piece (which is classified as a Mapleson E) (**Fig. 1.42**), Modified Jackson Rees (modified from an Ayre's T piece and classified as a Mapleson F) (**Figs. 1.43, 1.44**), Bain coaxial breathing circuit (classified as a Mapleson D) (**Fig. 1.45**), and Norman mask elbow.
- An advantage of the modified Jackson Rees non-breathing circuit is that it is easy to change the reservoir bag size (**Fig. 1.45**) without modifying the scavenging adapter for each size of bag, because the scavenging system is located proximal to the reservoir bag (**Fig. 1.44**). This is an important feature when carrying out face mask induction using an inhalant anesthetic agent. (See Chapter 5 for further information on inhalant anesthetic agents.)

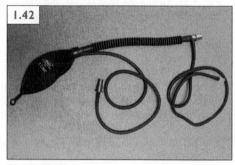

1.42

Fig. 1.42 A modified Ayre's T piece non-rebreathing circuit.

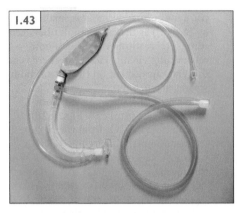

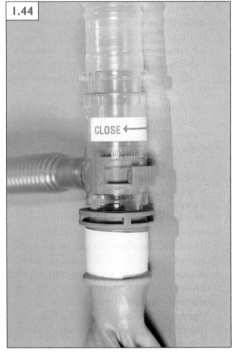

Figs. 1.43, 1.44 A modified Jackson Rees (modified from an Ayres's T piece) non-breathing circuit (1.43). The scavenging piece (1.44) is proximal to the reservoir bag. The fresh gas inlet hose (transparent oxygen tubing) is connected to the fresh gas outlet (see Fig. 1.21) of the anesthesia machine.

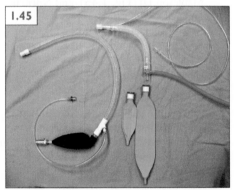

Fig. 1.45 Unlike the Bain circuit, the size of the reservoir bag on a modified Jackson Rees non-breathing circuit can be changed to any other size without modifying the scavenging piece. The metal scavenger adapter is located at the end of the reservoir bag in the Bain's circuit (left). Note the straight connectors, as opposed to a Y-piece, on the patient side of both non-rebreathing circuits.

- The key components of a non-rebreathing circuit are:
  - A **fresh gas inlet** (**Fig. 1.21**). This allows oxygen and anesthetic gas to enter the non-rebreathing circuit from either the common gas outlet of the anesthesia machine or from the anesthetic vaporizer outlet fitting (**Figs. 1.46, 1.47**).
- A **straight connector.** This is similar to the Y-connector (piece) used in a rebreathing circuit, but it is not Y-shaped (**Fig. 1.45**).
- A **reservoir bag.** The bag is attached to the non-rebreathing circuit and serves the same purposes as in the rebreathing circuit (i.e. to assist or control ventilation and meet the inspiratory demand of the gas volume).
- **Universal control arms** (**Fig. 1.48**). These are modified devices that can be used with a Bain's-type non-rebreathing circuit. It is equipped with a pop-off valve and a pressure manometer (as in a rebreathing circuit) to monitor circuit pressure and a reservoir bag to assist or control ventilation. Special mounting blocks are required to mount the universal control arm to the anesthesia machine (**Figs. 1.49–1.52**).

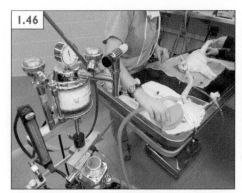

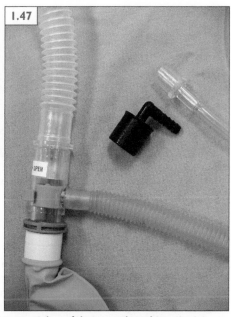

Figs. 1.46, 1.47 A cat maintained on a modified Jackson-Rees non-rebreathing circuit (**1.46**). The gas inlet of the non-rebreathing circuit is connected to the anesthetic vaporizer outlet fitting (**1.47**). This same adaptor is connected to the vaporizer outlet fitting on the lower portion of the machine next to the purple label of the isoflurane vaporizer (arrow, **1.46**). There are no rebreathing hoses connected to the inspiratory and expiratory limbs of the rebreathing circuit. The reservoir bag of the non-rebreathing circuit is green. This machine has a single CO_2 absorbent canister for soda lime or baralyme (**1.46**).

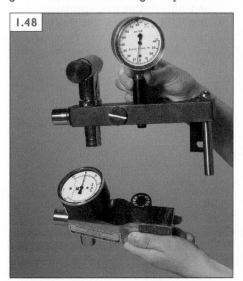

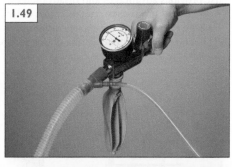

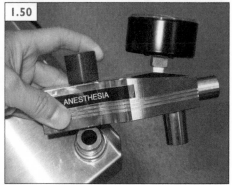

Fig. 1.48 Two different universal control arms are shown.

Figs. 1.49, 1.50 A universal control arm with a Bain non-rebreathing circuit. The configuration is similar to a rebreathing circuit, but without CO_2 absorbent. The fresh gas enters the non-rebreathing circuit through the transparent hose. The pressure manometer and pop-off valve are present to monitor circuit pressure and control or assist ventilation (**1.49**). A permanent mounting block is required to mount this device on the anesthesia machine (**1.50**).

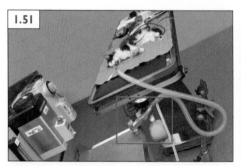

Fig. 1.51 A universal control arm (within the red box) with a Bain non-rebreathing circuit is being used in this cat.

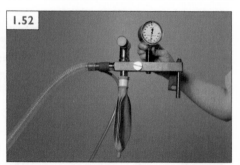

Fig. 1.52 Another type of universal control arm connected to a Bain non-rebreathing circuit is shown. This device uses a clamping mechanism to mount itself onto an existing anesthesia machine as opposed to the permanent mounting block required for the device in **Fig. 1.51**.

Modern human anesthesia machines for veterinary use

Recent trends show that more and more teaching hospitals and private practices are selecting modern human anesthesia machines with ventilator capacity for veterinary use. Their use provides advantages and disadvantages:

- Modern human anesthesia machines differ from conventional anesthesia machines because they integrate the use of electronics, software and hardware for cardiorespiratory monitoring, ventilation, and use of inhalant agents with high and low fresh gas flows.
- The machines usually come with all the bells and whistles, including pediatric and adult flowmeters, ventilator, ventilator monitor/control unit, cardiorespiratory monitors, drug/supply storage drawers, and a working station (**Figs. 1.53, 1.54**).

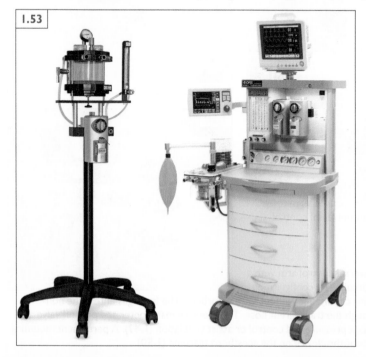

Fig. 1.53 A modern human anesthesia machine stands next to a modern veterinary anesthesia machine. The human machine comes with anesthetic monitor/ventilator hardware and software with storage draws and a mini-desk, whereas the veterinary machine contains the basic anesthetic components of 'FROGS'. (Images courtesy DRE Veterinary Medical Equipment *www. dreveterinary.com*).

- The fresh gases (oxygen, medical air, and nitrous oxide), pipelines, and electrical supply are usually integrated with the machine. It is therefore bulkier than a large size veterinary machine.
- The modern anesthesia machine's quality is usually excellent and frequently exceeds human anesthesia standards set by the American Society for Testing and Materials (ASTM) and have to be approved by the Federal Food and Drug Administration for using in humans.
- The machine is digitally integrated with many types of information, including anesthetic record, cardiorespiratory functions, and the machine performance data with fresh gas flow and inhalant anesthetic consumed over time. It can produce both an anesthetic record report and a financial report (the cost of inhalants over time).
- Modern anesthesia machines rely heavily on electricity. While they are equipped with battery backups, if there is a power outage, more complicated action needs to be taken place to operate them.
- Human anesthesia machines are usually much more expensive than veterinary anesthesia machines.
- Besides the bulky size, complex operation, and a steeper learning curve on operating a human anesthesia machine for

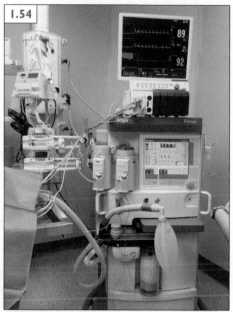

Fig. I.54 Modern human anesthesia machine equipped with various types of anesthetic monitors and is designed to be stationary. It is too bulky to be mobile. (Image courtesy of Dr Hsein-Chi Wang, National Chung Hsing University, Taiwan.)

veterinary patients, the main drawback is the cost of the machine. The machine is in general 10–20 times more expensive than a traditional veterinary anesthesia machine.

Selecting a breathing circuit

Patients smaller than 7–7.5 kg (15.4–16.5 lb) are suitable for use of a non-rebreathing circuit. Patients heavier than 7–7.5 kg should be maintained with a rebreathing circuit for economical reasons.

A non-rebreathing circuit minimizes the work of breathing for smaller dogs and cats because the circuit is designed to produce minimal resistance to breathing. In contrast, a rebreathing circuit contains one-way valves, CO_2 absorbents in a canister, and other constricting parts that all increase work and resistance to breathing. Small animals do

not have enough breathing force and tidal volume to overcome this resistance. In addition, most anesthetic agents, especially isoflurane, sevoflurane, and desflurane, induce muscle relaxation, which further reduces the ability of the respiratory muscles to overcome the resistance of a rebreathing circuit and breathe properly.

The advantages of a rebreathing circuit are reduced oxygen flow rate, which reduces the cost of inhalant anesthetic agent, and the preservation of heat and moisture from the patient.

Ambu bags

Key points relating to Ambu bags are listed below:

- Using an Ambu bag (**Fig. 1.55**) is an alternative method of providing positive-pressure ventilation to an animal with either room air or enriched oxygen without using an anesthesia machine and a breathing circuit.
- An Ambu bag is a self-expanding silicone bag with a one-way valve towards the patient and a flap valve near the oxygen delivery port (**Fig. 1.56**).
- The Ambu bag is connected to the endotracheal tube and the oxygen tubing.

With 100% oxygen provided to the reservoir bag, squeezing the silicone bag manually delivers oxygen to the animal's airway. Ambu bags can be used with just room air without a connection to 100% oxygen supply.

- An Ambu bag can be used to ventilate an animal through an endotracheal tube or a face mask, but the ventilation is more efficient when the animal is intubated.
- During expiration, the one-way valve of the Ambu bag, near the endotracheal tube, closes and the exhaled CO_2 is vented around the one-way valve to the atmosphere.

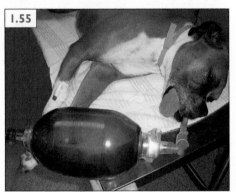

Fig. 1.55 This Ambu bag is part of a non-rebreathing circuit system. One end is connected to the endotracheal tube and the other is connected to the oxygen tubing with 100% oxygen provided into the silicone reservoir bag.

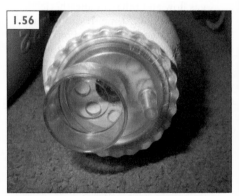

Fig. 1.56 One end of the Ambu bag is shown with a flap valve near the oxygen delivery port. The flap valve prevents inspiration of room air during positive ventilation when the bag is squeezed. The oxygen port allows oxygen into the rubber or silicone bag for delivery to the patient.

Ventilators

Five key points relating to ventilators are listed below (see also Chapter 11):

- Ventilators can be classified into two types: those with descending bellows (**Fig. 1.57**) and those with ascending bellows (**Fig. 1.58**). All ventilators have bellow housings.
- The ventilator acts like another pair of hands to help the veterinarian ventilate an animal under general anesthesia.

- Ventilators with ascending bellows should fill completely and raise the bellow to the top of the housing when the inspiratory hose is occluded during leak inspections.
- Ventilators with descending or hanging bellows should not fall when the patient port is occluded at the end of inspiration.
- Ventilators can be powered by oxygen, medical air, electricity, or batteries.

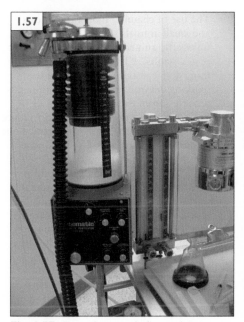

Fig. 1.57 A ventilator with descending bellows.

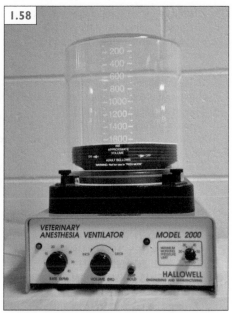

Fig. 1.58 A ventilator with ascending bellows. Both ascending and descending bellows are housed in the bellow housing.

Oxygen flow rates

The following factors and conditions determine the oxygen flow rates required for anesthetic induction and maintenance when using rebreathing and non-rebreathing circuits (see also Chapter 5).

THE OXYGEN CONSUMPTION REQUIREMENTS OF THE ANESTHETIZED ANIMAL

- Oxygen consumption rates in animals under inhalant anesthesia have been reported to range from 3 to 8 ml/kg/minute.
- When body temperature decreases (a common side-effect of general anesthesia), oxygen consumption decreases proportionally. As a result, the oxygen flow rate required to meet the oxygen consumption needs of the anesthetized patient is actually reduced. For example, a 50 kg dog requires an oxygen flow rate of 150–450 ml/minute to meet oxygen demand under general anesthesia.
- Providing a higher oxygen rate during anesthesia does not significantly influence hemoglobin saturation for oxygen (SpO_2) or partial pressure of arterial oxygen tension (PaO_2) when the oxygen demands are already met in healthy animals.

THE AMOUNT OF OXYGEN NEEDING TO CARRY INHALANT ANESTHETIC FROM THE VAPORIZER TO THE PATIENT

- Most modern vaporizers require a minimum flow rate of 200–350 ml/minute of oxygen (or fresh gas) to carry adequate anesthetic vapor to meet the accurate anesthetic concentrations set by the vaporizer.

AMOUNT OF OXYGEN FLOW REQUIRED TO REMOVE THE CO_2 EXHALED BY THE ANESTHETIZED ANIMAL FROM A NON-REBREATHING CIRCUIT

- Because a non-rebreathing circuit does not contain a CO_2 absorbent, it requires a higher oxygen flow rate to wash out or eliminate exhaled CO_2 from the animal and the non-rebreathing circuit.

- Therefore, when using a non-rebreathing circuit (for animals weighing <7 kg [15.4 lb]), a maintenance oxygen flow rate of about 200–250 ml/kg/min (approximately 100 ml/lb/min) is needed to ensure elimination of exhaled CO_2 and thus prevent rebreathing of the exhaled CO_2.
- For an averaged sized adult cat (approximately 4.5 kg [10 lb]), 1 liter/minute of oxygen flow is usually adequate for anesthesia maintenance.
- For a 1 kg (2.2 lb) Chihuahua, an oxygen flow rate of 500 ml is more than adequate when using a non-rebreathing circuit for anesthesia maintenance.

CHANGES TO THE SPEED OF INHALANT ANESTHETIC UPTAKE DURING THE TRANSITION FROM INTRAVENOUS INDUCTION TO INHALANT MAINTENANCE

- During the transition from intravenous induction to inhalant anesthetic maintenance, a higher oxygen flow rate and a higher vaporizer setting is required to change the anesthetic concentration within the re-breathing circuit quickly.
- The higher oxygen flow rate replaces the large volume of nitrogen within the breathing circuit as well as that expired by the animal during the initial anesthetic induction.
- The high oxygen flow rate, coupled with the higher vaporizer setting, also serves as an anesthetic agent carrier, allowing the anesthetic concentration to be changed within the volume barrier (mechanical space from the vaporizer to the breathing circuit to the patient's airway) relatively quickly. This provides a higher anesthetic concentration for the animal to uptake into the lungs.

CHANGES TO THE SPEED OF CHAMBER OR FACE MASK INDUCTION

- The larger the induction chamber size, the higher the oxygen flow rate required to denitrogenize the chamber rapidly and change the anesthetic concentration within a reasonable induction time.
- A long induction period and high anesthetic concentration for induction translate to higher costs when using inhalant anesthesia.

- The use of chamber induction for cats and small animals should be avoided unless the animal is impossible to handle (e.g. viscious). Chamber induction costs more and is also highly polluting to the working environment when the animal is retrieved from the chamber.
- Face mask induction can drastically reduce the cost of inhalant anesthesia induction due to the smaller mechanical volume barrier.
- Using a non-rebreathing circuit, especially with a modified Jackson Rees or Bain's circuit, instead of a rebreathing circuit will greatly reduce the time required for face mask induction. Again, this is due to the smaller mechanical volume barrier associated with the non-rebreathing circuit.
- When using a rebreathing circuit for face mask induction (**Fig. 1.59**), a higher oxygen flow rate is required to denitrogenize the volume rapidly and to change the anesthetic concentration

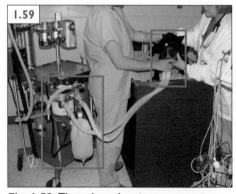

Fig. 1.59 The volume barrier represents mechanical space between the vaporizer and the breathing circuit and the patient's airway. In the example shown there is a total volume barrier of 8 liters between the vaporizer and the patient's airway made up of the entire rebreathing circuit (large green box: 1 liter breathing hose, 3 liter CO_2 absorbent canister, 3 liter rebreathing bag) and a 1 liter face mask (small green box). This volume space (barrier) acts as a barrier or obstacle to rapid anesthetic concentration change between the vaporizer and the dog's airway. Therefore, the higher the oxygen flow rate, the higher the anesthetic concentration from the vaporizer, and the more rapid the change in anesthetic concentration in this space volume barrier.

within the rebreathing circuit, which has a large volume barrier.

- 'Charging' the anesthesia machine and the rebreathing circuit with a high oxygen flow and a high vaporizer anesthetic percentage prior to starting face mask induction will smooth the induction, regardless of the inhalant anesthetic agent used.

IMPORTANT CONCEPT OF TIME CONSTANT FOR INHALANT ANESTHETIC DURING CHAMBER INDUCTION

- The time constant represents the volume of an induction chamber or breathing circuit (in liters) divided by the fresh gas flow rate (liters per minute).
- For example, a 10 gallon (44 liters) induction chamber with an oxygen flow rate of 10 liters per minute will take 4.4 minutes as one time constant.
- It takes four time constants to change an inhalant anesthetic concentration that is equal to the vaporizer output.

CHANGES TO ANESTHETIC DEPTH DURING ANESTHESIA MAINTENANCE

- During anesthesia maintenance, increasing the oxygen flow rate and the vaporizer percentage setting will increase the depth of anesthesia. These are important steps to prevent premature awakening during anesthesia for the animal maintained on a low oxygen flow rate.
- If the animal is too deep, the depth of anesthesia can be changed by increasing the oxygen flow rate or using the oxygen flush valve to introduce a large amount of oxygen into the rebreathing circuit. This, together with a decrease in the vaporizer percentage setting, reduces the anesthetic concentration in the mechanical volume barrier relatively quickly. Increasing alveolar ventilation with positive ventilation will decrease the inhalant anesthetic concentration in the physiologic volume barrier and quickly wash-out the anesthetic in the animal's brain.
- To avoid barotrauma, an oxygen flush valve should not be used with a non-rebreathing circuit (remember it is designed for small resistance and small volume barrier).

CONSERVATION OF THE PATIENT'S BODY TEMPERATURE AND AIRWAY MOISTURE

- Fresh oxygen is cold and dry. As it enters the airway, fresh oxygen bypasses the natural warming and moisturizing mechanisms and enters the trachea directly via the endotracheal tube.
- Using a higher than necessary oxygen flow rate decreases body temperature and dries the patient's airway.
- Using a lower oxygen flow rate for anesthesia maintenance preserves the animal's body temperature and airway moisture.

REDUCING THE COST OF A GIVEN INHALANT ANESTHETIC AGENT

- The cost of an inhalant anesthetic episode can be calculated using these four factors: fresh oxygen flow rate, duration of anesthesia, average vaporizer setting during anesthesia, and type and cost of inhalant anesthetic agent used. The equation below, which is used to calculate the cost of a given episode of anesthesia, is based on these four factors:

$$\frac{\text{Vaporizer dial setting (\%)}/100 \times \text{Oxygen flow rate (ml/min)}}{182.7 \text{ ml*}}$$

$$\times \text{Duration of procedure (min)}$$

$$\times \text{Cost of inhalant anesthetic/ml}$$

* 182.7 represents the amount (ml) of vapor to which 1 ml of sevoflurane liquid vaporizes at room temperature. For isoflurane, this value increases to approximately 190 ml.

- To give an example (using $USA), the surgical plane of sevoflurane is approximately 4%, so if 500 ml/minute of oxygen is used for maintenance, the duration of the anesthetic procedure is 30 minutes, and the cost of sevoflurane is $0.90 per ml, then the total cost is $2.95. The cost of a face mask induction with sevoflurane can be calculated using the same equation. With 8% sevoflurane, a 2 liters/minute oxygen flow rate, and a 3 minute induction, the cost is $2.36. Since sevoflurane is approximately 8–10 times more expensive than isoflurane, the previous calculation can be applied to isoflurane by dividing the answer

by a factor of approximately 10. As a result, 30 minutes of surgical plane of anesthesia with isoflurane costs $0.218.
- The above example emphasizes the fact that the cost of isoflurane anesthesia is relatively economical after investment in all of the equipment.
- A high oxygen flow rate increases cost by increasing the consumption of the inhalant anesthetic agent and the oxygen.
- In addition, excessive unused anesthetic waste gas consumes more charcoal absorber (if this method is used as waste gas management) over time, resulting in the charcoal absorber being changed more frequently and increasing costs further.
- It is also true that lower oxygen flow rates may increase the consumption of the CO_2 absorbent, but the cost of the CO_2 absorbent (soda lime or barium hydroxide lime) is approximately $0.01 per gram.
- It is clear that the cost of the inhalant, as well as, the oxygen flow rate, play the most influential roles in the cost of any given episode of inhalant anesthesia.

GLOBAL ISSUES, INCLUDING POLLUTION CONTROL AND ENERGY CONSERVATION
- Using a low, but appropriate, oxygen flow offers significant advantages that not only save costs and provide better patient care (less patient cooling and dehydration), but also reduce waste gas pollution.
- A leaking anesthesia machine or breathing circuit will mandate the use of an unnecessarily high oxygen flow rate, since part of the inhalant anesthetic escapes from the breathing circuit system before reaching the animal. It is important to service the anesthesia machine and perform leak checks on both the machine and the breathing circuit on a routine basis.
- Use of an unnecessarily high oxygen flow rate increases the waste of oxygen and inhalant anesthetic. These factors directly and indirectly increase the production of pollution in the global environment and the consumption of raw materials and energy to manufacture oxygen and anesthetic agents.

Endotracheal tubes

Several facts need to be understood with regard to endotracheal tubes.

TYPES OF ENDOTRACHEAL TUBES
There are three types of endotracheal tube: Murphy (**Fig. 1.60**), Magill (**Fig. 1.61**), and Cole's:
- Murphy endotracheal tubes contain a Murphy's eye (an escape hole) at the opposite end of the endotracheal tube opening. The Murphy's eye allows gas flow to bypass an obstruction in the patient end of endotracheal tube.
- Magill endotracheal tubes are similar to the Murphy's tube, but do not contain the Murphy's eye. Magill tubes can be a cuffed or plain (uncuffed).
- Cole's endotracheal tubes have a tapered end. There is no cuff; the airway is sealed with the tapered shoulder against the wall of endotracheal tube.

ENDOTRACHEAL TUBE CONSTRUCTION
Endotracheal tubes are constructed of different types of materials including polyvinyl chloride (PVC), silicone, or red rubber.

- The PVC endotracheal tubes are more rigid than either silicone or red rubber tubes and are therefore easier for intubation. Once the PCV endotracheal tubes are warmed by the body temperature, they soften and mold into the shape of the trachea. PVC endotracheal tubes have a radiopaque line running along their length, which enables them to be visible on radiographs.
- Silicone or red rubber tubes require a stylet to increase stiffness during intubation.
- Red rubber tubes are prone to crack over time, although they are designed for repeated use.
- Silicone tubes are expensive and, due to the high resistance of the outer wall on the airway, require significant lubrication on the outer wall during intubation.
- There is also an endotracheal tube called an armored or spiral metallic embedded reinforced tube (**Fig. 1.62**). The tube is made of silicone with a steel wire or nylon coil embedded in the wall. The embedded wire resists kinking or collapse when the neck or trachea is subjected to extreme

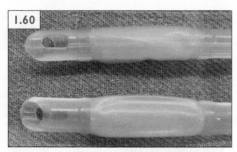

Fig. 1.60 A Murphy's eye on a Murphy's endotracheal tube. The eye is located on the opposite side of the endotracheal tube opening. Note the bevel of the endotracheal tube.

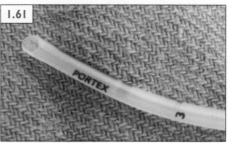

Fig. 1.61 An uncuffed Magill's endotracheal tube with no Murphy's eye.

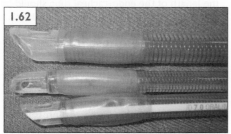

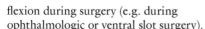

Fig. 1.62 An armored or spiral metallic embedded reinforced tube. The spiral metallic wire, which is embedded in the wall, prevents kinking or collapse.

flexion during surgery (e.g. during ophthalmologic or ventral slot surgery).
- Endotracheal tubes have a bevel at the patient end to facilitate viewing of the laryngeal opening by the anesthetist. They can be cuffed or uncuffed. Inflation of the cuff improves the airtight seal between the patient's tracheal wall and the tube and prevents aspiration of vomitus and secretions into the lungs.

ENDOTRACHEAL TUBE SELECTION
- Endotracheal tubes are available in different sizes (measured in internal and external diameter in millimeters) and lengths.
- Two methods are frequently employed to select an endotracheal tube:
  - The first is based on the width of the nasal septum of the dog's nose being equal to the outer diameter of the endotracheal tube (**Fig. 1.63**).
  - The second selects an endotracheal tube size based on palpation of the outer diameter of the animal's trachea in the mid-neck region (**Fig. 1.64**).

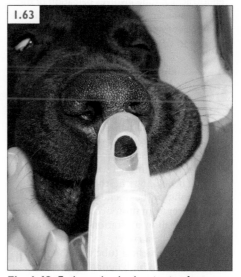

Fig. 1.63 Endotracheal tube size is often selected by comparing the width of the dog's nasal septum with the outer diameter of the endotracheal tube.

- A recent evaluation of these two methods found that direct palpation at the mid-neck region of the trachea is more accurate.
- The length of the endotracheal tube should be measured from the tip of the patient's nose to the tip of the shoulder (**Fig. 1.65**):
  - The marker number (in centimeters) on the wall of the endotracheal tube should be noted and insertion stopped when the marker is reached.
  - Placement too far into the patient intubates the patient's main stem bronchus, inducing one-lung ventilation, shunting, and hypoxia.

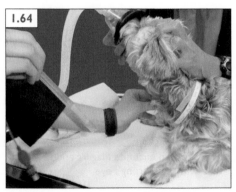

Fig. 1.64 Another method of selecting an endotracheal tube involves palpation of the outer diameter of the animal's trachea in the mid-neck region and comparing it with an estimated size of endotracheal tube.

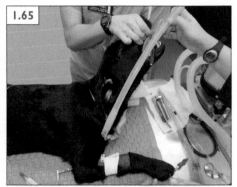

Fig. 1.65 To prevent bronchial intubation, the length of the endotracheal tube should be measured from the tip of the nose to the tip of the shoulder.

- The endotracheal tube cuff should be checked to make sure that it is airtight before induction. A leaky cuff can cause several problems:
  - The animal will not be properly anesthetized and will frequently wake up, because the anesthetic gas leaks from the animal's airway.
  - The leaking anesthetic gas also pollutes the operating room.
  - If regurgitation occurs, a leaky cuff may allow aspiration of regurgitant into the airway.
- The endotracheal tube cuff should be inflated to a high enough pressure to seal the trachea and prevent aspiration of any airway secretions as well as leakage of the airway gas. The cuff pressure should also be low enough to allow proper perfusion of the tracheal mucosal lining. Overinflation of the endotracheal cuff may result in tracheal necrosis due to poor perfusion of the tracheal mucosa over time, or tracheal bleeding, rupture, or post-extubation pain of the animal.
- A common way to check for proper cuff inflation is to continue to inflate the endotracheal tube cuff with a syringe until it no longer leaks during several positive-pressure breaths or manual ventilation at 15–20 cmH$_2$O measured by a pressure manometer in the breathing circuit. However, this method is not a guarantee for proper inflation of the cuff. The cuff

could be easily over- or underinflated, and more frequently overinflated.
- Endotracheal tube cuff inflation should be done carefully with a cuff pressure manometer (**Figs. 1.66, 1.67**) or with a syringe that has a pressure measuring device or indicator (**Fig. 1.68**) and inflated to a pressure not exceeding 20–25 cmH$_2$O. The cuff pressure should be part of the continuous monitoring during the entire intubation duration. Excessive inflation or underinflation of the cuff should be adjusted and the pressure measured again with a cuff pressure manometer.
- Both human and animal studies have demonstrated that lubricating the endotracheal tube cuff with water soluble gel before intubation helps prevent microaspiration of the airway or gastric secretions entering into the lungs by plugging the channels of the longitudinal folds (**Figs. 1.69, 1.70**) within the wall of a well inflated endotracheal tube cuff. The water soluble gel also facilitates intubation, especially when a silicone tube is used. Therefore, it is good practice to use water soluble gel to lubricate an endotracheal tube cuff prior to intubation.
- Too tight a cuff inflation exerts a high pressure on the tracheal wall and may result in tracheal rupture/tear or trachea mucosal ischemia, which leads to necrosis later if left in place for long periods.

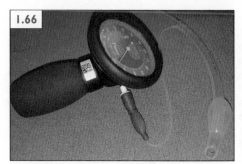

Fig. 1.66 An endotracheal tube cuff pressure manometer (black color) should be connected to an endotracheal tube pilot balloon (blue color) for continuous monitoring of endotracheal tube cuff pressure throughout the anesthesia. Changes in animal's body position, depth of anesthesia, or using positive-pressure ventilation all influence the endotracheal tube cuff pressure. When cuff pressure is under- or over-inflated, it can be immediately corrected via this manometer device. Note the manometer handle is actually a rubber bulb that can be used to inflate or deflate the cuff.

Fig. 1.67 The endotracheal tube cuff pressure should be measured continuously during the anesthesia. The cuff pressure is expressed as cmH_2O on the pressure manometer. This cuff was over-inflated and the pressure indicator on the manometer (shown by the white needle on the red zone) showed the cuff pressure was 90 cmH_2O. The cuff was deflated to the safe pressure as shown by the green zone on the device.

Fig. 1.68 An endotracheal tube cuff can be inflated with either a regular injection syringe (top), a commercial cuff inflation syringe with a digital cuff pressure indicator (middle), or another commercial syringe device that has a color-coded pressure indicator within the syringe barrel that detects the endotracheal cuff pressure (bottom; the pressure range for the red zone is 40–60 cmH_2O and the green zone is 20–30 cmH_2O in this device).

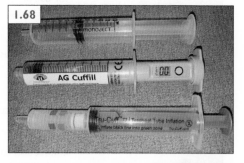

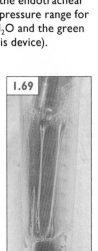
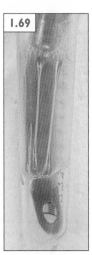

Fig. 1.69 The PVC endotracheal tube cuff can form a longitudinal fold, as shown here, even after it is well inflated. These longitudinal folds allow regurgitant fluid to seep into the trachea. This is called micro-aspiration. Notice the bubble on the top of the cuff; small bubbles also appear at the bottom of the cuff with a blue tinted solution.

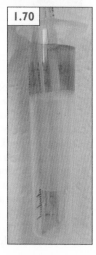

Fig. 1.70 A silicone endotracheal tube with cuff inflated was placed in a syringe case to simulate the endotracheal tube cuff inflation. Note the cuff does not form longitudinal folds as shown in **Fig. 1.69**, because of the elastic property of the silicone cuff. In this case, the cuff is inflated and no micro-aspiration occurred.

Laryngeal mask airway for cats

Laryngeal mask airways are an alternative to endotracheal tubes to protect the airway. One of the laryngeal mask designed for use in cats is called V-Gel (**Fig. 1.71**). It is designed to be inserted blindly into the pharyngeal area with the tip of the mask into the esophagus but the mask itself resting on the larynx the lumen of the mask directly faces the laryngeal opening. A cuff surrounded the mask can be inflated to seal the pharyngeal-laryngeal area and prevent the leakage of anesthetic gas.

- The advantage of using laryngeal masks in cats is that intubation can be rapidly achieved with inexperienced personnel and minimal trauma to the airway. The device also allows proper connection to capnography for monitoring of expired CO_2.
- The disadvantage of using a laryngeal mask is that if regurgitation occurs, it can result in macro- and microaspiration of regurgitant and secretions. Furthermore, the lumen of the mask itself is relatively narrow (**Fig. 1.72**) and could be obstructed by the mucus plug and airway secretion. The mask is also relatively expensive and can only be used a maximum of 40 times according to the manufacturer's suggestion.

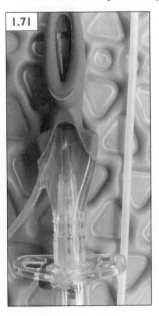

1.71

Fig. 1.71 A laryngeal mask designed for use in cats. The tip of the mask is inserted into the esophagus while the mask covers the laryngeal opening. Note the port is available for connection to a sidestream capnography.

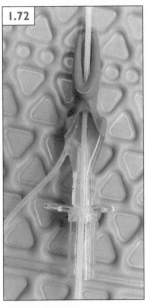

1.72

Fig. 1.72 An 8F size polypropylene stylet has been inserted into the lumen of the laryngeal mask to show the narrow size (~2.65 mm ID) of the lumen.

Laryngoscopes

- Laryngoscopes, which generally consist of a blade and a handle (**Fig. 1.73**), are used to assist endotracheal intubation. They are especially useful in brachycephalic dogs (**Figs. 1.74, 1.75**) or cats, or in upper airway obstruction cases where the glottis cannot be seen clearly.
- The blade, which can be straight or curved, has a light source and a flinch (**Fig. 1.76**). The light source is powered by a battery, which is usually housed in the handle. The blade either has a

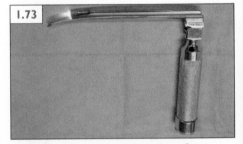

1.73

Fig. 1.73 A laryngoscope consists of a laryngeal blade and a scope handle.

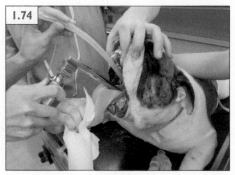
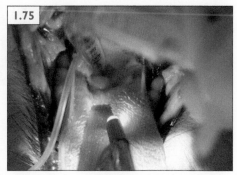

Figs. 1.74, 1.75 Laryngoscopes are a particularly useful aide for visualization of the laryngeal opening in a brachycephalic dog with a lot of redundant tissue in the upper airway.

light bulb screwed onto the blade or there is a bulb in the handle and light is transmitted via a fiberoptic to the tip of the blade (**Fig. 1.75**). The light source is used to visualize the laryngeal opening.

- The laryngeal blade manipulates the oral soft tissues, including the tongue, soft palate, and epiglottis, in order to facilitate intubation. Laryngeal blades appropriate for use in small animals range in size from 0 (small) to 5 (large). The two most common patterns of laryngeal blades are the Miller (straight blade) and the MacIntosh (curved blade) (**Fig. 1.76**), and there are many modifications based on these two patterns.

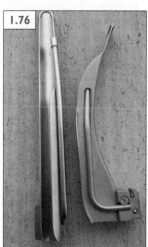

Fig. 1.76 The laryngeal blade contains a light source and a flinch to deflect the soft tissue of the tongue or larynx. Two commonly used laryngeal blades are the Miller (straight blade, left) and the MacIntosh (curved blade, right).

Induction chambers and face masks

INDUCTION CHAMBERS
- Induction chambers should be airtight, clear or transparent, and durable so that the animal can be seen clearly during induction (**Fig. 1.77**).
- Large chambers can be equipped with a partition (**Fig. 1.77**). A small sized animal can be placed in the partitioned off part the chamber and this will reduce the volume of anesthetic agents and minimize costs, as well as increase the speed of induction.
- The durability of the chamber prevents it from being broken or shattered during a rough induction.
- When performing a chamber induction, the chamber should be connected to a

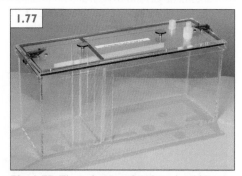

Fig. 1.77 The induction chamber should be transparent for observation of the animal during inhalant induction. Large chambers are sometimes equipped with a partition to reduce the chamber size for induction of a small animal.

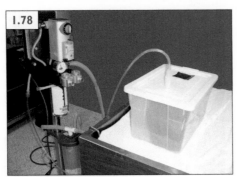

Fig. 1.78 When performing chamber induction, the chamber should be connected to a non-rebreathing circuit. This chamber is not as transparent, but it is still acceptable. Note that there is only one inlet for inhalant anesthetic gas and oxygen and no outlet for a scavenger hose or gas to exit, which facilitates induction. This is different to the chamber in **Fig. 1.79**, which is connected to both.

- non-rebreathing circuit (**Fig. 1.78**) and not to a rebreathing circuit (**Fig. 1.79**).
- When the chamber is connected to a rebreathing circuit, it increases the volume barrier and significantly slows the induction speed.
- If the chamber is connected directly to a non-rebreathing circuit or directly from a fresh gas line out of the common gas outlet, the space for denitrogenization, as well as changing anesthetic concentration, is reduced.
- Using only one inlet for the inhalant anesthetic gas and oxygen and no outlet for the scavenger hose or gas to exit (**Fig. 1.78**) minimizes the competition between the inhalant anesthetic gas going into the chamber and the scavenging vacuum

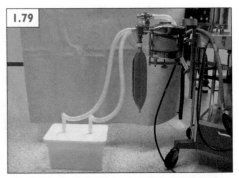

Fig. 1.79 An induction chamber connected to a rebreathing circuit significantly slows induction speed because of the increased mechanical volume barrier, which slows denitrogenization and equilibration of the vaporizer anesthetic concentration.

removing the inhalant anesthetic gas from the chamber. One study has shown that only minimal exhaled CO_2 from the animal builds up in the chamber during induction. The induction time is usually short and poses no danger to the animal if the chamber is not connected to a scavenging outlet.

FACE MASKS
- Face masks are used for induction of anesthesia or for providing oxygen to the animal.
- Face masks should be clear or transparent so that the animal's muzzle is visible (**Fig. 1.80**); it is critical to detect regurgitation when it occurs so that appropriate actions can be taken.
- Face masks are available in different sizes and shapes (**Fig. 1.81**).
- The size of the face mask is based on the animal's body size.

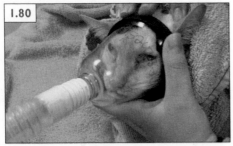

Fig. 1.80 A face mask should be transparent, so that the muzzle is visible, and fit tightly to prevent leaks.

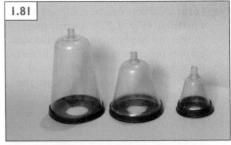

Fig. 1.81 Face masks come in different sizes. A tightly fitting face mask prevents leakage of the inhalant anesthetic agent during induction.

- Face mask that are too large increase the chance of leaks and prolongs the induction time.

- Face masks that are too small are not effective in inducing anesthesia.

Checking the accuracy of the flowmeter

Flowmeters should be periodically checked with a portable oxygen flowmeter (**Fig. 1.82**) to verify that the flow is accurate downstream from the flowmeter (**Fig. 1.83**). The portable oxygen flowmeter is a useful tool to diagnose a crack on the flowmeter of anesthesia machine or a leak downstream from the flowmeter. In these cases, the anesthesia machine flowmeter shows a different flow rate to the portable oxygen flowmeter (**Fig. 1.84**).

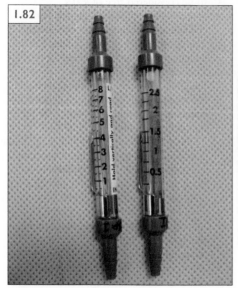

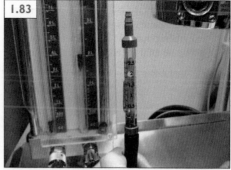

Fig. 1.83 This portable oxygen flowmeter is connected to a hose from the fresh gas outlet. When the oxygen flowmeter on the anesthesia machine is turned on, it should reflect the identical flow rate as the portable oxygen flowmeter. In this case, both flowmeters show an oxygen flow rate of 2 liters per minute.

Fig. 1.82 A portable oxygen flowmeter has a different scale for checking the accuracy of the oxygen flowmeter on the anesthesia machine. Note that the portable flowmeter on the left is designed to check a flow rate of between 1 and 8 liters per minute. The flowmeter on the right is designed to monitor an oxygen flow rate between zero and 2.5 liters per minute.

Fig. 1.84 A leak has been detected downstream from this anesthesia machine flowmeter. The portable oxygen flowmeter measures 1.25 liters per minute of oxygen flow at the fresh gas outlet and the machine flowmeter is turned off. Leaking oxygen will dilute the anesthetic concentration since the lost oxygen does not pass through the vaporizer. Note the position of the float in the flowmeter of the anesthesia machine (shown as 0) and in the portable oxygen flowmeter (shown as 1.25 liters per minute).

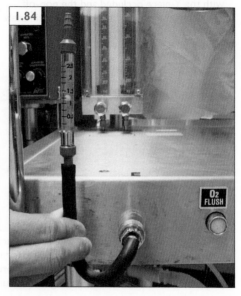

Checking the anesthesia machine and breathing circuit for leaks

Checking for leaks in the anesthesia machine and breathing circuit can be divided into positive-pressure and negative-pressure leak checks.

POSITIVE-PRESSURE LEAKS

- Checking the anesthesia machine and breathing circuit for leaks is easy and should be performed prior to each anesthesia case. A leaking machine or breathing circuit is not only inefficient for anesthetizing a patient properly, but it also pollutes the environment. An incorrectly connected anesthesia machine and breathing circuit could be fatal for the anesthetized animal.

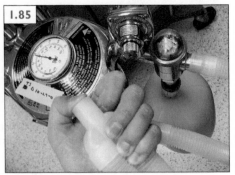

Fig. 1.85 Positive-pressure leak checking is being carried out on this rebreathing circuit with the Y-piece occluded and the pop-off valve closed and pressurized to approximately 30–40 cmH$_2$O; the oxygen flowmeter is turned off.

- To check for leaks, ensure that the anesthetic outlet fittings of the vaporizer are tightly in place and that the breathing hoses are connected to the anesthesia machine properly. The pop-off valve of the rebreathing circuit is closed, the 'y-piece' of the rebreathing circuit occluded, and the oxygen flowmeter turned on to pressurize the breathing circuit to 30 cmH$_2$O (Fig. 1.85). Once this pressure is reached, the flowmeter is turned off. The breathing circuit and the machine should hold this pressure for at least 10 seconds to be considered free of leaks.

- In a non-rebreathing circuit, the patient end of the breathing circuit is occluded. The non-rebreathing circuit does not contain a pressure manometer. However, a manometer can be placed between the reservoir bag and the breathing hose of the non-rebreathing circuit to perform a leak check in a similar fashion as for the rebreathing circuit (Figs. 1.86, 1.87). The pop-off valve is closed and oxygen flow continued until the pressure manometer reads 30 cmH$_2$O. The oxygen flow on the flowmeter is then turned off while continuing to occlude the breathing circuit system. If the pressure remains at 30 cmH$_2$O for 10 seconds, there are no leaks in the system. A breathing circuit is unacceptable if it leaks at ≥200 ml/minute.

- Do not use the oxygen flush valve to inflate the reservoir bag, but instead turn on the oxygen flowmeter. When the oxygen flush valve is depressed, oxygen bypasses the flowmeter and vaporizer and

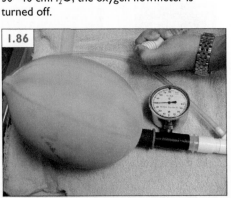
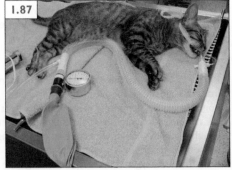

Figs. 1.86, 1.87 A pressure manometer attached between the breathing hose of the Bain's circuit and the reservoir bag is used to perform a leak check by occluding the scavenger until pressurized to 30 cmH$_2$O (1.86). This same pressure manometer can be used to monitor the pressure within the non-rebreathing circuit during spontaneous and controlled breathing (1.87).

goes directly into the reservoir bag via the fresh gas outlet. This allows a leak between the flowmeter and the vaporizer, or from the vaporizer to the fresh oxygen outlet, to remain undetected.

- If leaks are detected, several areas should be checked first. The priority areas are the reservoir bag itself, the corrugated breathing hoses and their connectors, the filler cap on the vaporizer, the end caps on either side of the vaporizer, and the CO_2 absorbent canister. A leak can be easily detected by spraying soapy water (use a diluted Nolvasan antiseptic soap solution) on these areas. The leak check procedure is repeated to pressurize the breathing circuit and look for bubbles in the soapy water (**Fig. 1.88**).

NEGATIVE-PRESSURE LEAKS

- Negative-pressure leak checks are primarily applied to the anesthesia machine and the vaporizer.
- Negative-pressure leak checks use a suction bulb attached to the common gas outlet of an anesthesia machine (**Fig. 1.89**). When the suction bulb is depressed, it creates negative pressure within the machine conduit system (**Fig. 1.90**). If there are

leaks along the conduit system (from the flowmeter to the vaporizer to the common gas outlet), the suction bulb will re-inflate. Some anesthesia machines have a check valve located between the machine and the common gas outlet. The negative-pressure leak check will not be accurate if this is the case. The location of the check valve always creates a negative pressure on the suction bulb when negative pressure is applied and, therefore, the purpose of the negative-pressure leak check on the machine is defeated.

- The negative-pressure leak check should also be applied to the vaporizer while the vaporizer dial is in the off position and the vaporizer turned on (**Figs. 1.91, 1.92**). The negative-pressure leak check detects cracks or leaks in the vaporizer. The filler

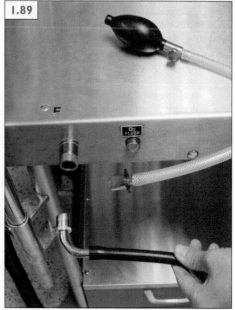

Fig. 1.89 The common gas outlet of an anesthesia machine is used for negative-pressure leak checking. The fresh gas inlet hose (black) of the rebreathing circuit is detached and white tubing with a suction bulb is connected to the common gas outlet to perform the negative-pressure leak checking. The oxygen flushing valve is located next to the common gas outlet and labeled 'O₂ flush'. When activated, the oxygen flushing valve allows oxygen (at 35 liters per minute) directly into the breathing circuit, bypassing the vaporizer.

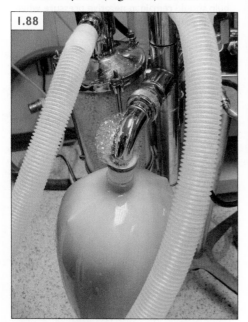

Fig. 1.88 Bubbles form when soapy water is sprayed on a leaking anesthesia machine or loose connection.

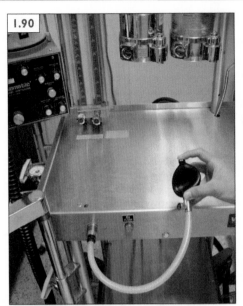

Fig. 1.90 When the suction bulb remains negative, there are no leaks in the passage between the flowmeter, the vaporizer, and the common gas outlet.

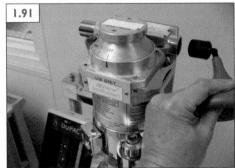

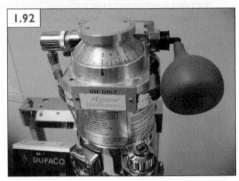

Figs. 1.91, 1.92 A suction bulb is applied to the vaporizer outlet to conduct a negative-pressure leak check on this vaporizer (**1.91**). The suction bulb should remain in negative pressure when the vaporizer is turned off or on (**1.92**).

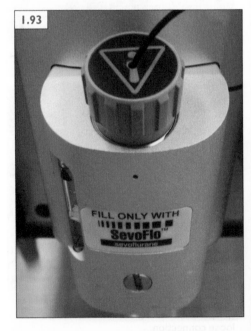

cap of the vaporizer is a common place for leaks if it is not tightened adequately. If a leak is detected, the filler cap (**Fig. 1.93**) of the vaporizer should be tightened and the negative-pressure leak check process repeated to rule out this problem.

- A loose filler cap on the vaporizer is a frequent cause of premature awakening of the animal during inhalant anesthesia. It also significantly slows the speed of a face mask or chamber induction. Sometimes, the leak from a loose vaporizer filler cap is so small that there is minimal smell of inhalant or bubbling of the inhalant anesthetic liquid, but it is enough that the animal frequently wakes prematurely.

Fig. 1.93 The filler cap of the vaporizer is one of the most overlooked places when evaluating leaks from the vaporizer. If it is not tightened (especially after filling the inhalant liquid), either the liquid anesthetic bursts out when the oxygen flowmeter is turned on and oxygen enters the vaporizer or, if the leak is small, the only symptom is continuous premature awakening of the animal during general anesthesia.

Checking the scavenging system for leaks and malfunctions

- The scavenging hoses should be properly attached at all connections (pop-off valve, waste gas collection, and charcoal absorbent canister).
- Charcoal canisters, when used for scavenging, should be changed at regular intervals.
- The vacuum active scavenging systems should be set appropriately to prevent over or under vacuum situations.
- Proper connection of the ventilator scavenging outlet to the scavenging system should be verified.
- The negative-/positive-pressure relief valve often malfunctions as a result of animal hair or dust accumulation inside the valve, therefore it should be cleaned periodically (**Fig. 1.94**).

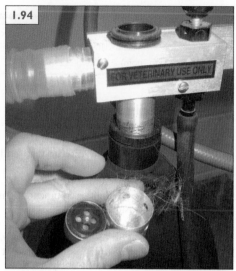

Fig. 1.94 The negative-/positive-pressure relief valve of the scavenger can attract hair and dust because of the continual negative pressure. If the valve is occluded with dust, it will malfunction. As a result, the scavenging active vacuum will compete with the anesthetic gas supply to the breathing bag or to the patient.

Monitoring of waste gas and pollution

Quantitative assessment of the effectiveness of a waste gas program can be done by measuring and monitoring trace-gas concentrations in the work zone. *Table 1.4* shows the two most commonly used methods of waste gas monitoring. Waste gas pollution limits in different countries will be set by the relevant authority. The maximum time-weighted average limits (in the USA) are consistent with recommendations from the National Institute of Occupational Safety and Health (NIOSH). These limits are based on a NIOSH study in 1978 examining the effect of halothane alone and halothane with nitrous oxide (*Table 1.5*). The same limits are anticipated for isoflurane and sevoflurane despite no study results from NIOSH being available.

Table 1.4 The two most commonly used methods of waste gas monitoring

	Real time monitoring	*Badge analysis*
Principles	Uses a real time monitor and detects waste gas concentration on the spot	Personnel wear a time-weighted averaging badge over a specific period of time and return the badge to the laboratory for analysis
Pros and cons	Real time reading allows immediate preventive action Value can be falsely high due to one-time measurement Real time monitoring is expensive and can be cost prohibitive to use	Time-weighted averaging is more representative for true exposure Individual calculations for waste gas exposure can be done since each person wears a badge Inconvenient to wear the badge Slowness in obtaining results delays immediate action to prevent exposure

Table 1.5 NIOSH maximum time-weighted average limits

NIOSH maximum allowed for time-weighted average limits	Halogenated hydrocarbons (halothane, isoflurane, sevoflurane)	Halogenated anesthetic agent when used with nitrous oxide
Parts per million (ppm)	≤2	≤0.5

Further reading

Al-Shaikh B, Stacey S (2013) *Essentials of Anaesthetic Equipment*, 4th edn. Churchill Livingstone, London.

American College of Veterinary Anesthetists (1996) Commentary and recommendations on control of waste anesthetic gases in the work place. *J Am Vet Med Assoc* **209**:75–7.

Dorsch JA, Dorsch SE (2008) *Understanding Anesthesia Equipment*, 5th edn. Lippincott Williams and Wilkins, Philadelphia, PA.

Hall LW, Clark KW, Trim CM (2001) *Veterinary Anaesthesia*, 10th edn. WB Saunders, London.

Hartsfield SM (1996) Anesthesia machines and breathing systems. In: *Lumb and Jones Veterinary Anesthesia*, 3rd edn. (eds JC Thurmon, WJ Tranquilli, GJ Benson) Williams & Wilkins, Baltimore.

Lish J, Ko JC, Payton ME (2008) Evaluation of two methods of endotracheal tube selection in dogs. *J Am Anim Hosp Assoc* **44**:236–42.

Spiegel JE (2010) Endotracheal tube cuffs: design and function. *Anesthesiology News: Guide to Airway Management* pp. 51–8.

Perioperative blood work and urine analysis

Jeff C Ko

Introduction

Medical history and physical examination of the patient help practitoners indentify the major concerns of the owner related to the patient's illness. Preoperative thoracic radiography, electrocardiography, and echocardiography help evaluate the patient's cardiopulmonary functions. Perioperative body fluid testing, including blood work, urine analysis, and other body secretions, helps practitioners verify/identify a deficit associated with a specific systemic dysfunction. These laboratory tests also help practitioners to formulate/modify anesthetic protocols and anesthetic management perioperatively. This chapter provides a quick reference and interpretation regarding body fluid testing that may have an impact on the anesthetic management of patients undergoing both diagnostic or surgical procedures.

Blood work

Depending on the patient's age, specific conditions, and procedures, blood work may include a simple packed cell volume (PCV), total protein (TP), serum or plasma glucose, or a complete blood count (CBC) with differential and chemistry profile.

- Venous blood can be collected from the jugular, cephalic, or lateral (in dogs) or medial (in cats) saphenous veins for hematologic tests.
- For over-all healthy and young animals, a simple PCV, TP, and blood glucose is all that is required before anesthesia.
- Blood collection tubes containing blood anticoagulants, such ethylenediaminetetraacetic acid (EDTA, purple rubber top tubes), heparin (green rubber top tubes), or sodium citrate (blue rubber top tubes), are used for different hematologic preference testing. EDTA is the most commonly used for cell morphology and hematologic studies. The blood samples can stay fresh for 2–12 hours if stored at −4°C. Heparin is good for immediate blood smear preparations. Sodium citrate is good for coagulation tests.
- A CBC may contain the following – PCV, hemoglobin concentration, TP, total red blood cell (RBC) count, erythrocyte indices (mean corpuscular volume [MCV], mean corpuscular hemoglobin concentration [MCHC], and mean corpuscular hemoglobin [MCH]), and total white blood cell (WBC) count with differential count and platelet estimation. Reference ranges are provided in *Table 2.1*.

Table 2.1 Hematology and biochemistry reference intervals in dogs and cats

Test	Dogs	Cats	Units
Hematology			
Eosinophils	0.1–0.125 (100–1,250)	0.1–0.15 (100–1,500)	× 10⁹/l (/μl)
Packed cell volume (PCV) (hematocrit, Hct)	0.35–0.55 (37.0–55.0)	0.3–0.45 (30.0–45.0)	l/l (%)
Hemoglobin	120–180 (12.0–18.0)	80–150 (8.0–15.0)	g/l (g/dl)
Lymphocytes	0.1–0.5 (1,000–5,000)	0.15–0.7 (1,500–7,000)	× 10⁹/l (/μl)
Mean corpuscular hemoglobin concentration (MCHC)	320–360 (32–36)	300–360 (30–36)	g/l (g/dl)
Mean corpuscular volume (MCV)	60–75 (60–75)	40–55 (40–55	fl (pg)
Monocytes	0.015–0.135 (150–1,350)	0.05–0.85 (50–850)	× 10⁹/l (/μl)
Neutrophils (band)	0–0.3 (0–300)	0–0.03 (0–300)	× 10⁹/l (/μl)
Neutrophils (segmented)	3–12 (3,000–12,000)	3–12 (3,000–12,000)	× 10⁹/l (/μl)
Platelets	200–500 (2–5)	200–500 (2–5)	× 10⁹/l (× 10⁵/μl)
Red blood cells (RBC)	5.5–8.5 (5.5–8.5)	5–10 (5–10)	× 10¹²/l (× 10⁶/μl)
White blood cells (WBC)	6–17 (6,000–17,000)	6–18 (6,000–18,000)	× 10⁹/l (/μl)
Biochemistry			
Albumin	23–39 (2.3–3.9)	27–39 (2.7–3.9)	g/l (g/dl)
Alanine aminotransferase (ALT)	3–69	20–108	U/l
Alkaline phosphatase (ALP)	20–175	23–107	U/l
Amylase	378–1,033	440–1,264	U/l
Blood urea nitrogen (BUN)	2.5–11.4 (7–32)	5.4–12.5 (15–35)	mmol/l (mg/dl)
Calcium	2.4–3.1 (9.7–12.3)	2.2–2.9 (9.0–11.7)	mmol/l (mg/dl)
Chloride	105–117	115–128	mmol/l (mEq/l)
Creatinine	44–132 (0.5–1.5)	80–203 (0.9–2.3)	μmol/l (mg/dl)
Glucose	3.7–7.3 (67–132)	4.2–7.4 (75–134)	mol/l (mg/dl)
Lipase	104–1,753	148–1,746	U/l
Phosphorus	0.7–2.6 (2.2–7.9)	0.8–2.8 (2.6–8.8)	mmol/l (mg/dl)
Potassium	3.5–5.0	3.5–5.1	mmol/l (mEq/l)
Sodium	138–148	148–157	mmol/l (mEq/l)
T4		30.9–59.2 (2.4–4.6)	nmol/l (μg/dl)
Total bilirubin	1.71–13.7 (0.1–0.8)	1.71–6.8 (0.1–0.4)	μmol/l (mg/dl)
Total protein (TP)	60–80 (6–8)	60–80 (6–8)	g/l (g/dl)

PACKED CELL VOLUME

- PCV, known as hematocrit (Hct), represents the percentage of RBCs in whole blood.
- PCV is important for anesthesia because it affects tissue oxygenation through hemoglobin concentration in the arterial blood oxygen content. Oxygen content largely depends on hemoglobin concentration, which is about one-third of the PCV. When the PCV is low, hemoglobin concentration is also low. Most of the anesthetic agents depress cardiac output. This together with low oxygen content results in reduction of tissue perfusion and oxygenation.
- Low PCV indicates anemia and may be caused by acute or chronic

blood loss. Acute blood loss may be due to tissue trauma or bleeding from a surgical site. A series of PCV tests should be performed to determine ongoing bleeding or blood clotting.

- Chronic blood loss may be due to cancer, parasites, or gastrointestinal ulceration. Hemoglobin can be either measured or estimated as one-third of PCV. The impact of low PCV on anesthesia is hypoxemia. In patients with a PCV <0.2 l/l (20%), anesthesia should be avoided because oxygenation of the tissue will be inadequate. Either whole blood transfusion or packed cells transfusion should be considered prior to surgery (see Chapter 8).
- For patients with a low PCV, anesthesia/sedation for bone marrow aspiration is usually required for diagnostic purpose. In this situation, while ideally a packed cell transfusion prior to the procedure is administered, providing 100% oxygen is necessary to improve oxygen content and the procedure should be as swift as possible.
- A high PCV may be due to dehydration, polycythemia, or splenic contraction in a stressed animal. A high PCV results in thick blood viscosity and slows blood flow, which also lead to poor tissue oxygenation. To improve blood flow and oxygen delivery and reduce blood viscosity in the polycythemic patient, a certain amount of blood can be removed via phlebotomy and replaced with the same volume of crystalloid fluid.

TOTAL PROTEIN

- Albumin, globulins, and fibrinogen constitute the three proteins in the plasma. Albumin is the main protein and is mainly produced in the liver. If albumin is low, total protein is low.
- TP plays a vital role in anesthetic drug distribution. Most anesthetic agents are highly protein bound. Low total protein increases a patient's sensitivity to anesthetic agents because protein-unbound anesthetics are active drugs and lack of plasma protein to bind the

anesthetic allows peak anesthetic activity to persist. The main plasma protein is albumin, which provides approximately 80% of the colloid oncotic pressure. A patient with low plasma proteins is at risk of fluid overload.

- In addition to the fluid balance mentioned, plasma protein should be assessed help to evaluate liver and kidney function:
  - Hypoproteinemia may be due to severe liver dysfunction, protein-losing nephropathy or enteropathy, malnutrition and malabsorption of the intestine, acute blood loss, or significant hemodilution if PCV is also low. When total protein is <35 g/l (3.5 g/dl) or albumin <15 g/l (1.5 g/dl), intravascular fluid starts to be lost into the pulmonary, pleural, abdominal, intestinal, or interstitial spaces and this results in pulmonary edema, pleural effusion, ascites, and distal limb edema. Plasma administration will help to improve hypoalbuminemia, despite the plasma containing a relatively small portion of albumin. Administering synthetic colloids (see Chapter 7) (hydroxyethyl starch) is beneficial since these fluids increase oncotic pressure and prevent fluid loss into the interstitial spaces. The TP measured by refractometry changes minimally after synthetic colloid fluid administration.
  - Hyperproteinemia may be due to dehydration or hypergammaglobulinemia induced by antigen.

BLOOD GLUCOSE

- Serum or plasma glucose levels (*Table 2.1*) serve as an indicator of glucose balance between production and utilization.
  - Hypoglycemia may be due to fasting, anorexia, insulin overdose, hepatic insufficiency, or portal systemic shunt. Hypoglycemic patients may have prolonged anesthesia recovery due to neuroglycopenia, and can be mistaken as having anesthetic overdose or increased anesthetic sensitivity. Blood glucose should be checked if

there is prolonged recovery in dogs and cats. Providing proper dextrose fluid support will facilitate recovery in these patients. Blood glucose levels can be improved by administering 5% dextrose to a hypoglycemic patient – add 100 ml of 50% (500 mg per ml) dextrose to 900 ml of fluid (normal saline or sterile water).

- Hyperglycemia may be due to diabetes or pancreatitis. It is important to correct dehydration in the hyperglycemic patient.
- Glucose should be carefully monitored in a diabetic patient undergoing anesthetic procedures (see Diabetic management in Chapter 10).

RETICULOCYTE COUNT

Reticulocyte (or polychromatic cells) count is used to differentiate bone marrow-responsive (regenerative) anemia from non-bone marrow-responsive (non-regenerative) anemia. An increased reticulocyte count indicates that the bone marrow is responsive to an anemic state.

- To classify types of anemia, RBC indices and morphology are necessary.
- Increased reticulocytes usually are not evident until days after the onset of anemia.

MEAN CORPUSCULAR VOLUME

- Refers to the size of the RBC.
- Macrocytic anemia is a bone marrow-responsive anemia because there are large-sized RBCs present and it is associated with increased MCV.
- Microcytic anemia is associated with decreased MCV and is frequently due to iron deficiency.
- If the MCV counts are normal (normocytic anemia), the anemia could be due to many different causes.

MEAN CORPUSCULAR HEMOGLOBIN CONCENTRATION

- Refers to the ratio of the weight of hemoglobin in each RBC.
- In iron deficiency or regenerative anemia, the MCHC is decreased (called hypochromic anemia).

- In normocytic anemia, the MCHC is normal.
- The MCHC does not increase.

WHITE BLOOD CELLS (OR LEUKOCYTES)

- The many forms of leukocytes include mature and immature neutrophils, lymphocytes, monocytes, eosinophils, and basophils.
- A differential count of the leukocytes should be performed because each type of WBC represents stress, stages of infection, and inflammation.
- Leukocytosis means there is an increase in WBC numbers. If the WBC count is $>50 \times 10^9/l$ (50,000 cells/µl), it indicates severe stress, infection, or inflammation.

NEUTROPHILS

- Neutrophils are generated by the bone marrow.
- Neutrophilia means there is an increase in neutrophils. Such an increase occurs because large amounts of mature neutrophils have been released from the bone marrow into systemic blood. Mild neutrophilia is frequently associated with excitement, stress, and corticosteroid administration. Bacterial, viral, and fungal infections may result in profound neutrophilia.
- Neutropenia means there is a decrease in neutrophils. This usually occurs with extreme infection. Infection-induced neutrophilia or neutropenia depends on the balance between bone marrow production and inflammatory tissue consumption of the neutrophils.

LYMPHOCYTES

- Lymphocytosis means increased numbers of lymphocytes. Lymphocytosis may occur in young (less than 3 years old), healthy, excited dogs and cats.
- Leukemia, lymphoma, or autoimmune diseases (colitis) may be the most common causes for dogs to have lymphocytosis; less commonly in dogs with hypoadrenocorticism (Addison's disease), *Ehrlichia* infection, or thymoma.
- Lymphopenia occurs because of slow release of lymphocytes by the lymphoid organs or increased lysis of lymphocytes

due to stress. Lymphopenia is frequently associated with a stress leukogram. In the stress leukogram, neutrophilia with lymphopenia and eosinopenia are strong indications of a cortisol-related stressful response.

EOSINOPHILS
- Eosinophilia (increased eosinophils from bone marrow production) is most commonly induced by parasite antigens (such as heart worms, cat lung worms) or allergens.
- Eosinophilia may also occur in hypoadrenocorticism.

PLATELETS AND COAGULATION TESTS
Platelets are also called thrombocytes. They play a vital role in blood clotting and patients undergoing surgery.
- If the platelet count is below $40-50 \times 10^9/l$ ($40,000-50,000/\mu l$) (called thrombocytopenia), the patient is prone to abnormal bleeding perioperatively.
- Coagulation tests assess the interaction between blood vessel walls, coagulation factors, and platelets to form a clot in a timely manner. A clot (consisting of platelets and fibrin) serves to indicate that both intrinsic (blood vessel) and extrinsic (tissue trauma) coagulation pathways are following their respective cascade successfully.

- The prothrombin time (PT) test measures blood clot formation time and represents assessment of the common clotting pathway and extrinsic activity. It evaluates clotting factors I, II, V, VII, and X.
- The partial thromboplastin time (PTT) test is an assessment of the intrinsic activity and common blood pathway of the blood clot. It evaluates factors I, II, V, VIII, IX, X, XI, and XII.
- The PT and PTT tests are frequently used together.
- Von Willebrand factor is a protein that helps platelets to adhere to the sites of blood vessel injury. This test is sometimes performed in bleeding dogs where there is a suspicion of deficiency of Von Willebrand's clotting factor.
- The buccal mucosal bleeding time (BMBT) test uses a spring-loaded blade inside a cassette to produce a small cut of precise depth on the mucosal membrane of the dog's lip. The test evaluates the ability of platelets to form a platelet clot. If the BMBT is prolonged, it indicates a decreased platelet function, which is seen in dogs with non-steroidal anti-inflammatory drug (NSAID) toxicity, uremia, thrombocytopenia, or von Willebrand's disease. The BMBT test should be used in dogs with thrombocytopenia.

Biochemistry profiles

Analyzing blood chemistry profiles provides an insight into liver, kidney, pancreas, and muscle function. In addition to enzyme analysis, serum electrolytes also provide vital information on fluid administration for assisting anesthetic management and treatment of cardiac arrhythmias.

LIVER FUNCTION TESTS
- The liver is responsible for the synthesis of plasma proteins, including albumin, clotting factors, and cholesterol. In addition, it is responsible for almost all anesthetic drug metabolism, detoxification of the body waste, and secretion of bilirubin.

- Alanine aminotransferase (ALT), formally known as SGPT (serum glutamate-pyruvate transaminase). Since the primary source of ALT is from the dog and cat's liver, increased ALT is a good indication of hepatocyte damage in these species.
- Aspartate aminotransferase (AST), formally known as SGOT (serum glutamate oxaloacetate transferase). AST is not liver specific since serum AST comes from more than one source within the body (skeletal and cardiac muscles, RBCs, pancreas, and kidneys), therefore an increased AST level only serves to indicate that there is liver or muscle damage.

- Arginase is a liver-specific enzyme. Increased arginase is indicative of liver dysfunction.
- The liver is also responsible for secreting bile, which passes through the gallbladder and the bile duct to the small intestines. When this bile flow pathway is obstructed (such as with bile duct obstruction) or there is a significant increase in bile synthesis within the liver, one of the liver enzymes (alkaline phosphatase [ALP]) leaks into the systemic circulation and can be detected via laboratory testing. ALP is frequently used to detect bile flow pathway disturbance (cholestasis). The reasons for cholestasis include hepatic inflammation, swelling, tumors, or bile duct obstruction, all of which cause ALP to increase.
- Increased ALP may also be induced by drugs used to treat seizure. This should be differentiated from pathologic cholestasis.
- When cholestasis occurs, another liver enzyme, gamma glutamyltransferase (GGT), also increases.
- Bilirubin is a by-product when hemoglobin breaks down in the liver. An increase in serum total bilirubin (both conjugated and unconjugated) concentrations may be due to jaundice, liver dysfunction, or cholestasis.
- Cholesterol is converted in the liver to bile acid, which is then stored in the gallbladder and secreted into the intestines to digest fat in dogs and cats. Normally, bile acid is cleared rapidly via first-pass blood circulation. When there is hepatic dysfunction, portal systemic shunt, or cholestasis, the bile acid increases in the systemic circulation and can be detected in the serum.
- Ammonia is a digestive product of protein via bacterial action in the intestine. Ammonia is rapidly absorbed from the lower gastrointestinal tract, cleared by the liver via the portal vein blood circulation, and converted to urea in the liver via the urea cycle. Elevation of ammonia is seen with hepatoencephalopathy, commonly associated with portal systemic shunt, and hepatic tumor. Normal values are usually 11.2–70.44 µmol/l (19–120 µg/dl).

An abnormal value is above 176 µmol/l (300 µg/dl).

- Canine hepatobiliary diseases can be largely divided into liver parenchymal itself-, biliary-, vascular-, or neoplastic-related diseases. Elevation of ALT, ALP, AST, and GGT enzymes are indicators of hepatobiliary injury. In order to confirm a significant hepatic impairment, additional liver function tests for measuring bilirubin, bile acids, and ammonia levels in blood are tested. However, all these biochemical indicators are not sufficient to specifically diagnose the underlying liver diseases.
- Recent development at the University of Edinburgh's Royal (Dick) School of Veterinary Studies reveals that using blood test screening for canine serum microRNA profiling (consisting of miR-21, miR-122, miR-126, miR-200c, and miR-222) can distinguish between parenchymal, biliary, and neoplastic hepatobiliary diseases. This blood test may become a vital tool in the near future for diagnosing a wide range of canine liver-related diseases.

KIDNEY FUNCTION TESTS

The kidneys are involved in body water and electrolyte balance in order to maintain body hemostasis (blood pH, blood pressure, absorption and excretion of various electrolytes), they produce important hormones (prostaglandins), and they excrete body wastes (urea and creatinine). The kidneys also excrete anesthetic drugs. An abnormal kidney function test implies that anesthetic drug excretion may be impaired.

- Blood urine nitrogen (BUN). The absorbed protein undergoes hepatic metabolism and produces ammonia. Ammonia is then converted to urea inside the liver via the urea cycle and excreted by the kidneys.
  - Measuring BUN provides information about the renal clearance rate of this protein.
  - Accumulation of BUN is called azotemia and can be classified as renal, pre-, or post-renal azotemia.
  - In cases of renal azotemia, it indicates that approximately 70–75% of nephrons

are dysfunctional, and the glomerular filtration rate (GFR) of the kidney is significantly reduced. The kidney is, therefore, unable to eliminate/reabsorb the urea, which leads to high BUN.
- Prerenal azotemia is usually associated with poor kidney perfusion due to poor blood pressure caused by severe dehydration or blood volume depletion. It could also be due to poor cardiac output due to cardiac dysfunction. All these conditions lead to poor elimination of BUN from the kidneys, resulting in accumulation of BUN in the blood.
- Postrenal azotemia is usually due to obstruction or dysfunction of the urinary tract, resulting in urea elimination deficiency.
- Creatinine is a metabolic product of the muscles and mainly eliminated via renal tubular filtration. Since creatinine is produced at a constant rate and predominantly eliminated by the kidney, increased creatinine indicates renal dysfunction. The normal plasma creatinine concentration is 44–88 µmol/l (0.5–1 mg/dl). It is a good estimation that for every 50% reduction in GFR, the creatinine concentration doubles.

PANCREATIC FUNCTION TESTS

The pancreas is responsible for lipid digestion and blood glucose balance. Amylase and lipase are produced by the pancreas and secreted into the intestines. The function of the pancreas can be assessed through measurement of serum amylase, lipase, and glucose.
- Body glucagon and starches are broken down by amylase. In cases of acute or chronic pancreatitis, or pancreatic duct obstructions, amylase is significantly increased. Sometimes renal and liver dysfunction or bowel obstruction unrelated to the pancreas may cause amylase to increase. Therefore, increased amylase alone does not indicate pancreatic dysfunction specifically.
- Lipase is mainly produced by the pancreas to digest lipids. In pancreatic dysfunctional animals, lipase may increase. However, lipase may also increase in other non-pancreatic

events including corticosteroid use or chronic renal disease. Both amylase and lipase should be measured to assess pancreatic function.

ELECTROLYTES

Interstitial, intra-, and extracellular fluids are full of positively-charged (cations) and negatively charged (anions) particles. Sodium and potassium are the main cations, whereas chloride is the main anion in these fluids.
- Sodium. It is the major cation of extracellular fluid (the interstitial fluid and plasma) and plays a major role in determining the fluid shift between intra- and extracellular spaces.
  - When hyponatremia (low sodium) occurs, fluids move from vascular space to intracellular space due to hypo-osmolality, resulting in hypovolemia in the vasculature and cellular edema. Hyponatremia is usually seen with diabetic ketoacidosis.
  - In contrast, when hypernatremia occurs, fluid shifts in the opposite direction. Hypernatremia occurs with water deprivation or prolonged administration of crystalloid fluid. Hypernatremia may cause cerebral edema.
- Chloride. Normal serum chloride concentrations range from 96 to 106 mmol/l (96–106 mEq/l). Chloride is the major extracellular anion. It is present to counterbalance sodium and therefore maintain equal positive and negative charges. When body chloride is lost, acidosis occurs and when chloride is retained, alkalosis occurs. Metabolic hyperchloremic acidosis is associated with dehydration, respiratory alkalosis, and loss of sodium bicarbonate. Hypochloremia can result from vomiting, diarrhea, renal dysfunction, or severe skin burn.
- Potassium. It is the major intracellular cation. Skeletal muscle weakness and paralysis occur when hypokalemia develops.
  - Hypokalemia <3 mmol/l (3 mEq/l) is associated with vomiting, diarrhea, chronic interstitial renal disease, or dogs that received loop diuretics.

Hypokalemia can induce muscle weakness and increase the risk of ventricular arrhythmias due to prolonged Q-T interval (prolonged repolarization) and lead to early afterdepolarizations. Because hypokalemia also hyperpolarizes the cardiac cell membrane, it interferes with lidocaine's effect in treating ventricular cardiac arrhythmias. During hypotension with exaggerated volume expansion using fluids, it can lead to hemodilution and hypokalemia. It is beneficial to add potassium chloride or phosphate to the crystalloid fluid to counteract hypokalemia. A rule of thumb is 20, 30, or 40 mmol/l (mEq/l) can be added to one liter of crystalloid fluid to counteract mild, moderate, or severe hypokalemia. However, the rate should not exceed 0.5 mmol (mEq)/kg/hour of potassium to avoid cardiac arrhythmias.

- Hyperkalemia frequently occurs with poor renal excretion of potassium. It may be associated with severe renal dysfunction, uroabdomen, urinary obstruction, acute kidney injury, or diabetic ketoacidosis. Hyperkalemia of >6 mmol/l (6 mEq/l) is considered life-threatening. Physiologic saline along with insulin and glucose should be administered to drive potassium back into the intracellular space. Blocked tom cats usually show hyperkalemia (7–7.5 mmol/l [7–7.5 mEq/l]) and this can result in serious cardiac arrhythmias and, ultimately, severe bradycardia and cardiac standstill (see Chapter 22).

- Calcium. It is the major ion for maintaining muscle contraction, blood coagulation, and neuromuscular excitability. Normal blood calcium is 2.25–2.75 mmol/l (9.0–11.0 mg/dl) in dogs. Blood calcium exists in both an ionized (active and not binding with albumin) and a non-ionized (inactive and albumin-bound) form. Measuring ionized calcium (iCa^{2+}) is more accurate than other forms of calcium since iCa^{2+} is a reflection of the physiologic calcium.

- Phosphorus. The majority (80%) of phosphorus is in the bone and less than 20% is in extracellular fluid. Plasma phosphorus is inorganic phosphorus and its concentration is mainly regulated by the kidneys. When the value is high, it is called hyperphosphatemia, which is due to decreased phosphorus excretion, as associated with hyperparathyroidism, or to increased renal phosphorus reabsorption because of hypoparathyroidism. Hyperphosphatemia also occurs in animals with hypothyroidism. Hypophosphatemia can be due to decreased intestinal absorption, increased renal phosphorus loss, or transcellular shift. Hypophosphatemia is common in diabetic ketoacidosis and is a result of excessive phosphorus loss in urine.

Urine analysis

Urine analysis pertaining to anesthesia mainly involves specific gravity (SG) because it is associated with kidney dysfunction. SG gives a good indication of renal function (i.e. the ability of renal tubules to concentrate urine). SG in dogs range from 1.001 to 1.070 and in cats can be up to 1.080. A SG of 1.030 or more in dogs and 1.035 or more in cats indicates that the urine is highly concentrated. Because such a high concentration of urine requires the majority of the functional nephrons to work properly, if high BUN and creatinine levels are present, there is a strong indication of pre-renal azotemia (due to dehydration or poor kidney perfusion).

Further reading

Desai N, Schofield N, Richards T (2017) Perioperative patient blood management to improve outcomes. *Anesth Analg* 2017 Oct 19 (Epub ahead of print) doi: 10.1213/ANE.0000000000002549.

Dirksen K, Verzijl T, Grinwis GC et al. (2016) Use of Serum microRNAs as biomarker for hepatobiliary diseases in dogs. *J Vet Intern Med* **30(6)**:1816–23.

Kumar A, Srivastava U (2011) Role of routine laboratory investigations in pre-operative evaluation. *J Anaesthesiol Clin Pharmacol* **27(2)**:174–9.

Oosthuyzen W, Ten Berg PWL, Francis B et al. (2018) Sensitivity and specificity of microRNA-122 for liver disease in dogs. *J Vet Intern Med* Aug 2 (Epub ahead of print) doi: 10.1111/jvim.15250.

Sharkey LC, Radin J (2010) *Manual of Veterinary Clinical Chemistry: A Case Study Approach*, 1st edn. Taylor & Francis, UK.

Zambouri A (2007) Preoperative evaluation and preparation for anesthesia and surgery. *Hippokratia* **11(1)**:13–21.

CHAPTER 3

Preanesthetic medication: drugs and dosages

Jeff C Ko

Introduction

The administration of drugs prior to anesthetic induction is called preanesthetic medication and is part of the general anesthetic procedure. Other parts of the anesthetic procedure include IV anesthetic induction, inhalant anesthetic maintenance, anesthetic recovery, and postoperative pain management.

Preanesthetic medication drugs, including tranquilizers/sedatives such as acepromazine, azaperone, diazepam, midazolam, xylazine, romifidine, medetomidine, and dexmedetomidine, have been used for sedation in dogs and cats (see *Table 3.1*). The clinical effects and reliability of these sedatives range from minimal to profound sedation. Preanesthetic medication drugs also include anticholinergics, such as atropine or glycopyrrolate, which are used to reduce salivation and airway secretions and prevent bradycardia. Other drugs used include opioids, dissociatives (ketamine or tiletamine) and non-steroidal anti-inflammatory drugs (NSAIDs). This chapter covers the route of administration, dosages, and the use of each drug alone or in combination for preanesthetic medication in dogs and cats.

Table 3.1 Preanesthetic drug classification and actions

Preanesthetic drug class	Drug	Sedative and other actions	Cardiovascular effects	Analgesia
Phenothiazine	Acepromazine	Mild to moderate sedation, no muscle relaxation	Vasodilation	None
Butyrophenone	Azaperone	Mild to moderate sedation, no muscle relaxation	Mild to moderate vasodilation but to lesser degree than acepromazine	None
Benzodiazepines	Diazepam, midazolam, zolazepam	Minimal to mild sedation in young and healthy animals. May induce profound sedation in geriatrics. Muscle relaxation	Minimal effects	None
Alpha-2 adrenergic agonists	Xylazine, romifidine, medetomidine, dexmedetomidine	Mild to profound sedation, muscle relaxation	Bradycardia, hypertension	Somatic and visceral
Dissociatives	Ketamine, tiletamine	Moderate dissociative sedation, increased muscle tone, increased salivation and airway secretions	Increase in heart rate and blood pressure	Somatic and mild visceral
Opioids	Mu receptor agonists: morphine, hydromorphone, fentanyl, pethidine (also called meperidine), methadone Mu receptor partial agonist: buprenorphine Kappa receptor agonist and mu receptor antagonists: butorphanol, nalbuphine	Mild sedation, no effect on muscle tone	Decrease in heart rate (except for pethidine, which has an anticholinergic effect) and no effect on the vasculature or cardiac contractility	Somatic and visceral
Anticholinergics	Atropine, glycopyrrolate	None	Increase in heart rate and decrease in salivation	None
Neuroactive steroidal anesthetics	Alfaxalone (although it is an IV induction agent, it can be administered IM as a sedative adjunct)	Mild sedation when given IM with muscle relaxation	Increase in heart rate	Minimal

Reasons for preanesthetic medication

The reasons for preanesthetic medication include:

- The provision of chemical restraint (i.e. sedation for IV catheterization and ease of animal handling).
- Reduction of anxiety in the animal, thereby reducing catecholamines and the risk of arrhythmias during anesthetic induction and maintenance.
- Reduction of the total required doses of induction and maintenance drugs.
- Provision of pre-emptive analgesia if an analgesic drug (including NSAIDs) is included as part of the premedication.
- Reduction of salivation and airway secretion or prevention of bradycardia induced by other drugs or the natural response of the animal.

Preanesthetic medication protocol

Various factors should be considered when formulating a preanesthetic medication protocol:
- The animal's health and its responses to procedures:
  - Animal's species, breed, sex, age, health status (cardiorespiratory, hepatic, renal, and other systemic functions), and weight.
  - Existing blood work and hydration status.
  - Animal's temperament and demeanor.
  - Concurrent medication of the animal.
  - Degree of painful stimulation.
  - Duration of the procedure and time of discharge.
- What is required and expected from the drugs used:
  - Degree and duration of sedation.
  - Degree and duration of analgesia.
  - Reduced salivation and airway secretions.
  - Anesthetic and analgesic side-effects (on the cardiorespiratory as well as other body systems) on the treated animal.

A flow chart for formulating a protocol and considering drug selection for preanesthetic medication is shown in **Fig. 3.1**.

A modification of the American Society of Anesthesiologists (ASA) physical status classification system can be used to evaluate the animal's health status (*Table 3.2*). This status, together with the temperament of the patient, is taken into account when formulating a

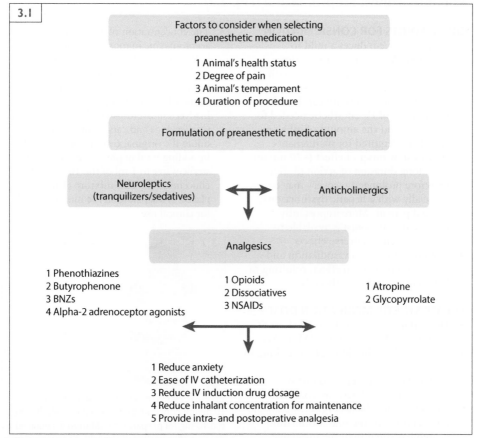

3.1

Factors to consider when selecting preanesthetic medication

1 Animal's health status
2 Degree of pain
3 Animal's temperament
4 Duration of procedure

Formulation of preanesthetic medication

Neuroleptics (tranquilizers/sedatives) ⬌ Anticholinergics

Analgesics

1 Phenothiazines
2 Butyrophenone
3 BNZs
4 Alpha-2 adrenoceptor agonists

1 Opioids
2 Dissociatives
3 NSAIDs

1 Atropine
2 Glycopyrrolate

1 Reduce anxiety
2 Ease of IV catheterization
3 Reduce IV induction drug dosage
4 Reduce inhalant concentration for maintenance
5 Provide intra- and postoperative analgesia

Fig. 3.1 Flow chart for formulating a preanesthetic plan and selecting a drug(s). BNZ, benzodiazepine; NSAID, non-steroidal anti-inflammaotory drug.

Table 3.2 American Society of Anesthesiologists physical status classification system

ASA classification	Animal health description
ASA I	Normal, healthy
ASA II	Mild to moderate systemic disease
ASA III	Severe systemic disease, but still active
ASA IV	Severe systemic disease and incapacitated
ASA V	Moribund, terminally ill
ASA-E	Emergency

protocol for using a tranquilizer/sedative alone or combined with an opioid.

- ASA I animals are considered to be normal and healthy overall.

- ASA II animals have mild to moderate systemic diseases.
- ASA III animals have severe systemic disease that limits activity but is not incapacitating.
- ASA IV animals have severe systemic disease that limits activity and is a constant threat to life.
- ASA V animals are moribund and are not expected to survive more than 24 hours with or without intervention. These animals are almost always hospitalized or terminally ill.
- ASA-E indicates an emergency operation of any physical status (i.e. ASA I-E for hit-by-a-car fracture surgery on an ASA I patient).

Phenothiazines: acepromazine (Fig. 3.2)

QUICK POINTS FOR CONSIDERATION

- Acepromazine induces a mild to moderate degree of sedation (some prefer the term tranquilization) with no analgesic property. However, acepromazine does significantly reduce the amount of IV anesthetic needed for induction and the amount of inhalant anesthetic required for maintenance.
- It has a slow onset of effect (~20 minutes), but a long duration of action (3–6 hours), therefore prolonged recovery may occur, especially with a hepatic dysfunctional or aged patient. More importantly, no specific antagonist is available to counteract these adverse effects.
- Acepromazine has a vasodilation and antithermoregulation effect, resulting in hypotension and hypothermia.

PREANESTHETIC MEDICATION DOSES

- Dogs: 0.02–0.05 mg/kg IV, IM, or SC
- Cats: 0.05–0.2 mg/kg IV, IM, or SC
- The total dose should not exceed 3 mg in large dogs.
- The oral dose of acepromazine is 0.5–1.0 mg/kg. There are commercial acepromazine tablets (**Fig. 3.2**) available for oral use, but the oral formulation is used less often than the injectable formulation for premedication.

- The concentration of injectable acepromazine in most countries is 10 mg/ml. The clinical dose is 0.02–0.05 mg/kg in dogs and slightly higher in cats, which is only a fraction of the labeled concentration. To avoid inadvertent overdosing of acepromazine in smaller dogs and cats, many veterinarians dilute the original concentration tenfold, by adding 9 ml of physiologic saline or sterile water to 1 ml of the 10 mg/ml concentration. This mixture (1 mg/ml) is placed in a separate sterile multidose vial for clinical use.

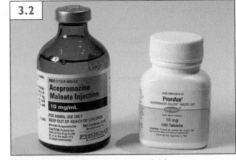

Fig. 3.2 Acepromazine is available as a 10 mg/ml concentration (also 2 mg/ml). If using the 10 mg/ml preparation, dilution is required to dose smaller patients properly. Acepromazine is also available in an oral tablet formulation.

- In countries where a less concentrated acepromazine injection is available (e.g. 2 mg/ml in the UK), dilution may not be necessary.

ADVANTAGES OF USING ACEPROMAZINE
- Acepromazine can be administered IV, IM, SC, or PO.
- The sedation effect is mild to moderate and is dose dependent. It is more reliable and profound than with benzodiazapines (BNZs), but less reliable than with alpha-2 adrenergic sedatives.
- Acepromazine has antiemetic and antiarrhythmic effects.
- The literature cautions against the use of acepromazine in dogs with a history of seizures because it is thought that it reduces the seizure threshold in these animals. However, a recent retrospective study reviewed the use of acepromazine in 36 dogs with a history of seizures of various origins. No seizures were reported within 16 hours of acepromazine administration. A small dose of acepromazine (0.02–0.05 mg/kg IM) is not likely to complicate the management of a patient with a history of seizures.
- Acepromazine has significant anesthetic induction- and inhalant-sparing effects despite its lack of analgesic property. When combined with other analgesic or sedative drugs, acepromazine synergistically enhances their actions. Anticipation of such reduction (sparing effects) of IV and inhalant anesthetic requirements are necessary to prevent anesthetic overdose.

DISADVANTAGES OF USING ACEPROMAZINE
- A slow onset of action, taking 20–30 minutes to reach peak efficacy.
- A long duration of action, lasting about 3–6 hours depending on the dose used. This is of benefit in long, involved procedures, but recovery from short procedures is prolonged. No specific antagonist is available for reversal in the event of a prolonged recovery.
- Minimal muscle relaxation or analgesic activities.
- Suppresses the sympathetic nervous system and also acts centrally to cause loss of vasomotor regulation, which can result in hypotension and hypothermia secondary to vasodilation. The alpha-1 adrenergic blockade activity peripherally further reduces blood pressure.
- Extensive metabolism by the liver, with the result that acepromazine should be used with caution in very young or very old patients, or patients with hepatic compromise to avoid a prolonged recovery.
- Although acepromazine has an antiemetic action, coadministration of acepromazine with opioids that have emetic actions (morphine, hydromorphone, and oxymorphone) still results in emesis during premedication. Administration of acepromazine should be given 15 minutes prior to the opioid to reduce, though not abolish, the incidence of vomiting.

Butyrophenone: azaperone

QUICK POINTS FOR CONSIDERATION
- Azaperone, a butyrophenone neuroleptic drug with sedative and antiemetic effects, was approved for use in pigs for sedation in the USA. It also has been used frequently in wildlife in combination with an opioid as a neuroleptic sedative.
- Azaperone can be used in dog and cats as an effective sedative in a similar fashion to acepromazine but with a shorter duration of action than acepromazine. This can be an advantage when a shorter duration of sedation is desired and profound long-lasting vasodilation is to be avoided.
- Azaperone is available in several countries outside of the USA.
- Azaperone can be used alone or in combination with various other sedatives (alpha-2 agonists and benzodiazepines) to enhance the overall sedative quality.

PREANESTHETIC MEDICATION DOSES
- Dogs: 0.2–0.4 mg/kg IV, IM or SC.
- Cats: 0.2–0.4 mg/kg IV, IM or SC.
- The sedation degree induced by azaperone is mild to moderate. However, when combined with medetomidine or dexmedetomidine, the sedative quality is profound and lateral recumbency can be achieved.
- The duration lasts about 1–2 hours.
- Azaperone can be used in a similar fashion to that of acepromazine.
- The side-effects and precautions of azaperone are very similar to acepromazine with less profound vasodilatory effect.

Benzodiazepines: diazepam (Fig. 3.3) and midazolam (Fig. 3.4)

QUICK POINTS FOR CONSIDERATION
- BNZs induce a mild degree of sedation only in animals.
- They have a relatively short duration of action with no analgesic property.
- BNZs have anticonvulsant activity.
- The effects of BNZs can be specifically antagonized by flumazenil.
- They have a minimal cardiorespiratory effect in animals.
- BNZs have a much less sparing effect on the requirement of IV and inhalant anesthetics.

PREANESTHETIC MEDICATION DOSES
- Dogs: 0.2–0.4 mg/kg IV or IM.
- Cats: 0.2–0.4 mg/kg IV or IM.
- Dogs and cats: oral dose is up to 2 mg/kg.
- Although diazepam can be administered IM, it is not the preferred route due to slow absorption. Furthermore, diazepam may cause pain on IM injection. Therefore, this route of administration should be avoided.
- Injectable diazepam and midazolam at 0.5–1 mg/kg administered rectally has been used to treat acute repetitive seizures in dogs. Diazepam gel is available commercially for treating cluster seizures in humans; it may also be used in dogs for a similar purpose.
- A study has shown that 0.2 mg/kg of diazepam (or midazolam) given IV as a preanesthetic medication 45 seconds before propofol induction reduces the induction dose by 26% when compared with propofol used alone. Increasing the dose of diazepam from 0.2 mg/kg to 0.4 mg/kg further reduces the propofol induction dose needed to achieve endotracheal intubation by 21–36%.

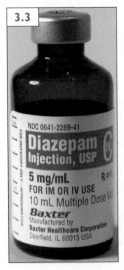

Fig. 3.3 Diazepam injectable formulation is available in a 5 mg/ml concentration.

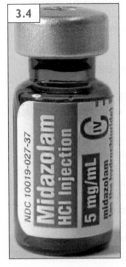

Fig. 3.4 Midazolam injectable formulation is available in a 5 mg/ml concentration.

Table 3.3 Differences between diazepam and midazolam

Differences	Diazepam (5 mg/ml)	Midazolam (5 mg/ml)
Formulation	Oily propylene glycol	Water soluble
Absorption	Rapid with IV injection, but slow with IM	Rapid with both IM and IV injection
Injection pain	Occurs with IM injection, but not IV	Occurs with IM injection, but not IV
Drug mixture	Will precipitate (with the propylene glycol formulation in the USA) when mixed with other anesthetic solutions in the same syringe	No precipitation when mixed with other anesthetic solutions
Cost	More expensive because less manufacturing production	Relatively cheap
Controlled substance	Yes	Yes

DIFFERENCES BETWEEN DIAZEPAM AND MIDAZOLAM (*TABLE 3.3*)

- Midazolam is a water soluble version of diazepam. If injected IM, it is absorbed relatively quickly and completely, therefore its effects are more predictable than those of diazepam.
- Diazepam can be administered IM, but absorption is slow and irregular. This is due to the propylene glycol base carrier.
- Because midazolam is water soluble, it can be mixed with many other anesthetic agents without precipitation. However, diazepam is produced in a propylene glycol carrier solution and causes immediate precipitation with other drugs, except ketamine. Diazepam should not be mixed in the same syringe with any other drugs.
- Previously, diazepam was less expensive than midazolam. From 2015 onward, fewer manufacturers were making diazepam, whereas midazolam manufacturing increased. Since this shift, midazolam is more readily available than diazepam and is less expensive than diazepam.

ADVANTAGES OF USING BENZODIAZEPINES

- Minimal cardiorespiratory depression, therefore suitable for use in geriatric, pediatric, or debilitated animals considered to be at higher anesthetic risk. The degree of sedation is more profound in geriatric patients than in younger ones.
- Enhances the anesthetic and analgesic effects of other drugs.
- Better choice for use in geriatric or debilitated patients or in combination with other sedative drugs, such as opioids, alpha-2 agonists, or ketamine, to optimize the sedative effects.
- The effects of BNZs can be specifically antagonized with flumazenil (0.02–0.1 mg/kg IV).

DISADVANTAGES OF USING BENZODIAZEPINES

- When administered alone, healthy dogs and cats exhibit minimal sedation, but sometimes exhibit paradoxical excitement or aggression instead.
- BNZs produce highly variable sedative responses among animals.
- They have no analgesic properties, but they do enhance the action of analgesic drugs when used in combination.
- They have a relatively short duration of action (<20 minutes).

Alpha-2 adrenergic agonists: xylazine (Fig. 3.5), romifidine, medetomidine, and dexmedetomidine (Fig. 3.6)

QUICK POINTS FOR CONSIDERATION

- Alpha-2 agonist sedatives induce a dose-dependent mild to profound degree of sedation including lateral recumbency.
- They have a rapid onset (~5 minutes) and moderate duration (~2 hours) of action, and analgesic and muscle relaxation properties.

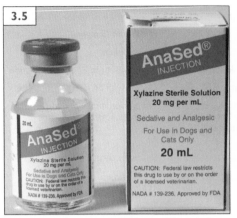

Fig. 3.5 Xylazine is available in a 20 mg/ml concentration for small animals and in a 100 mg/ml concentration for large animals.

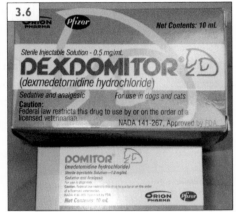

Fig. 3.6 Medetomidine (Domitor®) is available as a 1 mg/ml solution. Dexmedetomidine (Dexdomitor®) is available as a 0.5 mg/ml concentration solution.

- They have profound cardiovascular effects characterized by occasional second-degree heart blocks, bradycardia, and vasoconstriction.
- The drug effects can be specifically antagonized with alpha-2 receptor antagonists.

PREANESTHETIC MEDICATION DOSES
See *Table 3.4.*

DIFFERENCES BETWEEN THE VARIOUS ALPHA-2 ADRENERGIC AGONISTS
- Xylazine is the least potent and it has some alpha-1 adrenergic activity.
- Romidifidine has a potency somewhere between xylazine and medetomidine/dexmedetomidine.
- Medetomidine has two enantiomers (stereoisomers that are mirror images of each other but are not identical): dexmedetomidine and levomedetomidine. Dexmedetomidine is the dextro isomer of medetomidine and is approximately twice as potent as medetomidine.

- The clinical sedative and analgesic effects of medetomidine are a result of dexmedetomidine.
- At the clinically labeled dose, levomedetomidine is pharmacologically inactive.
- Dexmedetomidine requires less hepatic metabolism when compared with the raecemic mixture medetomidine. This is a result of the removal of levomedetomidine. Levomedetomidine has also been shown to slow down the metabolism of ketamine. Removal of levomedetomidine is likely to lead to a faster recovery when dexmedetomidine is used alone or is combined with other drugs such as ketamine (compared with medetomidine).
- Clinically, dexmedetomidine is almost twice as potent as medetomidine for clinical sedation of dogs and cats.
- Medetomidine and dexmedetomidine induce vasoconstriction with a duration that outlasts xylazine and results in a longer duration of hypertension.

Table 3.4 Premedication doses for xylazine, romifidine, medetomidine, and dexmedetomidine

Species	Xylazine	Romifidine	Medetomidine	Dexmedetomidine
Dogs	0.15–0.30 mg/kg IV, IM, or SC	5–10 µg/kg IV, IM, or SC	5–30 µg/kg IV, IM, or SC	2.5–20 µg/kg IV, IM, or SC
Cats	0.5–1.0 mg/kg IV, IM, or SC	20–40 µg/kg IV, IM, or SC	5–60 µg/kg IV, IM, or SC	10–40 µg/kg IV, IM, or SC

This hypertension also induces a reflex bradycardia that is more profound than seen with other alpha-2 agonists.

- Medetomidine or dexmedetomidine induce a longer duration of sedation than xylazine.
- Xylazine induces a bi-phasic blood pressure response in dogs. Blood pressure increases immediately after administration, peaking 5–10 minutes after IM administration. Blood pressure then decreases to below the baseline value for at least 90 minutes after administration. This response is likely to pose a danger to the animal during this stage when hypotension and bradycardia are present at the same time.
- The administration of an anticholinergic agent (atropine or glycopyrrolate) with an alpha-2 agonist is highly controversial and anesthestists are widely divided in their views/opinions on this point. Some consider that administration (either prior to, coadministered, or as a treatment after the animal has received an alpha-2 drug) is an absolute contraindication because it causes significant hypertension and increases the risk of arrhythmias and myocardial oxygen consumption. Others consider that lower doses of an anticholinergic agent (atropine at 0.02 mg/kg or glycopyrrolate at 0.005 mg/kg, IM) are more benign and tend to alleviate the anxiety of the practitioner worried about bradycardia, as well as treating for airway secretions. This author's view is that it is necessary when using xylazine; using an anticholinergic agent helps maintain blood pressure in the presence of bradycardia and hypotension in the later stages of a xylazine-containing protocol.
- This author considers that the use of anticholinergic agents with higher doses of medetomidine (>10 μg/kg) or dexmedetomidine (>5 μg/kg) is controversial since prolonged hypertension and a high heart rate may result in severe hypertension and possibly more arrhythmias. However, some anesthetists consider that giving low doses of atropine (≤0.02 mg/kg) or glycopyrrolate (≤0.005 mg/kg) with a lower dose of medetomidine (≤10 μg/kg) or dexmedetomidine (≤5 μg/kg) is acceptable. This is especially true when the vasoconstriction effect of medetomidine and dexmedetomidine starts to diminish (1 hour after administration), but their sympatholytic effect remains in action. In this author's opinion, the administration of an anticholinergic at this time is acceptable.
- One study has reported that doses of 80, 120, and 160 μg/kg of romifidine IM produce sedation in cats that is similar to that produced with 20 μg/kg of medetomidine IM.

ADVANTAGES OF USING ALPHA-2 ADRENERGIC AGONISTS

- Alpha-2 agonists have a wide range of effects including anxiolysis, calming, sedation, visceral and somatic analgesia, and mild to moderate muscle relaxation.
- Sedation is profound and reliable, with a fast onset of action.
- Reliable efficacy regardless of route of administration (IV, IM, or SC).
- Enhance the anesthetic or analgesic effects of other drugs.
- Alpha-2 agonists are reversible with yohimbine (**Fig. 3.7**), tolazoline (**Fig. 3.8**), and atipamezole (**Fig. 3.9**) (*Table 3.5*). (**Note:** In the UK, only atipamezole is available, therefore atipamezole is used for all alpha-2 agent reversals.)
- To reverse xylazine (0.25–0.5 mg/kg IM), the yohimbine dose is 0.1 mg/kg and the tolazoline dose is 0.5–1.0 mg/kg IM.

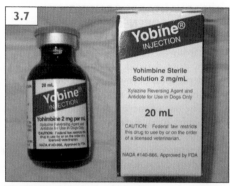

Fig. 3.7 Yohimbine (Yobine®) is a reversal agent or antagonist for xylazine.

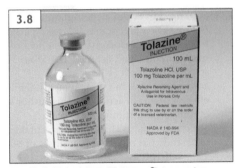

Fig. 3.8 Tolazoline (Tolazine®) is another antagonist for xylazine. This drug is approved for reversal of xylazine in horses only in the USA.

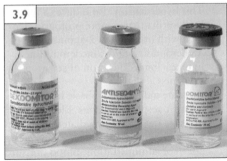

Fig. 3.9 Atipamezole (Antisedan®) is a reversal agent for medetomidine, romifidine, and dexmedetomidine.

Table 3.5 Reversal agents and their dose rate for alpha-2 agonists in dogs and cats

Alpha-2 antagonist	Dose
Atipamezole	Same volume as medetomidine and dexmedetomidine or 5–10 times the medetomidine and dexmedetomidine dose rate, IV, IM, or SC
Yohimbine	0.1–0.5 mg/kg IV, IM, or SC
Tolazoline	0.5–1 mg/kg IV, IM, or SC

- To reverse medetomidine or dexmedetomidine, the atipamezole dose is calculated to be an equal volume of the medetomidine or dexmedetomidine dose used (i.e. 5–10 times the calculated medetomidine or dexmedetomidine dose).
- Although yohimbine can be used to reverse medetomidine- or dexmedetomidine-induced sedation, dogs seem to experience a rougher recovery than when atipamezole is used for reversal.

DISADVANTAGES OF USING ALPHA-2 ADRENERGIC AGONISTS

- All alpha-2 drugs induce profound cardiovascular depression characterized by dose-dependent vasoconstriction, depression of myocardial contractility, and a reduction in cardiac output.
- The use of these drugs is associated with bradycardia, particularly medetomidine and dexmedetomidine in dogs. Bradycardia induced by medetomidine or dexmedetomidine is less common in cats.

- The respiratory depressive effects of alpha-2 agonists are minimal when the drugs are used alone, but when used in combination with opioids, ketamine, or tiletamine/zolazepam, profound respiratory depression may be induced in dogs and cats.
- A vomiting response is common following alpha-2 agonist administration, especially when low doses are administered SC. Cats are more susceptible to emesis than dogs. This vomiting response is unlikely to increase the risk of aspiration as the animals are still in light sedation and able to control their airway and swallowing.
- Myoclonic twitchings (involuntary twitches of the body or limbs) may occur with the use of alpha-2 agonists alone or in combination with other drugs. This is benign and no treatment is needed. However, these signs should not be interpreted as a light plane of sedation.

Dissociatives: ketamine and tiletamine

QUICK POINTS FOR CONSIDERATION
- Dissociative agents have a rapid onset of action (~5 minutes) and a moderate duration of effect (~2 hours).
- They have superior somatic but less visceral analgesia.
- Dissociatives stimulate sympathetic tone, therefore there is an increase in heart rate and blood pressure.
- They induce muscle rigidity with the animal maintaining swallowing and blinking reflexes.
- They tend to trigger seizure-like activity or muscle rigidity.
- They induce salivation and airway secretions.
- They cause pain on IM injection site due to their low pH.
- They may cause dogs to have emergence delirium, which consists of uncoordinated movements of the head and neck, vocalization, salivation, and agitation.

PREANESTHETIC MEDICATION DOSES
- Ketamine (**Fig. 3.10**) is usually combined with other sedatives (alpha-2 agonists, BNZs, azaperone, or acepromazine) when being used as a premedication:
  - Dogs: 1–3 mg/kg IV, IM, or SC.
  - Cats: 3–10 mg/kg IV, IM, or SC.
- Telazol® (**Fig. 3.11**) and Zoletil® are proprietary mixtures of tiletamine and zolazepam. This drug combination is not available in the UK and Canada, but it is available in other parts of Europe and is widely used in the USA:
  - Dogs: 6–8 mg/kg IM; 2–3 mg/kg IV.
  - Cats: 4–6 mg/kg IM; 2–3 mg/kg IV.

DIFFERENCES BETWEEN THE DISSOCIATIVES
- Tiletamine is chemically similar to ketamine, but is three times more potent and has a longer duration of effect.
- Tiletamine in combination with zolazepam (similar to diazepam and midazolam, but three times more potent) is marketed as Telazol or Zoletil (*Table 3.6*). The tiletamine and zolazepam proprietary combination

consists of a 1:1 weight to weight ratio in a lyophilized powder. This is reconstituted with sterile water to form 5 ml of a 100 mg/ml solution. Reconstituted Telazol can be stored at room temperature (20–25°C [68–77°F]) for 7 days or in a refrigerator for 56 days. Zoletil is also available as a 50 mg/ml solution when reconstituted.
- Zolazepam attenuates the muscle rigidity associated with tiletamine, producing a smoother induction and recovery. Telazol or Zoletil can be used as a premedicant, induction agent, or injectable anesthetic.

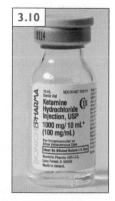

Fig. 3.10 Ketamine is a controlled substance in the USA as well as in some other countries.

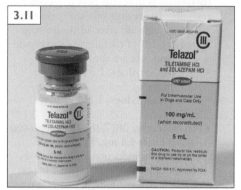

Fig. 3.11 Tiletamine/zolazepam (Telazol®) is marketed by Zoetis in the USA. Zoletil, marketed by Virbac, is available in Europe, Latin America, Asia, and the Pacific area. Zoletil is available in two concentrations, 50 mg/ml (Zoletil 50) and 100 mg/ml (Zoletil 100). Both Telazol and Zoletil are lyophilized powders that require sterile water for reconstitution.

Table 3.6 Differences between tiletamine and zolazepam

Telazol/Zoletil	Tiletamine	Zolazepam
Pharmacologic action	Dissociative anesthesia and analgesia	Sedation and muscle relaxation
Absorption	Rapid with IV injection, but slow with IM	Rapid with both IM and IV injection
Weight to weight ratio in the proprietary mixture	1	1
Species variation	Dogs metabolize zolazepam faster than tiletamine, therefore they have a prolonged rough recovery	Cats metabolize tiletamine faster than zolazepam, therefore they have a prolonged asleep recovery

- The dosages of tiletamine/zolazepam (Telazol) for dogs and cats recommended by the manufacturers are listed below. These dosages are higher than regular premedication when the drug is being used on its own:
  - Diagnostic: dogs, 6.6–9.9 mg/kg IM; cats: 9.7–11.9 mg/kg IM.
  - Minor surgical procedure of short duration (e.g. castration or laceration repair): dogs, 9.9–13.2 mg/kg IM; cats, 10.6–12.5 mg/kg IM.
  - The maximum allowable dose for supplementation of increment sedation or total anesthesia is 26.4 mg/kg IM for dogs and 72 mg/kg IM for cats.
- The metabolic half-life of tiletamine and zolazepam is different between dogs and cats. The results of a study on the metabolic half-life after administering 20 mg/kg IM of tiletamine/zolazepam in dogs and cats are shown below:
  - Tiletamine: dogs, 1.3 hours; cats, 2.5 hours.
  - Zolazepam: dogs, 1 hour; cats, 4.5 hours.
  - In November 2017, the FDA approved Telazol 2.2–4.4 mg/kg, IV as an intravenous induction agent for dogs. In the approval study, the half-life of tiletamine was 17–52 min, and was 5–25 minutes, following administration of 2.2 mg/kg IV of Telazol in the dogs.
- Dissociatives are usually combined with other sedatives, such as alpha-2 agonists (dexmedetomidine, medetomidine), BNZs (diazepam, midazolam), or phenothiazines (acepromazine), to induce better sedation and attenuate the side-effects.

ADVANTAGES OF USING DISSOCIATIVES
- Dissociatives produce strong somatic analgesia.
- They increase the sympathetic tone that typically accompanies higher heart rates and blood pressure.
- They have a relatively high margin of safety.
- At subanesthetic doses, dissociatives can be used as N-methyl D-aspartate (NMDA) receptor antagonists to prevent central sensitization (wind-up). This is usually through the use of continuous rate infusion (CRI) (see Chapter 24).

DISADVANTAGES OF USING DISSOCIATIVES
- When used alone at high doses, ketamine induces poor muscle relaxation and is associated with rough recoveries. It can also induce convulsions.
- The emergency delirium rough recoveries are characterized by paddling, repeated attempts to regain sternal recumbency, head-shaking, salivation, vocalization, sudden excitement, and movement.
- To eliminate these side-effects, ketamine is frequently used in combination with either diazepam, midazolam, xylazine, romifidine, medetomidine, dexmedetomidine, or other injectable anesthetics.
- The low pH of the solution causes pain on IM injection.
- Ketamine induces profuse salivation and airway secretions that are preventable with atropine or glycopyrrolate.
- Dissociatives frequently increase the heart rate and concurrent use of atropine or glycopyrrolate does not lead to a further increase in heart rate.

- Dose-dependent depression of the central nervous system (CNS) by dissociatives is characterized by analgesia and a light plane of anesthesia. The dog or cat may appear to be awake and conscious (thus, the term 'dissociative', meaning dissociated from the environment) even though they are sedated.
- Although the animal is dissociated from the environment, pharyngeal, laryngeal, corneal, and pedal reflexes persist and the eyes remain open.

- Continuous swallowing reflex with tight jaw tone during endotracheal intubation is a characteristic of dissociative agents and is very different from anesthesia induced by propofol or thiopental.
- All dissociatives cause an increase in intracranial pressure (ICP) and intraocular pressure (IOP). Therefore, their use should be avoided in animals with increased ICP or IOP.

Anticholinergics: atropine and glycopyrrolate (Figs. 3.12, 3.13)

QUICK POINTS FOR CONSIDERATION
- Anticholinergics are used for prevention of bradycardia, airway secretions, and salivation.
- Atropine has a shorter duration than glycopyrrolate.
- Neither drug has sedative activity.
- Low doses of atropine may induce bradycardia instead of increasing heart rate.
- Low doses of atropine may cause an increase in acetylcholine and act on presynaptic nerve ends (i.e. it acts like a cholinergic drug instead of an anticholinergic drug with low doses). Another proposed theory is that low concentrations of atropine may act on muscarinic-1 receptors and block sympathetic ganglia, resulting in a low heart rate.
- Iatrogenic tachycardia may occur when using anticholinergics.

PREANESTHETIC MEDICATION DOSES
- Atropine: dogs and cats, 0.03–0.04 mg/kg IM, 0.02 mg/kg IV.
- Glycopyrrolate: dogs and cats, 0.0075–0.01 mg/kg IM, 0.005 mg/kg IV.
- The use of atropine is generally not recommended in combination with medetomidine or dexmedetomidine

However, some practitioners do use a low dose of atropine in combination with these two drugs. Atropine can be used at its regular dose rate in combination with xylazine.

DIFFERENCES BETWEEN ATROPINE AND GLYCOPYRROLATE
See *Table 3.7.*

ADVANTAGE OF USING ANTICHOLINERGIC AGENTS
- Anticholinergic agents can be used for the treatment of intraoperative bradycardia, especially in the bradycardia-induced hypotensive patient, by administering an IV bolus or by IV titration.
- The titration method is to add the IV anticholinergic agent to 5 ml of physiologic saline and to give 1 ml every 30 seconds until the heart rate and blood pressure reach desirable levels. This method is useful to avoid the iatrogenic tachycardia induced by IV bolus administration of these anticholinergic agents.

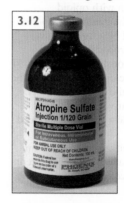
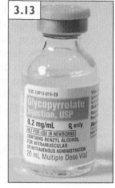

Fig. 3.12 Atropine is available in a 0.54 mg/ml concentration.

Fig. 3.13 Glycopyrrolate is available as a 0.2 mg/ml solution.

Table 3.7 Differences between atropine and glycopyrrolate

	Atropine	Glycopyrrolate
Onset of action after IV administration	2–3 minutes	2–3 minutes
Duration of action	45–60 minutes	80–120 minutes
Chronotropic effect	Tends to induce tachycardia	Less tachycardic response
Dromotropic effect	Facilitates electrical conductivity between the sinus node and the atrioventricular node, as well as other conduction pathways. More arrhythmogenic	Less arrhythmogenic
Purpose of use	Primarily for treatment of bradycardia or cardiac emergencies	Primarily used for prevention of salivation and bradycardia, but also used for longer cases due to the longer duration of action
Cost	Less expensive	More expensive
Blood–brain barrier and placental penetration	Crosses the blood–brain barrier and causes central nervous system excitement when grossly overdosed. Also crosses placental barrier and causes fetal tachycardia	Large molecule that does not cross the blood–brain barrier or the placental barrier

- Occasionally during titration, second-degree heart block may appear seconds to minutes before the heart rate increases. This is a normal response. The animal should be monitored closely, but no immediate treatment is needed. If the heart block persists, an additional dose of anticholinergic can be given to increase the heart rate.

Opioids

QUICK POINTS FOR CONSIDERATIONS

- Opioids produce strong analgesia, but are associated with bradycardia and respiratory depression.
- Vomiting and panting responses are commonly seen with opioid administration. The vomiting response may be attenuated by administering 1–2 mg/kg of maropitant (Cerenia-Zoetis) subcutaneously at 30 minutes to 1 hour prior to the opioid premedication.
- Opioids possess mild sedative activity. However, the sedative activity is not reliable and is far less than that induced by a sedative.
- There are profound sparing effects on induction and inhalant anesthetic agents when opioids are combined with other drugs.

- The sedative and analgesic effects can be reversed with specific opioid antagonists.

PREANESTHETIC MEDICATION DOSES AND PROPERTIES

- Opioids, such as morphine (**Fig. 3.14**), hydromorphone (**Fig. 3.15**), oxymorphone, methadone, fentanyl (**Fig. 3.16**), buprenorphine (**Fig. 3.17**), butorphanol (**Fig. 3.18**), and nalbuphine (**Fig. 3.19**), are commonly used for premedication and pain management in dogs and cats. The premedication doses of these opioids are listed in *Table 3.8*.
- Oxymorphone has largely been replaced by hydromorphone, which is significantly more expensive than hydromorphone (×10).
- Methadone has regained popularity among practitioners in recent years. It has several advantages over other opioids, including minimally induced nausea/vomiting and histamine release. Methadone is a NMDA receptor antagonist. When noxious stimuli are applied to the peripheral tissue, the excitatory neurotransmitter glutamate is released and activates NMDA receptors. Activation of the NMDA receptors results in hyperalgesia, neuropathic pain, and reduction of opioid receptor sensitivity. Methadone blocks NMDA receptors

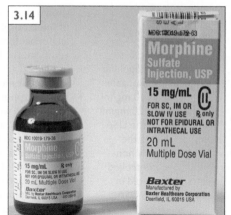

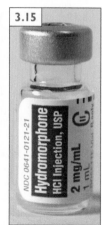

Fig. 3.14 Morphine is a full opioid mu and kappa receptor agonist.

Fig. 3.15 Hydromorphone is a full opioid mu and kappa receptor agonist; it is less expensive but just as effective, as oxymorphone.

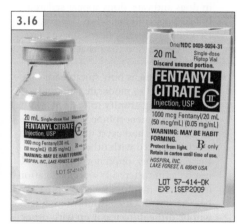

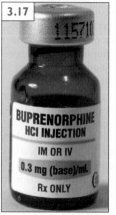

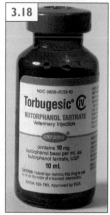

Fig. 3.16 Like morphine, fentanyl is a full opioid mu and kappa receptor agonist, but fentanyl is more potent than morphine. Injectable fentanyl is usually used as a constant rate infusion for pain management. Fentanyl is also available as a patch.

Figs. 3.17, 3.18 Buprenorphine is a partial mu receptor agonist. There are several commercial brands of buprenorphine. A veterinary commercial product approved for use in cats is available with high concentration at 1.8 mg/ml, instead of the human version of 0.3 mg/ml. Shown here is a multiple withdrawal vial of buprenorphine (3.17). Butorphanol is an opioid kappa receptor partial agonist and mu receptor antagonist. It is available in both injectable and oral tablet formulations (3.18).

and minimizes such pain. In humans, methadone has been used to improve analgesia when patients develop tolerance to other opioids.
- Methadone has been used in dogs as a premedicant (0.05–0.2 mg/kg). In a study in Greyhounds, 0.5 mg/kg IV methadone induced panting and defecation.
- Fentanyl has a rapid onset of action following IV or IM administration, but a relatively short duration of effect

(~30 minutes). Fentanyl is not commonly used IM. It is more commonly used IV followed by CRI.
- Pethidine and methadone are not commonly used as sedative/analgesics in dogs and cats. Pethidine is a synthetic opioid that has only one-fifth

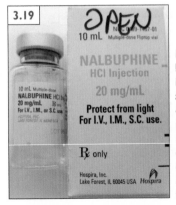

Fig. 3.19 Nalbuphine is available as 10 mg/ml or 20 mg/ml in the USA. It is the only non-controlled opioid in the USA.

to one-tenth the analgesic potency of morphine.

- Pethidine (also known as meperidine in the USA) is approved for IM injection at 3.3 mg/kg as a premedicant prior to a surgical procedure or for sedation, as an adjunct to sedation or anesthesia, or postoperatively as an analgesic in dogs and cats (in some European countries). Pethidine has an anticholinergic effect and is less likely to induce bradycardia than other opioids in dogs.
- Pethidine should not be administered IV as it is likely to cause histamine release and result in hypotension.
- A gross overdose or IV administration of pethidine may be associated with seizures and CNS excitement.
- Butorphanol has relatively good sedative activity when compared with other opioids. The sedative activity associated with low doses of buprenorphine is minimal.
- Butorphanol has a relatively short duration of action, whereas buprenorphine has a long duration of action. Butorphanol and buprenorphine are less likely to induce bradycardia than morphine, hydromorphone, or fentanyl.
- All opioids have a relatively poor bioavailability (<15%) following either oral or oral transmucosal (OTM) administration, except buprenorphine (~50% or more).
- The duration of buprenorphine action is dose dependent in dogs and cats. The higher the dose, the longer the duration tends to be. One study has

shown that a single dose (0.12 mg/kg) of buprenorphine OTM induces an analgesic duration of up to 24 hours. In addition, the higher dose seems to reduce individual variation as well as give a longer duration of action.

- Buprenorphine has been recently approved in the USA with a SC dose of 0.24 mg/kg q24 h in cats for postoperative analgesia up to 3 days. The same product can be used in dogs with a dose up to 0.12 mg/kg, IV, IM, SC, or OTM for postoperative pain management. This high dose of buprenorphine likely induces a prolonged sedative effect in dogs.
- The sedative response to high doses of buprenorphine seems to be different in dogs and cats: dogs appear sedated but cats appear euphorically active. In addition, dogs appear to have more profuse salivation than that observed in cats.
- Buprenorphine is only suitable for treating mild to moderate pain and it has a strong affinity to the opioid receptor. Buprenorphine will displace other opioids and exert its effects when coadministered with other opioids. Because of this, buprenorphine should not be administered as a premedication if a severely painful procedure is to be performed. Once administered, it will be difficult to top it up with other more potent opioids (such as morphine, hydromorphone, or fentanyl) to rescue pain due to the strong affinity of buprenorphine, which is only capable of treating mild to moderate pain.

DIFFERENCES BETWEEN THE VARIOUS OPIOIDS
See *Table 3.8.*

ADVANTAGES OF USING OPIOIDS
- Mild sedation when administered independently.
- Provide pre-emptive, intraoperative, and postoperative analgesia.
- Anesthetic-sparing effect on induction drugs and maintenance inhalant concentrations.
- Minimal impact on blood pressure and cardiac contractility.

Table 3.8 Differences between opioids and their dosages

Opioid	Class	Dose and route of administration (dogs and cats)	Duration of action	Side-effects and comments
Morphine	Mu–kappa agonist	0.25–1 mg/kg IM or SC; 0.25–0.5 mg/kg IV	2–4 hours	Bradycardia, respiratory depression, vomiting, panting
Hydromorphone	Mu–kappa agonist	0.05–0.2 mg/kg IV, IM, or SC	1–2 hours	Bradycardia, respiratory depression, less vomiting than with morphine, panting, may induce hyperthermia in cats
Fentanyl	Mu–kappa agonist	2–10 µg/kg IV only	15–30 minutes	Bradycardia, profound respiratory depression, apnea, panting
Buprenorphine	Partial mu agonist (or mu agonist and kappa antagonist)	20–50 µg/kg IV, IM, or SC; 40–120 µg/kg OTM (place the drug in the cheek pouch)	4–24 hours, dose dependent duration of analgesia; onset of action is slow (30 minutes)	Less bradycardia and respiratory depression in healthy dogs and cats even with very high doses (up to 0.12–0.24 mg/kg IV) due to its ceiling effect
Butorphanol	Mu antagonist and kappa agonist	0.2–0.4 mg/kg IV, IM, or SC	1–4 hours (dose dependent)	Less bradycardia and respiratory depression than other opioids, less panting response, ceiling dose is 0.8 mg/kg
Nalbuphine	Mu antagonist and kappa agonist	0.4–1 mg/kg IM or IV	1–2 hours	Less bradycardia and respiratory depression than other opioids. Used in the USA because it is the only non-controlled opioid available. Generally not available in other countries

DISADVANTAGES OF USING OPIOIDS

- Most opioids induce vagal tone and, therefore, cause various degrees of bradycardia and, at times, induce heart blocks (first or second atrioventricular blocks – see Chapter 22, ECG).

This bradycardia is responsive to anticholinergic intervention.
- While opioids induce minimal cardiovascular effects (except bradycardia), they do induce profound respiratory depression, even apnea.

Neuroleptic–analgesic combinations

OVERVIEW

- The combined use of a tranquilizer or a sedative with an analgesic agent for preanesthetic medication is referred to as a neuroleptic–analgesic combination. The modification of the ASA physical status classification system described earlier (see Preanesthetic medication protocol and *Table 3.2*) should be used to evaluate the patient's health status.

- The drugs should be drawn up separately and then combined into a single syringe for injection into the patient.
- Neuroleptic–analgesic combinations for elective surgical procedures (e.g. castration or ovariohysterectomy) and dental prophylaxis in healthy dogs (ASA I, II, I-E, II-E) are listed in *Tables 3.9, 3.10*, and *3.11*.

Table 3.9 Premedication, induction, and maintenance doses for a 4.5–22.7 kg (10–50 lb) dog using an opioid and medetomidine or dexmedetomidine combination

Drug	Weight of dog	Dose
Hydromorphone (2 mg/ml)	4.5–22.7 kg (10–50 lb)	0.5–2.5 ml IV or IM (0.22 mg/kg)
OR		
Butorphanol (10 mg/ml)		0.2–1.0 ml IV or IM (0.44 mg/kg)
OR		
Morphine (15 mg/ml)		0.2–0.1 ml IV or IM (0.66 mg/kg)
PLUS		
Medetomidine* (1 mg/ml [1,000 µg/ml]) OR Dexmedetomidine* (0.5 mg/ml [500 µg/ml])	4.5 kg (10 lb)	0.01 ml IV or IM (2.2 µg/kg)
	9 kg (20 lb)	0.02 ml IV or IM (2.2 µg/kg)
	13.6 kg (30 lb)	0.03 ml IV or IM (2.2 µg/kg)
	18.1 kg (40 lb)	0.04 ml IV or IM (2.2 µg/kg)
	22.7 kg (50 lb)	0.05 ml IV or IM (2.2 µg/kg)
AND/OR (some anesthetists discourage the concurrent use of atropine with this drug combination)		
Atropine (0.54 mg/ml)	4.5 kg (10 lb)	0.2 ml IV or IM (0.024 mg/kg)
	9 kg (20 lb)	0.4 ml IV or IM (0.024 mg/kg)
	13.6 kg (30 lb)	0.6 ml IV or IM (0.02 mg/kg)
	18.1 kg (40 lb)	0.8 ml IV or IM (0.02 mg/kg)
	22.7 kg (50 lb)	1.0 ml IV or IM (0.02 mg/kg)
Intravenous induction		
Propofol (10 mg/ml)	4.5–22.7 kg (10–50 lb)	3–5 ml IV or IM to effect (2.2–6.6 mg/kg)
OR Face mask induction		
Sevoflurane	4.5–22.7 kg (10–50 lb)	7–8% at 2 liters/minute O₂ flow for 3 minutes
OR		
Isoflurane		5% at 2 liters/minute O₂ flow for 3 minutes

*Medetomidine or dexmedetomidine are administered at the same volume in this combination.

- Some of the neuroleptic–analgesic combinations that can be used in dogs and cats are described below. The addition of atropine (0.04 mg/kg IM) or glycopyrrolate (0.01 mg/kg IM) is optional.
- The drugs to be combined should be mixed up in the same syringe and given as a single IM administration to induce a mild to moderate degree of sedation.
- Using neuroleptic–analgesic drug combinations will reduce the amount of

IV induction agent required as well as the inhalant used for anesthetic maintenance.

CONCEPTS OF USING TWO OR MORE SEDATIVES TOGETHER

- The sedatives mentioned in this chapter act on different receptor populations and trigger different mechanisms to induce sedation in the CNS. Through these different mechanisms, they generate various degrees of tranquilization and sedation. The degrees of sedation can be

Table 3.10 Premedication, induction, and maintenance doses for a 23.2–45.5 kg (51–100 lb) dog using an opioid and medetomidine or dexmedetomidine combination

Drug	Weight of dog	Dose
Hydromorphone (2 mg/ml) OR	23.2–45.5 kg (51–100 lb)	1–2 ml IV or IM (0.08 mg/kg)
Butorphanol (10 mg/ml) OR		0.5–1.0 ml IV or IM (0.2 mg/kg)
Morphine (15 mg/ml)		0.5–1.0 ml IV or IM (0.32 mg/kg)
PLUS		
Medetomidine (1 mg/ml [1,000 µg/ml]) OR	23.2–45.5 kg (51–100 lb)	0. 1 ml IV or IM (4.3–2.2 µg/kg)
Dexmedetomidine (0.5 mg/ml [500 µg/ml])		0. 1 ml IV or IM (2.2–1.1 µg/kg)

AND/OR
(some anesthetists discourage the
  concurrent use of atropine with this
  combination)		

Atropine (0.54 mg/ml)	23.2 kg (51 lb)	1.0 ml IV or IM (0.02 mg/kg)
	27.2 kg (60 lb)	1.2 ml IV or IM (0.02 mg/kg)
	31.8 kg (70 lb)	1.4 ml IV or IM (0.02 mg/kg)
	36.3 kg (80 lb)	1.6 ml IV or IM (0.02 mg/kg)
	90 lbs (40.9 kg)	1.8 ml IV or IM (0.02 mg/kg)
	45.5 kg (100 lb)	2.0 ml IV or IM (0.02 mg/kg)
Intravenous induction		
Propofol (10 mg/ml)	23.2–45.5 kg (51–100 lb)	5–6 ml IV or IM to effect (1.32–2.1 mg/kg)
OR Face mask induction		
Sevoflurane OR	23.2–45.5 kg (51–100 lb)	7–8% at 3 liters/minute O_2 flow for 3 minutes
Isoflurane		5% at 3 liters/minute O_2 flow for 3 minutes
Maintenance (adjust based on patient monitoring)		
Sevoflurane OR	23.2–45.5 kg (51–100 lb)	2–3% at 700 ml/minute on a rebreathing circuit
Isoflurane		1–1.5% at 700 ml/minute on a rebreathing circuit

Table 3.11 Premedication, induction, and maintenance doses for a 2.3–6.8 kg (5–15 lb) cat (average ~4.5 kg [10 lb]) using an opioid and medetomidine or dexmedetomidine combination

Drug	Weight of cat	Dose
Hydromorphone (2 mg/ml)	2.3–6.8 kg (5–15 lb)	0.2 ml (0.2–0.05 mg/kg) IM
OR		
Butorphanol (10 mg/ml)		0.1 ml (0.43–0.15 mg/kg) IM
OR		
Morphine (15 mg/ml)		0.1 ml (0.65–0.22 mg/kg) IM 0.2 ml (1.3–0.44 mg/kg)
PLUS		
Medetomidine (1 mg/ml [1000 µg/ml]) OR	2.3 kg (5 lb)	0.02 ml (medetomidine 8.8 µg/kg or dexmedetomidine 4.4 µg/kg) IM
Dexmedetomidine (0.5 mg/ml [500 µg/ml])	4.5 kg (10 lb)	0.04 ml (medetomidine 8.8 µg/kg or dexmedetomidine 4.4 µg/kg) IM
	6.8 kg (15 lb)	0.06 ml (medetomidine 8.8 µg/kg or dexmedetomidine 4.4 µg/kg) IM
Face mask induction		
Sevoflurane	2.3–6.8 kg (5–15 lb)	8% at 2 liters/minute O_2 flow on a rebreathing circuit for 3 minutes for intubation
OR		
Isoflurane		5% at 2 liters/minute O_2 flow on a non-rebreathing circuit for 3 minutes for intubation
OR Intravenous induction		
Propofol (10 mg/ml)	2.3–6.8 kg (5–15 lb)	1 ml (1.5–4.3 mg/kg) IV or IM to effect for intubation
Maintenance (adjust based on patient monitoring)		
Sevoflurane	2.3–6.8 kg (5–15 lb)	2–3% at 1 liter/minute on a non-rebreathing circuit
OR		
Isoflurane		1–1.5% at 1 liter/minute on a non-rebreathing circuit

enhanced when using several different classes of the sedative drugs together.

- Clinically, it is better to utilize smaller doses of two or more sedatives to induce a more profound degree of sedation and fewer side-effects than using a large dose of a single class sedative.
- For example, the degree of sedation induced by acepromazine (or azaperone) and midazolam is more profound than that with either drug used alone. The same applies to dexmedetomidine (or medetomidine) with midazolam (or with either azaperone or acepromazine).
- Possible sedative combinations are: acepromazine with midazolam, acepromazine with dexmedetomidine (or medetomidine), azaperone with dexmedetomidine (or medetomidine), acepromazine with midazolam and dexmedetomidine.

ASA I AND II DOGS
Acepromazine (0.02–0.04 mg/kg IM) or azaperone (0.2–0.4 mg/kg IM)
- Can be used in combination with one of the following opioids:
  - Morphine 0.25–1 mg/kg IM.
  - Hydromorphone 0.05–0.22 mg/kg IM.
  - Buprenorphine 0.02–0.12 mg/kg IM.
  - Butorphanol 0.2–0.4 mg/kg IM.
  - Nalbuphine 0.4–2 mg/kg IM.
  - Pethidine (meperidine) 2–3 mg/kg IM.
  - Methadone 0.05–0.5 mg/kg IM.

- The author's choice for inducing mild to moderate sedation in ASA I and II patients using one of the above combinations is:
  - Acepromazine (0.02 mg/kg IM) or azaperone (0.2–0.3 mg/kg IM) with either hydromorphone (0.05–0.2 mg/kg IM) or butorphanol (0.2–0.3 mg/kg IM) and without an anticholinergic agent. However, if the heart rate is low (<60 beats per minute), an anticholinergic, such as atropine or glycopyrrolate, should be administered to increase heart rate and maintain blood pressure.

Dexmedetomidine (5–8 μg/kg IM), medetomidine (8–10 μg/kg IM), romifidine (5–10 μg/kg IM), or xylazine (0.15–0.3 mg/kg IM)

- Can be used with one of the following opioids:
  - Morphine 0.25–0.5 mg/kg IM.
  - Hydromorphone 0.05–0.2 mg/kg IM.
  - Buprenorphine 0.02–0.10 mg/kg IM.
  - Butorphanol 0.2–0.4 mg/kg IM.
  - Nalbuphine 0.4–0.8 mg/kg IM.
  - Pethidine (meperidine) 2–3 mg/kg IM.
  - Methadone 0.05–0.2 mg/kg IM.
- Atropine (0.04 mg/kg IM) or glycopyrrolate (0.01 mg/kg IM) is likely to be beneficial in xylazine combinations, but is not recommended with the other alpha-2 sedatives.
- The author's choice for inducing mild to moderate sedation in ASA I and II patients using one of the above combinations is:
  - Dexmedetomidine (3–5 μg/kg IM) or medetomidine (6–10 μg/kg IM) with either hydromorphone (0.05–0.2 mg/kg IM) or butorphanol (0.2–0.4 mg/kg IM) and without an anticholinergic agent.

Tiletamine/zolazepam (5–8 mg/kg IM)

- Can be used with one of the following opioids:
  - Morphine 0.25–0.5 mg/kg IM.
  - Hydromorphone 0.05–0.1 mg/kg IM.
  - Buprenorphine 0.02–0.08 mg/kg IM.

- Butorphanol 0.2–0.4 mg/kg IM.
- Nalbuphine 0.4–0.8 mg/kg IM.
- Pethidine (meperidine) 2–3 mg/kg IM.
- Methadone 0.05–0.2 mg/kg IM.
- Atropine (0.04 mg/kg IM) or glycopyrrolate (0.01 mg/kg IM) is required to reduce the salivation and airway secretions induced by tiletamine.
- The author's choice for inducing a moderate to profound degree of sedation in ASA I and II patients using one of the above combinations is:
  - Tiletamine/zolazepam (5–7 mg/kg IM) with either hydromorphone (0.05–0.2 mg/kg IM) or butorphanol (0.2–0.4 mg/kg IM) and with an anticholinergic agent to reduce salivation and airway secretion. Lateral recumbency is likely to occur in 5 minutes after IM administration.

Use of two sedatives together

- Two sedatives can be combined to enhance the overall sedative quality when compared with a high dose of either sedative used alone.
- This strategy can be applied in either healthy or sick animals for better sedation with less cardiorespiratory depression.
- Examples of two sedative combinations:
  - Acepromazine 0.01 mg/kg with midazolam 0.2–0.4 mg/kg IM.
  - Acepromazine 0.01 mg/kg with dexmedetomidine (3–5 μg/kg) or medetomidine (6–10 μg/kg) IM.
  - Azaperone 0.1–0.2 mg/kg with midazolam 0.2–0.4 mg/kg IM.
  - Azaperone 0.1–0.2 mg/kg with dexmedetomidine (3–5 μg/kg) or medetomidine (6–10 μg/kg IM.
  - Midazolam 0.2–0.4 mg/kg with dexmedetomidine (3–5 μg/kg) or medetomidine (6–10 μg/kg) IM.
- All these two sedative combinations can be used with one of the following opioids:
  - Morphine 0.25–0.4 mg/kg IM.
  - Hydromorphone 0.05–0.1 mg/kg IM.
  - Buprenorphine 0.02–0.06 mg/kg IM.
  - Butorphanol 0.2–0.4 mg/kg IM.
  - Nalbuphine 0.4–0.8 mg/kg IM.
  - Pethidine (meperidine) 2–3 mg/kg IM.
  - Methadone 0.05–0.2 mg/kg IM.

SICK (ASA III, IV, V, III-E, IV-E, V-E), PEDIATRIC, OR GERIATRIC DOGS

- The following opioids can be used alone for preanesthetic medication of these patients:
  - Morphine 0.25–0.5 mg/kg IM.
  - Hydromorphone 0.05–0.1 mg/kg IM.
  - Buprenorphine 0.03–0.04 mg/kg IM.
  - Butorphanol 0.2–0.4 mg/kg IM.
  - Nalbuphine 0.4–0.8 mg/kg IM.
  - Pethidine (meperidine) 2–3 mg/kg IM.
  - Methadone 0.05–0.5 mg/kg IM.
- Atropine (0.04 mg/kg IM) or glycopyrrolate (0.01 mg/kg IM) is required to maintain an adequate heart rate in pediatric patients since their cardiac output is heart rate dependent.
- If additional sedation is required, one of the options below may be added:
  - A low dose of acepromazine (0.02 mg/kg IM).
  - A low dose of azaperone (0.1–0.3 mg/kg IM).
  - Diazepam or midazolam (0.2–0.4 mg/kg IM).
- A microdose of dexmedetomidine (2–4 µg/kg IM) or medetomidine (3–5 µg/kg IM) added to the opioid and diazepam or midazolam combination further enhances sedation.
- The author's choice for inducing a mild to moderate degree of sedation in these ASA III–V patients is:
  - Midazolam (0.3–0.4 mg/kg IM) with either hydromorphone (0.05–0.1 mg/kg IM) or butorphanol (0.2–0.3 mg/kg IM) and without an anticholinergic agent.
  - Alfaxalone (1–2 mg/kg IM [see Chapter 4]) may be added to the midazolam–opioid combination to enhance the sedation.

ASA I AND II CATS

- The following combinations can be used in healthy cats (ASA I, II, I-E, II-E) undergoing elective surgical procedures (castration or ovariohysterectomy) or dental prophylaxis.

Acepromazine (0.04–0.1 mg/kg IM), or azaperone (0.2–0.4 mg/kg IM)

- Can be given with one of the following opioids:

- Morphine 0.25–0.5 mg/kg IM.
- Hydromorphone 0.05–0.1 mg/kg IM.
- Buprenorphine 0.03–0.04 mg/kg IM.
- Butorphanol 0.2–0.4 mg/kg IM.
- Nalbuphine 0.4–0.8 mg/kg IM.
- Pethidine (meperidine) 1–2 mg/kg IM.
- Methadone 0.05–0.1 mg/kg IM.
- The use of atropine (0.04 mg/kg IM) or glycopyrrolate (0.01 mg/kg IM) is optional. Ketamine (3–5 mg/kg IM) can be added to enhance the sedation effect of an acepromazine–opioid combination.
- The author's choice for inducing mild to moderate sedation in ASA I and II patients with one of these combinations is:
  - Acepromazine (0.05 mg/kg IM) with either buprenorphine (0.03–0.04 mg/kg IM) or butorphanol (0.3–0.4 mg/kg IM) and with or without ketamine (3–5 mg/kg IM).

Dexmedetomidine (10–15 µg/kg IM), medetomidine (20–30 µg/kg IM), romifidine (20–30 µg/kg IM), or xylazine (0.25–0.5 mg/kg IM)

- Can be given with one of the following opioids:
  - Morphine 0.25–0.5 mg/kg IM.
  - Hydromorphone 0.05–0.1 mg/kg IM.
  - Buprenorphine 0.02–0.04 mg/kg IM.
  - Butorphanol 0.2–0.4 mg/kg IM.
  - Nalbuphine 0.4–0.8 mg/kg IM.
  - Pethidine (meperidine) 1–2 mg/kg IM.
  - Methadone 0.05–0.1 mg/kg IM.
- The use of atropine (0.02 mg/kg IM) or glycopyrrolate (0.005 mg/kg IM) is optional. Ketamine (3–5 mg/kg IM) can be added to enhance the sedation effect of the combination.
- In addition to ketamine, midazolam (0.2 mg/kg IM) can be used to enhance the overall quality of anesthesia (i.e. a combination of alpha-2 agonist–opioid–ketamine and midazolam).
- The author's choice for inducing a moderate to profound sedation using one of these combinations is:
  - Dexmedetomidine (10–15 µg/kg IM) or medetomidine (20–30 µg/kg IM) with either buprenorphine (0.03–0.04 mg/kg IM) or butorphanol (0.3–0.4 mg/kg IM) plus ketamine (3 mg/kg, IM) but without an anticholinergic agent.

Tiletamine/zolazepam (5–8 mg/kg IM)
- Can be given with one of the following opioids:
  - Morphine 0.25–0.5 mg/kg IM.
  - Hydromorphone 0.05–0.1 mg/kg IM.
  - Buprenorphine 0.02–0.04 mg/kg IM.
  - Butorphanol 0.2–0.4 mg/kg IM.
  - Nalbuphine 0.4–0.8 mg/kg IM.
  - Pethidine (meperidine) 1–2 mg/kg IM.
  - Methadone 0.05–0.1 mg/kg IM.
- Atropine (0.04 mg/kg IM) or glycopyrrolate (0.01 mg/kg IM) is necessary to reduce the salivation and airway secretions induced by tiletamine.
- The author's choice for inducing moderate to profound sedation with one of these combinations is:
  - Tiletamine/zolazepam (5 mg/kg IM) with either buprenorphine (0.03–0.04 mg/kg IM) or butorphanol (0.3–0.4 mg/kg IM) plus an anticholinergic agent (atropine, 0.04 mg/kg IM) for reducing salivation and airway secretions. Lateral recumbency is likely to occur within 5–8 minutes after IM administration.

Debilitated (ASA III, IV, V, III-E, IV-E, V-E), pediatric, or geriatric cats
- One of the following opioids can be used alone:
  - Morphine 0.25–0.5 mg/kg IM.
  - Hydromorphone 0.05–0.1 mg/kg IM.
  - Buprenorphine 0.01–0.03 mg/kg IM.
  - Butorphanol 0.2–0.4 mg/kg IM.
  - Nalbuphine 0.4–0.8 mg/kg IM.
  - Pethidine (meperidine) 1–2 mg/kg IM.
  - Methadone 0.05–0.1 mg/kg IM.
- Administration of atropine (0.04 mg/kg IM) or glycopyrrolate (0.01 mg/kg IM) is necessary in pediatric cats to maintain adequate heart rate, as cardiac output is heart rate dependent in these young animals.
- Additional options for use in ASA III–V-E cats include:
  - Low dose acepromazine (0.02 mg/kg IM) or azaperone (0.1–0.2 mg/kg IM).
  - Diazepam or midazolam (0.2–0.4 mg/kg IM).
  - Ketamine (1–2 mg/kg IM) enhances the sedation effects of an acepromazine-, diazepam- or midazolam–opioid combination.

- A microdose of dexmedetomidine (2–4 µg/kg IM) or medetomidine (3–5 µg/kg IM) further enhances the sedative effect of an opioid and diazepam or midazolam combination.
- The author's choice for inducing moderate to profound sedation in ASA III–V cats is:
  - Midazolam (0.3–0.4 mg/kg IM) with either buprenorphine (0.03–0.04 mg/kg IM) or butorphanol (0.2–0.4 mg/kg IM) and without an anticholinergic agent.
  - Midazolam (0.2–0.4 mg/kg) with an opioid (hydromorphone 0.1 mg/kg) and alfaxalone (1–2 mg/kg), with all three drugs mixed in the same syringe for a single IM injection.

ASA III or IV dogs and cats
- Additional options for preanesthetic medication in ASA III or IV dogs and cats are:
  - Premedication with hydromorphone, butorphanol, or morphine with a microdose of medetomidine or dexmedetomidine, followed by propofol or sevoflurane or isoflurane face mask induction, is a convenient and safe way to induce an ASA III or IV dog or cat.
  - In dogs premedicated with medetomidine and maintained on etomidate (CRI), the medetomidine significantly increases systemic vascular resistance (SVR) and decreases cardiac output, while the etomidate induces minimal changes in the hemodynamic status. The same scenario would be anticipated with dexmedetomidine.
  - Propofol infusion alleviates medetomidine- or dexmedetomidine-induced vasoconstriction due to its vasodilation effect.
  - Microdoses of medetomidine or dexmedetomidine can be combined with opioids, followed by IV propofol administration or sevoflurane (or isoflurane) face mask for anesthesia induction in dogs and cats. See *Tables 3.9–3.11* for doses.
  - Combine the opioid and medetomidine (or dexmedetomidine) in the same syringe and administer either IV or IM.

- If administered IV, wait 2–3 minutes before inducing with propofol or with sevoflurane or isoflurane via a face mask.
- If administered IM, wait 5–10 minutes before inducing with propofol or with sevoflurane or isoflurane via a face mask.
- To increase the speed of induction, face mask induction should be performed using a non-rebreathing circuit. If the patient is >7 kg (15 lb), switch back to a rebreathing circuit for inhalant maintenance after the transition is complete.
- After induction, but before any skin incision, administer carprofen (4.4 mg/kg SC), meloxicam (0.2 mg/kg SC), or robenacoxib (1–2 mg/kg SC) to give a 12–24-hour duration of analgesia in dogs or cats. (**Note:** Use these drugs only once in cats and not at all in animals contraindicated to NSAIDs.)

Case example

- 'Kiko' (**Fig. 3.20**), an 11-year-old spayed female Labrador Retriever weighing 25 kg (55 lb), was presented for laceration of the hindlimb. The dog was overall healthy.
- Signalment: PCV 0.46 l/l (46%); TP 70 g/l (7 g/dl); glucose 4.6 mmol/l (82 mg/dl); baseline heart rate 110 bpm; respiratory rate 26 bpm; temperature 39°C (102.3°F); nice temperament.
- Premedication (using the *Table 3.10* dose chart for a combination of dexmedetomidine and hydromorphone): dexmedetomidine 2.2 μg/kg plus hydromorphone 0.08 mg/kg, combined in the same syringe and administered as a single IM injection.
- Fifteen minutes post premedication the dog was moderately sedate and a venous catheterization was easily achieved under sedation (**Figs. 3.21**).
- Induction was with propofol (1.5 mg/kg IV) and the dog was successfully intubated (**Fig. 3.22**).
- Anesthesia was maintained with isoflurane (1–1.5% in oxygen) while the area was prepared for surgery (**Fig. 3.23**). Recovery was smooth and uneventful. The dog received carprofen (4.4 mg/kg SC) for additional pain management prior to surgery and a second dose of hydromorphone (0.05 mg/kg IM) postoperatively.

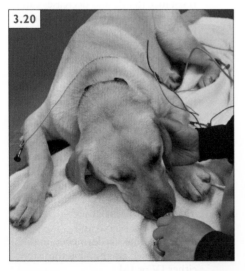

3.20

Fig. 3.20 An 11-year-old spayed female Labrador Retriever presented for repair of laceration of a hindlimb. The dog was premedicated with 2.2 μg/kg of dexmedetomidine and 0.08 mg/kg of hydromorphone. She was moderately sedated after premedication. Heart rhythm was monitored by electrocardiography and oxygen supplementation was provided prior to IV catheter placement.

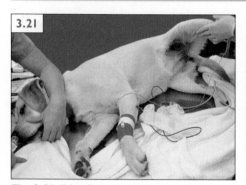

Fig. 3.21 IV catheterization was easily achieved under sedation. The hindlimb laceration site was inspected under sedation and prior to anesthesia induction. 100% oxygen was supplemented during this time via a flow-by method at the nose.

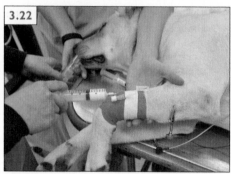

Fig. 3.22 Intubation was easily achieved after induction with propofol (1.5 mg/kg IV) to effect.

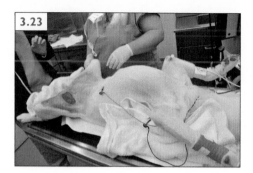

Fig. 3.23 Anesthesia was maintained with 1–1.5% isoflurane and blood pressure was well maintained while the laceration area was prepared for surgery.

Further reading

Bortolami E, Murrell JC, Slingsby LS (2013) Methadone in combination with acepromazine as premedication prior to neutering in the cat. *Vet Anaesth Analg* 40(2):181–93.

Grasso SC, Ko JC, Weil AB *et al.* (2015) Hemodynamic influence of acepromazine or dexmedetomidine premedication in isoflurane-anesthetized dogs. *J Am Vet Med Assoc* 246(7):754–64.

Hall LW, Clarke KW (1991) Principles of sedation, analgesia and premedication. In: *Veterinary Anaesthesia*, 9th edn. Baillière Tindall, London, pp. 51–79.

Ilbäck NG, Stålhandske T (2003) Cardiovascular effects of xylazine recorded with telemetry in the dog. *J Vet Med A Physiol Pathol Clin Med* 50:479–83.

Ko JC, Knesl O, Weil AB *et al.* (2009) FAQs – Analgesia, sedation, and anesthesia: making the switch from medetomidine to dexmedetomidine. *Compend Contin Educ Vet Pract* 31(suppl 1A):1–24.

Kukanich B, Borum SL (2008) The disposition and behavioral effects of methadone in Greyhounds. *Vet Anaesth Analg* 35:242–8.

Mair A, Kloeppel H, Ticehurst K. (2014). A comparison of low dose tiletamine-zolazepam or acepromazine combined with methadone for pre-anaesthetic medication in cats. *Vet Anaesth Analg* 41(6):630–5.

Monteiro ER, Coelho K, Bressan TF *et al.* (2016) Effects of acepromazine-morphine and acepromazine-methadone premedication on the minimum alveolar concentration of isoflurane in dogs. *Vet Anaesth Analg* 43(1):27–34.

Shah MD, Yates D, Hunt J *et al.* (2018) A comparison between methadone and buprenorphine for perioperative analgesia in dogs undergoing ovariohysterectomy.

J Small Anim Pract 2018 May 21 (Epub ahead of print) doi: 10.1111/jsap.12859.

Sheen MJ, Chang FL, Ho ST (2014) Anesthetic premedication: New horizons of an old practice. *Acta Anaesthesiol Taiwan* 52(3):134–42.

Tobias KM, Marioni-Henry K, Wagner R (2006) A retrospective study on the use of acepromazine maleate in dogs with seizures. *J Am Anim Hosp Assoc* 42:283–9.

Valverde A, Cantwell S, Hernández J et al. (2004) Effects of acepromazine on the incidence of vomiting associated with opioid administration in dogs. *Vet Anaesth Analg* 31:40–5.

CHAPTER 4

Intravenous injection techniques and intravenous anesthetic agents

Jeff C Ko

Introduction

This chapter builds on the preanesthetic medication drugs discussed in Chapter 3 and describes the IV anesthetic drugs used for induction of anesthesia and endotracheal intubation prior to inhalant anesthesia maintenance (**Fig. 4.1**). The chapter also covers the use of IV agents for short-term anesthesia maintenance. IV injection techniques are also described and the characteristics of each injectable anesthetic drug or drug combination are outlined. IV injectable combinations using medetomidine and dexmedetomidine are discussed in Chapter 9.

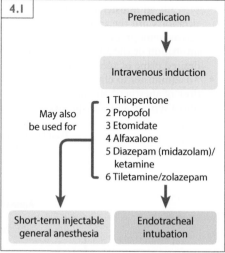

Fig. 4.1 Choices of intravenous induction agents with or without premedications in dogs and cats.

Intravenous injection techniques

INTRAVENOUS ANESTHETIC AGENTS

- IV anesthetic agents can be used in dogs and cats for inducing anesthesia prior to endotracheal intubation and maintenance with inhalant agents. They can also be used as a single bolus, as repeated intermittent boluses, or by constant rate infusion (CRI) for short-term chemical restraint or injectable anesthesia.
- When combined with other anesthetic agents, they can be used to achieve unconsciousness, analgesia, and muscle relaxation as part of a total intravenous anesthesia (TIVA) combination.
- The IV anesthetic agents traditionally used include thiopentone, propofol, diazepam (midazolam)/ketamine, etomidate, alfaxalone, and tiletamine/zolazepam. Other IV anesthetic agents used include medetomidine and dexmedetomidine in combination with ketamine, opioids, or diazepam (midazolam) (see Chapter 9 for doses and routes of administration).

INDUCTION OR SHORT-TERM RESTRAINT

- IV anesthetic agents used for anesthetic induction or short-term restraint are typically administered to effect by titration until the animal's jaw tone is relaxed enough to allow endotracheal intubation or the animal reaches the desired plane of anesthesia.
- To administer to effect, the full calculated dose of anesthetic should be withdrawn into a syringe and one-quarter to one-third of the dose administered at 5–10 second intervals until the desired plane of anesthesia is achieved or until the maximum calculated dose is used.
- Many dogs and cats suffer profound respiratory depression following rapid administration of an IV bolus, which results in overdose, cyanosis, and apnea. This is particularly true with drugs such as propofol, thiopental, etomidate, and alfaxalone.

ARM–BRAIN (CEPHALIC VEIN TO BRAIN) CIRCULATION TIME

- When administering an IV anesthetic induction agent, it is important to remember that it takes time (approximately 5–8 seconds) for the drug to be delivered from the cephalic vein (or saphenous vein) to the brain.
- The fact that the dog or cat is relaxed enough for endotracheal intubation or is in sternal or lateral recumbency is most likely the result of the anesthetic dose administered 5–8 seconds earlier.
- Administration of IV anesthetic agents as a single bolus induces apnea, which initiates a vicious cycle starting with a bad transition from IV induction to the maintenance phase and ending with apnea due to anesthetic use.

APNEA INDUCED BY INTRAVENOUS ANESTHETICS DURING INDUCTION

- A vicious cycle develops (**Fig. 4.2**) if the IV anesthetic agent is administered too quickly and/or apnea or hypoventilation occurs. Because the dog or cat is not breathing well, there is poor uptake of the maintenance

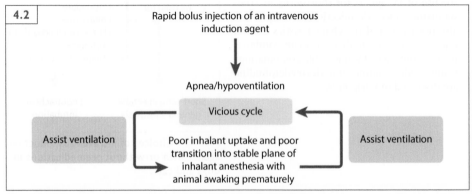

4.2

Rapid bolus injection of an intravenous induction agent

Apnea/hypoventilation

Vicious cycle

Assist ventilation

Poor inhalant uptake and poor transition into stable plane of inhalant anesthesia with animal awaking prematurely

Assist ventilation

Fig. 4.2 Schematic representation of the vicious cycle that follows intravenous induction agent-induced apnea or hypoventilation.

inhalant anesthetic agent during the period following IV induction. Once the IV induction agent is redistributed away from the brain, the animal begins to wake prematurely because the inhalant anesthetic concentration in the lungs (and, therefore, the brain) is low. When this occurs, the veterinarian either ventilates ('bags') the patient aggressively with higher doses of inhalant or immediately administers an additional IV anesthetic agent to reanesthetize the animal. This results in the patient becoming apneic again and another cycle begins.

- IV anesthetic agents should be administered slowly over a period of 60–90 seconds at the appropriate titration rate. If short-term chemical restraint is required, the agent can be administered as intermittent boluses. Apnea can be avoided using these techniques.
- If IV anesthetic agents are used to achieve a plane of anesthesia suitable for endotracheal intubation, they must not be given too slowly. Too slow an administration (i.e. over a period of 3–4 minutes) will result in the animal resisting intubation because the high plasma concentration of the agent needed to achieve the desired plane of anesthesia cannot be obtained.
- A balanced technique is required to ensure a smooth induction.

Characteristics of intravenous anesthetic agents used in dogs and cats

A summary of the dosages and cardiorespiratory side-effects of IV anesthetic agents is given in *Tables 4.1* and *4.2*.

Table 4.1 Dosages and cardiorespiratory effects of intravenous anesthetic agents in dogs and cats

Drug	Dosages for dogs	Dosages for cats	Cardiorespiratory effects and comments
Thiopentone	Non-premedicated: 15–20 mg/kg; premedicated: 8–10 mg/kg	Non-premedicated: 15–20 mg/kg; premedicated: 8–10 mg/kg	Not suitable for CRI due to drug accumulation and prolonged rough recoveries. Rapid injection causes apnea, cyanosis, and hypoventilation (less severe than propofol). Vasodilation, hypotension, premature ventricular contractions with bigeminy rhythm. Perivascular administration causes localized tissue necrosis
Propofol	Non-premedicated: 8–10 mg/kg; premedicated: 4–8 mg/kg; CRI: bolus with 2 mg/kg IV followed by 20–100 µg/kg/min	Non-premedicated: 8–10 mg/kg; premedicated: 4–8 mg/kg; CRI: bolus with 2 mg/kg IV followed by 20–100 µg/kg/min	Suitable for CRI due to its short metabolic half-life. Rapid injection will cause apnea and cyanosis. Vasodilation, hypotension, with an increased heart rate. Less arrhythmogenic than thiopentone. May cause pain on injection. Seizure-like phenomenon may occur in some dogs after induction or during propofol maintenance
Etomidate	Non-premedicated: 1.5–2.2 mg/kg; premedicated: 0.5–1.0 mg/kg; CRI: 50–100 µg/kg/min	Non-premedicated: 1.5–2.2 mg/kg; premedicated: 0.5–1.0 mg/kg; CRI: 50–100 µg/kg/min	Suitable for CRI due to short metabolic half-life. The propylene glycol formulation of etomidate is less desirable than other formulations due to severe hemolysis resulting from hyperosmolarity. Rapid injection causes apnea and cyanosis. Tends to induce vomiting, myoclonic twitching, and excitement in non-premedicated animals. Pain on injection

(Continued)

Table 4.1 (Continued) Dosages and cardiorespiratory effects of intravenous anesthetic agents in dogs and cats

Drug	Dosages for dogs	Dosages for cats	Cardiorespiratory effects and comments
Alfaxalone	Non-premedicated: 3 mg/kg; premedicated: 1–2 mg/kg; CRI non-premedicated: following induction, use 0.13–0.15 mg/kg/min; CRI premedicated: following induction, use 0.1–0.12 mg/kg/min; maintenance non-premedicated: intermittent bolus every 10 min at 1.3–1.5 mg/kg; maintenance premedicated: intermittent bolus every 10 min at 1.0–1.2 mg/kg Alfaxalone at 1–2 mg/kg can be administered IM as an adjunct to other sedatives	Non-premedicated: 5 mg/kg; premedicated: 2–4 mg/kg; CRI non-premedicated: following induction, use 0.16–0.18 mg/kg/min; CRI premedicated: following induction, use 0.11–0.13 mg/kg/min; maintenance non-premedicated: intermittent bolus every 10 min at 1.6–1.8 mg/kg; maintenance premedicated: intermittent bolus every 10 min at 1.1–1.3 mg/kg The IM dose of alfaxalone is the same for dogs and cats	Rapid injection causes apnea and cyanosis. Dose-dependent respiratory depression. Provide oxygen and/or intermittent positive-pressure ventilation to counteract the hypoxemia and hypercapnia. Use with care and reduce doses in the hepatic and renal compromised cases. Excitement or delirium may occur during recovery, especially after prolonged CRI When using as an IM sedative, alfaxalone adds sedation without adding cardiorespiratory depression to the existing sedative protocol. This is what makes alfaxalone attractive as a sedative adjunct
Diazepam (midazolam)/ ketamine	Non-premedicated: 0.27–0.3 mg/kg diazepam (midazolam) with 5.5–6.0 mg/kg ketamine; premedicated: 0.15 mg/kg diazepam (midazolam) and 4 mg/kg ketamine	Non-premedicated: 0.27–0.3 mg/kg diazepam (midazolam) with 5.5–6.0 mg/kg ketamine; premedicated: 0.15 mg/kg diazepam (midazolam) and 4 mg/kg ketamine	Collect both compounds into the same syringe and administer IV. Overdose may cause apnea and cyanosis. However, the likelihood is much lower than with propofol and etomidate. Tight jaw tone and swallowing on endotracheal intubation. Transit tachycardia immediately following induction. Ketamine hangover if duration of inhalant anesthesia is less than 30 minutes
Tiletamine/ zolazepam	Non-premedicated: 2.2–4.4 mg/kg; premedicated: 0.5–1.0 mg/kg	Non-premedicated: 2.2–4.4 mg/kg; premedicated: 1.0–1.5 mg/kg	Small injection volume. Quality of induction similar to diazepam (midazolam)/ketamine. Transit tachycardia may occur following induction. Repeated dosing will cause prolonged recovery

Table 4.2 Pharmacologic properties of intravenous anesthetic drugs in dogs and cats

Effects and clinical uses	Thiopentone	Propofol	Etomidate	Alfaxalone	Diazepam (midazolam)/ ketamine	Tiletamine/ zolazepam
Heart rate and arrhythmias	Increased, VPCs	May increase or decrease	No change	Increased rate, but no arrhythmias	Increased, VPCs	Increased, VPCs
Blood pressure	Decrease due to vasodilation	Decrease due to vasodilation	No change	Decrease due to vasodilation	Increase due to increase in heart rate	Increase due to increase in heart rate
Respiratory depression	Profound – apnea	Profound – apnea	Profound – apnea	Profound – apnea	Profound – apnea (less than other intravenous agents)	Profound – apnea (less than other intravenous agents)
Analgesia	None	None	None	None	Yes	Yes
Anticonvulsant	Yes	Yes	Yes	Yes	No	No

(Continued)

Table 4.2 (Continued) Pharmacologic properties of intravenous anesthetic drugs in dogs and cats

Effects and clinical uses	Thiopentone	Propofol	Etomidate	Alfaxalone	Diazepam (midazolam)/ ketamine	Tiletamine/ zolazepam
Metabolism	Slow hepatic	Rapid hepatic and extrahepatic, then renal	Rapid hepatic then renal	Rapid hepatic then renal	Slow hepatic and renal	Slow hepatic and renal
Route of administration	IV bolus	IV bolus or CRI	IV bolus or CRI	IV bolus or CRI	IV or IM	IV or IM
Pain on injection	No	Yes	Yes	No	No when IV and yes when IM	No when IV and yes when IM

CRI, constant rate infusion; VPC, ventricular premature contractions.

THIOPENTONE (THIOPENTAL) SODIUM
Overview
- Thiopentone sodium (**Fig. 4.3**) is a very short-acting barbiturate that largely replaced thiamylal in 1992. It is commercially available as a powder and is reconstituted to either a 2% (20 mg/ml) or 2.5% (25 mg/ml) solution.
- Thiopentone can be used in both dogs and cats.
- Thiopentone is no longer available in some countries (e.g. the USA) and the veterinary community generally has phased out its use for routine IV anesthetic induction.

Induction using thiopentone
- The induction dose of thiopentone in non-premedicated dogs and cats is 15–20 mg/kg.
- Induction is usually rapid, smooth, and excitement free.
- Premedication with acepromazine, xylazine, medetomidine, dexmedetomidine, diazepam or midazolam, opioids or tiletamine/ zolazepam reduces the induction dose to 6–10 mg/kg (see Chapter 3).
- A subinduction dose of thiopentone tends to cause excitement in non-premedicated dogs and cats. Therefore, when administering thiopentone for anesthetic induction, one-third to one-half of the calculated dose should be given rapidly to carry the animal through this excitement stage. The remainder is given by titration until the desired plane of anesthesia is reached.

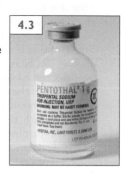

Fig. 4.3 Thiopentone is available as a powder and requires reconstitution with sterile water to a concentration of 2.0–2.5% depending on the volume of water added.

- The time from induction to walking normally following thiopentone administration is about 45 minutes in dogs and cats, compared with approximately 15 minutes following propofol administration. If a rapid recovery is required, propofol should be used instead of thiopentone.

Short-term immobilization using thiopentone
- A single dose of thiopentone results in a 5–8 minute duration of immobilization. This is appropriate for non-invasive procedures such as a laryngeal function examination in dogs and cats.
- The period of immobilization can be extended by giving additional intermittent boluses of 0.5–1.0 mg/kg over 3–4 minute intervals. However, repeated intermittent administration over a long period of time can result in prolonged rough recovery in dogs and cats.
- Premedication prior to a single bolus of thiopentone extends the duration of immobilization to 15 minutes.

- Thiopentone has minimal effect on laryngeal function, therefore it is usually used for laryngeal function examination in dogs. To perform this procedure, an IV catheter is placed in the dog's cephalic vein and its patency confirmed with a saline injection. Thiopentone (15–20 mg/kg) is then administered through the catheter as if for induction with the initial one-third administered quickly followed by slow administration of the additional titration boluses. The dog's jaw is opened carefully using a laryngeal scope and blade, taking care if the dog sneezes during induction. The rapid closing of the jaws can cause injury to the person intubating the dog. Titration is continued slowly until the jaws can be opened and the larynx clearly observed while the dog continues to breathe. If the dog becomes apneic, the animal should be intubated and ventilated with 100% oxygen until it resumes breathing. The endotracheal tube is then removed and the induction process repeated with thiopentone until the laryngeal examination is complete. The dog should be intubated at the end of the examination and allowed to recover spontaneously. Oxygenation before a laryngeal examination will help prevent immediate hypoxia should hypoventilation or apnea occur.

Other factors to take into consideration

- Thiopentone requires extensive liver metabolism. For this reason it is not an appropriate agent to use for a prolonged, repeated procedure requiring intermittent boluses or CRI given that it accumulates over time, leading to a prolonged, rough recovery.
- Thiopentone has a pH of 10 to 11. When administering thiopentone to dogs and cats, it should always be given via an IV catheter or butterfly catheter and not percutaneously. If thiopentone is accidentally injected perivascularly, it causes tissue irritation ranging from redness to various degrees of necrosis, depending on the volume injected. The skin and tissues may slough off a few days post perivascular injection. If perivascular injection does occur, the injection area should be immediately infiltrated with physiologic saline or saline with 2% lidocaine to dilute the concentration of thiopentone, minimize further tissue irritation, and provide some pain relief. The perivascular injection area should be compressed with a warm pack to facilitate drug absorption and reduce inflammation.

- Thiopentone has been known to increase the size of the spleen in dogs and cats following a single induction dose. If the size of the spleen becomes a problem during the surgery, a small amount of diluted epinephrine can be administered directly into the spleen to induce vasoconstriction and 'shrink' the spleen.

- The use of thiopentone should be avoided in sighthound breeds of dogs (e.g. Greyhounds, Afghan Hounds, Italian Greyhounds, Salukis) because of the prolonged rough recovery time, which is characterized by vocalization, paddling, repeated righting but unable to achieve sternal recumbency, salivation, and inability to stand.

- Thiopentone can potentially induce ventricular cardiac arrhythmias such as premature ventricular contractions or bigeminy (**Fig. 4.4**). If arrhythmias occur, they should be corrected immediately by intubating the animal and providing 100% oxygen via positive-pressure ventilation. The bigeminy usually subsides after ventilation with 100% oxygen. If the

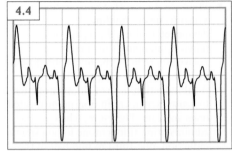

Fig. 4.4 During thiopentone induction, ventricular cardiac arrhythmias, such as ventricular bigeminy, may be observed. Note that there are four ventricular premature contractions in a roll in this trace.

arrhythmia persists, a bolus of lidocaine (2 mg/kg IV) should be administered.

- In one study, administrating thiopentone (11 mg/kg) and lidocaine (8.8 mg/kg) in combination did not induce bigeminy and had minimal effects on the cardiovascular system in dogs. Animals undergoing induction with any IV anesthetic agent should be monitored for arrhythmias using electrocardiography (ECG).

- Manufacturers recommend that unused portions of thiopentone should be discarded 24 hours after reconstitution; however, studies have shown that reconstituted thiopentone can be stored for up to 6 days at room temperature or 7 days in a refrigerator. Precipitation is likely to occur if the reconstituted drug is stored over time, and if this happens it should be discarded immediately.

- The availability of thiopentone is becoming an issue in some countries and most veterinary practitioners have switched to other IV induction agents for endotracheal intubation in dogs and cats.

PROPOFOL
Overview

- Propofol (**Figs. 4.5, 4.6**), 2,6-diisopropylphenol, is insoluble in water. It is most commonly formulated as an emulsion containing 10% soybean oil, 1.2% egg lecithin, and 2.25% glycerol with sodium hydroxide to adjust the pH to 7.0. The emulsion formulation of propofol does not contain preservatives and it promotes bacterial growth, therefore strict aseptic techniques must be enforced when withdrawing the drug. Any remaining emulsion should be discarded within 6 hours after opening. A new formulation of propofol containing benzyl alcohol (20 mg/ml) (PropoFlo™ 28) is available. The benzyl alcohol acts as a bacteriostatic agent and minimizes bacterial growth. As a result, there is a shelf-life of up to 28 days once the vial is opened. A water soluble propofol formulation (aquaFOL) is also available (**Fig. 4.5**).

- The use in cats of propofol containing benzyl alcohol has raised questions as to whether it may lead to benzyl alcohol-related toxicity. Current evidence indicates that a single induction dose of propofol containing benzyl alcohol (such as PropoFlo 28) is acceptable in cats and unlikely to have toxic effects. However, repeated injections or using CRI over time should be avoided.

- Perivascular injection of propofol does not cause tissue necrosis or skin sloughing if only a small volume is administered. However, if a large volume is inadvertently injected perivascularly, there is a risk of infection at the site.

- Propofol only works when administered IV; it is not effective when administered IM or SC.

- Propofol is a very versatile IV anesthetic. It can be used for induction, as a sedative for short-term immobilization, or as a CRI for anesthetic maintenance. Subinduction doses of propofol do not cause excitement in non-premedicated animals, therefore it can be used as a sedative at very low doses (0.5–1.0 mg/kg). Apnea or hypoventilation is very unlikely to occur when an animal is sedated with such a low dose.

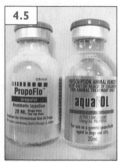
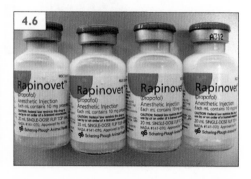

Figs. 4.5, 4.6 Propofol in an emulsion formulation is white in color. Several commercial brands of propofol are available. The water-soluble propofol formulation (aquaFOL, **4.5**) is transparent and has a longer shelf-life once opened.

Induction using propofol
- The induction dose of propofol in non-premedicated dogs and cats is 8–10 mg/kg.
- Premedication using sedatives/tranquilizers with or without opioids reduces the induction dose of propofol to 4–6 mg/kg.
- Intermittent boluses of propofol can be used to maintain anesthesia following initial bolus induction.
- Administering diazepam or midazolam (0.2–0.4 mg/kg), or medetomidine (1 µg/kg) or dexmedetomidine (0.5–1.0 µg/kg), or fentanyl (2 µg/kg) IV in dogs immediately prior to propofol induction spares propofol by approximately 33% when compared with propofol used alone.

Short-term chemical restraint using propofol
- A 0.5–1.0 mg/kg intermittent bolus injection at 2–4 minute intervals provides short-term chemical restraint in dogs

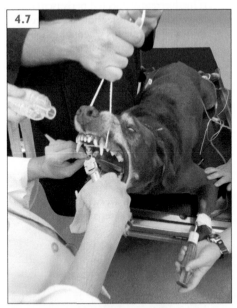

Fig. 4.7 Propofol has minimal effects on laryngeal function and is often used for laryngeal function examination in dogs. Note that the propofol is being titrated through a preplaced cephalic venous catheter while the dog's laryngeal function is being evaluated. Flow-by 100% oxygen is being provided via a breathing hose.

and cats and this can be extended as necessary.
- This technique is frequently used when performing bronchoscopy or a tracheal wash, where inhalant anesthesia may not be appropriate. The use of propofol allows the animal to be anesthetized without endotracheal intubation while providing a plane of anesthesia adequate for upper or lower airway diagnostic procedures.
- Short-term chemical restraint can be used for ECG, radiography, or other mildly invasive diagnostic procedures (e.g. joint tap, bone marrow aspiration) where an analgesic drug is concurrently provided. For example, premedicating with an opioid (such as butorphanol at 0.2 mg/kg IV or IM), following this with a loading bolus injection of propofol at 2 mg/kg IV and then giving 0.5–1.0 mg/kg at 3–4 minute intervals for as long as necessary, will provide up to 1 hour of chemical restraint. If the animal is not intubated, 100% oxygen should be provided via insufflation.
- As with thiopentone, propofol (and recently, alfaxalone) has minimal effects on laryngeal function and is often used for laryngeal function examination in dogs (**Fig. 4.7**) and cats. Several studies have shown that thiopentone is a better choice for assessing arytenoid motion in dogs than propofol, diazepam (midazolam)/ketamine, or premedication with acepromazine. However, propofol and thiopentone are both more effective in exposing the larynx for laryngeal function evaluation than diazepam (midazolam)/ketamine.
- A recent study has shown that regardless of the anesthetic agent(s) used, laryngeal function should be determined in conjunction with the respiratory rate and depth of respirations. Doxapram (up to 1 mg/kg IV) should be used to facilitate laryngeal exam if a dog is either apneic or has shallow respirations in order to accurately evaluate laryngeal function.

Total intravenous anesthesia using propofol
- Propofol can be given by CRI to maintain general anesthesia.
- The CRI dose of propofol ranges from 20 to 100 µg/kg/min. As this is a wide

dose range for CRI , it is recommended that a low dose is given initially and then increased as appropriate.

- A key advantage of giving propofol by CRI is its short metabolic half-life. Even after hours of CRI, the animal is still able to recover smoothly in a reasonable period of time, although this recovery may be a bit longer than that following inhalant anesthesia.
- If propofol is being used for an invasive procedure, analgesic agents (e.g. opioids, ketamine, alpha-2 agonists, or local anesthetics) should be considered for combination use with propofol infusion.
- Propofol solution is compatible with many different types of fluids (saline, balanced electrolyte fluids, lactated Ringer's solution [LRS], 5% dextrose), which can be mixed together for CRI administration or coadministered from the side injection port of the fluid infusion line (**Fig. 4.8**).
- Propofol is the preferred anesthetic agent for IV induction prior to cesarean section when compared with midazolam/ketamine, diazepam/ketamine, or tiletamine/zolazepam inductions. The neurologic reflexes of the puppies delivered are less depressed after propofol than with diazepam/ketamine or midazolam/ketamine, or thiopentone.

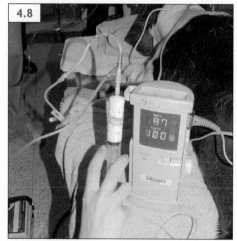

Fig. 4.8 Propofol is compatible with other fluids and can, therefore, be diluted with various fluids or coadministered via the side injection port of any intravenous fluid (lactated Ringer's solution or other balanced electrolyte) infusion line.

Other factors to take into consideration

- Propofol can be safely used in sighthounds because the recovery time is much shorter and smoother compared with thiopentone used alone.
- Propofol, when combined with acepromazine, produces minimal changes in spleen size during anesthesia in dogs.
- When using propofol for induction in cats and small dogs, it is preferable to use a 5 mg/ml solution instead of the current commercially available 10 mg/ml formulation. A 5 mg/ml propofol solution can be prepared by adding an equal volume of either a balanced electrolyte solution (e.g. LRS) or physiologic saline to the same volume of 10 mg/ml propofol.
- When propofol is administered in this way, a larger volume of injection is used (due to added fluids), slowing the speed of drug administration and minimizing the

potential for apnea and cyanosis in smaller animals.
- Cats typically take 15–20 minutes longer than dogs to recover from the same single induction or CRI dose of propofol.
- The cardiopulmonary effects of propofol and thiopentone are very similar, with both drugs inducing vasodilation and hypotension. Both drugs are equally capable of causing respiratory depression and apnea.
- While propofol induces unconsciousness and muscle relaxation and is used to treat seizures, occasionally it can induce a seizure-like phenomenon in dogs similar to that reported in humans. This seizure-like phenomenon is characterized by muscle rigidity in the front quarters of affected dogs; the neck region and forelimbs of the dogs may become stiff, while the hind quarters and hindlimbs remain relaxed. This stiffness tends to occur during or soon after anesthetic induction and into the early stages of the inhalant anesthesia maintenance. No treatment is required; the seizure-like activity disappears spontaneously after a few minutes. Administering diazepam (midazolam) or deepening the plane of inhalant anesthesia does not alleviate the phenomenon.

ETOMIDATE
Overview
- Etomidate (**Fig. 4.9**) is a unique IV anesthetic agent; it is neither a barbiturate nor a propofol, but is in a class of its own. Etomidate is available as a 2 mg/ml solution containing 35% propylene glycol (PG) by volume. It has a high osmolality of 4,965 mOsm/kg and a pH of 6.9. In some countries, etomidate may be available in formulations that do not contain PG.

Induction and maintenance using etomidate
- The induction dose of etomidate in dogs and cats is 1.5–2.2 mg/kg in non-premedicated animals and approximately 0.5–1.0 mg/kg in premedicated dogs and cats.
- In one study, a loading dose of 0.5 mg/kg IV, followed by 50 µg/kg/min CRI, was used without complication in healthy dogs premedicated with medetomidine (15 µg/kg IM).
- Like other injectable anesthetics, etomidate is administered by titration to facilitate endotracheal intubation or for anesthesia maintenance to avoid overdose and apnea.

Other factors to take into consideration
- Etomidate is considered the anesthetic induction agent of choice in critically ill patients given its minimal impact on the cardiovascular system.
- Etomidate itself induces minimal changes in heart rate and blood pressure, but the PG vehicle within the etomidate solution may be associated with arrhythmias, including bradycardia, ventricular premature contractions, and cardiac arrest, especially when a large amount of PG is administered IV at a relatively fast rate.
- Caution must be used when administering etomidate-PG to large dogs (>13.6 kg [30 lb]), as the low drug concentration (2 mg/ml) requires a large injection volume (the induction dose without premedication is 1–2 mg/kg IM).
- A large amount of PG causes excessive hyperosmolality of the blood (4,965 mOsm/kg, which is 16 times greater than blood osmolality), leading to hemolysis (**Fig. 4.10**) and hematuria soon after induction. The owner and veterinarian should monitor for hematuria post induction with etomidate.
- Etomidate given by CRI over a period of time is likely to reduce the PCV, which may be problematic in anemic dogs and cats.
- Use of the PG-free etomidate formulation is recommended.
- Respiratory depression associated with etomidate is similar to that seen with thiopentone, propofol, and alfaxalone. It can induce apnea and hypoventilation in dogs and cats at clinical doses if it is administered too rapidly or overdosed.
- Etomidate has an adrenocortical suppressive effect, which inhibits the stress response and induces immunosuppression for 1–2 weeks.
- Other disadvantages of etomidate include pain on injection, myoclonus, retching, and vomiting during or soon after induction in non-premedicated animals. The myoclonus and muscle twitching can

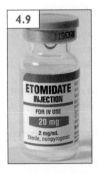

Fig. 4.9 Etomidate in a 35% propylene glycol solution.

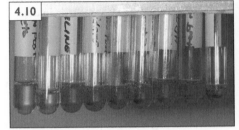

Fig. 4.10 Plasma collected before and after etomidate constant rate of infusion over a 1 hour period in a dog. Note the progressive increase (from left to right) in hemolysis over time from plasma samples.

be easily confused with a light plane of anesthesia. It is vital to differentiate these two situations carefully.

- Administering midazolam (0.2–0.4 mg/kg IV) 30 seconds to 1 minute prior to etomidate induction reduces the likelihood of the retching and muscle twitching associated with etomidate use alone. However, if the animal has been given a sedative or opioid as premedication, administration of midazolam prior to etomidate is not needed to avoid such side-effects.
- Etomidate is relatively expensive. The low concentration of the commercially available product (2 mg/ml) and the high induction dose (2 mg/kg in non-premedicated animals) make it a less desirable option than some of the other IV anesthetic agents.

ALFAXALONE
Overview

- Alfaxalone (3-alpha-hydroxy-5-alpha-pregnane-11,20-dione) is a neuroactive steroidal molecule with the properties of a general anesthetic agent. It is used for IV induction and maintenance of general anesthesia in dogs and cats.
- It is commercially available as a clear, aqueous, 10 mg/ml solution (**Fig. 4.11**). The alfaxalone molecule is solubilized using 2-alpha-hydroxypropyl beta cyclodextrin (HPBCD). HPBCD does not cause histamine release in dogs and cats.
- Alfaxalone induces anesthesia by modulating neuronal cell membrane chloride ion transport through the binding of alfaxalone to gamma-aminobutyric acid$_A$ (GABA$_A$) cell surface receptors.
- Alfaxalone can be administered as a single bolus for anesthetic induction, as repeated intermittent boluses, or by CRI for TIVA.

Induction and maintenance using alfaxalone

- The anesthetic induction doses of alfaxalone are:
  - Dogs: non-premedicated 3 mg/kg; premedicated 2 mg/kg.
  - Cats: non-premedicated 5 mg/kg; premedicated 4 mg/kg.

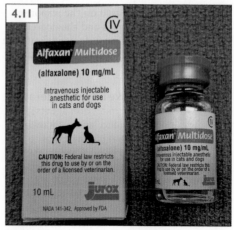

Fig. 4.11 Alfaxalone is a controlled (category IV) substance in the USA. Currently there are two formulations available. The picture shown here is a multidose formulation that allows 28 days of use after broaching. The other formulation only allows 6 hours of use after broaching.

- Premedication with drugs such as acepromazine, azaperone, alpha-2 agonists (medetomidine or dexmedetomidine), diazepam or midazolam, and opioids reduces the induction dose of alfaxalone.
- Alfaxalone should be administered slowly to effect over a period of 60 seconds with one-quarter of the total dose administered in each 15 seconds until endotracheal intubation is achieved.
- Alfaxalone CRI doses in dogs and cats are:
  - Dogs: non-premedicated 0.13–0.15 mg/kg; premedicated 0.1–0.12 mg/kg.
  - Cats: non-premedicated 0.16–0.18 mg/kg; premedicated 0.11–0.13 mg/kg.
- Alfaxalone dosages in dogs and cats for intermittent bolus administration following alfaxalone induction for every 10 minutes of maintenance anesthesia are:
  - Dogs: non-premedicated 1.3–1.5 mg/kg; premedicated 1–1.2 mg/kg.
  - Cats: non-premedicated 1.6–1.8 mg/kg; premedicated 1.1–1.3 mg/kg.

- Doses will vary based on the response of individual animals and the degree of stimulation. Clinical judgment should be exercised carefully and doses calculated accordingly.

Other factors to take into consideration

- As with other IV induction agents, alfaxalone may induce apnea following rapid induction and endotracheal intubation and oxygen supplementation with assisted ventilation should be instituted in these cases.
- Alfaxalone has a vasodilatory effect (although less than that of propofol) and so should be used with caution in hypotensive animals or those in shock.
- Heart rate usually increases after alfaxalone administration.
- Alfaxalone has a minimal analgesic effect.
- Alfaxalone has a relatively short plasma elimination half-life of 25 minutes using a 2 mg/kg dose in dogs and 45 minutes using a 5 mg/kg dose in cats.
- Alfaxalone does not accumulate and recovery is not prolonged. Alfaxalone can be considered an alternative anesthetic for injectable anesthesia maintenance, either through intermittent boluses or CRI, for procedures lasting up to 1 hour, without risk of drug accumulation and prolonged recovery.
- A small percentage of dogs and cats given alfaxalone may experience delirium, excitement, or a rough recovery. Recovering animals should be monitored closely.
- Alfaxalone, unlike propofol, can be given IM and is capable of inducing a sedative effect in dogs and cats.
  - The significant advantage of using alfaxalone with IM route as part of the sedative protocol is because it adds sedative effect without adding cardiorespiratory depression to the existing protocols.
  - On its own, alfaxalone's sedative effect is mild and its sedative quality is relatively poor.
  - The poor sedative quality is characterized by noise irritation, sensitivity to touch, and the animals maintaining their body position with slight head pressure. The quality of recovery is also poor, with tremors and vocalization.
- When alfaxalone (1–2 mg/kg IM) is combined with other sedatives (see Chapter 3) such as midazolam, dexmedetomidine, acepromazine or azaperone, the degree of sedation and recovery quality are significantly improved.
- Alfaxalone can be used with these sedatives with or without an addition of an opioid (butorphanol, buprenorphine, hydromorphone, or methadone) to enhance its sedative and analgesic qualities.
- In addition to combination with sedatives, and/or opioids, a small dose of ketamine (1–2 mg/kg) can be added as part of the IM administration to induce anesthesia.
- The use of IM alfaxalone is described in other chapters (see Chapters 10 and 17).

DIAZEPAM (MIDAZOLAM)/KETAMINE
Overview

- For many years, diazepam (midazolam) and ketamine (see **Figs. 3.3, 3.4,** and **3.10**) have been used in combination for IV induction of anesthesia in dogs and cats.

Induction and short-term immobilization using diazepam (midazolam)/ketamine

- The ratio of diazepam (midazolam) (5 mg/ml) to ketamine (100 mg/ml) used is 1:1 (volume to volume), administered IV at a dose of 1 ml/9 kg (20 lb) in both dogs and cats. This equates to diazepam (midazolam) at 0.28 mg/kg and ketamine at 5.6 mg/kg, combined in the same syringe.
- This combination allows dogs and cats to be induced and intubated within 1–2 minutes and it will provide short-term immobilization (8–10 minutes). The jaw tone and swallowing reflex of a dog or cat following diazepam (midazolam)/ketamine induction is stronger than that seen with propofol, thiopentone, etomidate, or alfaxalone induction.

Other factors to take into consideration

- While diazepam (midazolam)/ketamine use is a popular combination, it presents several potential challenges.
- Ketamine induces tachycardia (transient tachycardia of up to 220 beats per minute may be seen) shortly after induction with diazepam (midazolam)/ketamine.
- Ketamine is associated with rough recoveries in dogs receiving a short (<30 minutes) period of inhalant anesthetic maintenance. These rough recoveries are characterized by head shaking, salivation, and occasional vocalization and are caused by the slow metabolism of ketamine in dogs. Cats tolerate ketamine better than dogs, so this is not a clinical problem in cats.
- Ketamine is primarily metabolized through the liver before being excreted by the kidneys. This is a slow process. Dogs metabolize diazepam (midazolam) quickly with the result that dogs removed from inhalant anesthetic maintenance within 30 minutes of a diazepam (midazolam)/ketamine induction will have metabolized the diazepam (midazolam). The muscle relaxation associated with the inhalant is lost when inhalant anesthesia is terminated. The remaining ketamine dominates, causing the rough recovery.
- To avoid the ketamine hangover associated with a short duration of inhalant anesthesia, the ratio of diazepam (midazolam) to ketamine in the diazepam (midazolam)/ketamine combination can be modified from 1:1 (volume to volume) to 3:1 or 4:1 (i.e. 0.75 ml of diazepam (midazolam) and 0.25 ml of ketamine or 1 ml of diazepam (midazolam) and 0.25 ml of ketamine for a 9 kg [20 lb] dog) to enhance muscle relaxation and reduce the total amount of ketamine used (see *Table 4.3*).
- A microdose of medetomidine (5 µg/kg IV) or dexmedetomidine (2.5 µg/kg IV) administered with the 1:1 diazepam (midazolam)/ketamine combination minimizes the signs of ketamine hangover in dogs, inducing a better quality immobilization and a more relaxed muscle tone, including jaw tone.

Table 4.3 Different diazepam (midazolam)/ketamine mixture ratios for avoiding ketamine hangover (or carry-over) activity during recovery

Mixture ratio	Diazepam (midazolam) (5 mg/ml)	Ketamine (100 mg/ml)	Total intravenous volume (for a 9 kg [20 lb] dog)
1:1	0.5 ml	0.5 ml	1 ml
3:1	0.75 ml	0.25 ml	1 ml
4:1	1.00 ml	0.25 ml	1.25 ml

Tiletamine/zolazepam

OVERVIEW

- In the USA, tiletamine/zolazepam is sold under the trade name Telazol® (**Fig. 3.11**). In other countries it is sold as Zoletil® (approved for use in dogs and cats in the USA in 2017) and is available in two concentrations: 50 mg/ml after reconstitution and 100 mg/ml after reconstitution. The drug is not available in the UK and Canada.
- Tiletamine/zolazepam (100 mg/ml) is a 1:1 (weight to weight) combination of tiletamine (50 mg), a dissociative anesthetic, and zolazepam (50 mg), a benzodiazepine sedative and muscle relaxant.
- This combination is a rapid-acting injectable anesthetic for IV or IM use in dogs and cats. Immediate recumbency (<90 seconds) can be achieved following IV administration. A single induction dose of tiletamine/zolazepam does not result in a prolonged recovery. Tiletamine/zolazepam can also be administered IM for anesthetic induction and endotracheal intubation within 3–6 minutes (also see Chapter 9). Higher doses (single bolus or cumulative dose of >10–14 mg/kg) of tiletamine/zolazepam IV or IM have the potential to cause a prolonged recovery.

- Tiletamine/zolazepam is a versatile drug that can be used for sedation, induction, and TIVA. The anesthetic effects of tiletamine/zolazepam are dose dependent.
- In dogs, tiletamine/zolazepam is indicated for restraint and minor procedures requiring mild to moderate analgesia (e.g. radiography, orthopedic examination, dental treatment, laceration repair, draining an abscess, and wound debridement) of approximately 30 minutes duration.
- In cats, tiletamine/zolazepam is indicated for restraint or for anesthesia combined with muscle relaxation.
- Tiletamine/zolazepam can also be used for allergy skin testing and skin biopsy in dogs and cats because it does not induce histamine release and does not affect the results of allergy skin testing. In contrast to tiletamine/zolazepam, opioids, propofol, diazepam/ketamine, and many other IV drugs (except alpha-2 agonists), all induce either false-positive or false-negative effects on the allergy skin test.
- Tiletamine/zolazepam is compatible with many other anesthetic and analgesic agents. It is commonly combined with opioids (butorphanol, morphine, hydromorphone, buprenorphine) and other analgesics to produce profound analgesia for more painful surgical procedures.

INDUCTION AND IMMOBILIZATION
- Tiletamine/zolazepam alone can be used for anesthetic induction in dogs and cats followed by inhalant anesthetic maintenance with isoflurane or sevoflurane.
- Alternatively, a patient premedicated with acepromazine, xylazine, medetomidine, or dexmedetomidine, with or without opioids, can be induced with tiletamine/zolazepam IV for endotracheal intubation and maintained on an inhalant anesthetic agent. The IV induction dose of tiletamine/zolazepam in dogs and cats is 1–2 mg/kg in the premedicated animal and 2.2–4.4 mg/kg in the non-premedicated animal.

- IV use of tiletamine/zolazepam has recently been approved by the FDA as an IV induction agent in dogs. It has been employed by many practitioners as an alternative IV induction agent, especially when IV drugs, such as propofol, are not available. The main advantage of using tiletamine/zolazepam for IV induction is the small volume of drug required when compared with the diazepam (midazolam)/ketamine combination.
- Aggressive dogs or fractious cats can be rapidly immobilized or anesthetized following IM administration of tiletamine/zolazepam. A small volume of tiletamine/zolazepam IM eases the handling of the animals. The immobilization/anesthetic induction dose for dogs is 6–9 mg/kg IM and for cats it is 9–11 mg/kg IM (see also Chapter 3).

Other factors to take into consideration
- Unlike alpha-2 sedatives, tiletamine/zolazepam cannot be completely reversed with an antagonist (see later). Tiletamine/zolazepam does not constrict the blood vessels and greatly facilitates venous access for blood sampling, IV catheterization, or IV drug administration.
- As tiletamine/zolazepam is mainly metabolized by the liver and excreted by the kidneys, it is contraindicated in patients with significant liver dysfunction or renal impairment. It should not be used in dogs and cats with severe cardiac or pulmonary dysfunction and, because tiletamine/zolazepam crosses the placental barrier and produces respiratory depression in the newborn, it is also contraindicated for cesarean section.
- Dogs and cats metabolize tiletamine/zolazepam differently. Dogs metabolize tiletamine slowly. In addition, dogs metabolize zolazepam more rapidly than tiletamine. This allows tiletamine to dominate during the recovery phase and induce a typical dissociative recovery. This accounts for some of the rough recoveries, characterized by the salivation, vocalization, head shaking, muscle rigidity, and tremors seen in some dogs. If this occurs, clinical signs can be alleviated by administering diazepam

(midazolam) (0.2–0.4 mg/kg IM or IV) or medetomidine/dexmedetomidine (1–5 µg/kg IV or IM). In contrast to dogs, cats metabolize tiletamine more rapidly but metabolize zolazepam much more slowly. This accounts for the prolonged recovery following tiletamine/zolazepam administration. Although there is a specific zolazepam antagonist available (flumazenil), it is expensive and

it is not to practicable to keep this drug only for this purpose. The best way to avoid a prolonged recovery in cats is to use a smaller dose or to combine tiletamine/zolazepam with another anesthetic agent (e.g. opioid or alpha-2 agonist) to produce a tiletamine/zolazepam sparing effect.
- The use of tiletamine/zolazepam in combination with other drugs for injectable anesthesia is described in Chapter 31.

Further reading

Chiu KW, Robson S, Devi JL et al. (2016) The cardiopulmonary effects and quality of anesthesia after induction with alfaxalone in 2-hydroxypropyl-β-cyclodextrin in dogs and cats: a systematic review. *J Vet Pharmacol Ther* 39(6):525–38.

Covey-Crump GL, Murison PJ (2008) Fentanyl or midazolam for co-induction of anaesthesia with propofol in dogs. *Vet Anaesth Analg* 35:463–72.

Dodam JR, Kruse-Elliott KT, Aucoin DP et al. (1990) Duration of etomidate-induced adrenocortical suppression during surgery in dogs. *Am J Vet Res* 51:786–8.

Hatch RC, Clark JD, Jerigan AD et al. (1988) Searching for a safe, effective antagonist to Telazol® overdose. *Vet Med* 83:112–17.

Jackson AM, Tobias K, Long C et al. (2004) Effects of various anesthetic agents on laryngeal motion during laryngoscopy in normal dogs. *Vet Surg* 33:102–6.

Joubert KE, Picard J, Sethusa M (2005) Inhibition of bacterial growth by different mixtures of propofol and thiopentone. *J S Afr Vet Assoc* 76:85–9.

Ko JC, Nicklin CF, Melendaz M et al. (1998) Effect of micro-dose medetomidine on diazepam-ketamine induced anesthesia in dogs. *J Am Vet Med Assoc* 213(2):215–19.

Ko JC, Payton ME, White AG et al. (2006) Effects of intravenous diazepam or micro-dose medetomidine on propofol-induced sedation in dogs. *J Am Anim Hosp Assoc* 42:18–27.

Ko JC, Thurmon JC, Benson GJ (1993) Acute haemolysis associated with

etomidate-propylene glycol infusion in dogs. *Vet Anaesth Analg* 20:92–4.

Ko JC, Thurmon JC, Benson GJ et al. (1994) Hemodynamic and anesthetic effects of etomidate infusion in medetomidine-premedicated dogs. *Am J Vet Res* 55:842–6.

Luna SP, Cassu RN, Castro GB et al. (2004) Effects of four anesthetic protocols on the neurological and cardiorespiratory variables of puppies born by caesarean section. *Vet Rec* 154:387–9.

McKeirnan KL, Gross ME, Rochat M et al. (2014) Comparison of propofol and propofol/ketamine anesthesia for evaluation of laryngeal function in healthy dogs. *J Am Anim Hosp Assoc* 50(1):19–26.

Muir WW 3rd, Mason DE (1989) Side effects of etomidate in dogs. *J Am Vet Med Assoc* 194:1430–4.

O'Brien RT, Waller KR 3rd, Osgood TL (2004) Sonographic features of drug-induced splenic congestion. *Vet Radiol Ultrasound* 45:225–7.

Rawlings CA, Kolata RJ (1983) Cardiopulmonary effects of thiopental/lidocaine combination during anesthetic induction in the dog. *Am J Vet Res* 44:144–9.

Smalle TM, Hartman MJ, Bester L et al. (2017) Effects of thiopentone, propofol and alfaxalone on laryngeal motion during oral laryngoscopy in healthy dogs. *Vet Anaesth Analg* 44(3):427–34.

Thurmon JC, Ko JC, Benson GJ et al. (1994) Hemodynamic and analgesic effects of propofol infusion in medetomidine-premedicated dogs. *Am J Vet Res* 55:363–7.

Tracy CH, Short CE, Clark BC (1988) Comparing the effects of intravenous and intramuscular administration of Telazol®. *Vet Med* **83**:104–11.

Walder B, Tramèr MR, Seeck M (2002) Seizure-like phenomena and propofol: a systemic review. *Neurology* **58:** 1327–32.

Warne LN, Beths T, Whittem T *et al.* (2015) A review of the pharmacology and clinical application of alfaxalone in cats. *Vet J* **203(2):**141–8.

Wilson DV, Evans AT, Carpenter RA *et al.* (2004) The effect of four anesthetic protocols on splenic size in dogs. *Vet Anaesth Analg* **31:**102–8.

Inhalant anesthetic agents

Jeff C Ko

Introduction

Following preanesthetic medication and IV induction, the general anesthetic procedure enters the maintenance stage. Although injectable anesthesia is sometimes employed to maintain anesthesia, inhalant anesthesia is more commonly used, especially when a long duration (≥1 hour) of anesthesia is needed.

There are substantial differences between inhalant and injectable anesthesia maintenance. Inhalant anesthesia provides many advantages over injectable anesthesia. The pros and cons of inhalant and injectable anesthesia maintenance are listed in *Table 5.1.*

Inhalant anesthetic agents currently available for veterinary use are limited to isoflurane, sevoflurane, and desflurane (**Fig. 5.1**). Halothane has been discontinued in many parts of the world. Isoflurane is currently the main inhalant anesthetic agent on the veterinary market. Sevoflurane is also available for veterinary use. There are some potential advantages to using sevoflurane, but it is approximately 7–8 times more expensive than isoflurane, which limits its use. Desflurane is principally used in human anesthesia, but its advantages and disadvantages will also be discussed.

Table 5.1 Pros and cons of inhalant and injectable anesthesia maintenance

Pros and cons	Inhalant anesthesia	Injectable anesthesia
Supplementation of enriched oxygen	Definitely occurs because oxygen is frequently used as an inhalant anesthetic agent carrier	Additional step has to be taken to provide oxygen supplementation
Patient airway protection	Likely to occur because endotracheal intubation is part of the procedure, although face mask induction is sometimes used	Additional step has to be taken to intubate the animal in order to protect the airway

(Continued)

Table 5.1 (Continued) Pros and cons of inhalant and injectable anesthesia maintenance

Pros and cons	Inhalant anesthesia	Injectable anesthesia
Method of providing assisted or controlled ventilation	Anesthesia machine with a breathing circuit provides a method to assist or control ventilation of the anesthetized animal	Additional step has to be taken to use the anesthesia machine with a breathing circuit or Ambu bag to assist or control ventilation
Titration for depth of anesthesia	Easily adjustable	Difficult to adjust if administered via IM route or as an IV bolus
Duration of anesthesia	Accommodates long duration of anesthesia with minimal increase in metabolic burden	Limited to 1–2 hour duration due to significant increase in metabolic burden
Drug metabolism	Mainly eliminated through lungs via respiration and minimal burden on the liver and kidneys	Dependent on the liver and kidneys for excretion
Recovery speed	Relatively rapid	The longer the injectable anesthetic is used, the longer the recovery duration due to drug accumulation
Equipment and cost	Bulky and complex anesthesia machines and breathing circuits are required	Minimal equipment, such as needles and syringes
Pollution to operation environment	Waste gas management needed	Minimal pollution

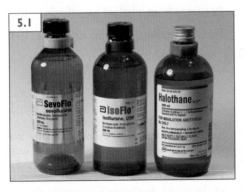

5.1

Fig. 5.1 Halothane (right, coded red) is no longer commercially available in most parts of the world. Isoflurane (middle, coded purple) is available in both the human and veterinary markets. It is available commercially in 100 ml or 250 ml packages. Each ml of isoflurane is vaporized into approximately 194 ml of isoflurane vapor at room temperature. Sevoflurane (left, coded yellow) is available only in a 250 ml plastic bottle for veterinary use. Each ml of sevoflurane vaporizes to approximately 182 ml of sevoflurane vapor at room temperature.

Uptake and distribution of inhalant anesthetic agents

A knowledge of how inhalant anesthetic agents are taken up and distributed is important in understanding the induction process and recovery from inhalant anesthesia. The process of uptake and distribution (i.e. the passage of the agent from the anesthesia machine to the animal's brain, **Fig. 5.2**) is described below:

- Oxygen from either the oxygen tank or pipeline source passes through the flowmeter. It carries the inhalant anesthetic vapor through the vaporizer and into the anesthesia machine conduit and the breathing circuit. The anesthetic vapor then passes into the endotracheal tube and the patient's airway, where it crosses the alveoli wall and enters the blood stream. Cardiac output delivers the anesthetic gas to all the body compartments or tissues, including the brain.
- The inhalant anesthetic agent is dissolved in various body tissues (compartments) including:
  - Vessel-rich tissues: brain, heart, lungs, liver, kidneys, and spleen, which receive a majority of the blood supply and, therefore, play a vital role in uptake, distribution, and elimination of the inhalant anesthetic agent.
  - Muscles.
  - Fat.

Fig. 5.2 The pathway of inhalant anesthetic agent from the anesthesia machine to the animal's brain with waste gas eliminated to the scavenging system. Oxygen from the pipeline or oxygen tank (1) passes through the oxygen flowmeter (2) into the isoflurane vaporizer (3) and carries isoflurane vapor based on the vaporizer dial concentration to the rebreathing circuit (4) with the CO_2 absorbent, reservoir bag, and breathing hose (5) before entering the endotracheal tube (6) and the lungs (7) where it is absorbed into the blood and eventually reaches the brain of the anesthetized dog. The unused isoflurane, oxygen, and CO_2 are vented back through the expiratory limb of the breathing hose (8) and enter the reservoir bag (9). Waste gas is eliminated through the scavenger (10), while CO_2 is removed by the CO_2 absorbent.

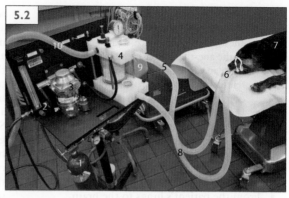

- Vessel-poor tissues (bones, cartilages, tendons, hairs). The fat and the vessel-poor tissues play a very small role in the uptake and distribution of an inhalant anesthetic agent.
- The goal of uptake inhalant anesthesia is to equilibrate the vaporizer anesthetic concentration to the alveolar anesthetic concentration, then the arterial blood anesthetic concentration, and, ultimately, the brain anesthetic concentration.

STAGE OF ANESTHESIA

- The level of anesthetic concentration induces the following stages of anesthesia within the CNS as the inhalant passes from the airway to the lungs and, eventually, to the brain:
  - Mild depression (sedation).
  - Involuntary excitement (including paddling, vocalization, muscle rigidity, defecation, and salivation).
  - Loss of consciousness (early stages of a light plane anesthesia).
  - Surgical plane of anesthesia.
  - Severe cardiorespiratory depression (deep plane of anesthesia).
- If the anesthetic plane is too deep (i.e. the anesthetic concentration is too high) for too long, the patient may die from low blood pressure, bradycardia, and apnea due to severe depression of the cardiorespiratory center of the brain and poor tissue perfusion.

- The most important concept is the recognition of the dose-dependent depression relationship of alveolar anesthetic concentration to the anesthetic concentration in the brain and other vital organs.
- The alveolar anesthetic concentration is a close approximation to the brain anesthetic concentration when they equilibrate.

ANESTHETIC PARTIAL-PRESSURE GRADIENT: INDUCTION PHASE

- The anesthetic partial-pressure gradient or partial-pressure difference varies from the outside environment to inside the patient and is determined by several factors during the equilibration process.
- From the anesthetic machine and breathing circuit to the patient's lungs, the anesthetic partial pressure is determined by:
  - Vaporizer percentage.
  - Oxygen inflow rate.
  - Total space volume or volume barrier of the rebreathing or non-rebreathing circuit, including the size of reservoir bag, double or single CO_2 canister, pediatric or adult sized hoses, and the patient's breathing.
- In general, the higher the vaporizer percentage, the higher the oxygen flow rate, the smaller the total space volume of the breathing circuit, the higher the respiratory rate, and the larger the respiratory tidal-volume, the more rapid the increase in the anesthetic partial pressure in the patient's lungs.

- To bring about a smooth transition from IV induction of anesthesia to inhalant anesthetic maintenance, a rapid change in the anesthetic agent concentration in an anesthetic machine with a rebreathing circuit is required. Ways of doing this are detailed in *Table 5.2*.
- If a non-breathing circuit is used, the oxygen flow rate is already high and the volume barrier is small (*Table 5.3*), therefore there is no need to increase the oxygen flow rate soon after IV anesthetic induction.
- From the patient's lungs to the brain, the anesthetic partial pressure is determined by:
  - The blood gas solubility of the agent (see Blood gas solubility).
  - The alveolar to arterial–venous anesthetic partial-pressure difference.
  - The patient's cardiac output.
  - A lower blood gas solubility inhalant (for example, sevoflurane) promotes the rapid increase of the partial pressure of sevoflurane gas concentrations in the lung and facilitate the equilibration of sevoflurane concentration between the lungs and the brain tissue, therefore, inducing a faster anesthesia induction and faster depth changes in the animals. Similarly, a debilitated animal with a low cardiac output (hence with a low pulmonary blood circulation),

results in a slow uptake of an inhalant anesthetic from the lung. This slow uptake resulted in a more rapid rise of an inhalant alveolar partial pressure in the lungs and since a greater proportion of the blood is supply to the brain than other body tissues, the induction of anesthesia is more rapid.

- Sevoflurane has a lower blood gas solubility than isoflurane and halothane, therefore sevoflurane concentrations increase more rapidly than isoflurane and halothane when other parameters are equal. Desflurane has the lowest blood gas solubility and the concentration of desflurane rises more rapidly than sevoflurane due to its lower blood gas solubility.

ANESTHETIC PARTIAL-PRESSURE GRADIENT: RECOVERY PHASE

- The recovery phase of anesthesia is the uptake and distribution of the inhalant anesthetic agent in reverse, such that the anesthetic flows from the patient's brain (and other vessel-rich compartments) to the lungs and out to the breathing circuit, eventually being eliminated from the scavenger system into the atmosphere.
- When the vaporizer is turned off, the anesthetic concentration gradient moves from the animal's brain (and other vessel-rich compartments) to the lungs

Table 5.2 Stepwise method of changing anesthetic concentrations within an anesthesia machine with a rebreathing circuit by adjusting the vaporizer volume % setting and oxygen flow rate over time

Vaporizer volume % immediately setting after IV induction	Oxygen flow rate (liters per minute)	Duration (minutes)
Isoflurane: 3% Sevoflurane: 5%	3	3
Isoflurane: 2% Sevoflurane: 4%	2	2
Isoflurane: 1% Sevoflurane: 3%	1	1
Maintenance to effect based on the depth of anesthesia required	0.5–1.0	To the end of the procedure unless the animal is awakening prematurely

Table 5.3 Volume barriers that slow down inhalant anesthetic concentration changes

	Mechanical volume barrier	Physiological volume barrier
Location	From the vaporizer to the animal's airway	From the animal's airway to its brain
Examples of barriers	Anesthetic breathing hoses, reservoir bag, CO_2 absorbents, face mask, endotracheal tube	The anatomic space from the trachea to the lungs, and the total blood volume

and the breathing circuit and exits via the scavenging system of the anesthesia machine.

- If a high oxygen flow rate is used to wash out the inhalant anesthetic within the machine and breathing circuit, the patient will recover faster due to the rapid decrease in the anesthetic partial pressure within the machine and breathing circuit and, therefore, the brain (and other vessel-rich) tissues.

TYPES OF VOLUME BARRIERS

- There are two kinds of volume barriers: mechanical and physiologic (*Table 5.3*):
  - The mechanical volume barrier applies to the barrier (obstacle volume space) between the vaporizer and the animal's airway for induction. The mechanical volume barrier includes the CO_2 absorbent and its canister (3–5 liters in volume), the hose (1 liter in volume), the rebreathing bag (reservoir bag: depends on size, but can be up to 3–5 liters in volume), and the face mask (0.5–1.0 liter in volume). This volume can be as much as 7–10 liters (**Fig. 5.3**). For these volumes to equilibrate with the partial pressure

of the inhalant agent (isoflurane or sevoflurane) will take time.

- The physiologic volume barrier applies to the anatomic space between the upper airway of the patient and the lungs and then from the lungs (via the blood) to the brain (i.e. the path the inhalant anesthetic agent travels from the nose to the brain).
- A smaller volume barrier allows the anesthetic concentration to build up relatively quickly, increasing alveolar ventilation and facilitating nitrogen washout from the patient's physiologic volume barrier. Certain techniques can minimize the volume barrier and facilitate the wash-in of the inhalant anesthetic and the washout of nitrogen (**Fig. 5.4**). The physiologic volume barrier cannot be physically changed, but it can be manipulated to facilitate delivery of the inhalant to the brain.

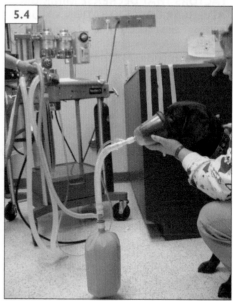

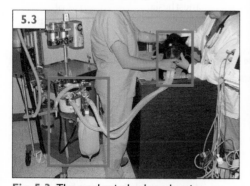

Fig. 5.3 The mechanical volume barrier includes the size of CO_2 absorbent, the space volume of the breathing hose, the volume of the reservoir bag (large green outlined box), and the size of the face mask (small green outlined box). Note the large (3 liters) reservoir (rebreathing) bag used on this small sized dog for face mask induction. This significantly increases the mechanical volume barrier between the vaporizer and the dog's airway. A smaller reservoir bag (1 liter/13.6 kg [30 lb] body weight) should have been used in this case.

Fig. 5.4 A non-rebreathing circuit (modified Jackson Rees) can be used for face mask induction of animals of all sizes. This drastically reduces the time from onset of induction to endotracheal intubation. The transparent oxygen hose only measures 15 ml in volume. The volume barrier of the 3 liter reservoir bag used in this large dog (31.8 kg [70 lb]) is still smaller than that of the entire rebreathing circuit for face mask induction.

Minimum alveolar concentration

- Minimum alveolar concentration (MAC) refers to the amount of anesthetic gas at 1 atmosphere that produces no gross purposeful movements in 50% of the animals subjected to supramaximal noxious stimulus (e.g. a skin incision or tail clamping). MAC is a measure of inhalant anesthetic potency. The lower the MAC, the more potent the inhalant agent. For example, halothane is more potent than isoflurane, and isoflurane is more potent than sevoflurane (*Table 5.4*).
- The surgical plane of anesthesia is 1.5–2 times the MAC of any inhalant anesthetic agent. Several factors influence the anesthetic concentration required to maintain an animal with inhalant anesthesia (see below).

FACTORS THAT DECREASE MINIMUM ALVEOLAR CONCENTRATION VALUES
- Dogs and cats with the conditions listed below require a lower anesthetic concentration (MAC) than normal to maintain general anesthesia using an inhalant anesthetic agent:
  - Hypothermia.
  - Metabolic acidosis.

- Severe hypotension.
- Severe hypoxia (PaO_2 <38 mmHg).
- Age (older animals require less anesthetic).
- Premedication with a sedative or tranquilizer, including opioids, alpha-2 agonists, or acepromazine.
- Local anesthetics.
- Pregnancy.
- Nitrous oxide.

FACTORS THAT INCREASES MINIMUM ALVEOLAR CONCENTRATION VALUES
- Dogs and cats with the conditions listed below require a higher anesthetic concentration (MAC) than normal to maintain inhalant anesthesia:
  - Hyperthermia.
  - Hypernatremia.

FACTORS THAT DO NOT AFFECT MINIMUM ALVEOLAR CONCENTRATION VALUES
- Factors that do not affect MAC include:
  - Metabolic alkalosis.
  - Hypertension.
  - The type of stimulation or duration of anesthesia.
  - Plasma potassium concentrations.

Table 5.4 Minimum alveolar concentration (volume %) for inhalant anesthetic agent used in dogs and cats

	Halothane	Isoflurane	Sevoflurane	Desflurane	Nitrous oxide
Dogs	0.87	1.28	2.1	7.2	188–297
Cats	1.14	1.63	2.58	9.8	255

Blood gas solubility

- The blood gas solubility (or partition coefficient) of an inhalant anesthetic agent dictates the speed at which it is absorbed into the animal's body compartments or tissues. A low blood gas solubility of an inhalant anesthetic agent achieves:
  - Unconsciousness more rapidly when inducing anesthesia via a face mask or an induction chamber.

- A more rapid change in the depth of anesthesia during anesthesia maintenance.
- A rapid recovery following anesthesia.
- The blood gas solubility of the various inhalant anesthetic agents are as follows:
  - Desflurane: 0.49.
  - Sevoflurane: 0.62.
  - Isoflurane: 1.27.
  - Halothane: 2.46.

- This suggests that when using desflurane, changes in anesthetic depth will be more rapid than with sevoflurane, isoflurane, or halothane, and the changes in anesthetic depth with sevoflurane will be more rapid than with isoflurane and halothane.

Pungency and airway irritation

- Pungency and airway irritation cause physical fighting and breath holding during face mask or chamber induction. Pungency and airway irritation also result in laryngeal spasm, salivation, and increased airway secretions.
- Pungency and airway irritation also impair alveolar ventilation and induce coughing, thus decreasing the anesthetic gas concentration in the lungs and causing a rough induction.

- Halothane and isoflurane are more pungent than sevoflurane and therefore tend to induce more breath holding than sevoflurane. Desflurane is more irritating to the airway than isoflurane or sevoflurane. As a result, induction of anesthesia using desflurane frequently induces coughing and is not practical for face mask or chamber induction in veterinary patients, despite its low blood gas solubility.

Isoflurane, sevoflurane, and desflurane

A summary of the properties of the modern inhalant anesthetic agents can be found in *Table 5.5*.

ISOFLURANE
- Does not contain preservatives.
- Is not broken down by sunlight.
- Has a pungent odor and tends to cause breath holding in non-premedicated animals.
- Depresses cardiovascular (reduction in cardiac output and induces vasodilation) and respiratory (reduces respiratory rate and tidal volume) functions in a dose-dependent manner.
- Is less arrhythmogenic than halothane.
- Is minimally metabolized (<1%) and thus alleviates the burden of hepatic metabolism.
- Is generally approximately 7–8 times cheaper than sevoflurane.
- The close similarity in vapor pressure between halothane and isoflurane

allows isoflurane to be administered in a halothane vaporizer once the halothane preservative (thymal) has been properly cleaned from the vaporizer.

SEVOFLURANE
- Has a lower blood gas solubility than isoflurane, resulting in a faster induction of anesthesia, changes in depth of anesthesia, and recovery from anesthesia.
- Is slightly less depressive on ventilation than isoflurane.
- The anesthetic index is the apneic inhalant anesthetic concentration divided by the MAC. The anesthetic index of sevoflurane in dogs is 3.45, while the index of isoflurane in dogs is 2.61. This indicates that sevoflurane is less likely to inhibit respiratory function than isoflurane at equal anesthetic concentrations.

Table 5.5 Properties of modern inhalant anesthetic agents

Property	Halothane	Isoflurane	Sevoflurane	Desflurane
Vapor pressure (mmHg) at room temperature (20°C [68°F])	244	240	170	681
Milliliters of vapor per ml of liquid at room temperature	227	194.7	182.7	209.7
Maximal vapor concentration (%) at sea level	32	32	22	89.6

- Has similar cardiovascular side-effects to isoflurane; both inhalants cause dose-dependent cardiovascular depression.
- It is less potent than isoflurane and is minimally metabolized (<3%) by the liver and kidneys.
- More sevoflurane is required per unit of time to induce the same plane of anesthesia as isoflurane (i.e. more sevoflurane liquid than isoflurane liquid is used per unit of time).
- Sevoflurane is more expensive than isoflurane.
- It may react with desiccated soda lime, causing chemical instability and heat production.
- Must be used with a vaporizer designed specifically for sevoflurane.

DESFLURANE

- Desflurane has a very high vapor pressure and therefore requires a special temperature-controlled, pressurized vaporizer to deliver an accurate anesthetic concentration to the patient.
- The vaporizer (**Fig. 5.5**) must be plugged into an electrical outlet to supply exogenous heat during operation. This is not always practical in veterinary medicine.
- Desflurane is the least potent of the modern anesthetic gases (apart from

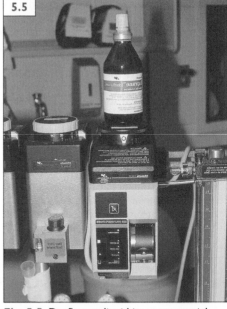

Fig. 5.5 Desflurane liquid in a commercial package with its vaporizer. Note that the desflurane vaporizer needs an external heat supply and therefore requires a power cord for an electric plug-in to provide heating.

nitrous oxide) with a MAC of 7.2% in dogs.
- It has similar cardiovascular side-effects to isoflurane.

Face mask and chamber induction with overpressurizing techniques

GENERAL PRINCIPLES

- Overpressurizing describes the delivery of a high anesthetic gas concentration in order to achieve a rapid change in anesthetic concentrations within a breathing circuit or induction chamber and, subsequently, a change in the anesthetic plane of the patient.
- To achieve overpressure and rapidly increase the anesthetic concentration, it is necessary to use a higher vaporizer concentration, to increase the oxygen flow rate, and to reduce the total volume barrier of the breathing circuit.
- Overpressurizing techniques should be used for face mask or chamber induction

or when a patient wakes up prematurely during surgery.

TECHNIQUE FOR FACE MASK INDUCTION

- A small reservoir bag (1 liter/13.6 kg [30 lb] body weight), an appropriately sized face mask, and a non-rebreathing circuit (e.g. a modified Jackson-Rees non-rebreathing circuit (**Fig. 5.6**) are required for face mask induction using overpressurizing (**Fig. 5.4**).
- A high oxygen flow rate (3–4 liters/ minute) is needed to denitrogenize the system during induction, especially if a rebreathing circuit (instead of a non-rebreathing circuit) is used.

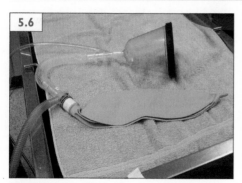

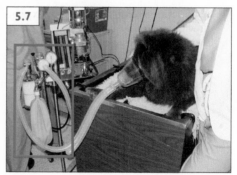

Fig. 5.6 A significant advantage to using a modified Jackson Rees non-rebreathing circuit is that the reservoir bag can be changed to any size without modifying the scavenging system. The scavenging system (blue tubing) and a valve are located proximal to the reservoir bag.

Fig. 5.7 A similar sized dog to the one shown in **Fig. 5.4** induced with isoflurane using a rebreathing circuit and face mask; this results in a slower induction time. This is due to a significantly larger mechanical volume barrier associated with a rebreathing circuit (green outlined box) than with a non-rebreathing circuit (7–10 liters versus 75 ml). This larger mechanical volume barrier requires more time for denitrogenation and equilibration of the anesthetic concentration.

- The highest vaporizer dial setting available (5% isoflurane, 8% sevoflurane) should be used to overpressurize the system (breathing circuit).
- A non-rebreathing circuit (**Fig. 5.4**) rather than a rebreathing circuit (**Fig. 5.7**) is used to reduce the total mechanical volume barrier of the breathing circuit and facilitate the speed of induction.
- After face mask induction with a non-rebreathing circuit, the animal is intubated and if the animal is heavier than 7.0–7.5 kg (15.4–16.5 lb), the non-rebreathing circuit should be changed to a rebreathing circuit for anesthesia maintenance. This allows a lower oxygen flow rate to be used for inhalant maintenance and is therefore more economical.
- If the animal is smaller than 7.0–7.5 kg (15.4–16.5 lb), the breathing circuit should not be changed; anesthesia should be maintained on the non-rebreathing circuit to minimize breathing resistance.
- Induction is achieved within 3 minutes using this method in non-premedicated dogs and cats. In premedicated animals, the time to induction is shorter.
- The animal is wrapped in a towel to effectively control its movement during induction.
- It is critical to monitor respiration during induction by watching the animal's chest

or the reservoir bag excursion on the non-rebreathing circuit.
- Initially, the animal may struggle for 3–10 seconds. When the animal is relaxed and breathing more regularly with a larger tidal volume, it is through the excitement phase and into a deeper plane of anesthesia. The toes should be finger pinched to assess the withdrawal response. If there is no response to the toe pinch, the jaw tone should be assessed for endotracheal intubation.
- Once larger animals (>7.5 kg [16.5 lb]) are connected to the breathing circuit, high oxygen flow rate (2–3 liters/minute) and vaporizer settings (isoflurane 3%, sevoflurane 4%) should be maintained in order to equilibrate the rebreathing circuit for about 3–5 minutes. If the vaporizer and oxygen flow are immediately reduced to maintenance levels, the animal is likely to wake prematurely.

TECHNIQUE FOR CHAMBER INDUCTION
- The chamber has a large space volume (e.g. a 10 gallon induction chamber has approximately 40 liters of space volume, see **Fig. 1.79**) that slows the change in

anesthetic concentration. A high oxygen flow rate (within vaporizer specification: usually <15 liters/minute) and a high vaporizer anesthetic concentration setting is necessary to maximize the speed of the change in anesthetic concentration within the chamber in order to anesthetize the animal with minimal excitement.

- A high oxygen flow rate (10–15 liters/minute) and the highest vaporizer anesthetic concentration setting should be used.
- An appropriately-sized chamber should be used. The larger the chamber, the slower the build up of inspired anesthetic concentration, which prolongs induction and results in extended rough struggling of the animal. See the important concept of chamber induction with time constant in Chapter 1.

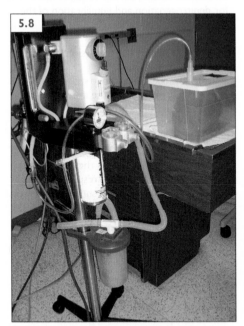

Fig. 5.8 The use of a single inflow induction chamber without an outlet significantly reduces the time for induction because the active scavenger system siphons the inhalant out of the chamber and prevents the build up of inhalant anesthetic within the chamber. Note that the outlet (scavenger port) of the chamber is blocked with a rubber cork (black color on the cover of the chamber).

- It is preferable to use a single inflow induction chamber without an outlet (**Fig. 5.8**).
- Some active scavenger systems attached to the chamber outlet siphon out the inhalant vapor more rapidly than the build up of inhalant anesthetic concentration within the chamber.
- The short duration of induction without an outflow will not drastically affect the CO_2 concentration within the induction chamber, but it will greatly facilitate induction speed. The CO_2 concentration within the chamber has only reached 45–50 mmHg by the time the anesthetic induces relaxation in the animal.
- Connecting the chamber to a rebreathing circuit for induction significantly increases the mechanical volume barrier and drastically slows the induction speed and results in a rough induction (**Fig. 5.9**).
- Chamber induction is used to induce profound sedation rather than achieve the depth of anesthesia required for endotracheal intubation. The animal should be removed from the chamber as soon as profound sedation is achieved (instead of waiting for a complete anesthetic induction) and a face mask used to complete the induction

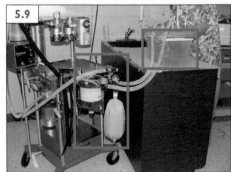

Fig. 5.9 Using an induction chamber with a rebreathing circuit significantly increases the duration of chamber induction. The mechanical volume barrier can reach 50 liters (40 liters of induction chamber [small green box] and 10 liters of rebreathing circuit [large green box]). The anesthetic concentration changes within the induction chamber are slower than those achieved using a non-rebreathing circuit (as shown in **Fig. 5.8**).

procedure prior to intubation. In this way, the animal's heartbeat, pulse quality, and rhythm can be monitored as soon as it is removed from the induction chamber, as well as during the face mask induction.

ADVANTAGES OF USING CHAMBER AND FACE MASK INDUCTION

There are several advantages in using the chamber followed by face mask induction technique. Also, there are several advantages in using face mask induction when compared with chamber induction:

- It is safer as the animal's pulse and heart rate can be palpated once the animal is removed from the induction chamber.
- The neck and head are less likely to be kinked (resulting in airway obstruction) as often happens inside an induction chamber.
- The duration of induction is shortened when using a face mask as there is less mechanical volume barrier with a non-rebreathing circuit.
- Costs are reduced because the oxygen flow rate and vaporizer settings are reduced for the face mask portion of the induction.

Inconsistencies during anesthesia maintenance

PREMATURE AWAKENING DURING A SURGICAL PROCEDURE

If the animal wakes prematurely on the surgery table, the inhalant anesthetic agent can be used to quickly and safely return the dog or cat to a surgical plane of anesthesia. The following steps can be used to manage premature awakening under general anesthesia:

- The vaporizer anesthetic concentration setting can be increased to a reasonably high percentage. It will take some time to change the anesthetic concentration within a rebreathing circuit, and the larger the volume of the rebreathing circuit, the longer it takes. However, the anesthetic concentration changes rapidly in a non-rebreathing circuit due to the smaller mechanical volume barrier. Therefore, the vaporizer setting should not be left too high for too long when using a non-rebreathing circuit, otherwise the animal will quickly become too deep and may experience respiratory or cardiac arrest due to an inhalant anesthetic overdose.
- If using a rebreathing circuit, increase the oxygen flow rate to 3–4 liters/minute as soon as premature awakening occurs.
- The animal can be manually ventilated ('bagged') to increase alveolar ventilation and increase the anesthetic concentration in the lungs and the brain. Often, the breathing pattern of a prematurely waking animal is characterized by rapid and shallow breathing. This results in dead space ventilation and does not assist gas exchange or rapid changing of the anesthetic concentration. Manually controlled ventilation increases the tidal volume of breathing and drives the higher anesthetic concentration into the caudal lung lobes to minimize the dead space ventilation via spontaneous breathing.

- If the animal is on a non-rebreathing circuit, the animal should be left to hyperventilate spontaneously and, often, the animal will become reanesthetized rapidly. This is because animals anesthetized with a non-rebreathing circuit are smaller and the anesthetic concentration can change relatively quickly despite shallow, rapid breathing.
- After the animal is reanesthetized, the vaporizer setting is reset to 0.5–0.75% higher than the previous setting when the animal was too light.

ANESTHETIC PLANE BECOMES TOO DEEP

The opposite situation to premature awakening can arise when the anesthetic plane is too deep. There are several steps that can be taken to reduce the anesthetic concentration rapidly and lighten an animal from a deep plane of anesthesia:

- Since 97–99% of modern inhalant anesthetic agents (isoflurane or sevoflurane) are eliminated via respiration, providing ventilation to an overly anesthetized animal while reducing the vaporizer setting will rapidly eliminate the excessive anesthetic concentration within the breathing circuit and drive the anesthetic gas out of the animal's lungs and body compartments. Therefore, the first action is to reduce the vaporizer volume percentage setting and then increase the oxygen flow rate.

- The oxygen flush valve can also be used to introduce a large amount of oxygen into the rebreathing circuit, but the oxygen flush valve should not be used with a non-rebreathing circuit, otherwise barotrauma may occur. The non-rebreathing circuit provides minimal resistance to breathing for animals smaller than 7 kg (15.4 lb). If an oxygen flushing valve (see Chapter 1) is activated, a large amount of oxygen (35–75 liters/minute at a pressure of approximately 58 psi [400 kPa]) could enter the lungs of a small animal with minimal resistance, which will result in barotrauma.

- The high anesthetic gas concentration in the mechanical volume barrier is reduced relatively quickly by the action of a high oxygen flow rate and a low anesthetic concentration.

- Increasing alveolar ventilation with positive ventilation (using a lower vaporizer volume percentage setting or with the vaporizer turned off) will help decrease the inhalant anesthetic concentration in the physiologic volume barrier and quickly wash out the high anesthetic concentration in the animal's brain and other body compartments.

- Once the anesthetic depth is reduced, the animal should be placed on a lower anesthetic vaporizer setting and its vital signs continually monitored.

Recovery from inhalant anesthesia

Similar principles and steps are applied in dogs and cats to reduce the anesthetic concentration and facilitate recovery from inhalant anesthesia:

- The anesthetic vaporizer should be turned off.
- Next, the oxygen flow rate should be increased to approximately 4–5 liters/minute to wash out the anesthetic from the breathing circuit to the scavenger system.
- Positive ventilation should be provided to the animal with the pop-off valve opened to facilitate the wash out of anesthetic from the lungs to the anesthesia machine and breathing circuits and from the breathing circuit to the machine's scavenging system. The endotracheal tube cuff should not be deflated at this time to prevent the escape of waste gas from the airway. Positive ventilation should be continued until the animal can be extubated or for approximately 3–5 minutes after the vaporizer has been turned off.

- This method minimizes pollution in the operating theatre since the anesthesia machine and breathing circuit are flushed with fresh oxygen and the residual waste gas from the animal's lungs and the anesthesia machine and breathing circuit are eliminated through the scavenging system.

Further reading

Abed JM, Pike FS, Clare MC et al. (2014) The cardiovascular effects of sevoflurane and isoflurane after premedication of healthy dogs undergoing elective surgery. *J Am Anim Hosp Assoc* **50(1)**:27–35.

Bennett RC, Fancy SP, Walsh CM et al. (2008) Comparison of sevoflurane and isoflurane in dogs anaesthetised for clinical surgical or diagnostic procedures. *J Small Anim Pract* **49**:392–7.

dos Santos PS, Nunes N, de Souza AP (2011) Hemodynamic effects of butorphanol in desflurane-anesthetized dogs. *Vet Anaesth Analg* **38(5)**: 467–74.

Hofmeister EH, Brainard BM, Sams LM et al. (2008) Evaluation of induction characteristics and hypnotic potency of isoflurane and sevoflurane in healthy dogs. *Am J Vet Res* **69**:451–6.

Lopez LA, Hofmeister EH, Pavez JC *et al.* (2009) Comparison of recovery from anesthesia with isoflurane, sevoflurane, or desflurane in healthy dogs. *Am J Vet Res* **70**:1339–44.

Lozano AJ, Brodbelt DC, Borer KE *et al.* (2009) A comparison of the duration and quality of recovery from isoflurane, sevoflurane and desflurane anaesthesia in dogs undergoing magnetic resonance imaging. *Vet Anaesth Analg* **36**:220–9.

Reed R, Doherty T (2018) Minimum alveolar concentration: Key concepts and a review of its pharmacological reduction in dogs. Part 1. *Res Vet Sci* **117**:266–70.

Soares JH, Brosnan RJ, Fukushima FB (2012) Solubility of haloether anesthetics in human and animal blood. *Anesthesiology* **117**(1):48–55.

Anesthesia monitoring and management

Jeff C Ko

Introduction

Monitoring anesthesia is vital to patient safety and contributes to a smooth recovery within a reasonable period of time; however, monitoring anesthesia itself presents no therapeutic value unless interventional action is taken to correct any deficit detected via such monitoring. This chapter describes which vital signs should be monitored and at what intervals, as well as how to intervene when vital signs are abnormal. Monitoring and proper intervention play a key role in the success of each anesthesia case. The American College of Veterinary Anesthesiologists (ACVA) has developed a set of guidelines for monitoring anesthetized patients. At a minimum, the following three parameters should be monitored at 3 minute intervals in all anesthetized patients (*Table 6.1*):

- Circulation.
- Oxygenation.
- Ventilation.

Other parameters that should be monitored include (*Table 6.2*):

- Signs of pain.
- Blood glucose, blood lactate, electrolyte balance, TP, and PCV.
- Core body temperature.
- Depth of anesthesia.
- Neuromuscular monitoring.

Table 6.1 Three major vital monitoring areas for ensuring tissues are perfused with well-oxygenated blood in the anesthetized animal

Monitoring areas/ techniques	Circulation (cardiovascular function)	Oxygenation (cardiorespiratory function)	Ventilation (respiratory function)
Basic (subjective)	Palpation of pulse. Assessing pulse rate, rhythm, and quality. Auscultation of heart sounds, capillary refill time	Assessing mucous membrane color	Observe chest excursion for respiratory rate, pattern, and depth
Advanced (objective)	ECG (rate and rhythms), blood pressure monitoring. Doppler ultrasound for blood flow and pressure. Blood lacate concentrations	Pulse oximeter for hemoglobin saturation. Blood gas analysis for PaO_2, inspired and expired end-tidal oxygen concentrations. Blood lactate concentrations	Capnography for end-tidal CO_2. Respirometery. Blood gas analysis for $PaCO_2$

Table 6.2 Other vital variables that require careful monitoring during the perioperative period

Other vital variable	Rationale
Signs of pain	Animal welfare, goal of anesthesia
Blood glucose	Management of diabetics, prevention of hypoglycemia in pediatric and liver failure patients, and in emaciated animals
Blood lactate	Assessing tissue perfusion status/prognosis and anaerobic metabolism
Blood electrolytes, total protein, and packed red cell volume	Assessing hydration and oncotic pressure status and oxygen carrying capacity
Body temperature	Homeostasis
Depth of anesthesia	Safety of anesthesia

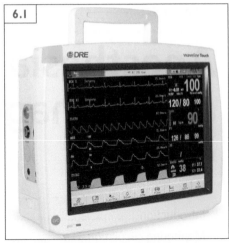

Fig. 6.1 The all-in-one monitor allows one to measure circulation (blood pressure), oxygenation (SpO$_2$) and ventilation (end-tidal CO$_2$). (Image courtesy DRE Veterinary Medical Equipment, www.dreveterinary.com.)

Where neuromuscular agents are used to paralyze skeletal muscles in ophthalmic surgery and thoracic surgery or to prevent fighting a mechanical ventilator by having continuous spontaneous breathing movements, proper neuromuscular monitoring should be executed to ensure that the patient is sufficiently anesthetized and recovers completely from the neuromuscular blockade when the procedure is complete.

The overall goals when monitoring anesthesia are to ensure adequate tissue perfusion with oxygenated blood, to facilitate a smooth, rapid recovery, and to minimize perioperative pain. Techniques for monitoring anesthesia are divided into subjective and objective monitoring. Subjective monitoring involves using an anesthetist's visual, tactile, and auditory senses to assess a patient's vital signs. Objective monitoring involves the use of equipment to asses a patient's vital signs. Modern technology allows monitoring of circulation, oxygenation, ventilation, and body temperature all combined into one piece of equipment (**Fig. 6.1**).

Monitoring circulation

Monitoring circulation focuses primarily on monitoring the cardiovascular function of the patient. Proper circulation of oxygenated blood is an indication of a functional cardiovascular system.

SUBJECTIVE ASSESSMENT OF CIRCULATORY FUNCTION
- Subjective assessments of the circulatory system that have been published by the ACVA include:
  - Palpation of the peripheral pulse provides a subjective feeling of the 'presence' or 'absence', 'strength' or 'weakness', and 'regularity' or 'irregularity' of the peripheral pulse.

When palpating the pulse, a progressively weakening pulse may correlate with decreased pulse pressure and reduced stroke volume (SV).
  - Palpation of heartbeats through the chest wall.
  - Auscultation of the heart using a regular stethoscope, esophageal stethoscope, or other audible heart sound monitor to assess the 'presence' or 'absence' and 'regularity' or 'irregularity' of the heartbeat.
  - Assessment of capillary refill time (CRT) provides a subjective evaluation of tissue perfusion. A prolonged CRT suggests poor tissue perfusion.

OBJECTIVE ASSESSMENT OF CIRCULATORY FUNCTION

- Objective methods used to monitor circulatory function include ECG, invasive or non-invasive blood pressure (BP) monitoring, and measuring blood flow by means of ultrasound Doppler blood flow.

Electrocardiography

- ECG evaluates the electrical activity of cardiac muscle and is useful for the detection of cardiac arrhythmias. An ECG also allows the anesthetist to evaluate the efficacy of antiarrhythmic treatment (also see Chapter 22).
- ECG should be used when performing IV induction in the debilitated or cardiac dysfunctional patient. Additionally, during anesthesia induction there are drastic changes in balance between the sympathetic and parasympathetic systems as the patient progresses from a conscious state to an unconscious state.
- An ECG only monitors the electrical activity of the heart (heart rate [HR]), not the mechanical activity (pulse rate and quality) and, as such, does not provide any other circulatory information (i.e. BP, SV, or cardiac output [CO]).
- ECG lead placement:
  - The use of ECG leads with alligator clips tends to cause skin pinching when placing them onto a conscious animal's skin, especially in thin-skinned dogs such as Greyhounds or other sighthounds. The recent development of loop wire ECG cables (**Fig. 6.2**) allows easy placement on both conscious and anesthetized animals during the perioperative period by simply sliding the loops onto the limbs. Alternatively, a small gauze pad soaked with alcohol or conduction gel can be placed on the skin and then alligator clips applied on the gauze with the skin, so that the pinch force is attenuated.
  - In small animals under general anesthesia a limb lead is frequently used. A limb lead II ECG is conducted by placing the ECG leads onto the limbs (left fore, right fore, and left

hind) with alligator clips. If the surgical procedure is to be performed on the hindquarters of the patient (e.g. castration or ovariohysterectomy), the left hindlimb lead creates an artifact due to surgery-induced motion. In this situation, a base-apex lead can be used instead.
- The base-apex lead is used by placing the right arm and left limb leads onto the right jugular furrow, and the left arm lead is placed on the left thorax, caudal to the heart (**Fig. 6.3**). It is important to have the left arm lead

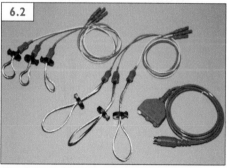

Fig. 6.2 A loop set wire ECG allows easy placement and monitoring of the cardiac rhythm on conscious dogs and cats during the perioperative period. The ECG wire loops slide onto the limbs (right and left forelimbs and left hindlimb) of the conscious dog or cat without the need for alligator clips, which cause painful skin pinching. (Image courtesy Paul Ulbrich, Vmed Technology.)

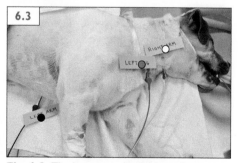

Fig. 6.3 The base-apex lead. Note the alligator clip placement of the right arm lead (white) and left leg lead (red) on the right jugular furrow, and the left arm lead (black) on the left thorax caudal to the heart.

placed caudal to the heart in order to obtain adequate electrical signals. When reading the base-apex lead, lead I or lead III should be selected to obtain a proper reading. In dogs and cats, the QRS complex is usually in positive deflection when lead I is selected (**Fig. 6.4**) and in negative deflection when lead III is selected. By using a base-apex lead, the hindquarters of the animal are completely free from ECG leads, minimizing artifact from surgery.

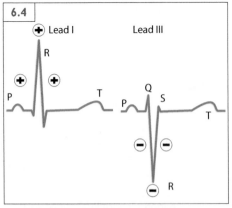

Fig. 6.4 Base apex leads I and III. This diagram shows positive and negative deflection of the QRS complex when using a base-apex lead. When lead I is selected, the QRS complexes in dogs and cats are in positive deflection. If lead III is selected, the QRS complexes are in negative deflection.

- The use of an esophageal ECG (**Figs. 6.5, 6.6**) provides an alternative way of monitoring electrical activity of the heart. An esophageal ECG must maintain contact with the mucosal area of the esophagus. The configurations and amplitude of an ECG obtained from an esophageal probe can change within a short period of time depending on the depth of the probe in the esophagus. As a result, esophageal ECG strips should be interpreted carefully. Esophageal ECG is best used to monitor heart rhythm.

Physiology of blood pressure monitoring

- Arterial BP provides information regarding blood flow to the tissues.
- The difference between the systolic and diastolic pressure is pulse pressure. Clinically, pulse pressure can be used to give a rough estimate of SV. However, pulse pressure should be interpreted with caution since it is a function of SV and the elasticity of the arterial tree. A good pulse pressure does not necessarily equal a mean arterial blood pressure (MAP) and, therefore, good tissue perfusion pressure. This can be illustrated by using two examples of systolic and diastolic BP to derive the same pulse pressure. However, the MAP (see the calculation

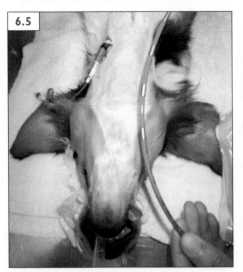

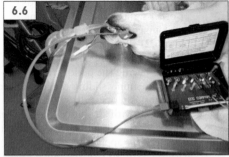

Figs. 6.5, 6.6 Esophageal electrocardiography. (**6.5**) The lead electrodes (metal) of an esophageal ECG are shown along the esophageal probes. (**6.6**) The probe (green color cable) is placed into the esophagus as shown. Note that the external ECG leads are connected to the conversion box on the right.

formulation below) from these two examples are drastically different:

- Systolic BP: 90 mmHg, diastolic BP: 30 mmHg, as seen in the patient with a patent ductus arteriosus with pulse pressure: 90 minus 30 = 60 mmHg. MAP = (systolic BP + 2 × diastolic BP)/3, therefore the MAP in this example is 90 +2 × 30)/3 = 50 mmHg, which is lower than the minimal requirement for organ perfusion pressure (60 mmHg).
- Systolic BP: 120 mmHg, diastolic BP: 60 mmHg, pulse pressure: 120 minus 60 = 60 mmHg. The MAP in this example is 120 + 2 × 60)/3 = 80 mmHg, which is sufficient for organ perfusion pressure.
- Pulse pressure can be felt through palpation of a large artery such as the femoral artery.
- BP is regulated by the sympathetic and parasympathetic nervous systems to maintain a balance between HR, myocardial contractility, and systemic vascular resistance (SVR).
- Physiologically, CO (**Fig. 6.7**) is a product of HR and SV (CO = HR × SV), while MAP is a product of CO and SVR (MAP = CO × SVR).
- HR is influenced by the autonomic nervous system. When parasympathetic nerves stimulate cardiac muscarinic receptors, HR decreases. When sympathetic nerves stimulate cardiac beta-adrenergic receptors on the myocardium, cardiac contractility increases, as well as HR.

- Three factors affect stroke volume: preload, afterload, and cardiac contractility of the heart:
  - Preload is determined by the blood volume and the amount of blood volume returning to the heart.
  - Afterload is primarily related to SVR and is controlled by the sympathetic nervous system.
  - Activation of sympathetic nerves causes increased arteriolar tone, reduced vascular diameter, and increased SVR.
- MAP is greatly affected by cardiac output and the effect of SVR.
- Routine monitoring of cardiac output (e.g. Doppler ultrasound monitoring via transthoracic, lithium dilution, or thermodilution techniques) is not practical and BP monitoring provides a close substitute for monitoring CO in a clinical setting.
- Clinically monitoring urine output (**Fig. 6.8**) in a patient without renal disease also serves as a good indication of intraoperative BP maintenance. Normal urine output is 1–2 ml/kg/hour. In dogs and cats, postoperative urine production of <1 ml/kg/hour suggests suboptimal renal perfusion and systemic hypotension. IV fluids (see Chapter 7) should be administered together with appropriate inotropic drugs to correct this deficit.
- Normal BP values and likely causes for variations in BP are listed in *Table 6.3.*

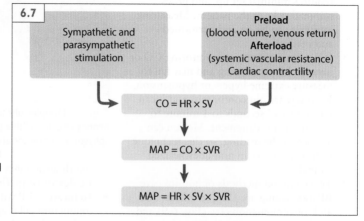

Fig. 6.7 Diagrammatic representation of blood pressure regulation. (For abbreviations see text.)

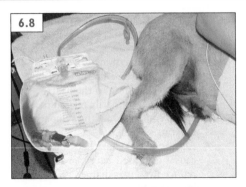

6.8

Fig. 6.8 Monitoring urine output is an important clinical method of validating renal perfusion and general tissue perfusion. If a dog or cat produces <1 ml/kg/hour of urine postoperatively, it is a strong indication of poor renal perfusion and systemic intraoperative hypotension. The deficit should be correctly immediately to prevent further deterioration of tissue perfusion. Urine output monitoring should be performed together with blood pressure monitoring.

Table 6.3 Normal range of arterial blood pressures and common causes for high and low blood pressures in dogs and cats

Blood pressure	Normal range (mmHg)	Causes for low blood pressure	Causes for high blood pressure
Systolic	90–140	Low cardiac output Low stroke volume Low venous return due to bleeding, dehydration or vasodilation Myocardial depression due to anesthesia, cardiac diseases Severe bradycardia or tachycardia Cardiac arrhythmias Deep plane of anesthesia	Patient is in pain or lightly anesthetized Higher heart rate and stroke volume due to use of inotropic or anticholinergic agents Dissociative agents, such as ketamine or tiletamine, might stimulate the sympathetic nervous system Use of epinephrine or norepinephrine or other inotropes such as ephedrine and phenylephrine (see text)
Mean	60–90	Low systolic blood pressure or low diastolic blood pressure	Light plane of anesthesia or high systolic and diastolic blood pressures
Diastolic	50–60	Vasodilation induced by certain anesthetics, such as acepromazine, propofol, alfaxolone, isoflurane, or sevoflurane Deep plane of anesthesia Septicemia	Light plane of anesthesia due to endogenous catecholamine induces vasoconstriction Alpha-2 sedatives (xylazine, romifidine, medetomidine, or dexmedetomidine) causing peripheral vasoconstriction Peripheral vasoconstriction agents, such as phenylephrine, or epinephrine will cause high diastolic pressure

Non-invasive blood pressure monitoring

- Non-invasive BP monitoring is easy, requires minimal set up, and poses minimal risks to the patient. Measuring intervals can be set and performed automatically.
- It is not as accurate as monitoring CO or invasive BP monitoring and may fail to measure extreme hyper- or hypotension. Readings are not continuous and it can take up to 45 seconds to 1 minute to record one measurement. Motion can also affect the reading, so this technique is difficult to use in non-anesthetized animals.
- Two common methods of non-invasive BP monitoring are Doppler ultrasound and sphygmomanometry (**Fig. 6.9**) and oscillometry (**Fig. 6.10**). The advantages

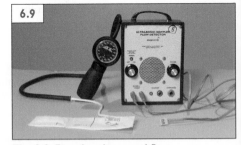

6.9

Fig. 6.9 Doppler ultrasound flow probes coupled with a pressure cuff and sphygmomanometer are commercially available.

and disadvantages of these two methods are described in *Table 6.4*.

- To measure BP with Doppler ultrasound, conduction gel is applied to the groove of the probe and the Doppler probe

Fig. 6.10 An automated oscillometric blood pressure monitor (BP-AccuGard) is being used on a dog undergoing castration surgery. The blood pressure cuff is placed on the left forelimb with tubing connected to the monitor. The systolic and diastolic blood pressures are shown on the screen of the monitor.

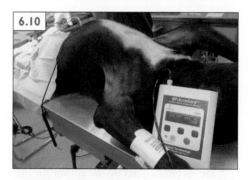

Table 6.4 Automated oscillometric blood pressure measuring devices compared with a Doppler ultrasonic flow detector

	Doppler ultrasonic flow detector	Automated oscillometric devices
Advantages	Can be applied to any sized animal (from a rat to a horse) Provides an audible signal of blood flow Relatively accurate during hypotension Equipment costs less	Requires neither experience nor input by the operator The automated measurement intervals can be adjusted from continuous to 120 minute intervals Measures systolic pressure and diastolic pressure and calculates mean arterial blood pressure for displacement Minimal hair clipping and no gel application is required
Disadvantages	Requires operator experience Does not work well when vasoconstriction is present Hair clipping and conduction gel application are required Measures systolic blood pressure only, although some authors claim that diastolic blood pressure can also be estimated	Less accurate or unreliable when used on a hypotensive or a small patient (<5 kg). However, newer models with better software are capable of measuring blood pressure on patients weighing <1 kg Sensitive to motion during the measurement Relatively expensive equipment

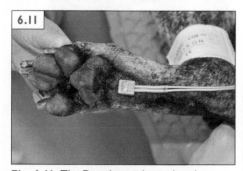

Fig. 6.11 The Doppler probe is placed on top of an artery with the blood pressure cuff proximal to the Doppler probe.

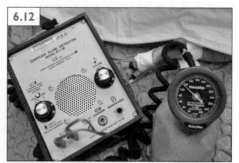

Fig. 6.12 The tubing of the blood pressure cuff is connected to the end of a sphyngomanometer. The blood pressure cuff is inflated with the sphyngomanometer until the Doppler noise disappear. The cuff is then gradually deflated until the noise reappears. At this time the pressure measured is the systolic blood pressure. Note that the probe is placed (taped) on top of the palmer digital artery with a ultrasound gel applied to increase the conductivity.

placed on top of an artery (Fig. 6.11). The BP cuff is placed proximal to the Doppler probe (Fig. 6.11). The tubing of the BP cuff is connected to the end of the sphygmomanometer and the cuff is inflated (Fig. 6.12) until there is no noise from the Doppler. This indicates that cuff pressure exceeds systolic BP. The cuff is gradually deflated until the first blood flow noise is audible through the Doppler unit. The pressure registered at this point is the systolic BP.

- Recent advances in technology have improved the accuracy and robustness of non-invasive BP monitors. Two units, the SunTech Vet20 and the BP-AccuGard (see **Fig. 6.10**), are reliable and consistent in measuring non-invasive BP. These monitoring units are recommended by the author for use in small patients. The SunTech Vet20 is not as convenient as the BP-AccuGard because it has to be manually started for measurement. There is no self-timer function for automatic measurement at a set time interval. The newer SunTech Vet30 has corrected these drawbacks. It has also added pulse oximetry and temperature measuring capacity to the newer unit (**Fig. 6.13**).

- A semi-automatic Doppler BP monitor, the Vet-DigiDop from Vmed Technology (**Fig. 6.14**), has recently being developed. This new Doppler eliminates sphygmomanometer use and the errors associated with reading from the pressure gauge. To operate this semi-automatic Doppler BP monitor simply push a button to initiate BP measurements and it automatically calculates and averages the readings.

- BP cuff placement:
  - The distal tibia, radial-ulna region, and tail base can all be used for BP cuff placement (**Fig. 6.15**).
  - The BP cuff should be positioned at the level of the heart.
  - To obtain the most accurate reading, the width of the BP cuff should be approximately 40% of the limb

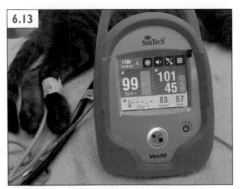

Fig. 6.13 The SunTech Vet30 is a newer version of Vet-20 and provides automated blood pressure measuring with various time intervals, and with added both pulse oximetry and body temperature measuring capacities.

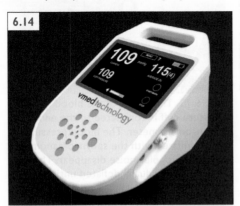

Fig. 6.14 This new Doppler blood pressure monitor eliminates sphygmomanometer use and automatically calculates and averages systolic blood pressure values.

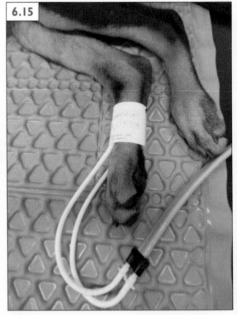

Fig. 6.15 A blood pressure monitor cuff placed on the distal tibia for measuring non-invasive blood pressure.

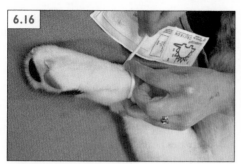

Fig. 6.16 The blood pressure cuff tubing can be used to estimate the circumference of the limb where the cuff will be placed.

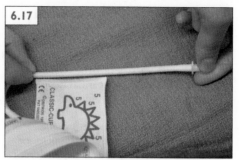

Fig. 6.17 The width of the blood pressure cuff should be approximately 40% of the limb circumference in order to obtain the most accurate blood pressure reading. In this case the tube of the blood pressure cuff was used to measure the circumference and the cuff width was then measured against it to approximately 40% of the limb circumference.

circumference (**Fig. 6.16**) at the site of placement (**Fig. 6.17**). Therefore, various sized cuffs should be available to accommodate different sized patients.

- Patient movement must be minimized when measuring BP.

Invasive (or direct) arterial blood pressure monitoring

- Arterial BP can be measured invasively by placing a catheter into an artery (**Fig. 6.18**) and connecting the catheter to a pressure transducer and monitor/recorder.
- This invasive method provides a continuous, beat-by-beat assessment (**Fig. 6.19**) of the patient's BP.
- Direct BP monitoring is more accurate than non-invasive monitoring in hypotensive or hypertensive situations.

- Because the arterial catheter is already in place, there is easy access to arterial blood for blood gas analysis.
- Invasive BP monitoring is less practical in a clinical setting because it requires more expensive equipment, personnel skilled in arterial catheter placement, and it increases the risk of infection and hematoma formation.

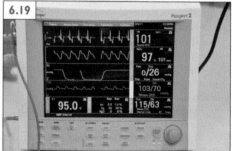

Fig. 6.19 Direct arterial blood pressure provides beat-by-beat measurement of blood pressure, as shown by the arterial wave form (red line in the bottom of the screen) on the ECG display (green line on the top of the screen). The heart rate of this dog was 101 beats per minute with direct arterial systolic blood pressure of 103 mmHg and diastolic blood pressure of 70 mmHg. Also there is a discrepancy between the direct and indirect blood pressure reading from this monitor. The indirect blood pressure (yellow color) reads 115 over 63.

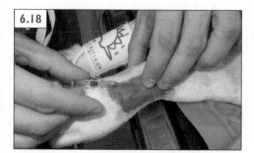

Fig. 6.18 Arterial blood pressure can also be measured invasively by placing a catheter into an artery percutaneously. In this case the catheter was placed in the dorsal pedal artery of the dog. Note that a blood pressure cuff has been placed on the other hindlimb in this animal.

Drug and surgical effects on blood pressure

- Common causes of the hypotension and hypertension are summarized in *Table 6.3*.
- Almost all anesthetic drugs have a direct dose-dependent myocardial depressant effect. Isoflurane, sevoflurane, tiletamine/zolazepam, ketamine, xylazine, medetomidine, dexmedetomidine, propofol, alfaxalone, and thiopentone all cause dose-dependent depression of myocardial contractility with associated reduction in CO.
- Sedatives such as acepromazine and azaperone reduce the sympathetic tone of the vascular system, resulting in vasodilation and hypotension.
- Acepromazine, azaperone, propofol, alfaxalone, thiopentone, isoflurane, and sevoflurane all decrease SVR, causing hypotension.
- Potent opioids, such as morphine, hydromorphone, and fentanyl, tend to cause bradycardia by activating parasympathetic tone (vagal tone), which results in bradycardia-induced hypotension.
- Xylazine and alpha-2 agonists, romifidine, medetomidine, and dexmedetomidine tend to cause bradycardia by inhibiting sympathetic tone. These drugs also induce peripheral vasoconstriction, which results in reflex bradycardia.
- High doses of local anesthetic drugs, acting like general anesthetic agents, can depress electrical conduction of the heart muscles, resulting in bradycardia and cardiac standstill or cardiac arrest.
- Epidural and spinal injection of local anesthetic drugs can lead to sympathetic blockade and cause marked arteriolar and venous dilation associated with severe hypotension.
- Severe blood loss during surgery can result in hypotension due to hypovolemia and reduction of venous return to the heart.
- Positive-pressure ventilation increases intrathoracic positive pressure, reducing venous return by compressing the great vessels. This, in turn, leads to reduced CO and lower BP.
- Overventilation is a common problem associated with the use of a mechanical ventilator. Overventilation results in low partial pressure of carbon dioxide ($PaCO_2$) and vasodilation due to reduced sympathetic nerve outflow. This leads to hypotension.
- In contrast, respiratory depression frequently occurs in spontaneously breathing patients leading to CO_2 build up and a higher $PaCO_2$. The elevated $PaCO_2$ increases sympathetic activity, which increases heart rate and CO to some extent.
- Response to surgical stimulation while in a light plane of anesthesia activates sympathetic tone and increases HR and BP.

Interpretation of blood pressure values

- *Table 6.3* outlines normal BP values and common causes of BP variations.
- Systolic BP is an approximate indicator of cardiac contractility:
  - A systolic BP of <80–90 mmHg is indicative of myocardial depression and an associated reduction in cardiac output/contractility. It can also suggest a lack of venous return.
  - A systolic BP >140 mmHg suggests a light plane of anesthesia with high sympathetic tone and CO. This is indicative of painful surgical stimulation in an anesthetized surgical patient.
- Diastolic BP is an approximate indicator of peripheral vascular resistance:
  - A diastolic BP of <50–60 mmHg indicates vasodilation or hypovolemia. Acepromazine sedated animals usually have a low diastolic BP due to vasodilation.
  - A diastolic BP >60 mmHg indicates peripheral vasoconstriction. Medetomidine or dexmedetomidine sedated animals usually have a high diastolic BP due to vasoconstriction.
- MAP should be at least 60–70 mmHg to maintain adequate tissue perfusion:
  - A MAP <60 mmHg suggests organ hypoperfusion.
  - A MAP >90 mmHg usually suggests a light plane of anesthesia.
  - MAP is a calculated value based on the following equation: MAP = (systolic BP + 2 × diastolic BP)/3. Various factors that induce a high systolic or diastolic pressure will result in a high MAP.

Managing blood pressure

- Hypertension occurs when an anesthetized animal is too light and reacts to surgical stimulation or has previously received a vasoconstrictive drug (e.g. medetomidine, dexmedetomidine, phenylephrine, or epinephrine). Rarely, disease-induced hypertension (e.g. pheochromocytoma) may be seen in dogs or in cats with hyperthyroidism, Cushing's disease, or kidney disease.
- Hypotension is the most common anesthesia/surgery-induced complication.
- Hypotension could be due to hypovolemia or inadequate cardiac function of various causes.
- Hypovolemia-induced hypotension can be largely classified into 2 categories:
  - Absolute hypovolemia due to acute blood loss or severe dehydration.
  - Relative hypovolemia due to anesthetic drugs or endotoxin (sepsis)-induced profound peripheral vasodilation.
- The inadequate cardiac function may be due to poor cardiac contractility, cardiac arrhythmias, or cardiac pathology.
- A balance between CO, blood volume, and vascular tone is important in maintaining appropriate BP under general anesthesia. There are several steps in managing hypotension:
  - First of all, if hypotension is due to absolute hypovolemia, it should be treated with fluid administration or blood transfusion accordingly (see Chapter 7). Ideally, the patient should be prepared for such treatment preoperatively.
  - With relative hypovolemia-induced hypotension, the first step is to lower the inhalant anesthetic concentration. Inhalant anesthetics induce dose-dependent myocardial depression and reduced vascular tone (hence lower vascular resistance). Reducing the inhalant concentration alleviates myocardial depression and associated vascular dilatory effect. This is the main advantage of inhalant anesthesia over injectable anesthesia, as the depth of anesthesia cannot be adjusted as readily once an injectable anesthetic has been administered.
  - If changing the plane of anesthesia is not effective at correcting hypotension, an increase in the intensity of stimulation is required. Often the patient is still being scrubbed for surgery and no active stimulation has been applied. A lighter plane of anesthesia allows for a better sympathetic systemic response to increased stimulation, with the release of adrenaline and associated improvement in the cardiovascular parameters.
  - The third step is to administer balanced IV electrolyte fluids to improve venous return. This should only be attempted if there are no contraindications to the short-term administration of a large volume of fluid (20 ml/kg/h). Alternatively, synthetic colloids (3 ml/kg bolus administration), such as 6% hydroxyethyl starch, can be used to improve BP and these are frequently more effective than using crystalloid fluids. Both methods increase intravascular volume and improve venous return, thus increasing cardiac output (see Chapter 7).
  - If hypotension is associated with bradycardia, administering an anticholinergic agent (e.g. atropine [0.02 mg/kg IV] or glycopyrrolate [0.005 mg/kg IV]) to increase HR will likely improve BP.
  - The relationship between HR and BP, with potential treatments in sedated or anesthetized animals, is listed in *Table 6.5*. This Table illustrates that simply monitoring HR without concurrent monitoring of BP can be misleading and lead to erroneous treatment for bradycardia or tachycardia.
- If all these steps fail to improve BP, then pharmacologic intervention with inotropic agents or vasopressors may be required to improve cardiovascular performance and ensure adequate tissue perfusion.

Table 6.5 Relationship between heart rate and blood pressure in sedated or anesthetized patients, with possible causes and treatments

Heart rate	Mean arterial blood pressure	Potential causes that lead to the situation	Potential treatments
Low	Low	Opioids High concentration of inhalant High vagal tone induced by diseases such as high cervical disease or intracranial disease Electrolyte imbalances Hypothermia	Anticholinergics for drug-induced bradycardia Treatment of underlying problems with pathophysiologic conditions
Low	High	Physiologic bradycardia (athletic animals) Alpha-2 agonist sedative (such as medetomidine and dexmedetomidine)-induced reflex bradycardia via peripheral vasoconstriction	Treatment not necessary unless blood pressure is becoming low
High	Low	Drug (acepromazine, propofol, inhalant anesthetics)-induced peripheral vasodilation Dehydration Hypovolemia due to blood loss or other causes Profound peripheral vasodilation due to septicemia or sepsis	Reduce anesthetic drug administration Appropriate fluid administration for replacement or resuscitation Peripheral vasoconstrictor drugs such as phenylephrine
High	High	Drug (such as dissociatives)-induced transitory effects Pain-induced sympathetic activation Hyperthyroidism Iatrogenic induced by inotropic drug overdose	Treating of underlying causes

Low heart rate = rate ≤60 bpm; high heart rate = rate ≥180 bpm.
Low MAP = pressure ≤60 mmHg; high MAP = pressure ≥90 mmHg.

Use of inotropic agents and vasopressors

- Both inotropes and vasopressors act on target receptors by stimulating the autonomic nervous system. Inotropes increase the contractile force of the myocardium, increasing CO, while vasopressors induce vasoconstriction, raising the BP. Several inotropes and vasopressors can be used for intraoperative management of BP. These include dopamine (**Fig. 6.20**), dobutamine (**Fig. 6.21**), ephedrine (**Fig. 6.22**), phenylephrine (**Fig. 6.23**), and epinephrine (**Fig. 6.24**).
- CRI is commonly used to administer dopamine and dobutamine. At low dose rates (2–10 µg/kg/min), both dopamine and dobutamine act on beta-1 adrenergic receptors to improve myocardial contractility and through beta-2 adrenergic receptors to induce vasodilation in skeletal muscles. At higher doses (10–20 µg/kg/min), both dopamine and dobutamine act on alpha-1 and alpha-2 adrenergic receptors to

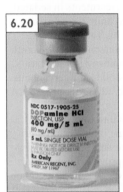

Fig. 6.20 Dopamine in an 80 mg/ml concentration.

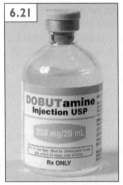

Fig. 6.21 Dobutamine in a 12.5 mg/ml concentration.

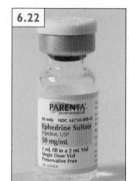

Fig. 6.22 Ephedrine is only available in a 50 mg/ml concentration. Dilution is required for use in smaller animals.

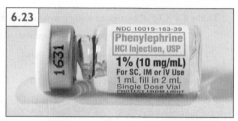

Fig. 6.23 Phenylephrine in a 10 mg/ml concentration.

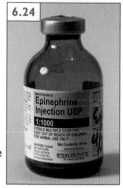

Fig. 6.24 Epinephrine in a 1:1,000 (1 mg/ml) concentration.

increase peripheral vascular resistance. Both dopamine and dobutamine are capable of inducing tachycardia via stimulation of beta-1 adrenergic receptors. At lower doses (<5 µg/kg/min) dopamine also acts on dopaminergic receptors to increase renal blood flow and potentially improve urine output.

- Ephedrine acts directly on beta-1 and beta-2 adrenergic receptors to improve myocardial contractility, but it also causes arteriolar and venous vascular constriction via noradrenaline release. In dogs and cats, ephedrine can be used as a small bolus injection at 0.15–0.25 mg/kg diluted with 5 ml of balanced electrolyte solution or saline and administered in small increments as IV boluses until the desired BP is achieved. This method is practical, convenient, and safe for clinics that perform daily surgeries of short duration, as it does not require the extensive set up of a CRI. Ephedrine can, however, also be administered as a CRI at 5–10 µg/kg/min in dogs and cats for surgeries of longer duration, or when intermittent bolus administration cannot maintain BP over time.
- Phenylephrine acts mainly on alpha-1 adrenergic receptors to increase peripheral vascular resistance and can be useful when the patient suffers profound vasodilation due to septic shock. Phenylephrine should be administered as a CRI at 2–10 µg/kg/min.
- Epinephrine can be used as a last resort for managing BP. Epinephrine at 1–10 µg/kg/min CRI dramatically increases BP. Epinephrine stimulates

alpha-1, beta-1, and beta-2 receptors activating both inotropic and vasopressor effects. Mydriasis can occur with epinephrine CRIs.

- Dopamine, dobutamine, ephedrine, and phenylephrine are capable of inducing cardiac arrhythmias, including bradycardia, ventricular arrhythmias, sinus arrhythmias, and tachycardia. Patients should be carefully monitored via ECG during the infusion. Should an arrhythmia occur, the CRI should be stopped. The effect of most of these inotropes is short lived and the arrhythmias subside rapidly once the CRI is discontinued.
- To maintain accuracy, inotropes and vasopressors should be administered using an infusion pump. However, not all clinics and hospitals will have an adequate infusion pump. *Table 6.6* provides a quick reference for an inotrope CRI using a 60 drops/ml drip set and a 100 ml fluid bag in place of an infusion pump. The key to using gravity flow instead of an infusion pump is to start the infusion slowly and then adjust the flow rate of the inotrope to effect based on the

Table 6.6 CRI of inotropes using gravity flow with a 60 drops/ml IV drip set

	Dopamine	Dobutamine	Ephedrine	60 drops/ml IV set
Concentration	80 mg/ml	12.5 mg/ml	50 mg/ml	
Volume needed in a 100 ml bag*	0.45 ml	2.8 ml	0.72 ml	
µg/ml after dilution	360 µg	360 µg	360 µg	
µg/drop with 60 drops/ml IV set	6 µg	6 µg	6 µg	
Body weight: (target dose rate 2–10 µg/kg/min)				
≤5 kg (11 lb)				1 drop every 30–60 seconds to start with, then adjust to effect based on monitored blood pressure
≤20 kg (44 lb)				1 drop every 20–30 seconds to start with, then adjust to effect based on monitored blood pressure
20–40 kg (44–88 lb)				1 drop every 2–3 seconds to start with, then adjust to effect based on monitored blood pressure
≥40 kg (88 lb)				1 drop every 2–3 seconds to start with, then adjust to effect based on monitored blood pressure

* Fluids can be a balanced electrolyte solution, normal saline, or 5% dextrose. If a fluid bag larger than 100 ml is used, the volume of inotrope or vasopressor should be multiplied by the appropriate amount. For example, if a 500 ml fluid bag is used, the volume of dopamine required is 0.45 ml multiplied by 5, so the total amount of dopamine should be 2.25 ml for a 500 ml bag with the same drip set and drip rate.

monitored BP. The flow rate of the inotrope should be carefully monitored and adjusted. If tachycardia or other types of arrhythmias (see below) occur due to overdose of inotrope infusion, then it should be stopped immediately and the patient monitored closely. If the desirable BP is not reached within 3–5 minutes of infusion, the flow rate speed should be adjusted to ensure inotropic effect occurs.
- Balanced electrolyte solutions (e.g. LRS or other commercially available crystalloid fluids such as Normosol), normal saline, or 5% dextrose in water can be used for CRI.

Assessing the effects of inotropes or vasopressors
- When using inotropes or vasopressors to maintain BP, it should be monitored using either a non-invasive method every 1 or 2 minutes or a direct arterial BP monitor until the desired pressure is reached (MAP of 70–90 mmHg or systolic blood pressure of 90–140 mmHg).

- Once the desired BP is reached, the inotrope or vasopressor CRI is adjusted to maintain the pressure.
- If an inotrope or vasopressor does not improve BP, another inotropic drug should be used. For example: start with dopamine or dobutamine (first choice) and if this does not achieve the desired pressure, then switch to ephedrine and phenylephrine, with epinephrine being the last choice. Clinics that prefer intermittent boluses instead of CRI for temporary BP improvement may use diluted ephedrine boli as their first choice drug.
- If cardiac arrhythmias (tachycardia, ventricular premature contractions, severe bradycardia, or ventricular arrhythmias) occur during an inotrope or vasopressor CRI, it should be discontinued immediately. Drug-induced arrhythmias are usually short lived and subside within minutes of termination or after bolus administration. Infusion should be resumed at a slower rate and careful monitoring exercised for the remainder of the CRI.

Monitoring fluid responsiveness using the plethysmographic variability index

The plethysmographic variability index (PVI) is a pulse oximeter (e.g. Masimo Radical 57 [**Fig. 6.25**] or Rainbow Radical 7)-derived index that allows evaluation of an individual's intravascular volume status. The perfusion index (PI) represents the strength of the pulse signal (plethysmographic change in volume) at the anatomic site of measurement from which the PVI is calculated using changes in the PI over respiratory cycles. An animal's response to fluid therapy under general anesthesia can be predicted using a PVI value.

- A common range of PVI is 5–43% with a median 18%.
- Research has shown that animals with a PVI value >18% are more likely to respond to fluid treatment than animals with a PVI value <18%.
- Together with invasive or non-invasive BP measurement, PVI provides a clinical method for goal-oriented fluid therapy under general anesthesia.
- A bolus of crystalloid (5–10 ml/kg over 5–8 min) or colloid fluid (3 ml/kg over 2–3 min) can be given to hypotensive animals with a PVI value >18%. Response to such treatment is reflected with a decrease in PVI value and an increase in BP.
- In animals with PVI values <18%, the bolus fluid treatment is not likely to work and fluid therapy is not the answer to treating hypotension. Adjusting the depth of anesthesia, using opioid adjunct therapy to further reduce the inhalant anesthetic depth and inotrope therapy is likely having a better outcome than giving a large amount of fluids and risk fluid overloading.
- Fluid therapy is based on the Frank–Starling law (mechanism), which states that administering fluids expands end-diastolic volume, thus increasing SV and CO.
- Not all animals respond to fluid-induced volume expansion of the heart. Cardiac dysfunctional, debilitated animals, or deep anesthetic depressed animals may not be able to respond to increased SV following fluid therapy. As a result, the PVI value will not decrease and the BP will not improve. On the other hand, if a high PVI value decreases and BP improves following the initial fluid bolus administration, then the fluid volume should be adjusted to reduce the possibility of fluid overload.

- In humans, PVI accurately predicts fluid responsiveness in anesthetized, mechanically ventilated patients with a normal sinus rhythm. In the anesthetized animal, mechanical ventilation can be replaced with assisted ventilation just a few minutes prior to and during the PVI measurement. Our study also showed that PVI values can be used in the spontaneous breathing animals with normal cardiac rhythms.

LIMITATION OF USING PVI AS A FLUID ADMINISTRATION GUIDE

- Because PVI is a non-invasive continuous hemodynamic estimation of pulse strength over respiratory cycles using a pulse oximeter, there are limitations to its accuracy.
- When pulse oximeter signal strength is affected by motion (i.e. significant movements from awake patients), vasoconstriction, or weak pulse quality, the reliability of PVI is reduced or not possible to use.

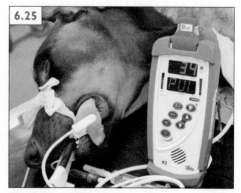

Fig. 6.25 A Masimo pulse oximeter equipped with software that allows the device to measure perfusion index and plethysmographic variability index (PVI). The PVI of this dog was 34, indicating that it would be a fluid responder.

- Other factors such as tachycardia, bradycardia, irregular heart rhythm, and spontaneously breathing (in humans) may also affect PVI accuracy because its algorithm requires a consistent photoplethysmograph derived from normal heart–lung interactions.
- PVI is not recommending in patients undergoing open chest or laparoscopic surgery.

Monitoring oxygenation

Oxygen is inspired and delivered to the tissues. Adequate BP is required to ensure appropriate tissue perfusion all over the body. If oxygenation is poor, either the respiratory or the cardiovascular systems (or both) are dysfunctional.

SUBJECTIVE ASSESSMENT OF OXYGENATION
- It is difficult to monitor oxygenation subjectively.
- Clinically, pink mucous membranes in an anesthetized patient are a subjective indicator of acceptable oxygenation.
- Oxygenation is difficult to assess in anemic patients or patients with marked peripheral vasoconstriction as these patients usually have very pale mucous membranes.
- Dogs or cats with pigmented mucous membranes are also difficult to assess.

OBJECTIVE ASSESSMENT OF OXYGENATION
- Hemoximetry measures the oxyhemoglobin saturation directly from arterial blood samples.
- Pulse oximetry measures hemoglobin saturation using a pulse oximeter placed on

the patient's tissue. This is a non-invasive method of monitoring oxygenation.
- PaO_2 is a measure of the portion of oxygen dissolved in the plasma of an arterial blood sample obtained via an invasive method.

HEMOXIMETRY AND PULSE OXIMETRY
- Both hemoximetry and pulse oximetry analyze hemoglobin saturation in arterial blood.
- Hemoximetry uses four wavelengths of light to identify and calculate the percentage of each of the four types of hemoglobin (oxyhemoglobin, reduced hemoglobin, methemoglobin, and carboxyhemoglobin) present in blood. An arterial blood sample and a blood gas machine equipped specifically to analyze all four types of hemoglobin are required for hemoximetry analysis.
- An alternative to expensive hemoximetry or a blood gas machine is to use a hand-held or other stationary blood gas analyzer for monitoring PaO_2 of arterial blood. There are several hand-held models of blood gas analyzers (**Figs. 6.25–6.27**).

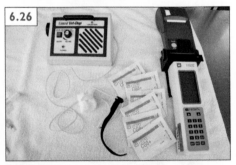

6.26

Fig. 6.26 A hand-held blood gas analyzer (i-STAT) with its printer is suitable for point of care use (right side of the picture). The appropriate cartridges have to be used for measurement of various variables. The Doppler unit is also shown (left side of the picture).

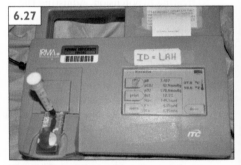

6.27

Fig. 6.27 A different blood gas analyzer model (IRMA). The arterial blood sample is injected into a cartridge, which is then placed into the blood gas analyzer for analysis. The results are available on a screen as well as a printout.

- Because methemoglobin and carboxyhemoglobin do not contribute to functional oxygen transport, pulse oximetry ignores these two two types of hemoglobin and uses only the two wavelengths (920–940 nm and 660 nm) required to detect oxyhemoglobin and reduced hemoglobin. Pulse oximetry, therefore, detects the percentage of hemoglobin that is saturated with oxygen (SpO_2) or the percentage of oxygenated hemoglobin.
- Pulse oximetry also provides non-invasive, continuous detection of pulsatile arterial blood in the tissue bed, calculates the percentage of oxyhemoglobin present in arterial blood, and also calculates the pulse rate of the monitored patient.

PLACEMENT OF THE PULSE OXIMETER PROBE

- There are several types of probes commercially available for pulse oximeters (**Fig. 6.28**).
- The most common probe is the lingual probe, which is placed on the tongue of the patient (**Fig. 6.29**).
- The lingual probe can also be placed on the toe web or pinna of an animal.
- A nasal probe can be placed on the nasal septum, toe web, or pinna.
- With reflectant probes (**Fig. 6.28**) the infrared and red light emitter and receiver are located on the same side of the probe. These probes can be placed on the cheek pouch, ventral tail base, or rectally to measure SpO_2.
- A human ear lobe probe can be placed at the tail base of an animal to measure SpO_2.

FACTORS THAT INFLUENCE PULSE OXIMETRY

- Motion (e.g. shivering or light plane of anesthesia).
- Ambient light (e.g. fluorescent light).
- Poor peripheral blood flow (secondary to hypotension or vasoconstriction).
- Electrical noise from electrocautery.
- Increased carboxyhemoglobin and methemoglobin levels in the blood.
- Hair, dark skin, or a pigmented tongue.

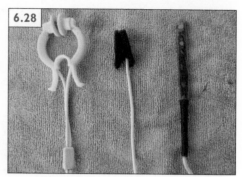

Fig. 6.28 Different pulse oximeter probes can be used in different anatomic locations. A nasal probe (left) can be placed on the nasal septum, toe web, or pinna of an anesthetized animal. A lingual probe (middle) can be placed on the tongue, toe web, or pinna, and a reflectant probe (right) can be placed in the cheek pouch, the ventral portion at the base of the tail, or rectally to measure the SpO_2.

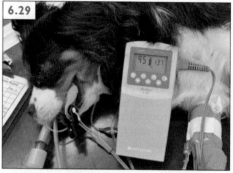

Fig. 6.29 A lingual probe placed on the tongue of a dog. The pulse oximeter is measuring both pulse rate (137 beats per minute) and hemoglobin saturation of oxygen (95%).

- Probe is too loose or too tight.
- Poor contact between the pulse oximeter lingual probe and lingual tissue results in artificially low readings. This can be minimized by using wet gauze together with the lingual probe (**Figs. 6.30, 6.31**). The water minimizes the air pocket and improves tissue contact and the gauze provides the probe with traction to the tissue.

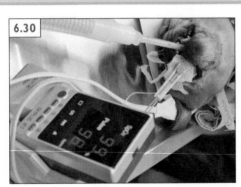
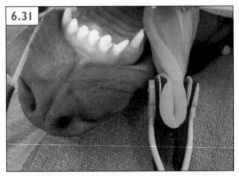

Figs. 6.30, 6.31 By placing the pulse oximeter probe on the tongue with some wet gauze (**6.30**), the air pocket between the probe and the tissue is minimized, thus improving the contact surface and reducing any artifact. Alternatively, double folding the tongue on itself (**6.31**) and placing the pulse oximeter probe on the folded tissue provides better contact between the tissue and the probe and maintains a consistent SpO_2 reading.

NORMAL VALUES FOR SpO_2

- Dogs and cats breathing 100% oxygen: the saturation value should be at least ≥95% and ideally maintained with 99–100%.
- Dogs and cats breathing room air (~21% oxygen): the saturation level should be at least ≥ 90% and ideally maintained with 95–99%.
- A SpO_2 value <90% is considered hypoxic.

NORMAL VALUES FOR PaO_2

- Dogs and cats breathing 100% oxygen (inspiratory fraction of oxygen, $F_iO_2 = 1$): 500–600 mmHg.
- To estimate the normal PaO_2 at different values of F_iO_2, assume that every 10% of inspired oxygen increases PaO_2 by 50–60 mmHg:
  - A dog or cat breathing room air (~21% oxygen, $F_iO_2 = 0.2$) should have a PaO_2 of between $(2 \times 50) = 100$ mmHg and $(2 \times 60) = 120$ mmHg.
  - A dog or cat in an oxygen cage breathing 40% oxygen ($F_iO_2 = 0.4$) should have a PaO_2 between $(4 \times 50) = 200$ mmHg and $(4 \times 60) = 240$ mmHg.
- Animals with PaO_2 values <60 mmHg are considered hypoxemic.

RELATIONSHIP BETWEEN SpO_2 (OR SaO_2) AND PaO_2

- A hemoglobin oxygen saturation (SaO_2) of 90% corresponds to a PaO_2 of 60 mmHg on the hemoglobin dissociation curve (**Fig. 6.32**).
- PaO_2 can be estimated from pulse oximetry by subtracting 30 from pulse oximeter readings of between 75% and 90%. This is because the hemoglobin dissociation curve has a linear relationship between 75% and 90%. For example, a pulse oximeter reading of 85% approximates to a PaO_2 of 55 mmHg (85 minus 30 = 55).
- The oxygen carrying capacity of an animal is expressed as oxygen content. Oxygen content is defined as the amount of oxygen carried by hemoglobin and the amount of oxygen dissolved in plasma.
- Oxygen content (ml/100 ml of blood) = 1.34 ml × hemoglobin concentration (approximately 1/3 of PCV) × oxygen saturation for hemoglobin (% SaO_2) + 0.0031 × PaO_2 (mmHg).
- Hemoglobin concentration can be measured with a portable device called Hemocue in approximately 1 minute using a small drop of blood. This provides a more accurate reading of hemoglobin concentration and is better than estimating using 1/3 of the PCV.
- Normally, oxygen content is approximately 20.3 ml/100 ml blood. Dissolved oxygen only occupies a very small amount of total oxygen content, normally 0.3 ml/100 ml or about 1.5% of the total oxygen content.

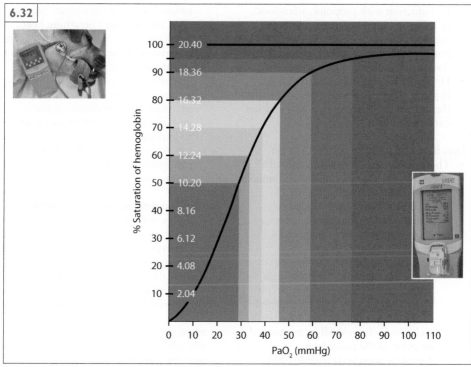

Fig. 6.32 A hemoglobin dissociation curve showing the relationship between SpO$_2$ (as measured clinically using a pulse oximeter) and PaO$_2$ (as measured clinically using a blood gas analyzer). Note that the shape of the curve is sigmoid. The numbers 2.04 to 20.40 on the left represent hemoglobin concentrations in oxygenated blood. The total amount of oxygen carried by the blood is a combination of the oxygen bound to the hemoglobin (SpO$_2$ or SaO$_2$, y axis) and the oxygen dissolved in the blood (PaO$_2$, x axis). (See text above for full equation.)

- Clinically, oxygen content can be increased by increasing hemoglobin oxygen saturation (SaO$_2$ or SpO$_2$), dissolving more oxygen in the blood (PaO$_2$), and increasing hemoglobin concentration (i.e. preventing blood loss or providing a blood transfusion).

HYPOXEMIA

- Hypoxia is defined as a deficiency in oxygen reaching the airway or lungs. Hypoxia can lead to hypoxemia, which can result in cyanosis. The physiologic causes of hypoxemia are listed in *Table 6.7*.

Hypoventilation

- Hypoventilation is defined by a high end-tidal CO$_2$ (ETCO$_2$) (>45 mmHg). Hypoventilation can be caused by IV

Table 6.7 Physiologic causes of hypoxemia

- Hypoventilation
- Low inspired concentration of oxygen
- Ventilation–perfusion abnormalities (shunting)
- Diffusion abnormalities from pulmonary parenchymal changes
- Low cardiac output
- Increased body metabolism for oxygen consumption
- Decreased arterial oxygen content due to anemia

induction agents, opioids, inhalant anesthetic agents, or a combination of these, leading to respiratory center depression and decreased respiratory rate, tidal volume, or both.

- The worst form of hypoventilation is apnea, which frequently occurs soon after

IV induction with propofol, alfaxolone, or thiopentone. The inhalant anesthetic agents isoflurane and sevoflurane are potent respiratory depressants and induce dose-dependent respiratory depression.

- Hypoventilation or apnea can lead to hypoxia and hypoxemia, especially when the animal is breathing room air and not enriched oxygen.

Low inspired oxygen concentration

- The hypoxic response associated with injectable anesthetic agents is attributable to hypoventilation and/or low CO induced by these agents. A hypoxic response in animals maintained on inhalant anesthesia may be due to a number of different causes:
  - Hypoxia can be induced by lack of oxygen supply to the anesthesia machine or to the breathing circuit. The oxygen supply may be depleted or the oxygen supply may have been accidentally turned off or not turned on prior to the procedure.
  - A broken anesthesia machine can go undetected and lead to hypoxia. For example, a crack in the oxygen flowmeter can cause a leak or the float inside may obstruct the outflow of oxygen though the flowmeter.
  - The oxygen flowmeter may have been inadvertently turned off.
  - The oxygen supply may be disconnected from the machine to the breathing circuit or from the breathing circuit to the patient's airway. The disconnection could be at the inlet or the outlet of the vaporizer (into the breathing circuit) or between the breathing circuit and the endotracheal tube.
  - If a ventilator is used, a disconnection or partial disconnection between the ventilator breathing hose and the breathing circuit can result in hypoxia.
  - If a ventilator is used, the pop-off valve on the breathing circuit may not be closed, leading to inadequate tidal volume or oxygen flow to the patient's airway.
  - The internal tubing of the breathing circuit can become disconnected or twisted between the oxygen supply hose and the outer breathing hose, resulting in a lack of supplied oxygen or reduced oxygen flow to the patient.
- Within a patient's airway, a twisted or obstructed endotracheal tube or an overinflated endotracheal tube such that the cuff obstructs the endotracheal tube outlet, can lead to hypoxia. An endotracheal tube inserted too far (i.e. endobronchial intubation) can also result in hypoxemia.

Ventilation perfusion abnormalities

- Excessive volume or pressure in the airway can cause barotrauma and lead to severe hypoxia.
- A damaged pressure regulator could, in theory, allow for excessively high oxygen or medical gas inflow into the breathing circuit, resulting in barotrauma.
- Pressing the oxygen flushing valve when using a non-rebreathing circuit will release a high volume of oxygen into the patient's airway and lungs, causing baro- or volutrauma. (See also Chapter 11.)
- Failure to open the pop-off valve can result in excessive waste gas build up with associated high airway pressure, leading to barotrauma.
- Obstruction of an exhalation one-way valve could also cause the circuit pressure to build up, resulting in barotrauma. This has been observed with a newly assembled anesthesia machine where the circular cardboard protector for the one-way valve was inadvertently left inside the dome of the valve.
- Obstruction of the outflow from the scavenging system can build up pressure in the circuit and the patient's airway and lungs, leading to barotrauma.
- A diaphragmatic hernia (**Fig. 6.33**) predisposes the patient to a ventilation perfusion mismatch.
- Laparoscopy (**Fig. 6.34**) or upper gastrointestinal endoscopy can greatly insufflate the stomach or abdomen, resulting in anterior displacement of the diaphragm, with associated hypoventilation and hypoxia.

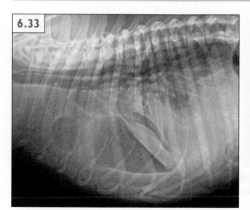

Fig. 6.33 Radiographic view of a diaphragmatic hernia that resulted in a severe ventilation–perfusion mismatch and low hypoxia. Note that the thoracic cavity is filled with abdominal viscera.

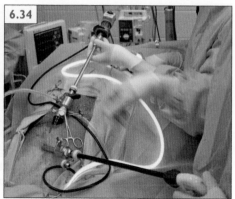

Fig. 6.34 Laparoscopy can insufflate the stomach or abdomen, leading to anterior displacement of the diaphragm and consequent hypoventilation and hypoxia.

Diffusion abnormalities from pulmonary parenchymal changes

- Pneumonia, lung torsion, pulmonary neoplasia, pulmonary edema, emphysema, and pneumothorax all impede oxygen diffusion.
- In these cases, oxygen cannot cross the thickened or otherwise pathologically changed alveolar wall to enter the capillary circulation. Therefore, the SpO_2 and PaO_2 will not improve significantly in these patients even with the provision of 100% oxygen.
- In cases of pneumothorax and tension pneumothorax, placing a chest tube and providing continuous negative pressure (via a suction pump) to evacuate the pleural air will improve oxygenation.

Low cardiac output

- Low CO, due to heart failure or severe cardiac arrhythmias, results in low cardiopulmonary and systemic circulation and hypoxia.
- Low CO due to the anesthetic agent is the most common cause of hypoxia under general anesthesia.
- Initiating measures to improve circulation (e.g. increasing BP) and reduce the depth of anesthesia are vital to restore oxygen perfusion to the tissues.

Increased body metabolism

- Fever or marked shivering increases oxygen consumption and results in low oxygen tension in the blood and the tissues.

Decreased arterial oxygen content

- Anemia or severe blood loss leads to low hemoglobin concentration with resultant low blood oxygen content.

Monitoring ventilation

Monitoring the respiratory functions of the patient is key.

SUBJECTIVE ASSESSMENT OF VENTILATORY FUNCTION

- Subjective assessments of respiratory efficiency include observation of chest wall movement and rebreathing bag excursions (if the patient is connected to an anesthesia machine).
- Auscultation of breathing sounds via an esophageal stethoscope or an audible respiratory monitor only provides a measure of respiratory rate and indicates the absence or presence of respiration.

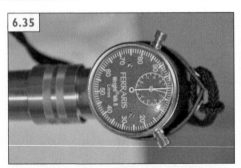

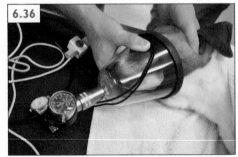

Figs. 6.35, 6.36 A respirometer (**6.35**) can be used to measure tidal volume and respiratory rate in an anesthetized or awake patient by attaching it to the breathing circuit/endotracheal tube or a face mask (**6.36**), respectively.

- All subjective assessments provide information about whether the patient is breathing and the rate and pattern of the breathing.
- Qualitative evaluation and monitoring of ventilation efficiency requires respirometry, blood gas analysis, or capnometry.

OBJECTIVE ASSESSMENT OF VENTILATORY FUNCTION

- Objective assessment of ventilatory function requires respirometry (**Figs. 6.35, 6.36**), $PaCO_2$ measurements, and capnometry.

Respirometry

- Respirometry assesses the tidal volume and minute volume of the anesthetized patient.
- Normal tidal volume in the anesthetized animal is approximately 10 ml/kg/min.
- Minute volume (MV) is the product of respiratory rate (RR) per minute and tidal volume (TV) of the patient (MV = TV × RR/minute).
- A respirometer measures the volume of expired gases.
- It is usually placed between the expiratory limb of an anesthesia machine and the anesthetic breathing hose. It can also be connected to a face mask (**Fig. 6.36**) and used to assess ventilation efficiency in a non-intubated anesthetized patient.
- Reduced RR and/or TV reduces the MV and reflects depressed ventilatory function.

Partial pressure of CO_2 in the arterial blood

- $PaCO_2$ may be used to assess and monitor ventilation efficiency.
- $PaCO_2$ is determined in a similar fashion to PaO_2, using a blood sample collected from a peripheral artery.
- Normal $PaCO_2$ in an anesthetized patient is 35–45 mmHg.
- A $PaCO_2$ >45 mmHg indicates respiratory inefficiency.
- $PaCO_2$ measurement is more accurate than a respirometer, but requires an expensive blood gas analyzer.

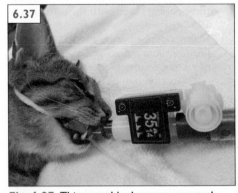

Fig. 6.37 This portable, battery operated mainstream EMMA II™ capnograph was connected to a cat's endotracheal tube. Note that a pediatric adapter (white color) is shown (immediately above the Bain breathing circuit [green color]). This design allows less dead space. The respiratory rate of this cat was 14 breaths per minute and the end-tidal CO_2 concentration was 35 mmHg.

Table 6.8 Differences between mainstream and sidestream capnography

	Mainstream	Sidestream
Definition	Patient's respiratory gases (oxygen, CO_2, inhalant anesthetic agents) pass through an adaptor that contains sensors for detecting inspiratory and expiratory gases	Actively pulls airway gases from the patient's airway or breathing circuit via an adaptor Long tubing connects to a remote sensor located in a monitor some distance from the patient's airway
Advantages	Faster response time to exhaled CO_2 gas Easier to clean Requires no scavenger on the sampled gas Can be calibrated on site without the need to use a reference gas cylinder Newly developed mainstream monitor has capacity of monitoring $ETCO_2$ and multiple anesthetic gases similar to those of sidestream monitors	Light weight and less drag on the patient's airway Can be used on MRI or CT patients with remote monitoring Automatically samples airway gases at a fixed rate: most have a sampling rate of 200 ml/min Has $ETCO_2$ and multiple anesthetic gases monitoring capacity Monitor can be remote from the patient when being used with CT or MRI and not cause interference
Disadvantages	Bulky and heavy and tends to drag on endotracheal tube and patient's airway, resulting in disconnection Tends to expose the delicate portion of the sensor to the water, secretions, and moisture when undertaking dental procedures Tends to have a bit more dead space	Slower (delayed) response to exhaled CO_2 gas due to the distance from sampling site to the sensor Prone to obstruction (with water or secretions) in the long sample tubing Requires scavenger for the sampled gas *Requires periodic calibration with a reference gas cylinder to maintain its accuracy Automatically samples (most machines) at a rate of 200 ml/min, which may be dangerous on a small patient with a small tidal volume. However, a newer model with microstream capacity samples at only 50 ml/min and can be safely used in small patients

* With sidestream capnography the CO_2 sensor must be calibrated against a reference CO_2 gas from a calibration cyclinder.

Capnography and capnometry

- Capnography (Emma™ II, **Fig. 6.37**) involves the measurement and displacement of the numerical value of CO_2 concentration and the depiction of the CO_2 in the inspired and expired air in wave form, during the respiratory cycle (inspiration and expiration). The waveform that is generated by the capnograph is called a capnogram.
- Capnometry refers to the measurement of CO_2 concentration without the capnogram. Capnometers lack the capnogram and, as such, cannot provide qualitative analysis or precise diagnosis of the morphologic changes of exhaled CO_2.
- Capnography can be further divided into mainstream and sidestream capnography. The differences between mainstream and sidestream capnography are described in *Table 6.8*.
- There are four distinct phases to a capnogram (**Fig. 6.38**):

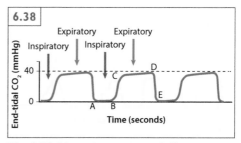

Fig. 6.38 Normal capnogram. A–B, inspiratory baseline; B–C, expiratory upstroke; C–D, expiratory plateau; D, end-tidal CO_2 concentration; D–E, expiratory down stroke and beginning of the inspiratory phase.

- Phase one is the inspiratory baseline. This phase represents fresh gas flow, anesthetic plus oxygen, past the CO_2 sensor during inspiration. The baseline should have a zero value otherwise the patient will be rebreathing CO_2.

- Phase two is the expiratory upstroke. This represents the arrival of CO_2 at the sensor just as exhalation begins. It is usually very steep.
- Phase three is the expiratory plateau, which represents exhaled CO_2. The peak of this exhaled CO_2 is called the $ETCO_2$.
- Phase four is the inspiratory downstroke. This is the beginning of the inhalation and is characterized by the CO_2 curve falling sharply to zero.
- There is only one normal capnogram shape. Any deviations from this shape require clinical investigation. Different capnogram shapes are shown in **Figs. 6.39–6.45**. Each represents a different clinical condition and can be used to aid diagnosis.

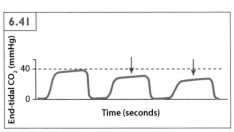

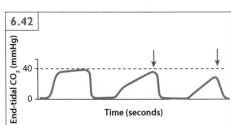

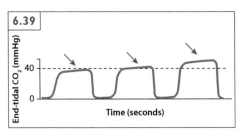

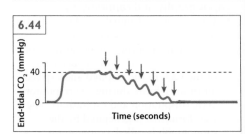

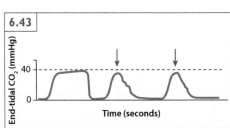

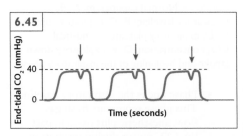

Figs. 6.39–6.45 Abnormal capnograms. **(6.39)** Increasing end-tidal CO_2 concentration as indicated by the arrows. **(6.40)** Rebreathing of CO_2. Note the CO_2 concentration did not return to zero during the inspiratory phase (arrows). **(6.41)** Decreasing end-tidal CO_2 concentration. **(6.42)** An obstructed airway due to kinking or obstruction of the endotracheal tube or breathing circuit. **(6.43)** A leak or inadequate seal around the endotracheal tube. **(6.44)** Capnogram showing cardiogenic oscillation (arrows), which occurs when the respiratory rate is slow and the expiratory phase is prolonged. **(6.45)** This capnogram shows that the animal is breathing against the ventilator during controlled ventilation.

End-tidal CO$_2$

- ETCO$_2$ is the PaCO$_2$ at the end of exhalation, and can be measured by a capnograph or capnometer.
- Normally, ETCO$_2$ reflects the PaCO$_2$ in the alveoli. The PaCO$_2$ concentration is, however, usually 5–10 mmHg higher than the ETCO$_2$. Differences between ETCO$_2$ and PaCO$_2$ may be due to an increased ventilation–perfusion mismatch or a leak in the sampling line around the endotracheal tube.
- ETCO$_2$ is commonly used for intraoperative monitoring of ventilation efficiency in an anesthetized patient. It is useful for determining optimal MV, hypoventilation, airway disconnection, or obstruction.
- ETCO$_2$ is increasingly being used in veterinary anesthesia, as it is a relatively inexpensive parameter to measure and provides a continuous method of documenting ventilation adequacy while limiting the need for invasive procedures such as arterial blood gas analysis.
- ETCO$_2$ concentrations between 35 and 45 mmHg are considered normal in anesthetized dogs and cats. In spontaneously breathing animals, an ETCO$_2$ of 25–30 mmHg is considered normal.

Interpretation of ETCO$_2$ concentrations

- In an anesthetized patient, a normal ETCO$_2$ concentration together with a normal capnogram indicates normal function of the patient's metabolism, circulation, and ventilation, and the anesthesia machine's breathing circuit. CO$_2$ is produced by tissue metabolism, carried to the lungs by the blood with adequate CO and pulmonary circulation, and subsequently exhaled by alveolar ventilation.
- Increases in ETCO$_2$ concentrations (>45 mmHg) (**Fig. 6.39**) may be due to impaired alveolar ventilation (anesthetic-induced respiratory depression), increased metabolism (malignant hyperthermia or sepsis), or the addition of CO$_2$ to the circulatory system as a result of rebreathing CO$_2$. Rebreathing CO$_2$ (**Fig. 6.40**) may also be due to soda lime or barium hydroxide lime exhaustion, an incompetent expiratory valve on the anesthesia machine (allowing exhaled

CO$_2$ to be reinhaled), or IV bicarbonate injection. The end-tidal CO$_2$ may also increase above 40–45 mmHg due to rebreathing of the CO$_2$.
- Decreased or abolished ETCO$_2$ (**Fig. 6.41**) concentrations may be seen with hyperventilation, low CO (low blood volume delivery to the lungs), respiratory arrest (no alveolar ventilation), or cardiac arrest (no circulation). Other situations, such as airway obstruction, may also decrease or abolish ETCO$_2$ (see below).
- Capnography in anesthetized patients provides vital information regarding the patient's airway patency and integrity. A depressed or absent capnogram may be due to an obstructed (**Fig. 6.42**) or dislodged endotracheal tube, a misplaced endotracheal tube (i.e. esophageal intubation), an obstructed endotracheal tube or airway, a leak around the endotracheal tube cuff (**Fig. 6.43**), or disconnection of the endotracheal tube from the anesthesia machine. Qualitative analysis of capnogram morphology can help detect and diagnose patient and anesthesia machine abnormalities.
- A cardiogenic oscillation capnogram (**Fig. 6.44**) is considered to be normal when the heart is beating against the lungs and inducing an oscillation of the exhalation CO$_2$ wave.
- An animal breathing against a ventilator can also be detected using capnography (**Fig. 6.45**).

Managing abnormal ETCO$_2$

- Respiratory depression from inhalant and injectable anesthetics causes ETCO$_2$ to increase above 45 mmHg. Reducing the concentration of inhalant and injectable anesthetic will correct this situation. This should be coupled with assisted or controlled ventilation to drive the ETCO$_2$ to 35–45 mmHg.
- If a non-rebreathing circuit is used, the oxygen flow rate may not be high enough to wash out the CO$_2$. This may be due to human error or a problem with the flowmeter, and results in rebreathing of exhaled CO$_2$ from the non-rebreathing circuit. This can be corrected by increasing the oxygen flow rate to properly wash out exhaled CO$_2$.

- If the one-way valve, especially the exhalation one-way valve, in a rebreathing circuit is open or absent, significant dead space in the rebreathing circuit will cause rebreathing of CO_2 from the breathing circuit. This situation can be prevented by routinely cleaning one-way valves and ensuring that they are functional before and during anesthesia.
- A disconnected oxygen supply tube (the inner tube of the coaxial non-rebreathing circuit system) can also result in high inspired CO_2, leading to a high $ETCO_2$ concentration. The breathing circuit and its tube should be properly inspected before each use.
- A common problem is exhausted or too tightly packed CO_2 absorbent (either soda lime or baralyme). This allows most of the CO_2 to pass through, so

that the patient inhales the expired CO_2. When this happens, all the CO_2 absorbent should be discarded and the canister refilled with a new batch.
- Decreased $ETCO_2$ concentrations are most often due to hyperventilation or overventilation during controlled ventilation. This can be corrected by adjusting the TV or RR, or both, in the controlled ventilated patient. If spontaneous hyperventilation occurs, the ventilation should not be adjusted unless the animal is too lightly anesthetized.
- Low CO (low blood volume delivered to the lungs) also causes a reduction in $ETCO_2$. This situation is managed in the same way as you would hypotension.

Use of multigas (anesthetic gas) monitors

- A multigas monitor (**Fig. 6.46**) is usually combined with a capnograph, and the monitor displays values of inspired and expired anesthetic gas (isoflurane, sevoflurane, desflurane) as well as oxygen and CO_2 concentrations (**Fig. 6.47**). As with a capnograph, multigas monitors have both mainstream (**Fig. 6.48**) and sidestream devices.

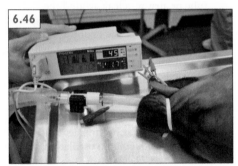

Fig. 6.46 A mainstream multigas monitor in use. The adapter is connected directly to the endotracheal tube of an anesthetized dog. The multigas monitor also serves as a capnograph. The $ETCO_2$ is 45 mmHg and the inspiratory isoflurane concentraton is 1.7%.

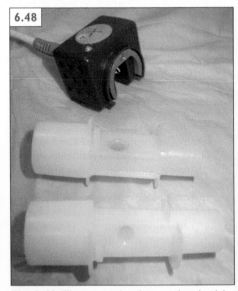

Fig. 6.48 The inspired and expired end-tidal gases are analyzed as they pass through the adapter. Note the small, transparent window on the adapter to detect the gas. The gas is analyzed in the blue part of the adapter.

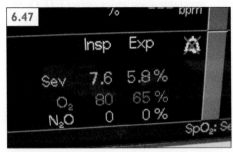

Fig. 6.47 This multigas monitor shows an inspired sevoflurane concentration of 7.6% and expired sevoflurane of 5.8%. It also shows inspired oxygen of 80% and expired oxygen of 65%.

- The advantages of using a multigas monitor to monitor inspired and expired anesthetic gases are:
  - Detection of inspired and expired anesthetic gas concentrations in the animal or within the breathing circuit. This information can be used to assist in anesthetic depth assessment.
  - Display of the rate of change in inspired anesthetic concentration within the breathing circuit.

- Detection of a malfunctioning anesthetic vaporizer.
- Detection of mixed anesthetic agents when two vaporizers with different agents are turned on simultaneously or a vaporizer that has been filled with two different inhalant anesthetics.
- Detection of leaks in the anesthesia machine or breathing circuit downstream from the vaporizer.

Monitoring other vital parameters

Low body temperature, abnormal blood glucose concentrations, and abnormal electrolyte levels, PCV, and plasma TPs all cause complications during anesthesia and prolong recovery. Monitoring these variables helps to clarify the patient's condition so that appropriate/timely intervention can be applied as necessary.

MONITORING BODY TEMPERATURE
- Body temperature should be monitored perioperatively at 5 minute intervals. This allows for detection of hypo- or hyperthermia in anesthetized and recovering patients.
- Hypothermia is defined as mild (36.6–37.7 °C [98–99.9 °F]), moderate (35.5–36.6 °C [96–98 °F]), severe (33.3–35.5 °C [92–96 °F]), or critical (<33.3 °C [92 °F]). Hyperthermia is defined as a body temperature higher than 39.2 °C (102.5 °F).
- Hypothermia is a common consequence of general anesthesia due to cutaneous heat loss or heat lost from the surgical site (abdomen or thorax). There is also significant heat loss from the airway due to the inhalation of cold oxygen.
- Hypothermia correlates with clinical signs of mental dullness, decreased HR and RR, decreased MAP, central nervous depression, and increased mortality rates.
- Hyperthermia can occur as an adverse reaction to inhalant or injectable anesthetic agents. It is not uncommon for Greyhounds to develop a malignant hyperthermic response to diazepam (midazolam)/ketamine induction or halothane (or, occasionally, isoflurane and sevoflurane) gas anesthetic.

- The body temperature of long-haired dogs or cats under a surgical drape with an exogenous heat source can elevate during surgery.
- A temperature sensor placed on the tympanic membrane can be used to monitor blood flow.
- A temperature sensor placed in the lower one-third of the esophagus measures the temperature of aortic blood.
- Rectal body temperature measures local changes in temperature that depend on regional blood flow and other factors. It may be different from core temperature, but is a useful and convenient way of monitoring relative changes in body temperature.

Management of hypothermia and hyperthermia
- Hypothermia prolongs recovery and delays wound healing.
- Active warming with a forced hot-air warmer (**Fig. 6.49**), a water circulating heating blanket, towels around the patient, or socks placed on the paws helps to provide external heat to the patient and prevent further heat loss. Rice socks (**Figs. 6.50, 6.51**) and warm saline bags can also be used to provide an exogenous heat source.
- Warm IV fluids or blood, warm saline lavages, or warm water enemas can also be used to warm a patient internally. All of these methods decrease heat loss.
- To manage hyperthermia induced by inhalant anesthesia, the animal should be removed from the anesthesia machine and provided with oxygen from another

source to minimize possible continuous triggers with residual inhalant in the system. An IV injection of dantrolene (7–10 mg/kg) can be used to lower the body temperature and counteract malignant hyperthermia.

- To manage other causes of hyperthermia, the animal should be removed from all exogenous heat sources, cold balanced electrolyte fluids administered, ice packs placed over the body surface, and 100% oxygen provided through a face mask to reduce body heat. An alcohol bath or wet hair exposed to an electric fan will cool body temperature quickly.

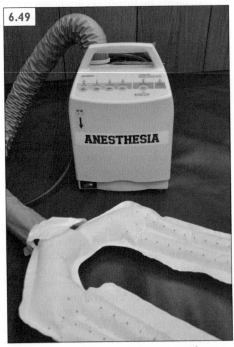

Fig. 6.49 A forced hot-air warmer with a blanket connected to the hot air hose. Note the mini-holes on the blanket that allow hot air to vent to the patient.

MONITORING BLOOD GLUCOSE LEVELS

- Hypoglycemia or severe hyperglycemia prolongs anesthetic recovery.
- Pediatric patients fasted before general anesthesia can become hypoglycemic before, during, and after anesthesia.
- Diabetic dogs and cats require regular monitoring of their blood glucose level before, during, and after anesthesia to maintain appropriate levels. Insulin administration should be continued at the full dose or reduced to one-half the regular dose until induction of anesthesia. Thereafter, the blood glucose level should be monitored every 30 minutes or more frequently if the levels are not within the normal range.
- Patients with conditions such as liver failure, portal systemic shunt, emaciation, insulinoma, and septic shock all potentially having hypoglycemia and

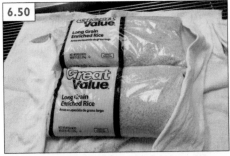

Fig. 6.50 A stockinette or sports sock can be filled with raw rice to make a rice sock. The sock is heated in a microwave oven for approximately 30 seconds to 1 minute on high power to generate sufficient heat for use as an external heat source. Care should be taken not to place a very hot rice sock on an anesthetized animal; severe skin thermal injury can occur.

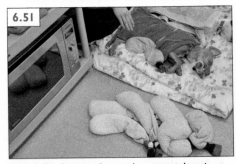

Fig. 6.51 Rice socks can be warmed up in a microwave oven within minutes. A heated rice sock can be used to provide additional heat besides a warm towel to keep a recovering dog warm.

require regular monitoring of their blood glucose level perioperatively.

- Capillary blood from the toe nails, blood vessels, or ears of dogs and cats can be used to monitor blood glucose levels.
- Commercial glucose test kits (**Fig. 6.52**) are available for intraoperative glucose monitoring.
- A target blood glucose concentration of between 3.9 and 10.0 mmol/l (70 and 180 mg/dl) is normally acceptable in an anesthetized patient.
- Blood glucose values <3.9 or >13.3 mmol/l (<70 or >240 mg/dl) require intervention.
- If blood glucose falls below 3.9 mmol/l (70 mg/dl), 5% dextrose solution should be administered, together with a balanced electrolyte solution, until the blood glucose level returns to normal. Alternatively, 50% glucose can be added to a balanced electrolyte solution and administered simultaneously until the blood glucose level returns to the normal range.

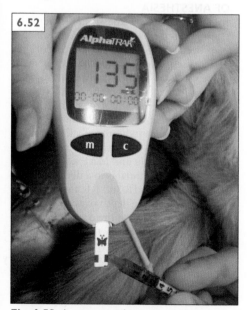

6.52

Fig. 6.52 A commercial veterinary glucose testing kit designed for use in dogs and cats is available. A small drop of blood is all that needed to determine the glucose level. The glucose level is displayed as 7.5 mmol/l (135 mg/dl).

- If hyperglycemia occurs (>13.3 mmol/l [240 mg/dl]), an additional dose of insulin should be given to prevent a potential hyperglycemic coma and the blood glucose should continue to be monitored at a regular interval to see if any further treatment is warranted.

MONITORING BLOOD LACTATE

- Measuring blood lactate is important for the critically ill patient before, during, and after major surgery.
- Serial blood lactate measurements will guide treatment and provide a prognosis. As tissue perfusion decreases, blood lactate levels will increase. High blood lactate levels are associated with morbidity and mortality.
- Decreased tissue perfusion leads to anaerobic metabolism as an alternative for energy production and results in hyperlactatemia.
- Three factors determine optimal tissue perfusion: CO, hemoglobin concentration, and arterial oxygen content.
- Serial measurement of blood lactate concentration has more prognostic value than a single measurement.
- Normal blood lactate values are ≤2 mmol/l (18 mg/dl).
- Mild hypoperfusion is typically associated with blood lactate values of 3–5 mmol/l (27–45 mg/dl).
- Moderate hypoperfusion is associated with blood lactate values of 5–7 mmol/l (45–63 mg/dl).
- Severe hypoperfusion is associated with blood lactate values >7 mmol/l (63 mg/dl).
- Efforts must be taken to investigate why the lactate level is increased and proper therapeutic intervention instituted. All the monitoring techniques and intervention therapeutics mentioned in this chapter are vital in preventing further deterioration of tissue hypoperfusion with poorly oxygenated blood. Measuring blood lactate may serve as a prognostic tool for success or failure of a given treatment.
- A single drop of blood is needed for lactate measurement (**Fig. 6.53**). Studies have shown that there is no significant

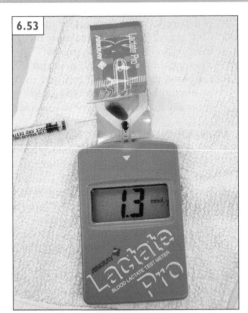

Fig. 6.53 A portable human blood lactate monitor, which has been validated for use in dogs, is handy for measuring blood lactate concentration in critically ill dogs undergoing major surgery and in assessing overall tissue perfusion.

difference in blood lactate concentrations whether using arterial or venous blood.

- Some human portable blood lactate monitors (**Fig. 6.53**) have been validated for use in animals and results are similar to stationary blood lactate monitors.

MONITORING BLOOD ELECTROLYTES, TOTAL PROTEIN, AND PACKED CELL VOLUME

- While plasma electrolytes, TP, and PCV are routinely measured, these variables are of vital importance if intraoperative bleeding is severe or if the values were abnormal prior to surgery.
- The minimal acceptable TP level is 40 g/l (4 mg/dl) and PCV is 0.2 l/l (20%). When TP is <40 g/l (4 g/dl), the albumin is also likely to be low (<15–20 g/l [1.5–2.0 g/dl]). Low albumin affects osmotic pressure and predisposes patients to pulmonary or body edema. Low albumin also affects the patient's ability to bind and transport anesthetic agents, enzymes, and free radicals. Oxygen content is significantly affected if the PCV

decreases to <0.2 l/l (20%). This affects the hemoglobin concentration and oxygen carrying capacity.

- If the TP value or the packed RBC volume value falls below these levels, a patient's recovery may be compromised, necessitating a blood or plasma transfusion.
- Hyponatremia (≤135–145 mmol/l [135–145 mEq/l]) and hypocalcemia (ionized calcium <1.2 mmol/l [5 mg/dl]) are associated with muscle weakness and prolonged recovery. Supplementation of these electrolytes may be necessary during general anesthesia.
- Normal serum potassium concentrations for dogs and cats range from 4.2 to 5.9 mmol/l (4.2 to 5.9 mEq/l). Elevated serum potassium concentrations are associated with ECG changes (see Chapter 10), which cause bradycardia and arrhythmias and lead to hypotension during the perioperative period. Preanesthetic electrolyte monitoring is vital to treat and prevent fatal arrhythmias.

MONITORING THE DEPTH OF ANESTHESIA

- The depth of anesthesia should be monitored closely during anesthetic procedures. BP is considered one of the most sensitive indicators of anesthetic depth under normal circumstances. In anesthetized dogs and cats without an inotropic agent on board, systolic BP >140 mmHg or MAP >90 mmHg is considered an indicator of a lighter plane of anesthesia. In contrast, systolic BP <80–90 mmHg and MAP <60 mmHg indicate the animal is in a deep plane of anesthesia. HR and RR also serve as indicators of the depth of anesthesia.
- Other indicators of the depth of anesthesia include jaw tone (**Fig. 6.54**), eye signs and reflexes (palpebral and corneal reflexes, **Fig. 6.55**), and voluntary movement in response to surgical stimulation. A tight jaw tone and eyes that are centered with a strong palpebral reflex, with or without spontaneous movements, indicate that the animal is in a light plane of anesthesia. Loose jaw tone, eyes rotated to a ventral position with only the sclera visible (**Fig. 6.56**), no palpebral reflex, mild corneal reflex,

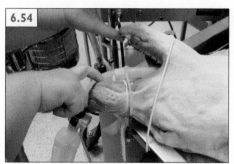

Fig. 6.54 The jaw tone of an anesthetized dog is being subjectively assessed. This serves as an indication of the depth of anesthesia.

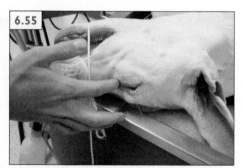

Fig. 6.55 The palpebral and corneal reflexes of this dog are being evaluated as indications of the depth of anesthesia.

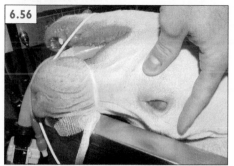

Fig. 6.56 The eye rotated to a ventral position with only the sclera visible indicates a surgical plane of anesthesia.

and no spontaneous movements suggest a surgical plane of anesthesia.

- The vaporizer settings over the previous 10–20 minutes also serve as a good indication of depth of anesthesia when evaluated together with other vital signs.
- Recent developments in monitoring human consciousness under general anesthesia have lead to the development of the bispectral index (BIS) monitor. The BIS monitor is a device that measures the signal from an electroencephalogram (EEG) of a patient and computes it to a number between zero and 100. This serves as an indicator of the effects of anesthesia on a patient's level of consciousness, the number correlating with the level of consciousness. At 100, the patient is wide awake; under 60, the patient is considered unconscious. The BIS monitor has been adapted for use in dogs and cats in an academic setting, but is not practical for daily use. When used

properly, the change in the BIS value is a reliable method of evaluating the depth of anesthesia in dogs and cats under isoflurane anesthesia.

PAIN MANAGEMENT

- Acute pain management is discussed in Chapter 24. Continuous monitoring of pain during the perioperative period is vital to successful anesthesia care. Assessment of pain following analgesic therapy should be continued at set intervals postoperatively.
- While pain assessment is relatively subjective, pain scales can be useful for continuous monitoring of and assessment of pain. The visual analog scale (VAS) and the numerical rating scale (NRS) are two commonly used simple methods for monitoring the degree of pain (*Table 6.9*).
- When an animal is found to be in pain, using a pain scale during the postoperative period, proper intervention with rescue analgesic drugs should be administered in a more consistent manner.
- All hospital personnel caring for the animal perioperatively should be trained in the appropriate use of a uniform pain scoring system. Staff should also know how to provide analgesic therapy when pain is detected during the monitoring process. Pain assessment should be continued after administration of analgesic therapy in order to assess the efficacy of the pain management. Additional analgesic treatment is needed if pain is not adequately alleviated. (See Chapter 24 for further details.)

Table 6.9 Visual analog scale and numerical rating scale

Visual analog scale:

Uses a 10 cm line for observers to record their impression of the degree of pain experienced by the dog or cat. After marking the scale, the distance between the beginning (0 cm, no pain) and the end of the mark (all the way to 10 cm as worst pain possible) is measured and recorded in the patient record as degree of pain severity.

0 cm (no pain)   10 cm (worst pain possible)

Numerical rating scale:

Uses an equally divided line marked with numbers ranging from 0 to 10. The observer marks the scale just like the visual analog scale and the resulting number is recorded in the animal's record as degree of pain severity before and after an analgesic therapy. A more comprehensive scale may add an animal's expected behavior as descriptions at each number along the line to facilitate the observation of the pain severity.

No pain   Worst possible pain

0	1	2	3	4	5	6	7	8	9	10

Neuromuscular monitoring

- When neuromuscular blocking agents (NMBAs) are used, the degree and duration of neuromuscular blockade should be monitored to ensure that an adequate blockade is achieved, determine when additional NMBAs are required, and facilitate a full and safe recovery from the blockade. It is important to recognize that NMBAs do not provide any anesthetic or analgesic actions; they simply immobilize the patient. It is, therefore, absolutely imperative to provide adequate anesthesia and analgesia in these cases and to ensure that an appropriate depth of anesthesia is achieved.

- The most commonly used NMBAs in veterinary medicine are non-depolarizing neuromuscular blocking agents, which include atracurium, vecuronium, and pancuronium. The use of depolarizing neuromuscular blocking agents, such as succinylcholine, is limited in modern veterinary anesthesia due to their rapid onset and short duration of action.

- Non-depolarizing NMBAs compete with acetylcholine (ACh) at the ACh receptors located in the postsynaptic neuromuscular junction, preventing the depolarization of the muscle fibers required for muscle contractions.

- Depolarizing NMBAs act directly at the neuromuscular junction by binding to postsynaptic ACh receptors, causing transient muscle fasciculations and persistent depolarization of the muscle fibers. This has a rapid onset and short duration of action. The succinylcholine action is terminated by plasma cholinesterase.

- Among the non-depolarizing NMBAs, atracurium and vecuronium have an intermediate duration of action of 20–30 minutes, while pancuronium has a duration of action of approximately 30–45 minutes.

- Atracurium is metabolized by Hoffmann elimination, an action based on the blood pH and body temperature for enzymatic ester hydrolysis and non-enzymatic alkaline hydrolysis. Vecuronium is mainly metabolized by the liver, with a very small amount excreted through the kidney. Pancuronium is principally metabolized by the kidneys.

- Clinical doses for NMBAs are:
  - Atracurium, 0.1–0.2 mg/kg IV.
  - Vecuronium, 0.1 mg/kg IV.
  - Pancuronium, 0.05–0.1 mg/kg IV.

- The degree of neuromuscular blockade can be monitored with a peripheral nerve stimulator (**Fig. 6.57**).

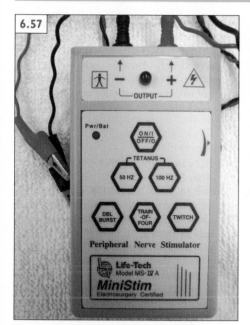

Fig. 6.57 A peripheral nerve stimulator. The electrodes are on the left. The train-of-four and the tetanus set at 50 Hz and 100 Hz are two stimulations.

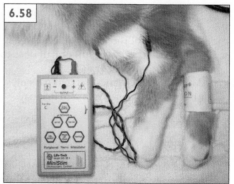

Fig. 6.58 Electrodes (red and black leads) attached to either side of the peroneal nerve in the hindlimb of a cat for monitoring neuromuscular blocking activity.

- 'Train-of-four' stimulation from a peripheral nerve stimulator delivers four electrical impulses at a frequency of two per second (2 Hz). The rate of attenuation of muscle twitching can be evaluated by comparing the fourth twitch to the first twitch. When a non-depolarizing NMBA starts to paralyze the muscle fibers, the twitch disappears from the fourth, then the third, then the second, and eventually the first twitch. As the NMBA is metabolized, twitching returns from one to four. A strength ratio of the fourth twitch to the first twitch >0.7 indicates adequate recovery of muscle strength.
- Tetanic stimulation is delivered at a frequency of 50 or 100 per second (50 or 100 Hz) (**Fig. 6.58**) and induces a tetanic muscle response characterized by tonic muscle contractions. This tetanic stimulation is painful, and if an animal is not properly anesthetized, it will be roused from general anesthesia. Tetanic stimulation is a more accurate method of evaluating neuromuscular

block function than 'train-of-four' stimulation. When completely blocked, the tetanic stimulation induces no muscle contractions at the site.
- The patient should be recovered under close supervision for any kind of muscle weakness or residual paralysis, especially if non-depolarizing NMBAs are not antagonized at the end of the procedure. In human anesthesia, a sustained head-lift test indicates the patient has sufficient overall muscle strength, including adequate diaphragmatic and respiratory muscle function, to sustain breathing. The same can be applied to animal patients. If a dog or cat can lift its head, then the endotracheal tube can be removed as the animal is not likely to have residual paralysis.
- As an alternative, non-depolarizing NMBAs can be antagonized with either neostigmine, pyridostigmine, or edrophonium to reverse the blockade. These drugs restore neuromuscular function by inhibiting acetylcholinesterase and allowing the build up of ACh at the neuromuscular junction.
- When antagonizing a non-depolarizing NMBA, atropine or glycopyrrolate should be administered IV prior to reversal to prevent bradycardia and significant airway secretions due to a surge of ACh activity when neostigmine, pyridostigmine, or edrophonium are administered.

- During neuromuscular monitoring, an increase in twitching indicates a second dose of the same NMBA can be administered at either full or half dose to extend the muscle paralysis.
- An inadequately anesthetized patient under the influence of a NMBA may not be able to move or breathe rapidly when subjected to painful stimulation, although the HR and RR will increase accordingly. Anesthesia should be increased to ensure these animals are not in pain while under neuromuscular blockade.

Further reading

American College of Veterinary Anesthesiologists (1995) Suggestions for monitoring anesthetized veterinary patients. *J Am Vet Med Assoc* **206**:936–7.

Bednarski R, Grimm K, Harvey R *et al.* (2011) AAHA Anesthesia Guidelines for Dogs and Cats. *J Am Anim Hosp Assoc* **47**:377–85.

Chen HC, Sinclair MD, Dyson DH (2007) Use of ephedrine and dopamine in dogs for the management of hypotension in routine clinical cases under isoflurane anesthesia. *Vet Anaesth Analg* **34**:301–11.

Cullen LK (1996) Muscle relaxants and neuromuscular blocks. In: *Lumb and Jones' Veterinary Anesthesia*, 3rd edn. (eds JC Thurmon, WJ Tranquilli, GJ Benson) Williams & Wilkins, Baltimore, pp. 337–64.

Darovic GO (1987) Cardiovascular anatomy and physiology. In: *Hemodynamic Monitoring: Invasive and Noninvasive Applications.* (ed GO Darovic) WB Saunders, Philadelphia, pp. 33–61.

de Papp E, Drobatz KJ, Hughes D (1999) Plasma lactate concentration as a predictor of gastric necrosis and survival among dogs with gastric dilatation–volvulus: 102 cases (1995–1998). *J Am Vet Med Assoc* **215**:49–52.

Dorsch JA, Dorsch SE (1994) Gas monitoring. In: *Understanding Anesthesia Equipment, Construction, Care and Complications.* (eds JA Dorsch, SE Dorsch) Williams & Wilkins, Baltimore, pp. 547–607.

Hughes D, Rozanski ER, Shofer FS *et al.* (1999) Effect of sampling site, repeated sampling, pH, and PCO_2 on plasma lactate concentration in healthy dogs. *Am J Vet Res* **60**:521–4.

Robertson RA, Gogolski SM, Pascoe P *et al.* (2018) AAFP Feline Anesthesia Guidelines. *J Feline Med Surg* **20(7)**:602–34.

Stoelting RK, Miller RD (1994) Monitoring. In: *Basics of Anesthesia*, 3rd edn. (eds RK Stoelting, RD Miller) Churchill Livingstone, New York, pp. 201–15.

Thorneloe C, Bédard C, Boysen S (2007) Evaluation of a hand-held lactate analyzer in dogs. *Can Vet J* **48**:283–8.

Tremper KK (1992) Oximetry, capnography and other non-invasive wizardry. In: *Review Course Lectures. Supplement to Anesthesia & Analgesia.* International Anesthesia Research Society, pp. 136–41.

CHAPTER 7

Fluid therapy

Ann B Weil and Jeff C Ko

Introduction

This chapter describes the different types of fluid available for administration to anesthetized patients, including crystalloids, colloids, and blood products. It also contains information about fluid selection and indications for fluid therapy in a variety of clinical conditions.

Composition and fluid distribution within animals

- An animal's body water is approximately 60% of the adult body weight, blood volume being about 7% of the body weight.
- Body fluid compartments can be divided into intracellular (two-third of the total body water) and extracellular compartments (the remaining one-third of the total body water).
- The extracellular fluid compartment is composed of the intravascular, interstitial, and transcellular (the fluids outside of the cellular membrane barriers, such as cerebrospinal fluid, synovial fluid, and pleural fluid) compartments.

- Water moves between compartments primarily through the process of osmosis, whereby net movement of water (solvent) occurs by moving down solute concentration gradients across a semi-permeable membrane.
- Electrolytes are chemical particles that dissociate in solutions to form electrically-charged particles or ions.
- Sodium is the primary extracellular cation and bicarbonate and chloride are the predominant extracellular anions. Potassium is the primary intracellular cation. Electrically-neutral plasma proteins help maintain intravascular volume.

Indications for fluid therapy under general anesthesia

- Fluid therapy is a vital tool to help provide the stable conditions required for cardiovascular support.

- Inhaled anesthetics cause a dose-dependent vasodilation of the peripheral vessels and reduction in cardiac output.

Table 7.1 Sensible and insensible loss of body fluids

Sensible fluid loss	Insensible fluid loss
Vomiting and diarrhea	Fluid loss through airway during inhalant anesthesia
Blood loss during surgery or trauma	Water vapor loss through respiration and panting
Ascites	Evaporation through open body cavity during surgery
Urination under normal conditions	Third spacing of fluid loss is due to sequestration of body fluids during the perioperative period and includes fluid accumulated in the lumen or bowel wall, peritoneum, and other traumatized tissues. Burn patients also suffer such fluid loss

Fluid administration is essential to counter hypotension and ensure optimal oxygen delivery to tissues.

- Animals are exposed to both sensible and insensible fluid loss (*Table 7.1*) in the perioperative period and are unable to compensate for these losses without proper fluid administration.

2013 American Animal Hospital Association/American Association of Feline Practitioners Fluid Therapy Guidelines for Dogs and Cats

- The new guidelines challenge the old practice of giving 10 ml/kg/hour or higher of fluids to healthy dogs and cats undergoing general anesthesia.
- The new guidelines suggest an initial dose of balanced crystalloid fluids at 3 ml/kg/hour in cats and 5 ml/kg/hour in dogs during general anesthesia.
- When vasodilation-induced hypotension occurs:
  - The first step is to decrease anesthetic depth by adjusting inhalant concentration.
  - Then administer an IV bolus of an isotonic crystalloid such as lactated Ringer's solution (LRS) at 3–10 ml/kg. Repeat the same amount once when necessary.
  - Use colloid fluids (such as VetStarch or Hetastarch) if crystalloid fluid fails to correct the hypotension. The colloid fluid should be titrated to effect at a relatively slow rate of 5–10 ml/kg for dogs, and 1–5 ml/kg for cats to minimize the risk of fluid overload.
- If crystalloid and/or colloid boluses are unable to correct the hypotension, (and the patient is not hypovolemic), other methods such as vasopressors or balanced anesthetic techniques using opioids or local anesthetics to reduce inhalant concentrations should be sought to improve blood pressure.
- Hypotonic solutions should be used with caution to correct hypovolemia because such hypotonic fluid bolus can lead to hyponatremia and water intoxication.

Fluid classification

- Careful evaluation of each patient preoperatively will help establish the proper course of fluids required during the anesthetic period.
- Fluids are most commonly administered IV for replacement needs, but may also be delivered SC or interosseously.
- Fluids administered during general anesthesia are predominantly classified as crystalloid, colloid, or blood products.

CRYSTALLOIDS
- Normal saline (**Fig. 7.1**), hypertonic saline (**Fig. 7.2**), LRS (**7.3**), and Plasma-Lyte A (**Fig. 7.4**) are all crystalloid fluids.
- An ideal balanced crystalloid should have the following characters: (1) contains appropriate main electrolyte concentrations, including Na^+, Cl^-, Ca^{2+}, K^+, and Mg^{2+}; (2) be able to maintain or normalize acid–base balance; and

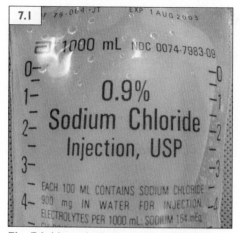

Fig. 7.1 Normal saline contains 0.9% NaCl.

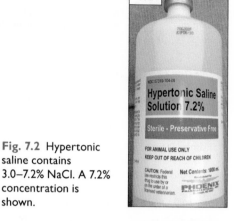

Fig. 7.2 Hypertonic saline contains 3.0–7.2% NaCl. A 7.2% concentration is shown.

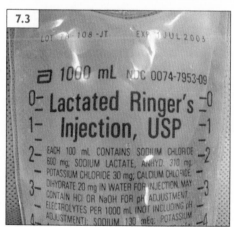

Fig. 7.3 Lactated Ringer's solution is a crystalloid fluid.

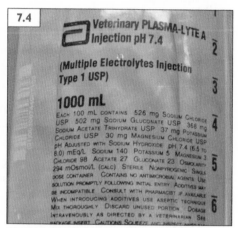

Fig. 7.4 Plasma-Lyte A solution is a balanced crystalloid fluid that resembles plasma in its content of electrolytes, osmolality, and pH.

(3) be isosmotic and isotonic so that it does not cause inappropriate fluid shifts.

- They contain small particles that are osmotically active and can pass through capillary membranes. Crystalloids disseminate throughout the body fluid spaces, while colloids tend to remain within the intravascular spaces.

- Based on tonicity, crystalloids can be further divided into hypotonic (<270 mOsm/l), isotonic (270–300 mOsm/l), and hypertonic (>300 mOsm/l) fluids. Tonicity of a fluid compares the osmolality (concentration of solute per unit of solvent) of the fluid with the intracellular osmolality.

- Based on their usage, crystalloid fluids can also be classified as maintenance or replacement fluids and these differ in their electrolyte concentration:
  - **Maintenance fluids** represent the fluid requirements to meet the metabolic needs of an animal and are used to meet daily insensible (respiratory and transcutaneous losses – ~15 ml/kg/ day) and sensible fluid losses (urinary and fecal fluid losses – ~25 ml/kg/ day). Daily sensible and insensible fluid losses are about 40–60 ml/kg/ day. The fluids are usually hypotonic, containing lower sodium and higher

Table 7.2 Composition of various crystalloid fluids

Solution	Na+ (mmol/l)	K+ (mmol/l)	Cl- (mmol/l)	Ca++ (mmol/l)	Mg++ mmol/l)	Buffer (mmol/l)	Calories Kcal/l	Osmolality (mOsm/l)
Dextrose 5% in water	-	-	-	-	-	-	170	252
Dextrose 2.5% in 0.45% saline	77	-	77	-	-	-	85	280
Lactated Ringer's solution	130	4	109	3	-	Lactate 28	9	274
Ringer's solution	147	4	156	4	-	-	-	310
Plasma-Lyte A	140	5	98	-	3	Acetate 27 Gluconate 23	21	294
Normosol-R	140	5	98	-	3	Acetate 27 Gluconate 23	15	294
Normosol-M	40	13	40	-	3	Acetate 16	-	364
Dextrose % in Ringer's lactate	130	4	109	3	-	Lactate 28	179	525
Normal saline (0.9%)	154	-	154	-	-	-	-	308
Dextrose 50%	-	-	-	-	-	-	1700	2525
Dextrose 5% in saline (0.9%)	154	-	154	-	-	-	170	-
Hetastarch	154	-	154	-	-	-	-	309
VetStarch (6% hydroxyethyl starch 130/0.4)	154	-	154	-	-	-	-	308

potassium concentrations (such as Plasma-Lyte A, Normosol-M, or 0.45% NaCl with KCl; see Normosol-M versus Normosol-R in *Table 7.2* for details of their compositions).

- **Replacement fluids** are usually isotonic and are considered balanced as they have similar electrolyte composition and tonicity to plasma. They are suitable for rapid volume restoration. Replacement fluids are most commonly used during general anesthesia, because they are isotonic and can be given rapidly IV to expand intravascular compartment. Replacement crystalloid fluid rates are commonly given at 3–10 ml/kg/hour during anesthesia.

Advantages of crystalloid fluids
- Can be used for volume replacement for normal patients undergoing general anesthesia.
- Can be administered at high rates for patients in hypovolemic shock. Roughly one blood volume is delivered per hour: 90 ml/kg/hour in dogs and 60 ml/kg/hour in cats.
- Cost effective.
- Rapid onset of effect.
- Long shelf life.
- Easily obtained and available.

Disadvantages of crystalloid fluids
- Dilution of plasma proteins and red blood cells.
- Need three times equivalent volume to replace lost blood and lack oxygen carrying capability.
- Can create hypothermia if large volumes are administered at room temperature.
- Relatively short duration of effect. Only 10% of administered volume remains in the intravascular space after 1 hour.

Types of crystalloid fluids and their clinical indications
Lactated Ringers solution and Normosol-R (Plasma-Lyte A)
- These are balanced isotonic fluids.
- They contain acetate, lactate, or gluconate, which serve as alkalinizing

agents to maintain acid–base balance (see *Table 7.2*).

- Commonly used as replacement solutions under general anesthesia at a rate of 5–10 ml/kg/hour.
- Fluids with additional potassium chloride supplementation should not be used during general anesthesia in case large volumes must be administered rapidly. Life-threatening hyperkalemia may occur with bolus administration of potassium.

Hypertonic saline

- Hypertonic saline has an osmolality of 2400 mOsm/l, which classifies it as hypertonic.
- The advantage of using hypertonic saline is that it uses the least amount of infused fluid to achieve the most cardiovascular benefit within a short time.
- It is commercially available as 3–7.5% solutions of sodium chloride.
- It is used primarily to treat severe hypovolemic shock, including hemorrhagic shock. In dogs, the shock dose of hypertonic saline is 4–5 ml/kg and in cats 2–4 ml/kg.
- It exerts beneficial effects primarily through improvement in intravascular volume and reduction in afterload as the solute load draws fluid from the intracellular compartment. Vital organ blood flow is, therefore, improved.
- The intravascular effect of hypertonic saline is transient and lasts approximately 30–60 minutes. Thereafter, the osmotic pressure between the intra- and extravascular spaces equilibrate. Regular isotonic crystalloid solutions must be administered in order to replace the interstitial fluid loss.
- Contraindicated in patients with hypernatremia, risk of volume overload, renal insufficiency, or severe dehydration.

Dextrose added to fluids

- Dextrose can be added to crystalloid solutions at a variety of concentrations, with 2.5% and 5% commonly used in small animal practice.
- Dextrose 5% in water is considered isotonic, but the glucose is rapidly metabolized by cells such that the

remaining free water is hypotonic, resulting in electrolyte abnormalities in the extracellular fluid if large volumes are bolused rapidly.

- If dextrose administration is desired, dextrose can be added to LRS or Normosol-R, resulting in a hypertonic solution initially, but once the dextrose is metabolized, the solution will be isotonic. For example, to make 2.5% dextrose in LRS, 50 ml of LRS is removed from a 1 liter bag and replaced with 50 ml of 50% dextrose.
- Indications for adding dextrose to crystalloid fluids:
  - Pediatric patients.
  - Geriatric patients.
  - Patients with severe liver dysfunction.
  - Diabetic patients undergoing anesthesia but receiving insulin where blood glucose could be low during the perioperative period. (See Chapter 10 for information on anesthesia in animals with specific diseases.)

Normal saline

- Does not contain any bicarbonate precursors.
- Considered an acidifying solution.
- Large volumes administered rapidly will dilute plasma bicarbonate, causing a dilutional acidemia.
- Indications for use of normal saline:
  - Patients with metabolic alkalosis (e.g. a patient with pyloric obstruction).
  - Patients with hyperkalemia (e.g. dogs with Addison's disease).
  - Dogs or cats with a ruptured bladder.
  - Tom cats with a blocked urethra.

COLLOIDS

- Colloid fluids may be naturally occurring (plasma, albumin, whole blood) or synthetic (dextrans, hydroxyethyl starch, gelatins).
- Colloid solutions are aqueous solutions containing particles with large molecular weights.
- Some of these particles can diffuse through capillary membranes, but many cannot and remain within the intravascular space. This tends to increase intravascular oncotic pressure, which retains fluid within the intravascular space and also draws some fluid in from the interstitial space.

Indications for colloid fluid therapy

- Use when crystalloids alone are not sufficient to maintain intravascular volume (e.g. moderate to severe hypovolemic shock).
- Rapid volume replacement with less redistribution to interstitial space.
- Low plasma proteins.
- Increased capillary permeability (e.g. systemic inflammatory response syndrome).
- Hypovolemia with cerebral or pulmonary edema.
- Patients with third-space losses.

Contraindications for colloid fluid therapy

- Potential for volume overload, as the fluid stays primarily within the intravascular space.
- Potential for coagulopathies with synthetic colloids.
- Potential for allergic reaction with natural colloids.
- More costly to administer than crystalloids.

Types of colloid fluids and their clinical indications

Hetastarch (Fig. 7.5)

- Synthetic polysaccharide, with starch molecules of varying molecular weights.
- Long-lasting vascular expansion (up to 24 hours).
- Store at room temperature.
- Dose is 20 ml/kg/day in dogs; 10 ml/kg/day in cats.
- Under general anesthesia the fluid can be administered at a dose of 3 ml/kg/hour for alleviating hypotension.

VetStarch (Fig. 7.6)

- Each 100 ml contains 6 g of hydroxyethyl starch 130/0.4 in isotonic 0.9% sodium chloride injection solution.
- It is a plasma volume substitute indicated for the treatment and prophylaxis of hypovolemia.
- Frequently, a 3 ml/kg IV bolus in dogs and cats with normal cardiac function can rapidly correct hypotension.
- It can be used at 3 ml/kg/hour as a CRI together with 3 ml/kg/hour of other balanced crystalloid fluids to prevent hypotension from occurring.
- Overdose may lead to fluid overload, especially in pulmonary edema and congestive heart failure patients.
- Caution should be taken when administering to renal azotemic patients that are not hypovolemic.
- It should not be used in patients in dialysis treatment.
- It should not be used in severe hypernatremia or severe hyperchloremia.
- It also should be used with caution in the patients with intracranial bleeding since it might interfering with blood clotting.

Dextran-70

- A similar product to VetStarch is Dextran-70 in 0.9% NaCl. It can be used in a similar fashion to Hetastarch, but has a shorter duration.

BLOOD PRODUCTS

- Blood products can be natural or synthetic. The natural blood products include fresh

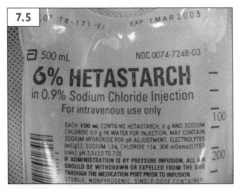

Fig. 7.5 Hetastarch is a colloid fluid.

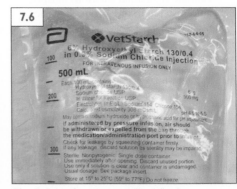

Fig. 7.6 VetStarch is a colloid fluid.

or stored whole blood, fresh, fresh frozen or frozen plasma, and packed blood cells. Synthetic products in veterinary medicine are not currently available.

- Patients requiring blood products before general anesthesia include:
  - Patients with severe blood loss or with anemia (PCV <0.2 l/l [20%]).
  - Hypoproteinemic patients with TP <40 g/l (4 g/dl) or albumin <20 g/l (2 g/dl).
  - Patients with bleeding disorders (e.g. coagulopathies or thrombocytopenia).
- Whole blood is the best replacement for acute blood loss, when both PCV and TP levels are low.
- Packed red cells are used to treat anemic patients who have normal protein levels.
- Plasma (**Fig. 7.7**) is used to treat protein loss when RBCs remain adequate.
- Patients with PCV equal to or less than 0.2 l/l (20%) or an anticipated blood loss of 20% of blood volume. A dog's blood volume is 80–90 ml/kg and a cat's is 60–70 ml/kg.

Cautions when administering natural blood products

- A filtered blood administration set should be used when administering blood or blood products (**Fig. 7.8**).
- Whole blood should be warmed to body temperature prior to administration.
- Dogs should be cross-matched if they have had a prior transfusion or a litter of puppies.
- All cats should be blood typed due to naturally occurring alloantibodies. Hemolytic transfusion reactions can occur in cats that have never received a transfusion.

Dose rates of whole blood

- 10–22 ml/kg.
- 2.2 ml of whole blood/kg body weight (or 1 ml/lb body weight) raises PCV by 0.01 l/l (1%), provided the donor's PCV is approximately 0.4 l/l (40%). If the donor's PCV is >0.4 l/l (40%) (e.g. Greyhounds with a PCV of 0.6 l/l [60%]), less blood volume is needed to raise the PCV.
- Administer slowly initially (5 ml/kg/hour for 30 minutes; monitor for transfusion reaction).

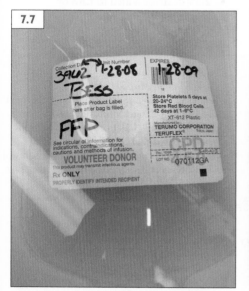

Fig. 7.7 Fresh frozen plasma is available for plasma transfusion in dogs and cats. It must be thawed to room temperature before administration.

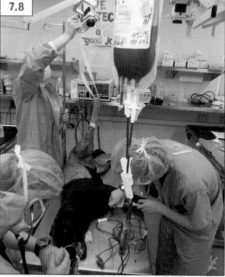

Fig. 7.8 A filter set should be used for whole blood transfusion.

Signs of transfusion reaction (under general anesthesia)

- Tachycardia.
- Tachypnea or dyspnea.
- Increased body temperature.
- Hypotension.
- Urticaria.
- Edema.

Case examples

HEALTHY PATIENT UNDERGOING GENERAL ANESTHESIA FOR ELECTIVE PROCEDURE

- Balanced, isotonic, replacement fluid.
- LRS or Normosol-R (or Plasma-Lyte A) (both 5 ml/kg/hour).

PATIENT WITH SUSPECTED PORTOSYSTEMIC SHUNT REQUIRING GENERAL ANESTHESIA

- PCV = 0.42 l/l (42%); TP = 40 g/l (4 g/dl).
- Normosol-R (or Plasma-Lyte A) with 2.5% dextrose added at 3 ml/kg/hour plus VetStarch at 3 ml/kg/hour.

PATIENT WITH HEMOLYTIC ANEMIA TO BE ANESTHETIZED FOR BONE MARROW ASPIRATION

- PCV = 0.14 l/l (14%); TP = 68 g/l (6.8 g/dl).
- Packed RBCs at 5 ml/kg/hour plus Normosol-R (or Plasma-Lyte A) at 5 ml/kg/hour.

- Since lactated Ringer's solution contains calcium, it should not be administered in the same IV line to prevent clotting of the blood product.

PATIENT WITH BLEEDING ABDOMINAL MASS PRESENTED FOR SURGERY

- PCV= 0.12 l/l (12%); TP = 38 g/l (3.8 g/dl).
- Packed RBCs at 5 ml/kg/hour plus VetStarch at 5 ml/kg/hour.
- Whole blood transfusion at 5–10 ml/kg/hour.

PATIENT WITH RUPTURED BLADDER PRESENTING FOR BLADDER REPAIR

- 0.9% NaCl at 5 ml/kg/hour.

TWO- TO THREE-MONTH-OLD MALE PUPPY PRESENTED FOR LACERATION REPAIR

- 2.5% dextrose added to LRS or Normosol-R.

Further reading

Aarnes TK, Bednarski RM, Lerche P *et al.* (2009) Effect of intravenous administration of lactated Ringer's solution or Hetastarch for the treatment of isoflurane-induced hypotension in dogs. *Am J Vet Res* **70**:1345–53.

Kudnig ST, Mama K (2002) Perioperative fluid therapy. *J Am Vet Med Assoc* **221**:1112–21.

Lanevschi A, Wardrop KJ (2001) Principles of transfusion medicine in small animals. *Can Vet J* **42**:447–54.

Mama K (2002) Fluid therapy. In: *Veterinary Therapy and Pain Management Secrets.* (ed SA Greene) Hanley & Belfus, Philadelphia, pp. 31–5.

Muir WW 3rd (2017) Effect of intravenously administered crystalloid solutions on acid–base balance in domestic animals. *J Vet Intern Med* **31(51)**:1371–81.

Muir WW 3rd, Wiese AJ (2004) Comparison of lactated Ringer's solution and a physiologically balanced 6% Hetastarch plasma expander for the treatment of hypotension induced via blood withdrawal in isoflurane-anesthetized dogs. *Am J Vet Res* **65**:1189–94.

Rizoli S (2011) PlasmaLyte. *J Trauma* **70(5 Suppl)**:S17–18.

Seeler DC (2007) Fluid, electrolyte, and blood component therapy. In: *Lumb and Jones' Veterinary Anesthesia and Analgesia*, 4th edn. (eds WJ Tranquilli, JC Thurmon, KA Grimm) Blackwell Publishing, Ames, pp. 183–202.

CHAPTER 8

Blood components and transfusion therapy

Paula A Johnson and J Catharine Scott-Moncrieff

Introduction

Canine and feline patients suffering from critical illness trauma or undergoing invasive surgical procedures often require treatment with blood products. As the quality of care provided to veterinary patients has grown exponentially, so has the technology and complexity associated with transfusion therapy. Appropriate screening of donors and recipients to minimize risks, and tailoring of therapy for specific needs has become the standard of care.

This chapter will describe commonly utilized blood products in small animal medicine including fresh whole blood, packed red blood cells (pRBCs), fresh frozen plasma (FFP) and frozen plasma (FP), cryoprecipitate, platelet products, and albumin products. For each product, preparation, proper storage, indications for use, dosing recommendations, and administration protocols will be discussed. This chapter will also review safe transfusion practices including blood typing, cross matching, transfusion monitoring, diagnosis and treatment of transfusion reactions, and safe sources of blood products including use of autologous blood transfusions. The benefits and complications associated with massive blood transfusions are also discussed.

Blood products

FRESH WHOLE BLOOD
Preparation
Whole blood should be collected aseptically from a prescreened donor into a sealed gas-diffusible blood collection bag containing an appropriate anticoagulant preservative such as citrate–phosphate–dextrose–adenine (CPDA-1). Whole blood collected to be utilized immediately is drawn into a single unit bag whereas blood collected with the intention to separate the pRBCs from the plasma for future use is drawn into a three bag collection system (**Fig. 8.1**). The single unit bag (the single blood bag) is for whole blood collection and contains CPDA-1 solution. It is available in various capacity sizes. The three bag collection system (so called the triple blood bag) is designed to separate freshly whole blood into three blood components, namely pRBC, plasma, and platelets through the process of centrifugation and extraction. During the preparation of the pRBC, it also removes much of the needed nutrients for RBCs maintenance during storage. Preserving solutions and additives are added to the RBCs after removal of plasma and

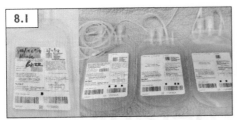

Fig. 8.1 Left: Single unit blood collection bag. Right: three bag blood collection system (Terumo Corporation, Tokyo, Japan).

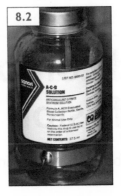

Fig. 8.2 Anticoagulant citrate dextrose solution USP Formula A (Sanofi, Paris France).

platelets. With the triple blood bag collection system, the primary bag contains CPD (as anticoagulant) and a satellite bag contains SAGM (saline, adenine, glucose, and mannitol, as additives). If the blood is being collected into a syringe, anticoagulant citrate dextrose (ACD) is used (**Fig. 8.2**). The ratio of anticoagulant to blood should be: 1 ml of anticoagulant to 7 ml of blood.

Storage

If whole blood is kept at room temperature, it should be utilized within 4 hours. If not utilized immediately, whole blood can be stored in a blood bank refrigerator designed to keep blood products at the appropriate temperature. It is important to realize that platelets begin to lose their activity once refrigeration occurs. Whole blood can be stored in CPDA-1 for up to 28–37 days.

Indications

Whole blood is recommended when a patient has suffered massive blood loss of multiple or all blood components (RBCs, plasma, and platelets). When there is loss of

>30–40% of the blood volume, resuscitation with whole blood to replace all components is recommended. (See *Table 8.1* for classes of hemorrhage, clinical signs, and recommended treatment.) Whole blood may also be indicated when there is a need for platelets and other platelet products are not readily available.

Dosing

Whole blood can be administered at a dose of 10–20 ml/kg of body weight (BW) or the amount of whole blood to administer can be calculated based on the target PCV for the patient utilizing the following formula:

Transfusion amount in (ml)=

$$\frac{(PCV\ desired - PCV\ current)}{PCV\ donor\ \times\ blood\ volume\,(ml/kg)\ \times\ BW\,(kg)}$$

PCV, packed cell volume; BW, body weight
Blood volume for canine = 90 ml/kg; feline = 60 ml/kg

Table 8.1 Classes of hemorrhage, clinical signs, and recommended therapy

Class of hemorrhage	% blood loss	Clinical signs	Treatment recommendations
I	<15	Typically no change in vital signs	Fluid resuscitation usually not required
II	15–30	Tachycardia, pale mucous membranes, cool extremities, early signs of behavior or mentation change	Volume resuscitation with crystalloids is recommended.
III	30–40	Hypotension, tachycardia, prolonged CRT, pale mucous membranes, cool extremities, further deterioration of mental status	Fluid resuscitation with crystalloids and blood transfusion is usually necessary
IV	>40	Severe hypotension, tachycardia that can progress to bradycardia, arrhythmias, coma	Aggressive resuscitation with crystalloids and blood products required to prevent death

CRT, capillary refill time.

In general, administration of 2 ml whole blood/kg BW will raise the PCV by 1%.

Administration

Blood products containing RBCs, including whole blood and pRBCs, should be administered IV or via an intraosseous catheter. Strict sterility must be maintained when handling blood products and connecting the component bag or syringe to the infusion set or patient catheter. Whole blood and pRBCs should be administered at room temperature. Red cell-containing products should be administered using a dedicated blood administration set with a 170 micron inline filter (**Fig. 8.3**) or for smaller patients a standard extension set with an inline filter attached, such as a hemonate filter (**Fig. 8.4**) can be used. Fluids that contain calcium or dextrose or are not isotonic can cause lysis of RBCs if administered in the same infusion line and catheter. If simultaneous administration of fluids other than isotonic saline is necessary, this should be done using a separate line and catheter. To ensure that any clinical

signs associated with a transfusion reaction can be attributed to the transfusion administration, other medications and feeding the patient should be avoided while the transfusion is being given. More details regarding transfusion reactions is discussed later in this chapter.

Not all fluid pumps are safe for administration of blood products because of the risk of lysis of the RBCs. Administration via gravity flow is recommended if the fluid pump has not been demonstrated to be safe for RBC administration. The rate of administration is dependent on the patient's immediate need and clinical status. Ideally, transfusion of any blood product should be started at a slow rate (0.5–1.0 ml/kg/h) for the first 15–30 minutes to allow for monitoring for transfusion reactions. After this, if no signs of a reaction have occurred, the rate can be adjusted in order to complete the transfusion in the desired time frame. A rate of 5–10 ml/kg/hour is recommended; however, it is important to ensure the patient can tolerate this rate and volume. Blood products should not remain at room temperature for >4 hours because there is increased risk of exponential bacterial growth beyond this time period.

PACKED RED BLOOD CELLS
Preparation

In dogs, a unit of fresh whole blood is drawn aseptically into a three bag collection system containing CPDA-1. After collection, the bag of whole blood is centrifuged at 5,000 g for 5 minutes at 6°C. The RBCs are then separated from the plasma. A unit of pRBCs is approximately 200–250 ml, which can be divided into one-half units each containing approximately 125 ml of pRBCs. For cats, a unit of pRBCs contains approximately 25 ml of cells (**Fig. 8.5**).

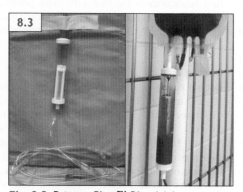

Fig. 8.3 Primary Plum™ Blood Administration Set (Hospira, Lake Forrest, Illinois).

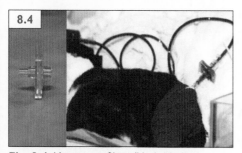

Fig. 8.4 Hemonate filter (Utah Medical Products, Midvale, Utah).

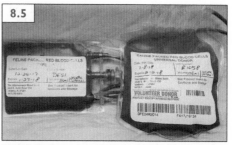

Fig. 8.5 One unit of feline pRBCs, half unit of canine pRBCs.

Storage

pRBCs are stored in anticoagulant nutrient solution at a temperature between 1° and 6°C. The bags should be stored in an upright position with adequate space between bags. The shelf life is up to 37 days.

Indications

pRBCs are administered when patients are anemic (lack of RBCs or hemoglobin) due to blood loss, hemolysis, or bone marrow dysfunction. pRBCs can be simultaneously administered with plasma when volume replacement is also needed.

Dosing

The 'transfusion trigger' is the hemoglobin level at which a patient demonstrates clinical signs of decreased oxygen carrying capacity and poor tissue perfusion. Clinical signs include pale mucous membranes, exercise intolerance, weakness, tachypnea, tachycardia, and hypotension. There are no studies that define an appropriate transfusion trigger in veterinary patients; however, in human medicine transfusions are recommended when the hemoglobin concentration is <70 g/l (7 g/dl) (PCV <0.21 l/l [<21%]). It is important to clinically assess each patient individually, because there are situations in which a patient may require a transfusion sooner. Patients for which general anesthesia is planned would fall in this category. A typical dose for administration of pRBCs is 5–10 ml/kg. Alternatively, the dose can be calculated in order to reach a target PCV utilizing the following formula when the pRBCs have a PCV of approximately 0.6 l/l (60%):

1.5 ml × desired % increase in PCV × BW (kg)

In general, the administration of 1 ml of pRBCs/kg BW will raise the PCV by 1%.

Administration

pRBC administration follows the same guidelines as for whole blood (see above).

FRESH FROZEN PLASMA/FROZEN PLASMA
Preparation

After separation, plasma should be rapidly frozen. If plasma is frozen less than 6 hours from the time of collection it is deemed FFP. If the plasma is not frozen within 6 hours it is classified as FP. One unit of canine FFP or FP is approximately 250 ml.

Storage

FFP should be stored between –20°C and –70°C, and can be stored for up to 1 year. After 1 year of storage, due to the decrease in stability of the labile coagulation factors V and VIII, FFP is reclassified as FP. If maintained at appropriate temperatures, FP can be stored for up to 5 years. Frozen plasma is used to provide albumin, and the vitamin K-dependent clotting factors II, VII, IX, and X. Bags of FFP and FP should be stored in a protective box in order to prevent damage to the product (**Fig. 8.6**).

Indications

The most common indications for use of FFP/FP include treatment of coagulopathies and hypoalbuminemia. The use of FFP/FP to treat the hypocoagulable phase of disseminated intravascular coagulopathy (DIC) is controversial. The current human literature recommends treating DIC with plasma only if there is evidence of active hemorrhage. The use of FFP to treat pancreatitis is also controversial.

Dosing

Recommended dosing for FFP/FP is 10–20 ml/kg. If FFP/FP is being used to increase the albumin concentration in patients with severe hypoalbuminemia, a dose of 45 ml/kg is required to increase the albumin concentration by 10 g/l (1 g/dl). Because of the need for such a high volume, this is not practical based on the total volume needed, risk of volume overload, and cost.

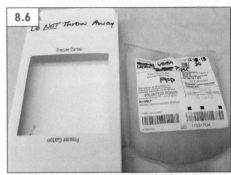

Fig. 8.6 One unit of FFP and the protective freezer carton.

Administration

Plasma must be thawed prior to administration. Once the product is removed from the freezer it should be allowed to sit within its protective box for 10–15 minutes at room temperature before beginning the warming process. This is to prevent damage to the bag, which is susceptible to cracking or other damage. Once the plasma product is removed from its outer covering it should be placed in a plastic Ziploc bag and then in a warm water bath for thawing. The FFP/FP should not be immersed in water that is >37°C (**Fig. 8.7**). Plasma products should be administered using a blood administration set with a 170 micron inline filter (**Fig. 8.3**) or, for smaller patients, a standard extension set with an inline filter attached, such as a hemonate filter (**Fig. 8.4**). Once the product is thawed it should be used within 4 hours in order to reduce the risk of loss of labile clotting factors and to avoid the increased risk of exponential bacterial growth. The rate of plasma administration is dependent on the patient's immediate need and clinical status; however, the initial rate should be 0.5–1.0 ml/kg/hour to monitor for signs of a reaction. The rate can then be increased to complete the transfusion in the desired time-frame keeping in mind the product should not be at room temperature for longer than 4 hours.

CRYOPRECIPITATE AND CRYOPRECIPITATE-DEPLETED FRESH FROZEN PLASMA (CRYOSUPERNATANT)
Preparation

Cryoprecipitate is prepared by thawing 1 unit of FFP at 4°C and centrifuging it again at 5,000 g for 5 minutes. The centrifuged solution can be separated into precipitated component and cryo-depleted plasma. The precipitated component contains factors VIII, XI, XII, von Willebrand factor, and fibrinogen and is rapidly refrozen and called cryoprecipitate. After the cryoprecipitate is separated, the remaining thawed plasma is called cryo-depleted plasma or cryosupernatant. The factors in the cryoprecipitate are significantly reduced in the cryosupernatant. The cryosupernatant can be used to treat animals with hemophilia B (factor IX deficiency). The remaining precipitate product containing factors VIII, XI, XII, von Willebrand factor, and fibrinogen is rapidly refrozen.

Storage

Cryoprecipitate can be stored at between –20°C and –70°C for up to 1 year.

Indications

Cryoprecipitate is indicated in patients that have von Willebrand's disease, hemophilia A, and hypofibrinogenemia. One advantage to using cryoprecipitate as opposed to whole blood or FFP is the smaller volume required (**Fig. 8.8**).

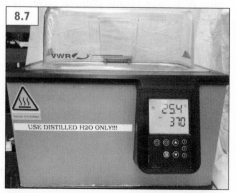

Fig. 8.7 General purpose water bath (VWR, Radnor, Philadelphia).

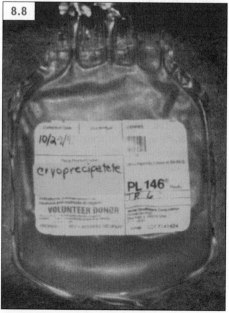

Fig. 8.8 Unit of cryoprecipitate.

Dosing

The recommended dosing for cryoprecipitate is 12–20 ml/kg or 1 unit/10 kg BW. Dosing can be repeated until active bleeding is controlled.

Administration

Cryoprecipitate should be administered similarly to other plasma-containing products as previously indicated.

PLATELET PRODUCTS
Indications

Indications for platelet transfusion include patients with severe thrombocytopenia (platelet counts <20,000/µl) or thrombopathia that are actively bleeding. Platelet transfusions may also be administered to prevent life-threatening hemorrhage in patients with severe thrombocytopenia or thrombopathia that are scheduled to undergo surgical procedures or interventions. Patients receiving massive transfusions (i.e. transfusion of a volume of blood greater than the patient's blood volume in less than 24 hours or transfusion of a volume half that of the patient's blood volume in less than 3 hours) are also candidates for platelet transfusion.

Administration

Administration of lyophilized platelet products should be performed following the recommended product guidelines. This includes handling with aseptic technique and strictly following appropriate reconstitution instructions. Administration of platelet products other than the lyophilized product is the same as administration of other blood products, including the use of a proper filter and monitoring for any signs of a transfusion reaction. Patients should be monitored for evidence of transfusion reactions during administration. (See later section on transfusion reactions for more details.)

See *Table 8.2* for more details on various platelet products, storage, shelf-life, and dosing recommendations.

ALBUMIN PRODUCTS
Preparation

Both canine and human albumin (**Fig. 8.9**) are obtained from pooled plasma.

Indications

Use of albumin is indicated in patients with severe hypoalbuminemia (albumin <10 g/l [1 g/dl]), septic patients, and hypotensive patients that have hypoalbuminemia and require fluid resuscitation.

Dosing

The albumin dose should be calculated based on the patient albumin deficit (see *Table 8.3*).

Administration

Albumin products should be administered using a filtered blood administration set or a standard IV fluid set with an inline filter such as a hemonate filter. The initial rate should be between 0.5 and 1.0 ml/kg/hour for the first 15–30 minutes to monitor for signs of a transfusion reaction. If there are no signs of a transfusion reaction, the rate can be increased such that the transfusion is completed within the desired time. Because albumin products have such a high colloid oncotic pressure it is important to monitor patients receiving this product for signs of volume overload. If the decision is made to administer human serum albumin to a canine patient, it is critical that one realizes this should be done one time and one time only. There are significantly increased risks of canine patients having severe, even anaphylactic reactions if they are administered a human serum albumin product a second time. The risks are increased as the canine develops antibodies. Currently there are very few studies and very limited information available on the administration of human serum albumin products to

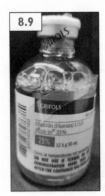

Fig. 8.9 25% Human serum albumin (Grifols, Barcelona, Spain).

Table 8.2 Characteristics of available platelet products

	Fresh whole blood	Fresh platelets	Chilled platelets	Frozen platelets	Cryopreserved platelets	Lyophilized platelets
Storage conditions	Room temperature	22°C, with continuous gentle agitation	4°C	−20 to −30°C	6% DMSO, −80°C	−80°C
Shelf life	4 hours	5 days	8–10 days	6 months	1 year	2 years
Dosing recommendations	10 ml/kg (expected to raise platelet count 10,000/µl)	1 unit per 10 kg body weight	1 unit per 10 kg body weight	1 unit per 10 kg body weight	2.5 units per 10 kg body weight	Based on the concentration of the product and goal platelet count
Advantages	Readily available	Optimal post-transfusion platelet recovery, survival, and function	Decreased risk of bacterial proliferation during storage	Decreased risk of bacterial proliferation during storage; commercially available	Long-term storage; commercially available	Long-term storage; sterility (result of paraformaldehyde stabilization)
Disadvantages	No shelf life; must be used immediately	Short shelf life; limited availability; risk of bacterial proliferation during room temperature storage	Rapidly cleared from circulation; limited availability; short shelf life	Rapidly cleared from circulation	Reduced post-transfusion platelet recovery and half-life; impaired in-vitro function, although evidence of hemostatic efficacy in vivo	Short in-vivo life span of platelets; use limited to control of active hemorrhage; commercial availability of canine product is limited

Table 8.3 Characteristics of canine and human serum albumin products

	5% or 16% canine lyophilized albumin	25% human serum albumin (Fig. 8.9)
Storage conditions	1–26°C	20–24°C
Shelf life	Unreconstituted, 2 years; reconstituted, 6 hours	3 years
Dosing recommendations	Albumin deficit (g) = 10 × (desired albumin g/dl − patient albumin g/dl) × BW (kg) × 0.3 Target albumin is most commonly 2.0 g/dl	Albumin deficit (g) = 10 × (desired albumin g/dl − patient albumin g/dl) × BW (kg) × 0.3 Target albumin is most commonly 2.0 g/dl
Advantages	Less immunogenic for canine patients; commercially available	Commercially available
Disadvantages	Not recommended for use in cats	Greater risk of allergic reaction when compared with canine albumin

feline patients. As a result, administration of human serum albumin should be considered with great caution. There are currently no feline-specific albumin products available.

Transfusion monitoring

Following the recommended guidelines for proper handling and administration of blood products is imperative to minimize the chance of adverse events.

- Baseline information, including, temperature, pulse, pulse quality, respiratory rate, capillary refill time (CRT), mucous membrane color, blood pressure, and pretransfusion PCV/total solids (TS), should be obtained and recorded (**Fig. 8.10**).
- The initial rate should be slow, as indicated above. Temperature, pulse, respiratory rate, CRT, and mucous membrane color should be recorded every 5 minutes for the first 15 minutes, at 30 minutes, and then hourly until the transfusion is complete.
- Monitoring should be continued for 2 hours after the transfusion is complete. Clinical signs of transfusion reactions include fever, increase in body temperature >2°C, tachycardia, hypotension, vomiting, diarrhea, discolored urine, urticaria, and acute changes in respiratory status. These findings should be interpreted in light of the patient's initial clinical status.
- Once the transfusion is successfully completed a PCV/TS should be obtained

1–2 hours post transfusion. Patients receiving plasma-containing products for a coagulopathy should also have clotting

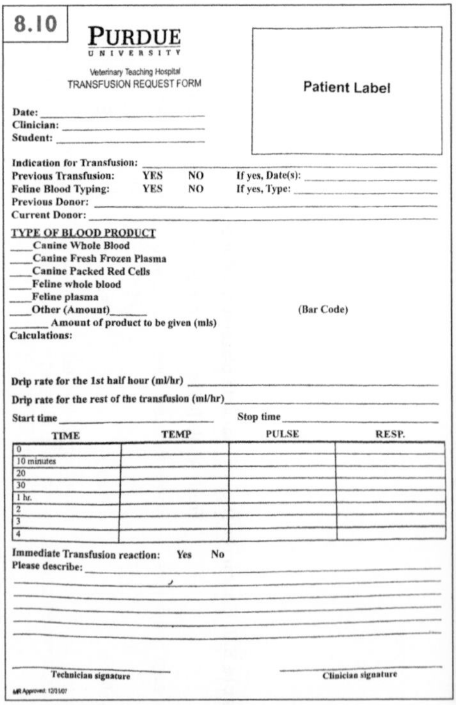

Fig. 8.10 Transfusion recording form.

times re-evaluated. Patients should continue to be monitored closely for 24–48 hours after transfusion to identify delayed reactions.

TRANSFUSION REACTIONS

Types of transfusion reactions, clinical signs, and recommended treatment for transfusion reactions are shown in *Table 8.4.*

Table 8.4 Transfusion reaction types, timing of reaction, clinical signs, and recommended therapies

	Reaction type	Timing from start of transfusion	Clinical signs	Treatment
Immunologic reactions	Allergic, type I hypersensitivity; mild, moderate, severe	Immediate, up to 4 hours after	Tachypnea, dyspnea, bronchospasm, tachycardia, hypotension, fever, cardiac arrhythmia, vomiting, urticarial, pruritus, angioedema, erythema, vomiting	Mild: stop transfusion, diphenhydramine, can usually restart transfusion within 15–30 minutes at slower rate Moderate: stop transfusion, fluids, diphenhydramine, corticosteroids, can try restarting transfusion at slower rate Severe: stop transfusion, fluids, diphenhydramine, corticosteroids, epinephrine, CPR is warranted
	Acute hemolytic	Immediate, up to 24 hours after	Tachypnea, dyspnea, hypotension, tachycardia, fever hemoglobinemia, hemoglobinuria, collapse, shock	Stop the transfusion, administer corticosteroids, IV fluids, vasopressor therapy may be needed to help maintain blood pressure if reaction is severe
	Febrile non-hemolytic transfusion reaction	Immediate, up to 4 hours after	Fever, vomiting, tachypnea, rigors, chill	Stop the transfusion; if signs resolve quickly, the transfusion can be restarted with continued monitoring
	Transfusion-related acute lung injury	Within 2–6 hours	Tachypnea, dyspnea, chills, fever, hypotension	Stop transfusion, oxygen supplementation, some patients may require ventilator support
Non-immunologic reactions	Sepsis/microbial infection	Immediate or can be delayed	Tachypnea, tachycardia, fever, vomiting, shock, collapse	Stop transfusion, remove all suspected contaminated lines and catheters, culture blood and urine from recipient and donor, start broad-spectrum antibiotics, IV fluids, if warranted utilize blood products from different donor
	Citrate toxicity/hypocalcemia	During, up to 6 hours after	Signs associated with hypocalcemia: tremors, fever, cardiac arrhythmias, vomiting, seizures	Stop transfusion, supplement with 10% calcium gluconate and monitor ECG, restart transfusion, monitor calcium* and continue supplementation if warranted

(Continued)

Table 8.4 (Continued) Transfusion reaction types, timing of reaction, clinical signs, and recommended therapies

	Reaction type	Timing from start of transfusion	Clinical signs	Treatment
Non-immunologic reactions	Transfusion-associated circulatory overload	Within 2 to 6 hours	Tachypnea, dyspnea, tachycardia, jugular venous distention, nasal discharge, pulmonary crackles/edema	Stop transfusion, administer diuretics with or without vasodilators, can try restarting transfusion at slower rate if appropriate or choose different blood product
	Hypothermia	Immediate, up to 4 hours after	Depression, shivering, low body temperature	Stop transfusion, begin external warming, administer warm fluids, administer warm blood products (not beyond 37°C) when restarting transfusion
	Hypophosphatemia	During, up to 6 hours after	Clinical signs associated with anemia as a result of destruction/lysis of red blood cells	Stop transfusion, supplement phosphorus using sodium phosphate or potassium phosphate and monitor phosphorus
	Hyperkalemia	During, up to 4 hours after	Bradycardia, cardiac arrhythmias, ECG changes	Stop transfusion, administer 0.9% NaCl IV, dextrose and insulin, monitor potassium

* Most ideal to monitor ionized calcium.

Safe transfusion practices

Although transfusions may be lifesaving, there are inherent risks. Blood products should be obtained from sources that screen donors appropriately and blood typing and cross matching should be utilized to reduce the risk of potential complications associated with transfusion administration. Autologous blood transfusions can also be considered as a viable option.

BLOOD TYPING
- Dogs have more than 12 different blood type groups referred to as dog erythrocyte antigens (DEAs). (See *Table 8.5* for a list of the most common canine blood types.) Canine erythrocytes are either positive or negative for each DEA.
- In dogs, DEA 1.1-positive is the most common blood type. Dogs with DEA 1.1-negative blood are considered 'universal' donors. Conversely, dogs with DEA 1.1-positive blood type are considered universal recipients. Acute hemolysis may result if the blood type

is transfused incorrectly. Luckily, in dogs naturally-occurring antibodies against DEA 1.1 are rare; therefore, severe antigen–antibody reactions are less likely to occur on initial transfusion. Blood typing cards are available for DEA 1 typing of dogs (DMS Laboratories, Flemington, New Jersey); however, false positives may occur. There is also a non-chromatographic strip-based test (Alvedia, Lyon, France) for in-clinic use that has been reported to be more reliable.
- Testing for the other blood type groups requires sending blood samples to outside laboratories (Animal Blood Resources International, Dixon, California). Cross matching can be very helpful when blood typing for other blood groups is not available.
- Cats have three blood types: A, B, and AB. Type A is most common. Cats have naturally-occurring antibodies, which means that cats that are blood type A have anti-type B antibodies, and vice versa.

Table 8.5 Most common canine blood types

Dog erythrocyte antigen	Incidence (%)
1.1	42
1.2	20
3	6
4	98
5	23
6	98–99
7	45
8	40

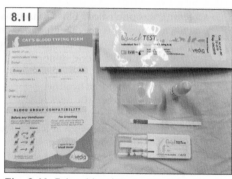

Fig. 8.11 Feline blood typing kit (Alvedia, Lyon, France).

As a result, transfusing a type A cat with type B blood or a type B cat with type A blood may result in a severe acute hemolytic reaction that could result in death. For this reason, it is imperative that every cat is blood typed prior to receiving a blood transfusion.

- Cats that have type AB blood are considered universal recipients. If type specific blood is not available, type AB cats should receive type A blood. To facilitate the ease of blood typing there are rapid blood typing cards available for use in practice (**Fig. 8.11**).
- It is important to remember that blood typing does not negate the need to perform a cross match.

CROSS MATCHING

- This test allows establishment of serologic compatibility between the transfusion recipient and the blood donor in order to decrease the risk of a transfusion reaction.
- Cross matching identifies the presence of alloantibodies. A major cross match tests for alloantibodies in the recipient's plasma against the donor's RBCs, and a minor cross match tests

for alloantibodies in the donor's plasma against the recipient's RBCs.
- A major cross match is therefore most important when transfusing RBCs. A major and minor cross match is recommended if whole blood is being transfused. A minor cross match is recommended for plasma transfusions; however, this is rarely performed.
- The most common method is a manual procedure that includes washing steps and an incubation step, but the procedure is not standardized between laboratories. Recently, a tube gel method (DMS Laboratories) and a strip (Alvedia) cross match method have become available. These methods are still undergoing evaluation. To date there is no definitive recommended gold standard for cross match procedures in veterinary patients.
- Cross matching is recommended in dogs and cats if the transfusion history is unknown, if the animal has received a previous transfusion more than 7 days before, or if a hemolytic reaction is known to have occurred with a previous transfusion. It should also be performed in dogs if the donor blood type is unknown (donor is not a universal donor).

Safe sources of blood products

Canine and feline blood products can be obtained from commercial blood banks, practice blood banks, or healthy clinic patients. All pets should be appropriately screened before becoming blood donors.

BLOOD DONORS

- In 2016, an update on the 2005 American College of Veterinary Internal Medicine (ACVIM) Consensus Statement on blood donor infectious disease screening was published. This Consensus Statement intends to provide guidance on appropriate blood-borne pathogen testing for canine and feline blood donors in North America.

- Blood donors should be healthy adult animals between the ages of 2 and 7 years. Dogs should be at least 30 kg and cats should weigh at least 5 kg. Prospective donors should never have received a blood transfusion and should be up to date on routine vaccines.
- Screening should include gathering a history including travel history, a physical examination, blood typing, CBC, chemistry profile, urinalysis, and fecal flotation. Infectious disease testing depends on the geographic area and the pet's travel history.
- Standard testing in dogs includes *Anaplasma* spp., *Babesia* spp., *Bartonella* spp., *Ehrlichia* spp., *Hepatozoon canis/americanum, Leishmania donovani, Mycoplasma* spp., *Neorickettsia risticii, Rickettsia felis, Trypanosoma cruzi, Brucella canis* (breeding animals). Recommended testing for cats includes feline leukemia virus, feline immunodeficiency virus, feline infectious peritonitis, *Mycoplasma haemofelis, Anaplasma* spp., *Cytauxzoon felis, Ehrlichia canis, Hemoplasmas,* and *Bartonella* spp.
- While in the program, each animal should have a complete physical examination, routine vaccination, and minimum database evaluated at least once a year, as well as follow-up disease testing.
- Donors should be fed a complete and balanced diet and supplemented with ferrous sulfate if donating more frequently than every 6–8 weeks. Prior to blood collection the donor should have a brief physical examination and a PCV/TS.
- Indications to postpone blood collection include a fever (temperature >39°C [102.5°F]), PCV <0.4 l/l (40%), TS <130 g/l (13 g/dl), or any other new findings on physical examination.

AUTOLOGOUS BLOOD TRANSFUSION

- Autologous blood transfusions may be considered in emergency situations when blood products are limited or unavailable.
- The advantages of autotransfusion include immediate availability, the decreased risk of transfusion reactions, and decreased cost. Patients that have sustained trauma, have postoperative hemorrhage, or those with a coagulopathy resulting in hemorrhage into a body cavity (hemoabdomen, hemothorax) are the best candidates for autotransfusion.
- Ideally patients suffering from a coagulopathy should be treated for the coagulopathy prior to harvesting the blood and auto transfusing, although this is not an absolute requirement as long as the patient is being treated appropriately (i.e. receiving FFP/FP for therapy simultaneously). It is not recommended to autotransfuse patients with blood that may be contaminated with urine, feces, bile, bacteria, purulent material, or neoplastic cells.
- Blood should be collected from the patient aseptically and handled aseptically at all times up to and including reinfusion to the patient. After collection it can be placed in a bag for delivery or delivered directly from the syringe.
- The blood should be reinfused IV through a proper blood filter as described earlier. The filter may need to be changed frequently during reinfusion as blood clots often occlude the filter. Anticoagulant may be needed if the patient is actively bleeding; however, no anticoagulant may be required if the blood being syphoned from the patient has been present in the body cavity for at least an hour.
- There are several techniques described in the literature including the use of cell salvage collection systems. However, a simple and efficient technique described utilizes a two-syringe technique. Blood is removed from the body cavity utilizing a 60 ml catheter tip syringe making removal easier and the blood is then transferred to a standard luer-lock syringe by inserting the end of the luer tip into the catheter tip. The blood can be reinfused as rapidly as needed, particularly if the patient is critically unstable.

- Autologous transfusions can be pre-emptively planned. Blood can be obtained from a patient and stored 2–4 weeks prior to a planned surgical procedure or intervention that places the patient at risk for significant blood loss.

MASSIVE TRANSFUSIONS

- Patients that suffer loss of blood volumes close to or equal to their total blood volume require massive transfusions as a life saving measure.
- The term 'massive transfusion' has been defined in a number of ways including:
  - transfusion of a volume of whole blood or blood products that is equal to or exceeds the patients total blood volume within 24 hours;
  - replacement of ½ a blood volume in 3–4 hours, and lastly;
  - infusion of 1.5 ml/kg/minute of blood products within a 20 minute time period. Though giving a massive transfusion can be a lifesaving measure, it also comes with a plethora of potential complications that can contribute to creating life-threatening pathologic changes. (See *Table 8.6* for a list of complications associated with large volume blood transfusions.)
- The pathology associated with massive transfusions has been well documented in the human literature. Massive hemorrhage (volume loss) leads to severe anemia, which leads to poor oxygen carrying capacity, poor tissue perfusion, and hypotension resulting in the 'lethal triad' (hypothermia, coagulopathy, and acidosis).
- Occurrence of the lethal triad is well documented to be associated with increased mortality. Infusion of crystalloids and large volumes of blood products can cause and worsen dilutional coagulopathy, thrombocytopenia, and the various metabolic derangements and hypothermia, perpetuating a vicious cycle.
- Recommendations for management of massive transfusions in humans include administration of blood products (RBCs, plasma, and platelets) in a 1:1:1 ratio. (See *Table 8.7* for a list of suggested monitoring and targets for patients receiving massive transfusions.)

Table 8.6 Complications associated with massive or large-volume blood transfusion

Electrolyte abnormalities	Hypocalcemia Hyperkalemia Hypokalemia Hypomagnesemia
Hyperammonemia	
Hemostatic defects	Thrombocytopenia Secondary coagulopathy Hyperfibrinolysis Factor VIII deficiency
Hypothermia	
Acid–base status	Metabolic acidosis Metabolic alkalosis
Transfusion reactions	Allergic Acute or delayed hemolytic Febrile non-hemolytic transfusion reaction
Transfusion-related acute lung injury	
Transfusion-related immunomodulation	Immunosuppression
Transfusion-associated circulatory overload	
Bacterial contamination	
Infectious disease transmission	

Table 8.7 Recommended monitoring and targets for massive transfusion-treated patients

Temperature	>35°C (95°F)
Acid–base status	pH >7.2, base excess <–6, lactate <4 mmol/l (36 mg/dl)
Ionized calcium	>1.1
Hemoglobin	This should not be used alone as the transfusion trigger, but should be interpreted in context with hemodynamic status and organ and tissue perfusion
Platelet count	>50,000 × 10^9/l (500 × 10^5/µl)
PT/aPTT	<1.5 × normal
International normalized ratio	<1.5
Fibrinogen	>10 g/l (1 g/dl)

aPTT, activated partial thromboplastin time; PT, prothrombin time.

Further reading

Beer KS, Silverstein DC (2015) Controversies in the use of fresh frozen plasma in critically ill small animal patients. *J Vet Emerg Crit Care* **25(1)**:101–6.

Davidow B (2013) Transfusion medicine in small animals. *Vet Clin North Am Sm Anim Pract* **43(4)**:735–6.

Giger U (2015) Transfusion therapy. In: *Small Animal Critical Care Medicine*, 2nd edn. (eds. D Silverstein, K Hopper) Elsevier, St. Louis, pp. 327–32.

McMichael M (2015) Prevention and treatment of transfusion reactions. In: *Small Animal Critical Care Medicine*, 2nd edn. (eds. D Silverstein, K Hopper) Elsevier, St. Louis, pp. 333–7.

Pham HP, Shaz BH (2013) Update on massive transfusion. *British J of Anaesth* **111(suppl 1)**:i71–82.

Robinson DA, Keifer K, Quandt J (2016) Autotransfusion in dogs using a 2-syringe technique. *J Vet Emerg Crit Care* **26(6)**:766–74.

Savage WJ (2016) Transfusion reactions. *Hematol Oncol Clin N Am* **30**:619–34.

Wardrop KJ, Birkenheuer A, Blais MC *et al.* (2016) Update on canine and feline blood donor screening for blood-borne pathogens – Consensus Statement. *J Vet Intern Med* **30**:15–35.

Zenithson Y Ng, Stokes J E, Alvarez L *et al.* (2016) Cryopreserved platelet concentrate transfusions in 43 dogs: a retrospective study. *J Vet Emerg Crit Care* **26(5)**:720–8.

Injectable sedative and anesthesia–analgesia combinations in dogs and cats

Jeff C Ko

Introduction

Injectable anesthesia is an alternative to inhalant anesthesia. It differs from inhalant general anesthesia because it combines the steps of premedication, induction, and maintenance together without using inhalant equipment and inhalant anesthetic agents. However, doses of injectable anesthetic agents can be calculated that will induce various degrees of sedation sufficient to achieve both invasive and non-invasive procedures. (**Note:** Injectable anesthesia can also be used as a premedication prior to IV induction and inhalant anesthesia [see Chapter 3].) In addition, it can be used to induce general anesthesia that is suitable for surgery. As with inhalant anesthesia, injectable anesthesia for surgical procedures should achieve three specific goals: unconsciousness, muscle relaxation, and analgesia. An ideal injectable anesthetic combination should achieve these three goals, but also allow a rapid and smooth recovery in dogs and cats.

Injectable sedative–anesthetic–analgesic combinations can be broadly divided into two pharmacologic groups. One group uses dexmedetomidine or medetomidine as the primary drug, while the other group uses tiletamine/zolazepam as the primary drug. This chapter covers both sedative and injectable anesthesia and includes a review of various sedative–anesthetic combinations with indications, contraindications, and the dosages of these combinations in dogs and cats.

Dexmedetomidine (and medetomidine)-based protocols

Both dexmedetomidine and medetomidine have brand and generic products available worldwide. Dexmedetomidine and medetomidine can be either used alone or be combined with other sedatives or analgesics to produce mild, moderate, or profound sedation. They can also extend a surgical plane of anesthesia when the appropriate dose rates of these combinations are used. The sedative protocols usually involve lower dosages than the injectable anesthetic combinations. The analgesic effects of dexmedetomidine and medetomidine last approximately 1 hour into the postoperative period if the drugs are not reversed with the antagonist atipamezole.

Dexmedetomidine (or medetomidine) and ketamine are suitable for use in generally healthy, exercise-tolerant dogs and cats for sedation or chemical restraint during clinical examination, for radiography, and for minor surgical procedures. These anesthetic combinations can also be used to achieve a surgical plane of anesthesia for rapid immobilization, non-invasive procedures, or for a wide range of invasive surgical procedures (e.g. ovariohysterectomy, castration, wound repair, dental procedures, orthopedic examinations and surgeries, soft tissue or bone biopsies). When microdoses of dexmedetomidine (or medetomidine) are used, these drugs can be combined with diazepam, midazolam, or opioids for sedation or chemical restraint of sick or diseased dogs and cats.

DEXMEDETOMIDINE (OR MEDETOMIDINE)–KETAMINE COMBINATIONS

- The dexmedetomidine–ketamine and medetomidine–ketamine combinations that can be used in dogs and cats are listed in *Tables 9.1* and *9.2*.

Patient selection, purpose of use, dosages, and route of administration

- Dexmedetomidine (medetomidine)–ketamine injectable combinations can be used in generally healthy, exercise-tolerant dogs and cats <12 years old (and for giant breed dogs <6 years old). Geriatric animals should receive either reduced doses of

Table 9.1 Medetomidine–ketamine combinations in dogs and cats

Species	Medetomidine (µg/kg)	Ketamine (mg/kg)
Dog	10–20 IV 30–40 IM	1–2 IV 3–4 IM
Cat	30–50 IV 40–80 IM	2–3 IV 3–5 IM

Table 9.2 Dexmedetomidine–ketamine combinations in dogs and cats

Species	Dexmedetomidine (µg/kg)	Ketamine (mg/kg)
Dog	5–10 IV 15–20 IM	1–2 IV 3–4 IM
Cat	15–25 IV 20–40 IM	2–3 IV 3–5 IM

dexmedetomidine or medetomidine or another drug combination.
- Low-dose combinations induce profound sedation suitable to facilitate radiographic procedures such as hip radiographs. Alternatively, the low dose can be used as a preanesthetic medication to induce sedation and facilitate catheterization, reduce stress, and facilitate IV induction for endotracheal intubation.
- High-dose combinations induce a surgical plane of anesthesia suitable for castration, ovariohysterectomy, and other abdominal or soft tissue surgical procedures. This is particularly useful in trap–neuter–release clinics where feral cats and stray dogs need chemical immobilization prior to surgery. The duration of the surgical plane of anesthesia is approximately 20–25 minutes following a single IM administration.
- These combinations induce a rapid onset of lateral recumbency (5–8 minutes if IM and 1–2 minutes if IV) following administration and are useful for reliable IM immobilization of an aggressive dog or cat.
- IV doses induce a more rapid onset of action with a more intense effect and slightly shorter duration of surgery (10–15 minutes), with an associated quick recovery.

- Endotracheal intubation is consistently achieved within 5–8 minutes of IM administration of the high-dose combinations, with the animal reaching a surgical plane of anesthesia immediately after lateral recumbency. As such, the combination should not be administered until a few minutes before planned surgery. The animal should be intubated and maintained with 100% oxygen on an anesthesia machine or a similar device, as oxygenation is desirable. If an animal under injectable anesthesia shows signs of premature awakening, one-half of the original dose of dexmedetomidine–ketamine or medetomidine–ketamine can be administered either IM or IV to extend sedation or anesthesia for an additional 5–10 minutes. Alternatively, isoflurane (1%) or sevoflurane (2%) can be supplemented at a lower percentage to extend the surgical plane of anesthesia if an anesthesia machine is available.
- Due to the endogenous catecholamine release stimulated by ketamine, heart rate (HR) remains between 70 and 100 beats per minute during anesthesia with the dexmedetomidine–ketamine or medetomidine–ketamine combinations in dogs. While a pronounced sinus arrhythmia may occur as the ketamine is metabolized, HR remains higher than during anesthesia with a dexmedetomidine–butorphanol (or medetomidine–butorphanol) combination in dogs.
- Cats being given these combinations maintain a relatively normal HR because they are less sensitive to the cardiovascular effects of dexmedetomidine or medetomidine than dogs, and the HR does not decrease as much as in dogs receiving the same combination.
- This combination induces excellent muscle relaxation and is suitable for orthopedic examinations and also provides analgesia during moderately painful surgical procedures.
- While this drug combination induces excellent muscle relaxation once it takes full effect, occasionally dogs highly sensitive to ketamine may

have seizure-like activity. If this does occur, a supplement of a half-dose of dexmedetomidine or medetomidine can be given IM to counteract the ketamine effect. Alternatively, diazepam or midazolam (0.2–0.4 mg/kg IV) can be administered to resolve the issue and proceed with the planned anesthetic event.
- Since dexmedetomidine and medetomidine act on alpha-2 adrenoreceptors in the peripheral vasculature, blanching of the mucous membranes is apparent when using these combinations and the blood pressure tends to be high, with all three pressures (systolic, mean, and diastolic) in the 90–140 mmHg range.

Reversal of dexmedetomidine–ketamine and medetomidine–ketamine combinations with atipamezole

- Dexmedetomidine–ketamine and medetomidine–ketamine combinations are reversible with atipamezole. (**Note:** In dogs, reversal with atipamezole should not be attempted until at least 40 minutes after the administration of ketamine [higher than 3–4 mg/kg].)
- Reversal is achieved with the same volume of atipamezole (or 10 times the milligram dose of dexmedetomidine or 5 times medetomidine).
- Ketamine provides a degree of postoperative analgesia following reversal of dexmedetomidine or medetomidine, but it also has a side-effect of hangover (see below).
- If not reversed, the animal remains in lateral recumbency for approximately 1.5 hours, walking normally within 2.5 hours of the initial IM drug administration. With IV administration, the recovery is approximately 30 minutes shorter.
- Ketamine undergoes extensive hepatic biotransformation in dogs. Ketamine 'hangover' (carry-over) effect will occur if reversal of dexmedetomidine takes place earlier than 40 minutes after the administration of the dexmedetomidine–ketamine combination. This hangover

effect is characterized by typical dissociative signs with salivation, head shaking/bobbing, tongue flicking, vocalization, muscle rigidity, and sometimes seizures. If this situation occurs, the animal should be treated with diazepam or midazolam (0.4 mg/kg IV) to alleviate these hangover signs. Repeated injections of diazepam or midazolam may be necessary to attenuate these severe side-effects.

- Cats metabolize ketamine differently to dogs (more quickly – relatively unconjugated in the liver and excreted through the kidney), so these combinations can be reversed at any time in cats without significant signs of a ketamine hangover.
- Hypothermia can occur if an animal is not reversed and not kept warmed. It is necessary to provide a towel or blanket with an exogenous heat source (e.g. water heating blanket or forced hot air warmer) during recovery. (See Chapter 6 for more information on managing body temperature.)

Differences between dexmedetomidine–ketamine and medetomidine–ketamine

- Medetomidine is a racemic mixture containing levomedetomidine. Studies have shown that levomedetomidine interferes with the hepatic metabolism of ketamine. As a result, dexmedetomidine–ketamine treated animals recover faster than those treated with medetomidine–ketamine.
- While the recovery time is faster with dexmedetomidine–ketamine, the total duration of surgical anesthesia is as long or longer than with medetomidine–ketamine.

DEXMEDETOMIDINE (MEDETOMIDINE)–BUTORPHANOL

- Doses for the dexmedetomidine–butorphanol and medetomidine–butorphanol combinations that can be used in dogs and cats are listed in *Tables 9.3* and *9.4*.

Table 9.3 Medetomidine–butorphanol combinations in dogs and cats

Species	Medetomidine (µg/kg)	Butorphanol (mg/kg)
Dog	10–20 IV	0.1–0.2 IV
	30–40 IM	0.3–0.4 IM
Cat	30–50 IV	0.2–0.3 IV
	40–80 IM	0.3–0.4 IM

Table 9.4 Dexmedetomidine–butorphanol combinations in dogs and cats

Species	Dexmedetomidine (µg/kg)	Butorphanol (mg/kg)
Dog	5–10 IV	0.1–0.2 IV
	15–20 IM	0.3–0.4 IM
Cat	15–25 IV	0.2–0.3 IV
	20–40 IM	0.3–0.4 IM

Patient selection, purpose of use, dosages, and route of administration

- Similar patient selection criteria as with the of dexmedetomidine–ketamine and medetomidine–ketamine combinations.
- These drug combinations can be mixed in the same syringe and administered to a dog or a cat as a single injection either IV or IM.
- The combination induces a rapid onset of lateral recumbency (within 5–8 minutes of IM administration or within 1–2 minutes of IV administration).
- As with the dexmedetomidine–ketamine (and medetomidine–ketamine) combination, this combination also provides rapid, reliable immobilization of aggressive dogs or cats. The muscle relaxation is profound and is suitable for radiography, orthopedic examination, bandage changes, and wound or laceration repair.
- Depending on the dose selected (*Table 9.3* or *9.4*), the sedated dogs and cats can be intubated and a light plane of anesthesia suitable for minor surgical procedures achieved for a duration of 20–25 minutes.
- Dogs and cats sedated with this combination have a lower HR than those anesthetized with a dexmedetomidine (medetomidine)–ketamine combination, but the blood pressure is similarly high with both combinations.

Reversal of dexmedetomidine–butorphanol and medetomidine–butorphanol combinations with atipamezole

- Unlike the dexmedetomidine–ketamine or medetomidine–ketamine combinations, dexmedetomidine– or medetomidine–butorphanol can be reversed at any time after the completion of the procedure.
- Reversal is achieved with the same volume of atipamezole (or 10 times the milligram dose of dexmedetomidine or 5 times medetomidine).
- Butorphanol provides a degree of postoperative analgesia following reversal. The same dose of butorphanol can be given to provide additional analgesia.
- If not reversed, the animal remains in lateral recumbency for approximately 1 hour and is walking normally within 2 hours from the initial drug administration.
- Hypothermia can occur if exogenous heat is not provided and should be addressed by providing a towel or blanket with an exogenous heat source (e.g. circulating water heating blanket or forced hot air warmer) during the recovery.
- Note that the higher doses of this combination are associated with greater cardiorespiratory depressive effects than doses at the lower end of the range.
- As with other injectable combinations, a low dose of isoflurane (1%) or sevoflurane (2%) will extend the duration of the surgical plane of anesthesia if required.

Differences between dexmedetomidine (medetomidine)–ketamine and dexmedetomidine (medetomidine)–butorphanol

- There are minimal differences in the analgesia, blood pressure, and respiratory rates associated with these two combinations. However, pharmacologically, dexmedetomidine (or medetomidine)–butorphanol is considered only a sedative combination instead of an injectable general anesthetic combination because neither the alpha-2 agonists nor the opioid is a general anesthetic agent.
- HR remains higher (average 30 beats higher per minute) with the ketamine combinations than with the butorphanol combinations.
- Butorphanol combinations can be reversed with atipamezole at any time in dogs, but ketamine combinations should not be reversed within 40 minutes of administration in dogs.

DEXMEDETOMIDINE (MEDETOMIDINE)–BUTORPHANOL–MIDAZOLAM (OR DIAZEPAM) SEDATIVE COMBINATION

- The dosages for dexmedetomidine (and medetomidine)–butorphanol–midazolam and dexmedetomidine (and medetomidine)–butorphanol–diazepam combinations in healthy dogs and cats are listed in *Table 9.5*.

Patient selection, purpose of use, dosages and route of administration

- This combination reduces the dose required for dexmedetomidine or medetomidine by replacing it with

Table 9.5 Dosages for dexmedetomidine (medetomidine)–butorphanol–midazolam combinations in healthy dogs and cats

Species	Dexmedetomidine (medetomidine) (μg/kg)	Butorphanol (mg/kg)	Midazolam (diazepam) (mg/kg)
Dog	2.5–5 IV (5–10 IV) 5–10 IM (10–20 IM)	0.2 IV 0.3 IM	0.2 IV 0.4 IM
Cat	10–15 IV (20–30 IV) 20–25 IM (40–50 IM)	0.2 IV 0.3 IM	0.2 IV 0.4 IM

Note: All of these drugs can be collected in one syringe for a single injection unless a diazepam with propylene glycol formulation is being used, in which case the diazepam must be administered in a separate syringe.

midazolam or diazepam. It is preferred in patients that cannot tolerate higher doses of dexmedetomidine or medetomidine.

- It provides analgesia equivalent to the dexmedetomidine (medetomidine)–butorphanol combinations, but induces less cardiorespiratory depression since less dexmedetomidine (medetomidine) is used.
- Following IM injection, dogs or cats can be intubated and they reach a profound sedation that lasts 20–25 minutes. If the combination is administered IM, the animal can be intubated and maintained on 100% oxygen only. If a deeper plane of anesthesia is required for surgery, it can be extended by using a low concentration of isoflurane (1%) or sevoflurane (2%), increasing the vaporizer volume percentage as needed.
- The sedation and muscle relaxation seen with this combination is attributable to both dexmedetomidine's (or medetomidine's) effects on alpha-2 adrenergic receptors and midazolam's (or diazepam's) effects on gamma aminobutyric acid (GABA) receptors in the CNS.
- As with the butorphanol combinations discussed above, bradycardia is seen, but is typically less profound since less dexmedetomidine (medetomidine) is used.
- Diazepam is often available combined with a propylene glycol (PG) vehicle. Precipitation will occur when mixing this formulation of diazepam with any of the drugs in this combination, and the diazepam should be administered separately from the other anesthetic agents. Midazolam is water soluble and does not precipitate when mixed in the same syringe with any of these agents.

DOG-SPECIFIC DEXMEDETOMIDINE COMBINATIONS
Dexmedetomidine–butorphanol–ketamine (also called 'doggie magic', Table 9.6)

- This is a combination using dexmedetomidine, butorphanol (10 mg/ml) and ketamine. As an alternative to butorphanol, the same volume of morphine (15 mg/ml) or hydromorphone (2 mg/ml) can be used

in the same combination, despite their different concentration.

- The advantages of adding ketamine to the dexmedetomidine and butorphanol combination when compared with just dexmedetomidine–butorphanol are better analgesia with a higher HR and a more consistent level of sedation/anesthesia.
- The drugs in this combination are mixed in the same syringe and administered as a single IM injection. Depending on the dosage selected, this drug combination rapidly induces a degree of anesthesia ranging from mild sedation to a surgical plane of anesthesia. Guidelines for IM dosing rates of dexmedetomidine, based on the body surface area, range from 62.5–500 $\mu g/m^2$, which approximates to 2.5–20 $\mu g/kg$ (*Table 9.7*):
  - 62.5 and 125 $\mu g/m^2$ of dexmedetomidine with the same volume of butorphanol (10 mg/ml) and ketamine (100 mg/ml) provides mild sedation. Alternatively, it can be used as a premedication prior to IV induction and inhalant anesthesia maintenance.
  - 250 $\mu g/m^2$ of dexmedetomidine with the same volume of butorphanol (10 mg/ml) and ketamine (100 mg/ml) provides profound sedation for suture removal, positioning for hip radiographs and minor surgical procedures such as joint taps and simple laceration repair.
  - 375 and 500 $\mu g/m^2$ of dexmedetomidine with the same volume of butorphanol (10 mg/ml) and ketamine (100 mg/ml) provides a surgical plane of anesthesia for procedures lasting 30–40 minutes (e.g. ovariohysterectomy).
- Dexmedetomidine doses are based on an animal's body surface area (m^2) to minimize variations in sedative and analgesic effects. (See *Table 9.6* for IM dosages based on body weight.) The weight range and sedation desired is selected to determine the volume of drugs required. For IV administration, the volume is reduced by one-half of the IM dose, thus decreasing the total dose.

Table 9.6 Drug volumes (ml) for dexmedetomidine alone or in combination with butorphanol, ketamine, or butorphanol and ketamine for various degrees of sedation–anesthesia in dogs

Weight (kg) (lb)	Minimal sedation (62.5 µg/m²)	Mild sedation (125 µg/m²)	Moderate sedation (250 µg/m²)	Surgical anesthesia (375 µg/m²)	Surgical anesthesia (500 µg/m²)
1–2 (2–4)	0.01	0.02	0.04	0.06	0.075
2–3 (4–7)	0.02	0.04	0.08	0.12	0.15
3–4 (7–9)	0.025	0.05	0.10	0.15	0.20
4–5 (9–11)	0.035	0.07	0.14	0.20	0.30
5–10 (11–22)	0.05	0.10	0.20	0.29	0.40
10–13 22–29)	0.065	0.13	0.26	0.38	0.50
13–15 (29–33)	0.075	0.15	0.30	0.44	0.60
15–20 (33–44)	0.085	0.17	0.34	0.51	0.70
20–25 (44–55)	0.10	0.20	0.40	0.60	0.80
25–30 (55–66)	0.115	0.23	0.46	0.69	0.90
30–33 (66–73)	0.125	0.25	0.50	0.75	1.00
33–37 (73–81)	0.135	0.27	0.54	0.81	1.10
37–45 (81–89)	0.15	0.30	0.60	0.90	1.20
45–50 (99–110)	0.165	0.33	0.66	0.99	1.30
50–55 (110–121)	0.175	0.35	0.70	1.06	1.40
55–60 (121–132)	0.19	0.38	0.76	1.13	1.50
60–65 (132–143)	0.20	0.40	0.80	1.19	1.60
65–70 (143–154)	0.21	0.42	0.84	1.26	1.70
70–80 (154–176)	0.225	0.45	0.90	1.35	1.80
>80 (>176)	0.235	0.47	0.94	1.42	1.90

Select the body weight to determine the drug volume according to the degree of sedation required. If using dexmedetomidine in combination with butorphanol (10 mg/ml), with or without ketamine, use the same volume for each drug.

All injections given IM. For IV injection reduce the calculated volume by half.

Medetomidine can be used to replace dexmedetomidine in this Table.

Table 9.7 Degree of sedation associated with the various dosages of dexmedetomidine in healthy dogs. The dose rate expressed with body surface area (µg/m²) is shown to approximate with body weight in µg/kg

Dose rate (µg/m²) ~ (µg/kg)	Degree of sedation
62.5 ~ 2.5	Very mild (suitable for geriatric and sick dogs, but does not induce reliable sedation for young, healthy dogs)
125 ~ 5	Mild
250 ~ 10	Moderate
375 ~ 15	Profound
500 ~ 20	Profound sedation suitable for mildly invasive procedures

- To calculate the dose for the weight of dog listed in *Table 9.6*, look up the body weight in kg or lb, decide what degree of sedation or anesthesia needed, and then select the value listed that matches up with the body weight as each drug volume. For example, a 13 kg (29 lb) dog presented for an abdominal surgical procedure should receive 0.38 ml of dexmedetomidine, 0.38 ml of butorphanol, and 0.38 ml of ketamine IM. All three drugs are administered at the same volume as a single injection. If this 13 kg dog is more excited and restless, a slightly high dose rate, using *Table 9.6*, can be administered. Therefore, instead of using volumes of 0.38 ml of dexmedetomidine, butorphanol, and ketamine, by moving the body weight to the next level (i.e. 13–15 kg, see *Table 9.6*), 0.44 ml of dexmedetomidine, 0.44 ml of butorphanol, and 0.44 ml of ketamine can be given.

- Dexmedetomidine is twice as potent as medetomidine. The current formulation of dexmedetomidine (0.5 mg/ml) allows it to be used in place of medetomidine (1 mg/ml) at the same volume. Therefore, *Table 9.6* can also be used to calculate the dose for the medetomidine–butorphanol–ketamine combination.
- Following IV administration of this combination (at the dose rate of 250 µg/m² or higher), anesthesia occurs within 2–3 minutes and endotracheal intubation can be achieved at that time.
- Placing an IV catheter may pose a slight challenge due to the associated vasoconstriction of alpha-2 drugs (dexmedetomidine or medetomidine). Vasoconstriction is more pronounced during the surgical plane of anesthesia when dexmedetomidine activity reaches a peak.
- The surgical plane of anesthesia (doses of 375–500 µg/m²) is achieved within 5–8 minutes following IM administration and is maintained for approximately 30–40 minutes after drug administration.
- The dog can be intubated, allowed to breathe room air, or, for best results, provided with 100% oxygen.
- For painful procedures lasting >30–40 minutes, it is important to provide supplemental isoflurane or additional injectable anesthetic combination (give one-half of the original injectable combination volume IV or IM for a 15 minute extension) to prevent 'sudden awakening'. Isoflurane can be started immediately on induction of anesthesia if a long duration of anesthesia is

anticipated. The isoflurane is started at 0.5%, increasing it by 0.25% every 15 minutes until 1.75% is reached. Similarly, sevoflurane can be provided immediately at 1.5–2.0%, increasing it by 0.5% every 15 minutes until 3.75% is reached. A surgical plane of anesthesia can the be maintained with 1.5–1.75% isoflurane or 3.75–4.0% sevoflurane.

- Apnea is the hallmark of an anesthetic overdose and can occur when injectable and inhalant anesthetic agents are used in combination if their combined dose-sparing effects are not taken into consideration:
  - If apnea occurs while an inhalant anesthetic agent is being used, the vaporizer off should be turned off and the animal ventilated (4–6 times per minute) until it resumes spontaneous breathing. If the apnea occurs after injectable anesthetic combinations, the animal should be intubated and ventilated until spontaneous breathing resumes. Ideally, providing 100% oxygen with ventilation is the best practice.
  - Ventilating an apneic animal induced by an inhalant anesthetic agent eliminates the majority (97–99%) of the inhalant, allowing the animal to return to a lighter plane of anesthesia.
  - Once spontaneous breathing has resumed, reinstate the inhalant anesthetic concentration at a vaporizer dial setting of 0.5–0.75% less than that of the vaporizer dial setting before the apnea occurred.
- Atipamezole can be used to reverse the dexmedetomidine component of the combination. If not reversed with atipamezole, recovery to walking will take approximately 2.5 hours from the time of drug administration at the 375 and 500 µg/m² dose rates. A recovery time of 1.5 hours occurs after administration at the 250 µg/m² dose rate.
- As this combination contains ketamine, dogs should not be reversed within 45 minutes of ketamine administration.

Advantages of the 'doggie magic' anesthetic combination

- All three components of this combination provide analgesia acting at different mechanism of the pain pathway, contributing to true multimodal analgesia for surgery.
- The alpha-2 agonist (dexmedetomidine or medetomidine) acts on the alpha-2 agonist receptors to induce sedation, muscle relaxation, and analgesia.
- The opioid (butorphanol) acts on the kappa receptors to induce analgesia. As a sole agent, butorphanol is only capable of treating mild to moderate pain, but when combined with the other anesthetic agents in this combination, it acts synergistically to enhance the analgesia of the other two agents and profound analgesia is induced. Using butorphanol rather than a more potent opioid, such as morphine or hydromorphone, reduces the risk of profound respiratory depression, panting, bradycardia, and vomiting response. However, either morphine or hydromorphone can be used to replace butorphanol at the same volume with dexmedetomidine plus or minus ketamine (see *Table 9.6*).
- Ketamine provides profound somatic analgesia and mild to moderate visceral analgesia. When used in this drug combination, it also works synergistically with the other two sedative–analgesic drugs.
- The release of endogenous catecholamines and the cardiac stimulatory effects of ketamine act to counter the dexmedetomidine-induced bradycardia, resulting in a higher HR.
- Additional analgesia can be provided with the addition of an injectable NSAID (e.g. carprofen) soon after the dog is anesthetized, prior to starting the procedure. Injectable meloxicam or other injectable NSAIDs can also be used.

Dexmedetomidine–butorphanol

- *Table 9.6* is a flexible dose rate table. It provides dose rates for combinations such as dexmedetomidine–butorphanol–ketamine,

dexmedetomidine–butorphanol, or dexmedetomidine–ketamine. Alternatively, it can be used for dexmedetomidine use alone.
- Dexmedetomidine can be combined with the same volume of butorphanol without the use of ketamine (see *Table 9.6*). The volume required is based on the degree of sedation desired. For example, a 13 kg (29 lb) dog presented for a minor laceration repair should receive 0.38 ml of dexmedetomidine and 0.38 ml of butorphanol IM. All the drugs are administered at the same volume, regardless of which drugs are used in the combination.
- Butorphanol can be replaced with the same volume of morphine (15 mg/ml) or hydromorphone (2 mg/ml) (see *Table 9.6*).
- Combining buprenorphine with dexmedetomidine is not recommended because of the different onsets of peak action. Dexmedetomidine is a rapid-onset sedative, while buprenorphine does not reach its peak until 20–30 minutes after administration. Buprenorphine can be administered either 15 minutes prior to dexmedetomidine or used as a postoperative analgesic agent after another dexmedetomidine–opioid combination.

Dexmedetomidine–ketamine

- As with the dexmedetomidine–butorphanol combination, dexmedetomidine can be combined with the same volume of ketamine (100 mg/ml) (see *Table 9.6*).
- The dexmedetomidine and ketamine volumes required are based on the degree of sedation–anesthesia desired. All the drugs are administered at the same volume.

Dexmedetomidine used alone for sedation using *Table 9.6* dose chart

- The dose rates approved for use in dogs are 125 µg/m² IM, 375 µg/m² for both IM and IV, and 500 µg/m² IM. *Table 9.6* also outlines the 62.5 and 250 µg/m² dose rates to broaden the application.
- The degrees of sedation associated with these doses are described in *Table 9.7*.

- The degree of sedation is more reliable when combined with the same volume of butorphanol (or with morphine or hydromorphone) or ketamine, rather than using dexmedetomidine alone.

CAT-SPECIFIC COMBINATIONS
Dexmedetomidine–butorphanol–ketamine

- This combination of drugs is often referred to as 'kitty magic' or 'DBK combination'.
- The IM dosages for this combination are listed in *Table 9.8*. The weight range of the cat and the sedation desired are selected and the volumes of the drugs determined. The doses listed are used for sedating cats (low doses) or anesthetizing them for surgery (high doses).
- The same volume of medetomidine can be used in place of dexmedetomidine.
- Following IM injection, the onset of sedation occurs within 3 minutes and lateral recumbency within 5 minutes. Intubation is possible after 5–6 minutes and a surgical plane of anesthesia lasting 35–45 minutes is achieved.
- Atipamezole (same volume as dexmedetomidine or medetomidine) can be used to antagonize the dexmedetomidine or medetomidine. Unlike in dogs, in cats the residual ketamine effect following antagonism of dexmedetomidine with atipamezole

is minimal. Therefore, reversal of dexmedetomidine or medetomidine can be achieved at any time.
- The cat can be intubated, allowed to breathe room air, or started on 100% oxygen (best practice) following the high doses of the 'kitty magic' combination.
- For painful procedures in cats lasting longer than 30–40 minutes, it is important to provide supplemental isoflurane or additional injectable anesthetic agent to prevent 'sudden awakening'. As in dogs, isoflurane can be started immediately on induction of anesthesia at 0.5%, increasing it by 0.25% every 15 minutes until 1.75% is reached. Similarly, sevoflurane can be provided immediately at 1.5–2%, increasing it by 0.5% very 15 minutes until 3.75% is reached. A surgical plane of anesthesia can then be maintained with 1.5–1.75% of isoflurane or 3.75–4.0% sevoflurane. Alternatively, an additional one-half of the original injectable anesthetic combination volume can be given either IM or IV to extend the surgical plane of anesthesia (for an additional 15 minutes).
- Apnea is the hallmark of an anesthetic overdose in kitty magic-anesthetized cats and can occur soon after drug injection or when inhalant anesthetics are used together if their combined dose-sparing effects are not taken into consideration.

Table 9.8 Drug volumes (ml) for dexmedetomidine alone or in combination with butorphanol, ketamine, or butorphanol and ketamine for various degrees of sedation in cats

Weight (kg) (lb)	Mild sedation	Moderate sedation	Profound sedation/ minor surgery	Surgery
1–2 (2–4)	0.006	0.013	0.03	0.05–0.08
2–3 (4–7)	0.012	0.025	0.05	0.1–0.15
3–4 (7–9)	0.025	0.05	0.1	0.2–0.25
4–6 (9–13)	0.05	0.1	0.2	0.3–0.35
6–7 (13–15)	0.1	0.2	0.3	0.4–0.45
7–8 (15–18)	0.15	0.3	0.4	0.5–0.55
8–10 (18–22)	0.2	0.4	0.5	0.6–0.65

Select the body weight to determine the drug volume of dexmedetomidine (500 μg/ml) according to the degree of sedation required. If using dexmedetomidine in combination with butorphanol (10 mg/ml), with or without ketamine, use the same volume for each drug.
All injections given IM. If given IV, reduce the calculated volume by half.
Medetomidine can be used to replace dexmedetomidine in this Table.

- If apnea occurs when used in combination with an inhalant, the vaporizer should be turned off and the cat ventilated until it resumes spontaneous breathing.
- Ventilating the animal in this situation eliminates the majority (97–99%) of the inhalant agent, allowing the animal to return to a lighter plane of anesthesia.
- Once spontaneous breathing has returned, reinstate the inhalant anesthetic concentration at a vaporizer dial setting of 0.5–0.75% less than that of the vaporizer dial setting before the apnea occurred.
- If apnea occurs soon after 'kitty magic' administration, the cat should be intubated and ventilated with either room air or 100% oxygen until spontaneous breathing resumes.

Dexmedetomidine used together with butorphanol for sedation in cats

- As with dogs, if butorphanol is combined with dexmedetomidine, sedation in cats is more reliable than when dexmedetomidine is used alone. Furthermore, the dose of dexmedetomidine can be reduced and the same level of sedation achieved compared with using a higher dose of dexmedetomidine alone.
- Various dose rates for dexmedetomidine can be combined with butorphanol (with the same injection volume of both drugs) based on the desired level of sedation and the health status of the cat (*Table 9.8*).
- Dexmedetomidine–butorphanol can be used when ketamine is not suitable (kidney disease or hypertrophic cardiomyopathy).

Dexmedetomidine used together with ketamine for sedation/anesthesia in cats

- Various dose rates of dexmedetomidine can be combined with ketamine (with the same injection volume of both drugs) based on the desired level of sedation/anesthesia and the health status of the cat (*Table 9.8*).
- Low doses should be used in cats with systemic dysfunctions.

Dexmedetomidine used alone for sedation in cats

- The dose rate of dexmedetomidine approved for preanesthetic and sedation–analgesia use in cats (in the USA) is 40 µg/kg IM.
- The various dose rates, based on the desired level of sedation and health status of the cat, are listed in *Table 9.8*.
- In general, cats with systemic illness should be given lower dose rates for premedication. The lower the dose, the less the sedative effect.

Dexmedetomidine (medetomidine)–butorphanol–ketamine–midazolam (or diazepam)

- This combination presents an alternative to the 'doggie or kitty magic' protocols discussed above and may be used for castration or ovariohysterectomy of healthy dogs or cats.
- The dosages for this combination are listed in *Table 9.9*.
- The surgical duration provided is 30–40 minutes and intubation can occur within 5–8 minutes of drug administration.

Table 9.9 Dexmedetomidine (or medetomidine)–butorphanol–ketamine–midazolam (or diazepam) combinations in dogs and cats

Route of delivery	Species	Dexmedetomidine (or medetomidine) (µg/kg)	Butorphanol (mg/kg)	Ketamine (mg/kg)	Midazolam or diazepam (mg/kg)
IV	Dog	8 (10)	0.2	1.5	0.2
	Cat	20 (30)	0.2	2	0.2
IM	Dog	15 (20)	0.2	3	0.4
	Cat	30 (60)	0.3	4	0.4

Note: All of these drugs can be collected in one syringe for a single injection unless a diazepam with propylene glycol formulation is being used, in which case the diazepam must be administered in a separate syringe.

- The surgical plane of anesthesia can be extended in a similar fashion to that described for the 'doggy and kitty magic' protocols.
- Postoperative pain management can also be extended by using NSAIDs or buprenorphine (or other types of opioid) at the conclusion of the surgery.
- Buprenorphine can be administered at a dose of 20–40 µg/kg IM, IV, or SC.
- The peak of action of buprenorphine is 20–30 minutes after administration and, as such, it is unlikely to interact with the residual butorphanol in this combination.
- Advantages of this drug combination include:
  - Profound analgesia with muscle relaxation.
  - The midazolam or diazepam further enhances muscle relaxation and hypnosis.

Advantages of midazolam over diazepam in this combination

- Midazolam can be mixed with the other drugs in the same syringe, allowing for the administration of a single injection.
- Midazolam is absorbed more completely when administered IM.
- Diazepam should not be mixed in the same syringe with any of the other drugs in this combination if the PG formulation is used. The PG vehicle can cause precipitation. In this case, diazepam should be administered separately. If midazolam or a water-soluble diazepam is used, the combination can be drawn up in the same syringe and administered as a single injection.

ALTERNATIVE INJECTABLE ANESTHETIC COMBINATIONS AND TECHNIQUES FOR GIANT BREED DOGS

- Giant breed dogs (e.g. Great Danes, Saint Bernards, Newfoundlands, Borzoi, Great Pyrenees, Irish Wolfhounds, Scottish Deerhounds, Greyhounds, various Mastiffs) are unique in many ways, but primarily because they have a heavy body weight.
- Some of the giant breed dogs may have occult dilated cardiomyopathy.

- Dexmedetomidine or medetomidine is designed to be dosed ideally according to body surface area, not to body weight. Using the full dose of an alpha-2 agonist based on body weight is likely to cause excessive cardiovascular depression in these giant breed dogs.
- To avoid potential overdoses in these large dogs, a lower dose of dexmedetomidine or medetomidine should be given, calculated using body surface area rather than body weight (see *Table 9.6*).
- IV administration is preferred over IM administration in these dogs, as IV administration allows for the dosage of each drug to be reduced while still achieving the same surgical plane of anesthesia. The duration of surgical anesthesia is shorter when the anesthetic combination is administered IV.
- The IV anesthetic combination outlined in *Table 9.10* can be used for minor surgical procedures lasting no more than 10–15 minutes. These might include laceration repair, chemical immobilization for hip radiographs, ear examination, arthrocentesis, small skin mass removal. The combination is also useful for providing IV anesthetic induction with analgesia.

Table 9.10 In giant breed dogs the following intravenous anesthetic combination can be used for minor surgical procedures lasting no more than 10–15 minutes

Drug	Intravenous dose
Dexmedetomidine or medetomidine	2–3 µg/kg or 3–4 µg/kg
Ketamine	0.5–1 mg/kg
Butorphanol or morphine or hydromorphone	0.1–0.2 mg/kg or 0.15–0.25 mg/kg or 0.025–0.05 mg/kg
Methadone	0.5–1.0 mg/kg
Diazepam or midazolam	0.2–0.4 mg/kg or 0.2–0.4 mg/kg

Note: All of these drugs can be collected in one syringe for a single injection unless a diazepam with propylene glycol formulation is being used, in which case the diazepam must be administered in a separate syringe.

- Inhalant anesthetic agents can be used to extend the duration of anesthesia.

CHEMICAL RESTRAINT COMBINATIONS FOR ANIMALS WITH SYSTEMIC ILLNESS OR GERIATRIC DOGS AND CATS

- Systemically ill dogs or cats are defined as animals having cardiac, respiratory, liver, or renal dysfunction.
- Geriatric dogs or cats have been defined recently as dogs or cats that have completed 75–80% of their anticipated life span (i.e. most of the giant breed dogs >6 years old; toy breed dogs >12 years old; cats >14 years old) before they are considered geriatric. Old age in itself is not a disease, but anesthetic combinations and dosages should be reduced in elderly patients as aging reduces the margins of cardiorespiratory tolerance and increases the brain sensitivity to the anesthetic agent, therefore increasing the anesthetic risk.

Dexmedetomidine–midazolam (diazepam)-based combinations

- Dogs:
  - IM sedative injection combination: dexmedetomidine–opioid–midazolam (*Table 9.11*).

- Midazolam can be replaced with diazepam at the same dose rate, but the diazepam (with PG formulation) must be administered separately, as stated previously.
- Butorphanol can be replaced with either morphine or hydromorphone in this combination.
- Cats.
  - IM sedative injection combination: dexmedetomidine–butorphanol–midazolam (*Table 9.12*).
  - Midazolam can be replaced with diazepam at the same dose; however, since diazepam cannot be mixed with other drugs due to precipitation caused by the PG, it should be administered in a separate syringe.
  - This is a useful combination for sedation and anesthesia of obstructed tom cats (urolithiasis).

Advantages of the dexmedetomidine–midazolam (diazepam)-based combinations

- Reliable sedation with less cardiorespiratory depression.
- Provision of pre-emptive analgesia.
- Small volume to administer.
- Rapid recovery.

Table 9.11 Intramuscular drug doses for systemically ill dogs or geriatric dogs when using a dexmedetomidine–butorphanol–midazolam combination. Medetomidine can be used instead of dexmedetomidine; morphine, hydromorphone or methadone instead of butorphanol; and diazepam instead of midazolam

Drug	Intramuscular dose
Dexmedetomidine or medetomidine	3–5 µg/kg or 4–6 µg/kg
Butorphanol or morphine or hydromorphone	0.1–0.2 mg/kg or 0.15–0.25 mg/kg or 0.025–0.05 mg/kg
Methadone	0.5–1.0 mg/kg
Midazolam or diazepam	0.2–0.4 mg/kg or 0.2–0.4 mg/kg

Note: All of these drugs can be collected in one syringe for a single injection unless a diazepam with propylene glycol formulation is being used, in which case the diazepam must be administered in a separate syringe.

Table 9.12 Intramuscular drug doses for systemically ill cats or geriatric cats when using a dexmedetomidine–butorphanol–midazolam combination. Medetomidine can be used instead of dexmedetomidine and diazepam instead of midazolam

Drug	Intramuscular dose
Dexmedetomidine or medetomidine	5–8 µg/kg or 8–10 µg/kg
Butorphanol	0.2–0.4 mg/kg or
Midazolam or diazepam	0.2–0.4 mg/kg or 0.2–0.4 mg/kg

Note: All of these drugs can be collected in one syringe for a single injection unless a diazepam with propylene glycol formulation is being used, in which case the diazepam must be administered in a separate syringe.

- Both the opioid and dexmedetomidine or medetomidine are reversible.
- Midazolam and diazepam can be antagonized with flumazenil, but the short duration of action of these drugs usually means that reversal is not required.

Other considerations with the dexmedetomidine–midazolam (diazepam)-based combinations
- Enriched oxygen (i.e. 100%) should be provided perioperatively.
- Dexmedetomidine can be reversed with the same volume of atipamezole IM.
- If necessary, dexmedetomidine or medetomidine can be either completely or partially reversed with atipamezole via titration (by diluting atipamezole in saline and administering it IV to effect).
- The use of atropine or glycopyrrolate should be avoided in dexmedetomidine- or medetomidine-treated animals to avoid arrhythmias (e.g. bradycardia via peripheral vasoconstriction through the baroreceptor reflex) and excessive hypertension.

Microdose dexmedetomidine (medetomidine) and propofol combinations in dogs and cats with systemic illness
- An IV catheter should be placed to facilitate easy administration of propofol intermittent boluses.
- Each bolus of propofol provides approximately 3–5 minutes of immobilization.

- Propofol intermittent boluses can be administered as frequently as required and do not require an infusion pump for administration.
- Butorphanol and dexmedetomidine or medetomidine provide analgesia.
- Butorphanol can be replaced by hydromorphone (0.025–0.05 mg/kg), morphine (0.15–0.5 mg/kg), or nalbuphine (1–2 mg/kg), with the lower doses administered IV and the higher doses IM.
- Dogs:
  - Butorphanol, 0.2 mg/kg IV or IM (given IM if sedation is required prior to IV catheterization).
  - Dexmedetomidine, 3–5 µg/kg IV or medetomidine 4–6 µg/kg (lower doses) or IM (higher doses).
  - Propofol (10 mg/ml) at 1 mg/kg IV in intermittent boluses every 3–5 minutes as needed. 100% oxygen supplementation is best practice in these animals.
- Cats:
  - Butorphanol, 0.2 mg/kg IV or IM.
  - Dexmedetomidine, 4–8 µg/kg IV or medetomidine 8–10 µg/kg (IV lower doses; IM higher doses).
  - Diluted propofol (5 mg/ml) instead of full strength propofol (10 mg/ml) at 1 mg/kg IV in intermittent boluses every 3–5 minutes as needed. (More information about propofol dilution can be found in Chapter 4.)
  - 100% oxygen supplementation is best practice in these animals.

Tiletamine/zolazepam-based protocols

TILETAMINE/ZOLAZEPAM–BUTORPHANOL–DEXMEDETOMIDINE (MEDETOMIDINE)
- Telazol–Torbugesic–Dexdomitor (TTDex) and Telazol–Torbugesic–Domitor (TTD) combinations are versatile and suitable for use in dogs and cats for premedication, chemical restraint, or surgery.
- TTDex and TTD combinations are composed of tiletamine/zolazepam powder reconstituted with 2.5 ml of butorphanol (Torbugesic, 10 mg/ml) and 2.5 ml

dexmedetomidine (Dexdomitor, 500 µg) or medetomidine (Domitor, 1,000 µg) instead of the sterile water typically used to reconstitute tiletamine/zolazepam (*Table 9.13*).
- The total volume following reconstitution is 5 ml.
- The final concentration contains 100 mg/ml tiletamine/zolazepam, 5 mg/ml butorphanol (or other opioids such as morphine or hydromorphone), and 250 µg/ml of dexmedetomidine or 500 µg/ml medetomidine (*Table 9.14*).

Table 9.13 Reconstitution of the TTDex and TTD combinations using tiletamine/zolazepam (Telazol or Zoletil, 100 mg/ml) with butorphanol and dexmedetomidine or medetomidine

TTDex	TTD
Telazol or Zoletil-100 powder	Telazol or Zoletil-100 powder
Torbugesic 2.5 ml (butorphanol 10 mg/ml)	Torbugesic 2.5 ml (butorphanol 10 mg/ml)
Dexdomitor 2.5 ml (dexmedetomidine 0.5 mg/ml)	Domitor 2.5 ml (medetomidine 1 mg/ml)

Table 9.14 Contents of each milliliter of the TTDex and TTD combinations

TTDex and TTD individual drug components	Each ml contains
Tiletamine/zolazepam	100 mg
Butorphanol or morphine or hydromorphone	5 mg or 7.5 mg or 1 mg
Dexmedetomidine or medetomidine	250 μg or 500 μg

- Alternatively, the tiletamine/zolazepam can be diluted as instructed on the package with sterile water and each of the three drugs in the combination can be drawn up separately and mixed into one syringe for administration as a single IM or IV injection.
- If more potent analgesia is desired, the butorphanol in the TTD combination can be replaced with 2.5 ml of morphine (15 mg/ml) or hydromorphone (2 mg/ml) and dosed at the same rate as TTDex or TTD in dogs and cats. Alternatively, additional opioids can be given during the surgical procedure or for postoperative pain management. (**Note:** Giving morphine or hydromorphone within 30 minutes of administration of a TTDex mixture that contains butorphanol will weaken the analgesic effect, since the residual butorphanol [an opioid kappa receptor agonist and a mu receptor antagonist] tends to antagonize the morphine or hydromorphone [both are opioid mu and kappa agonists]. Ideally, additional morphine or hydromorphone should not be given until at least 60 minutes after initial TTDex administration.)
- If morphine or hydromorphone is used instead of butorphanol in the TTDex (or TTD) combination, vomiting and panting responses tend to occur much more frequently than with TTDex and butorphanol.
- Depending on the desired effect, TTDex and TTD may be given at 0.01–0.04 ml/kg IM for premedication,

immobilization, and up to a surgical plane of anesthesia.
- Small volumes of TTDex or TTD require the use of an insulin syringe for drug administration for accuracy. 0.01 ml of TTDex is equal to one unit volume when using U-50 (50 units) or U-100 (100 units) insulin syringes. 0.03 ml of TTDex is equal to 3 units of volume when using these syringes.

Premedication using TTDex or TTD in dogs and cats
- The TTDex or TTD mixture should be given at 0.01 ml/kg IM. Dogs and cats are dosed at the same rate. (See also *Tables 9.15, 9.16,* and *9.17.*)
- The combination can be administered IV for a faster onset and more intense level of sedation.
- Onset of sedation occurs within 8–10 minutes of IM administration.
- This drug combination provides excellent pre-emptive analgesia as it contains tiletamine, butorphanol, and dexmedetomidine or medetomidine as analgesic agents.
- When used as a premedicant, the TTDex/TTD combination reduces the IV induction agent required (e.g. thiopentone or propofol) by 60–70%. It also spares the amount of inhalant agent required for anesthetic maintenance in the first 20–30 minutes of inhalant anesthesia. The usual inhalant concentration required for maintenance post TTDex/TTD premedication is approximately 1% isoflurane or 2% sevoflurane.

Table 9.15 Dose of each individual component of the TTDex and TTD combinations at the various dose rates based on the level of sedation/anesthesia desired

TTDex and TTD individual drug components	Premedication (0.01 ml/kg)	Profound sedation (0.02 ml/kg)	Surgical plane of anesthesia (0.03–0.04 ml/kg)
Tiletamine/zolazepam	1 mg/kg	2 mg/kg	3–4 mg/kg
Butorphanol or morphine or hydromorphone	0.05 mg/kg or 0.075 mg/kg or 0.01 mg/kg	0.10 mg/kg or 0.15 mg/kg or 0.02 mg/kg	0.15–0.2 mg/kg or 0.23–0.3 mg/kg or 0.03–0.04 mg/kg
Dexmedetomidine or medetomidine	2.5 µg/kg or 5 µg/kg	5 µg/kg or 10 µg/kg	7.5–10 µg/kg or 15–20 µg/kg

Table 9.16 Dosage of the TTDex and TTD combinations using tiletamine/zolazepam (100 mg/ml) with butorphanol and dexmedetomidine or medetomidine for premedication, profound sedation, and surgery in dogs and cats

Level of sedation required	TTDex or TTD (ml/kg IM)	TTDex or TTD (ml/kg IV)
Premedication (mild-moderate sedation)	0.01 ml/kg	0.005 ml/kg
Chemical restraint (profound sedation)	0.02 ml/kg	0.01 ml/kg
Surgical plane of anesthesia	0.03–0.035 ml/kg	0.0175 ml/kg
Surgical plane of anesthesia for more aggressive animals or more painful surgery	0.04 ml/kg	0.02 ml/kg

Table 9.17 Dose chart (in ml) for TTDex or TTD for sedation and anesthesia. To create TTDex, add 2.5ml dexmedetomidine (Dexdomitor) and 2.5 ml butorphanol (Torbugesic, 10 mg/ml) to one bottle of tiletamine/zolazepam (Telazol or Zoletil, 100 mg/ml) powder. To create TTD, add 2.5ml medetomidine (Domitor, 1 mg/ml) and 2.5 ml butorphanol (Torbugesic, 10 mg/ml) to one bottle of tiletamine/zolazepam (Telazol or Zoletil, 100 mg/ml) powder

Weight (kg) (lb)	Mild sedation 0.05 ml/kg	Moderate sedation 0.01 ml/kg	Profound sedation 0.02 ml/kg	Surgical anesthesia 0.035 ml/kg	Surgical anesthesia 0.04 ml/kg
1–2 (2–4)	0.005	0.01	0.02	0.035	0.04
2–3 (4–7)	0.013	0.025	0.05	0.09	0.12
3–4 (7–9)	0.018	0.035	0.07	0.12	0.15
4–5 (9–11)	0.023	0.045	0.09	0.16	0.19
5–10 (11–22)	0.038	0.075	0.15	0.26	0.37
10–13 (22–29)	0.06	0.12	0.24	0.40	0.48
13–15 (29–33)	0.07	0.14	0.28	0.49	0.58
15–20 (33–44)	0.09	0.18	0.36	0.61	0.78
20–25 (44–55)	0.12	0.23	0.46	0.79	0.98
25–30 (55–66)	0.14	0.28	0.56	0.96	1.25
30–33 (66–73)	0.16	0.32	0.64	1.1	1.3
33–37 (73–81)	0.18	0.35	0.7	1.2	1.45
37–45 (81–99)	0.21	0.41	0.82	1.44	1.7
45–50 (99–110)	0.24	0.48	0.96	1.66	1.95

(Continued)

Table 9.17 (*Continued*) Dose chart (in ml) for TTDex or TTD for sedation and anesthesia. To create TTDex, add 2.5ml dexmedetomidine (Dexdomitor) and 2.5 ml butorphanol (Torbugesic, 10 mg/ml) to one bottle of tiletamine/zolazepam (Telazol or Zoletil, 100 mg/ml) powder. To create TTD, add 2.5ml medetomidine (Domitor, 1 mg/ml) and 2.5 ml butorphanol (Torbugesic, 10 mg/ml) to one bottle of tiletamine/zolazepam (Telazol or Zoletil, 100 mg/ml) powder

Weight (kg) (lb)	Mild sedation 0.05 ml/kg	Moderate sedation 0.01 ml/kg	Profound sedation 0.02 ml/kg	Surgical anesthesia 0.035 ml/kg	Surgical anesthesia 0.04 ml/kg
50–55 (110–121)	0.26	0.53	1.1	1.84	2.2
55–60 (121–132)	0.29	0.58	1.2	2.0	2.3
60–65 (132–143)	0.32	0.63	1.3	2.18	2.5
65–70 (143–154)	0.34	0.68	1.4	2.36	2.7
70–80 (154–176)	0.38	0.75	1.5	2.63	3.0
>80 (>176)	0.4	0.8	1.6	2.8	3.2

- It is vital to provide additional opioids or other analgesic agents (e.g. local anesthetics or NSAIDs) for additional analgesia when using TTDex (or TTD) as a premedication. This is because the opioid dose in the TTDex (or TTD) at this dose rate is low and will not last for longer than 1 hour.

Profound sedation using TTDex or TTD for minor surgical or radiographic procedures

- The TTDex or TTD mixture should be given at 0.02 ml/kg IM. Dogs and cats are dosed at the same rate. (See also *Tables 9.15, 9.16,* and *9.17.*)
- Lateral recumbency occurs within 5–8 minutes following a single IM injection.
- This drug combination provides excellent muscle relaxation and is suitable for taking pelvic radiographs (particularly for hip scoring schemes).
- Some dogs or cats sedated with this dose of TTDex or TTD may allow for intubation without any other anesthetic induction drugs.
- This sedative dose is also induction and inhalant sparing: 80–90% for IV induction agents and 60–70% for inhalant agents for anesthesia maintenance.
- Some dogs or cats can be castrated using this dose, but the anesthesia provided is inadequate for ovariohysterectomy or other more painful surgeries.

- Spontaneous recovery from injection to walking is approximately 2 hours following IM injection.
- As with premedication using TTDex (or TTD), it is vital to provide additional opioids or other analgesic agents (e.g. local anesthetics or NSAIDs) for additional analgesia/postoperative pain relief when using these doses of TTDex (or TTD) for surgery.

Surgical plane of anesthesia using TTDex or TTD

- The TTDex or TTD mixture should be given at 0.03–0.04 ml/kg. Dogs and cats are dosed at the same rate. (See also *Tables 9.15, 9.16,* and *9.17.*)
- This dose is sufficient for surgical procedures such as castration, ovariohysterectomy, and feline abdominal procedures. The duration of anesthesia is 30–40 minutes.
- In aggressive dogs or cats, TTDex or TTD at 0.035–0.04 ml/kg IM induces recumbency within 3–5 minutes and allows oral-tracheal intubation.
- The IV dose is one-half of the IM dose.

Other considerations

- TTDex and TTD combinations are effective and economical for use in dogs and cats.
- They provide better sedation, muscle relaxation, and analgesia in cats than

previous combinations (e.g. Telazol–ketamine–xylazine, TKX).

- At the end of the procedure, the dexmedetomidine or medetomidine can be reversed with atipamezole to speed up recovery in cats. For dogs, because of the dissociative hangover, it is not advised to reverse the dog until at least 40–60 minutes after TTDex or TTD administration.

TILETAMINE/ZOLAZEPAM–DEXMEDETOMIDINE (OR MEDETOMIDINE) COMBINATION WITHOUT OPIOIDS

- Dogs and cats can be anesthetized with a combination of tiletamine/zolazepam (2 mg/kg and dexmedetomidine (20 µg/kg) (or medetomidine [30 µg/kg]) administered in a single IM injection.
- The advantage of this drug combination is that in some countries tiletamine/zolazepam is not a controlled substance and not using an opioid in this drug combination allows the combination to be controlled substances free and minimizes record keeping for inspection.
- A surgical plane of anesthesia can be induced for 30 minutes with this drug combination.
- Anesthesia can be extended (15 minutes) by administering additional dexmedetomidine (5–8 µg/kg) or medetomidine (10–20 µg/kg) IV.
- Atipamezole can be used to reverse the dexmedetomidine or medetomidine.
- The same precautions for reversal-induced tiletamine hangover are applied in dogs being given this drug combination.

TILETAMINE/ZOLAZEPAM–OPIOID COMBINATIONS WITHOUT DEXMEDETOMIDINE/MEDETOMIDINE

- Dogs can be anesthetized with tiletamine/zolazepam (5–6 mg/kg) plus either butorphanol (0.2–0.4 mg/kg), morphine (0.5–1.0 mg/kg), or hydromorphone (0.05–0.1 mg/kg) administered IM as a single injection.
- Cats can be anesthetized with tiletamine/zolazepam (8–9 mg/kg) plus either butorphanol (0.2 mg/kg), morphine (0.5–1.0 mg/kg) or hydromorphone (0.05–0.1 mg/kg) administered IM as a single injection.
- Lateral recumbency occurs within 5–8 minutes.
- Dogs and cats are easily intubated.
- This combination provides a shorter duration (10–15 minutes) of surgical plane anesthesia than TTDex (or TTD).
- The total anesthetic duration from initial injection to full recovery (walking) is approximately 2 hours.
- Isoflurane (starting 0.75–1%) or sevoflurane (starting 2–3%) can be used to extend the duration of general anesthesia.
- NSAIDs can be administered preoperatively for additional analgesia.
- This drug combination can induce hypoxemia, so supplemental oxygen should be provided during the first 5–10 minutes post injection.
- The disadvantages of this combination are the longer recovery time and shorter analgesic duration than with the TTDex or TTD combinations.

Case examples

- Using 'doggie magic' as a premedication in a dog following propofol induction and isoflurane for maintenance for surgery (**Figs. 9.1–9.4**).
- Using 'doggie magic' IM as a profound sedation for hip radiography in a dog (**Figs. 9.5–9.7**).
- Using 'kitty magic' IM for castration in a cat (**Figs. 9.8–9.11**).
- Using TTDex combination in a dog for orthopedic device removal (**Figs. 9.12, 9.13**).

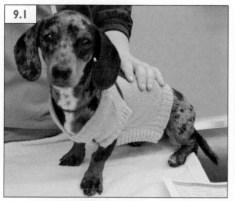
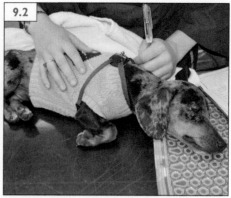

Figs. 9.1, 9.2 (**9.1**) A 2-year-old docile male Miniature Dachshund weighing 10 kg presents for castration. Blood work and physical examination are all within normal range and the ASA status is I. The dog is premedicated with 'doggie magic' (*Table 9.6*) at a profound dose rate made up of dexmedetomidine 0.2 ml (10 µg/kg), butorphanol 0.2 ml (0.2 mg/kg), and ketamine 0.2 ml (2 mg/kg) mixed in the same syringe and administered as a single IM injection. (**9.2**) The dog shows profound signs of sedation and assumed lateral recumbency within 5 minutes of injection.

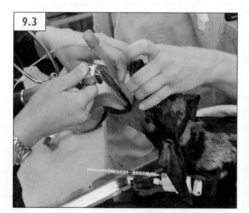
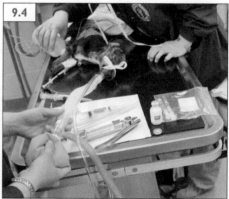

Figs. 9.3, 9.4 (**9.3**) IV catheter placement is easily achieved. The dog is induced with 1 mg/kg of propofol and intubation is easily accomplished approximately 8 minutes after the initial IM injection. (**9.4**) The dog is maintained on 100% oxygen and approximately 1% isoflurane for the first 20 minutes. Additional analgesic drugs were given including more butorphanol (0.2 mg/kg IV) and carprofen (4.4 mg/kg SC) for postoperative pain management.

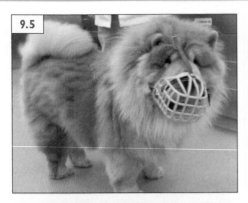

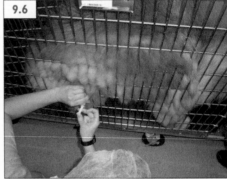

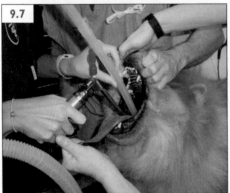

Figs. 9.5–9.7 (**9.5**) A 6-year-old Chow presents for hip radiography. The animal is difficult to handle for such a procedure and a muzzle is placed. The dog is overall healthy. (**9.6**) A single IM injection of 375 μg/m² of dexmedetomidine–butorphanol–ketamine ('doggie magic') is administered with the dog restrained in a squeeze cage. (**9.7**) The drug combination has taken effect 5 minutes after injection and the Chow is in a stage of anesthesia such that it can now be intubated. The dog was maintained on oxygen only for the hip radiography. The dog recovered to a walking state 2 hours after the injection.

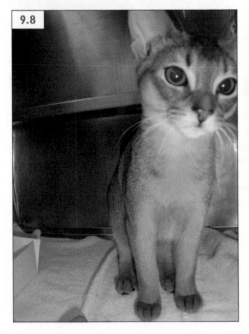

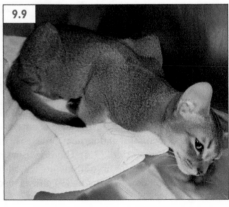

Figs. 9.8, 9.9 (**9.8**) A healthy, 8-month-old Abyssinian cat is presented for castration surgery. (**9.9**) A surgical dose of dexmedetomidine–butorphanol–ketamine ('kitty magic') is administered as a single IM injection.

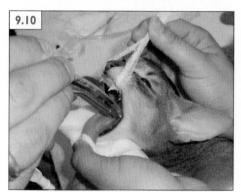

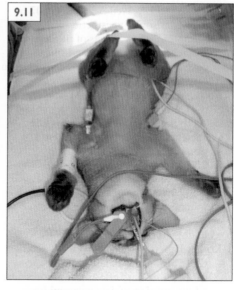

Figs. 9.10, 9.11 (9.10) Five minutes later a stage of anesthesia has been induced such that the cat is able to be intubated. (9.11) Surgery is performed while the cat is breathing room air (in this case 100% oxygen should be provided for best practice). Various cardiorespiratory monitors are applied to the cat including a pulse oximeter for hemoglobin saturation for oxygen, electrocardiograhy for an electrocardiogram, capnography for end-tidal CO_2, and blood pressure measurement.

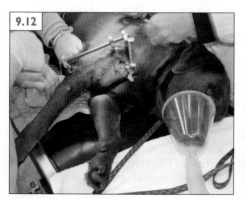

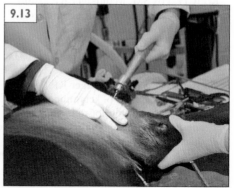

Figs. 9.12, 9.13 (9.12) An overall healthy (ASA-II), 4-year-old Labrador Retriever weighing 40 kg (88 lb) is presented for removal of an orthopedic device following a fracture repair. The dog is given tiletamine/zolazepam–butorphanol–dexmedetomidine (TTDex) IM at a dose rate of 0.02 ml/kg. The dog could not be intubated, but 100% oxygen via face mask is provided during the procedure. (9.13) Sedation and analgesia are profound and suitable for removal of the device. The dog recovered spontaneously within 2 hours following injection.

Further reading

Barletta M, Austin BR, Ko JC *et al.* (2011) Evaluation of dexmedetomidine-ketamine with opioids as injectable anesthetic combinations for castration in dogs. *J Am Vet Med Assoc* **238**:1159–67.

Grasso SC, Ko JC, Paranjape V *et al.* (2015) The hemodynamic impact of acepromazine or dexmedetomidine premedication on isoflurane anesthetized dogs. *J Am Vet Med Assoc* **246**(7):754–64.

Ko JC, Abbo LA, Weil AB *et al.* (2007) A comparison of anesthetic and cardiorespiratory effects of tiletamine-zolazepam-butorphanol and tiletamine-zolazepam-butorphanol-medetomidine in cats. *Vet Ther* **8**:164–76.

Ko JC, Austin BR, Barletta M *et al.* (2011) Evaluation of dexmedetomidin-ketamine with opioids as injectable anesthetic combinations for castration in cats. *J Am Vet Med Assoc* **239(11)**:1453–62.

Ko JCH, Bailey JE, Pablo LS *et al.* (1996) Comparison of sedative and cardiorespiratory effects of medetomidine and a medetomidine-butorphanol combination in dogs. *Am J Vet Res* **57**:535–40.

Ko JC, Barletta M, Sen I, Weil AB *et al.* (2013) Influence of ketamine on the cardiopulmonary effects of intramuscular administration of dexmedetomidine-buprenorphine with subsequent reversal with atipamezole in dogs. *J Am Vet Med Assoc* **242(3)**:339–45.

Ko JCH, Fox SM, Mandsager RE (2000) Sedative and cardiorespiratory effects of medetomidine, medetomidine-butorphanol, and medetomidine-ketamine in dogs. *J Am Vet Med Assoc* **216**:1578–83.

Ko JCH, Fox SM, Mandsager RE (2001) Anesthetic effects of ketamine or iso-flurane induction prior to isoflurane anesthesia in medetomidine-premedicated dogs. *J Am Anim Hosp Assoc* **37**:411–19.

Ko JC, Knesl O, Weil AB *et al.* (2009) FAQs: Analgesia, sedation, and anesthesia: making the switch from medetomidine to dexmedetomidine. *Compend Contin Educ Pract Vet* **31(suppl 1A)**:1–24.

Ko JCH, Mandsager RE, Lange DG *et al.* (2000) Cardiorespiratory responses and plasma cortisol concentrations in dogs treated with medetomidine before undergoing ovariohysterectomy, *J Am Vet Med Assoc* **217**:509–14.

Ko JCH, Nicklin CF, Melendaz M *et al.* (1998) Effect of micro-dose medetomidine on diazepam-ketamine induced anesthesia in dogs. *J Am Vet Med Assoc* **213**:215–19.

Ko JC, Payton M, Weil AB *et al.* (2007) Comparison of anesthetic and cardiorespiratory effects of tiletamine-zolazepam-butorphanol and tiletamine-zolazepam-butorphanol-medetomidine in dogs. *Vet Ther* **8**:113–26.

Ko JCH, Payton ME, Whiter AG *et al.* (2006) Effects of intravenous diazepam or micro-dose of medetomidine on propofol induced sedation in dogs. *J Am Anim Hosp Assoc* **42**:18–27.

Ko JCH, Thurmon JC, Benson GJ *et al.* (1993) An alternative drug combination for use in declawing and castrating cats. *Vet Med* **88**:1061–5.

Krimins RA, Ko JC, Weil AB *et al.* (2012) Evaluation of anesthetic, analgesic and cardiorespiratory effects in dogs after intramuscular administration of dexmedetomidine-butorphanol-tiletamine-zolazepam or dexmedetomidine-tramadol-ketamine drug combination. *Am J Vet Res* **73(11)**:1707–14.

Krimins, RA, Ko JC, Weil AB *et al.* (2012) Hemodynamic effects of tiletamine/zolazepam-butorphanol-dexmedetomidine and ketamine-butorphanol-dexmedetomidine in dogs. *Am J Vet Res* **73(9)**:1363–70.

Anesthetic considerations for specific diseases

Ann B Weil and Jeff C Ko

Introduction

This chapter provides a brief overview of anesthetic protocols that may be appropriate in animals affected by various disease syndromes that are not covered in the previous chapters.

Hepatic dysfunction

Specific hepatic disease-induced dysfunctions relating to anesthesia are listed in *Table 10.1*.

GENERAL CONSIDERATIONS

- Liver dysfunction impairs drug metabolism and prolongs recovery from anesthetics. Nearly all anesthetic drugs undergo biotransformation by the liver.
- Patients with liver dysfunction are prone to hypoglycemia. The liver plays a central role in the formation, storage, and release of glucose.
- Patients with hepatic compromise may be unable to generate adequate body heat, predisposing them to hypothermia and slow metabolism and resulting in prolonged recovery.
- Hemostasis. The liver produces coagulation factors, plasminogen, and antithrombin and is responsible for metabolism of many activators of the coagulation and plasmin cascades. Surgery in patients with hepatopathies may be complicated by poor blood clotting ability. Liver failure may result in disseminated intravascular coagulation (DIC). Hemostasis (prothrombin time [PT], partial thromboplastin time [PTT], buccal mucosal bleeding time) should be evaluated (see Chapter 2)

Table 10.1 Specific hepatic disease-induced dysfunctions relating to anesthesia

Disease-induced abnormality	Consequences	Management
Drug metabolism	Prolonged recovery	Use drugs that have a short metabolic half-life
Glycogenesis	Hypoglycemia Unable to general adequate body heat/ hypothermia	Provide glucose and exogenous heat source
Protein synthesis	More free unbound anesthetic/increased drug sensitivity and slow drug metabolism Low oncotic pressure leads to edema	Avoid repeat dosing of injectable anesthetics Use a drug that avoids liver metabolism and use lower doses with titration technique Use of colloid fluids
Clotting factors	Oozing and difficult for blood to clot	Plasma transfusion

prior to surgery in all patients with compromised liver function.

- Protein synthesis. The liver is the primary site of plasma protein synthesis (except for gamma globulins and factor VIII). Plasma albumin values are one of the best indicators of liver function. Many anesthetics bind with plasma proteins such that the drug is divided into active versus bound (inactive) fractions. If plasma albumin is low, higher concentrations of the active component accumulate, resulting in a more profound patient response to the anesthetic. This predisposes the animal to an anesthetic overdose at normal dose ranges. Additionally, albumin is important for producing plasma oncotic pressure, which retains fluid within the intravascular space. If albumin is low (<15–20 g/l [1.5–2.0 g/dl]), fluid may redistribute, predisposing patients to edema of the body cavities, (including pulmonary effusion and abdominal ascites) and extremities. If perioperative fluid administration is not monitored carefully, these animals may also develop iatrogenic pulmonary edema.
- Biodegradation. The liver biodegrades and excretes endogenous and exogenous substances, including anesthetic drugs. Using high doses of long-acting sedatives or anesthetic agents (e.g. acepromazine) in these patients may result in significantly prolonged anesthesia or delayed anesthetic recovery.

Any anesthetic or sedative drug dependent on the liver for metabolism and excretion may last longer in animals with hepatic compromise.

- Serum chemistry (e.g. serum alanine aminotransferase [ALT], see Chapter 2), can be used as a sensitive indicator of liver cellular damage. Other enzymes, such as alkaline phosphatase (ALP) and blood urine nitrogen (BUN), also serve as indirect indicators of hepatic integrity. Elevation in these enzymes indicates potential liver dysfunction.
- The liver receives approximately 20% of cardiac output (CO). Systemic hypotension during general anesthesia results in poor hepatic perfusion, potentially damaging the liver and leading to acute liver failure.
- Causes of liver dysfunction can be largely classified into hepatic parenchymal disorders, those of biliary tract origin, and vascular abnormalities (i.e. portocaval shunt). Patients with severe liver dysfunction may also have multiorgan dysfunction, encephalopathy, and severe metabolic derangements.

ANESTHETIC MANAGEMENT AND PHARMACOLOGIC CONSIDERATIONS

- If the patient has elevated levels of ammonia, lactulose should be administered orally and by enema to reduce ammonia levels (see Chapter 2) prior to general anesthesia.

- Further hepatic damage can be minimized by properly maintaining blood pressure to preserve liver perfusion.
- Anesthetic drugs with a short half-life, that depend on pathways other than liver metabolism for termination of anesthetic action (e.g. propofol has extrahepatic metabolism in addition to regular hepatic metabolism), or are reversible, should be used.
- The use of acepromazine and alpha-2 adrenergic agonists should be avoided in patients with moderate to severe liver disease. Benzodiazepines (BNZs) should be avoided in patients with severe liver disease, hepatic encephalopathy, or suspected portocaval shunts. BNZs increase gamma aminobutyric acid (GABA) neurotransmission, which may exacerbate mental stupor.
- Anesthetic drugs, such as opioids, can be used to provide analgesia and reduce general anesthetic requirements. A more profound sedation may occur from opioid administration if the patient has significant liver disease.
- Propofol and alfaxalone are excellent IV induction agents for patients with liver disease, as redistribution and metabolism are extremely rapid after a single injection. Propofol is also eliminated from the body by extrahepatic mechanisms. Etomidate is also a good alternative for patients with liver disease.
- Dogs primarily metabolize ketamine and tiletamine via the liver and administration in patients with severe liver dysfunction leads to a prolonged recovery. Although cats still require ketamine to be metabolized by the liver to nor-ketamine, the majority of nor-ketamine is excreted unchanged in the urine without going through oxidation by the liver. Ketamine and tiletamine are therefore less impacted in liver dysfunctional cats.
- Inhalant anesthetic agents are the best choice for maintenance anesthesia in patients with liver dysfunction. They can also be used to induce anesthesia via face mask (see Chapter 5).
- Fluid administration must be carefully managed to prevent fluid overload, which leads to the dilution of serum protein (TP and albumin). Patients with a low TP require a plasma transfusion or colloids. (See Chapter 7 for more details on fluid therapy of anesthetized patients.)

EXAMPLES OF ANESTHETIC PROTOCOLS FOR DOGS WITH LIVER DYSFUNCTION
Premedication
- Use an opioid alone or in combination with a low dose of a sedative if appropriate (e.g. acepromazine 0.01–0.02 mg/kg; azaperone 0.1–0.2 mg/kg; dexmedetomidine/medetomidine 3–5 µg/kg; midazolam/diazepam 0.2–0.4 mg/kg) in fractious patients.
- Opioids:
  - Butorphanol 0.2–0.4 mg/kg IV or IM or
  - Hydromorphone 0.05–0.1 mg/kg IV or IM or
  - Buprenorphine 0.04–0.06 mg/kg, IV or IM or
  - Morphine 0.25–0.5 mg/kg IV or IM.
  - Methadone 0.2–0.3 mg/kg IV or IM.
- Sedatives: avoid the sedatives listed below in dogs with severe liver dysfunction. However, they may be used judiciously in dogs with mild-to-moderate liver dysfunction.
  - Low doses of acepromazine (0.01–0.02 mg/kg IV or IM).
  - Low doses of azaperone (0.1–0.2 mg/kg, IV or IM).
  - Low doses of dexmedetomidine (2–4 µg/kg) or medetomidine (4–8 µg/kg) IV or IM.
  - Low doses of diazepam or midazolam (0.2–0.4 mg/kg IV or IM).
  - Alfaxalone at 1–2 mg per kg IM can be added to other sedative and opioid combinations to enhance the sedative effect. An example of this combination would be midazolam 0.2 mg/kg, butorphanol 0.2 mg/kg, and alfaxalone 2 mg/kg all in one syringe for IM injection as a premedication combination.

Induction
- Propofol 6 mg/kg IV or
- Etomidate 2–3 mg/kg IV or
- Alfaxalone 2–3 mg/kg IV or
- Face mask induction with isoflurane or sevoflurane.

Maintenance

- Maintain anesthesia using isoflurane or sevoflurane.

ANESTHETIC PROTOCOLS FOR CATS WITH LIVER DYSFUNCTION

- The same premedication and IV agents as described above for dogs can be used.
- Avoid using BNZs (midazolam or diazepam) in severe liver dysfunctional patients.
- For cats, a small dose of ketamine (0.5–1 mg/kg, IM) can be added to the sedative combination to enhance sedative quality, e.g.:
  - Midazolam 0.1–0.2 mg/kg, butorphanol 0.2–0.4 mg/kg, and ketamine 1 mg/kg and alfaxalone 2 mg/kg. These drugs can be administered either IM or IV.
- Alternatively, the cat can be anesthetized with an inhalant anesthetic agent (e.g. isoflurane or sevoflurane) using a face mask or induction chamber.
- Maintain on isoflurane or sevoflurane.

OTHER CONSIDERATIONS

- Perioperative supportive care with glucose, plasma, appropriate fluids, and inotropes may be required in some cases.
- Opioids and local anesthetics should be used for pain management. NSAIDs should be avoided in these cases.

Cardiac dysfunction

Specific cardiac disease-induced dysfunctions relating to anesthesia are listed in *Table 10.2*. There are a variety of acquired or congenital cardiac dysfunctions in dogs and cats. These cardiac dysfunctional patients may require sedation or general anesthesia for cardiac or non-cardiac-related procedures. The following describes considerations for hemodynamic and anesthetic managements of these patients.

GENERAL CONSIDERATIONS

- Dogs and cats with cardiovascular disease (with or without concurrent respiratory disease) are at higher risk during general anesthesia than other diseased animals. This is due to:
  - Increased likelihood of cardiac failure and death due to pre-existing cardiovascular dysfunction.
  - Less tolerance of anesthetic-induced cardiovascular depression and cardiac arrhythmias.
- Adverse effects on other organ systems due to decreased tissue perfusion secondary to poor CO.
- Dogs and cats with left-sided congestive heart failure (hypertrophic and dilated cardiomyopathy) are likely to develop compensatory tachycardia in order to increase CO.
- Poor cardiac response to hemodynamic stability drugs (inotropes, fluids).
- Difficult resuscitation when cardiac compensation occurs.
- Commonly occurring cardiac diseases in dogs and cats are summarized in *Table 10.3*.

HYPERTROPHIC CARDIOMYOPATHY

- Hypertrophic cardiomyopathy is common in cats, especially in cats with hyperthyroidism. It is less common in dogs.
- The principle pathology is increased thickness and stiffness of the left

Table 10.2 Specific cardiac disease-induced dysfunctions relating to anesthesia

Disease-induced abnormality	Consequences	Management
Poor cardiac contractility	Hypotension, reduction of cardiac output, less tolerance for extreme blood pressure and heart rate changes	Thorough physical examination, cardiac medication and prepare animals prior to general anesthesia Avoid drugs that cause extreme heart rates and excessive cardiac depression Avoid hypercapnia and hypoxemia
Arrhythmias	Hypotension and increased anesthesia risk for more serious arrhythmias	Treat arrhythmias Avoid drugs that increase cardiac arrhythmias

Table 10.3 Pathology and anesthetic management of commonly occurring cardiac diseases in dogs and cats

Cardiac diseases	Principle pathology	Anesthetic management
Hypertrophic cardiomyopathy	Increased thickness of the ventricular septal wall Reduction in ventricular filling volume	Avoid anesthetic agents that increase cardiac contractility and heart rate Avoid conditions that decrease ventricular filling (e.g. vasodilation, increased airway pressure, tachycardia and hypovolemia)
Dilated cardiomyopathy	Ventricular enlargement with mitral regurgitation Marked reduction in cardiac contractility	Avoid further reductions in cardiac contractility Tachycardia and bradycardia are both detrimental
Mitral valve regurgitation	Decrease in stroke volume, secondary to regurgitation, through an incompetent mitral valve	Avoid bradycardia, excessive decreases in contractility, and increased systemic vascular resistance Bradycardia is associated with left atrium volume overload
Tricuspid valve regurgitation	Swelling of the right ventricle or injury of the tricuspid valve Tricuspid valve does not close properly, causing blood to leak back into the right atrium during ventricular contraction	Maintain ventricular filling with fluid administration Minimize intermittent positive-pressure ventilation and drug-induced vasodilation

ventricular septum and wall. The coronary circulation to the thickened myocardium is reduced and easily leads to myocardial ischemia. The ventricular filling volume is also reduced due to stiffer wall with less compliance.

- Drugs or events that result in tachycardia and/or increased myocardial work significantly increase myocardial oxygen consumption and reduce ventricular chamber filling time for the blood, resulting in significant CO reduction and myocardial tissue perfusion impairment.
- Hypertrophic cardiomyopathy patients may have symptoms that include atrial fibrillation, aortic stenosis (see below Aortic stenosis section), and congestive heart failure with pulmonary edema and pleural effusion.
- Hemodynamic management of such patients should be directed at avoiding drugs or events that result in obstruction of the left ventricular outflow tract. This includes tachycardia and an increase in myocardial contractile work or decrease in ventricular filling volume.
- Anesthetic management should be directed at avoiding anesthetic drugs such as ketamine, tiletamine/zolazepam, atropine/glycopyrrolate, and inotropes that increase heart rate (HR) and

cardiac contractility. Avoid events such as stress, anxiety, pain, and inadequate depth of anesthesia that lead to release of catecholamines.

- Conditions such as anesthetic-induced vasodilation, positive-pressure ventilation that increases airway pressure, acute blood loss, or dehydration-induced hypovolemia all worsen ventricular filling volume.
- Many cats may be on heart medications such as propranolol (a beta-blocker to reduce HR) and furosemide (a diuretic to reduce potential pulmonary edema). These medications should be continued until anesthetic induction to allow hemodynamic stability. The beneficial effect of beta-blocker medication is to reduce the HR so that the ventricular blood filling time and volume can be increased during diastole, as well as simultaneously decreasing myocardial oxygen consumption.

DILATED CARDIOMYOPATHY

- Both dogs and cats can be affected by dilated cardiomyopathy. It is most commonly seen in giant breed dogs, and less commonly in cats.
- Dilated cardiomyopathy is characterized by ventricular enlargement with associated mitral regurgitation and

impaired systolic work of the ventricles (more commonly occurs in the left ventricle). Increased left atrial pressure also results in left atrial enlargement in affected animals and is frequently associated with atrial fibrillation. The enlarged heart results in a marked reduction in cardiac contractility.

- Hemodynamic management of animals with dilated cardiomyopathy is to minimize reduction in cardiac contractility by maintaining a relative faster HR while avoiding severe tachycardia, which drastically increases myocardial oxygen consumption.
- Anesthetic management should be directed at avoiding bradycardia due to limited stroke volume. Care should be taken to avoid fluid overload on the dilated heart. Using reasonable doses of ketamine and tiletamine/zolazepam are helpful in ensuring a higher HR while maintaining adequate cardiac contractility. Dopamine or dobutamine CRI may be necessary to maintain the cardiac contractility.
- Animals on digoxin and diuretics should be kept on these drugs until anesthesia induction to maintain hemodynamic stability.

MITRAL VALVE REGURGITATION (OR INSUFFICIENCY)

- Mitral valve regurgitation is often seen in geriatric dogs and occasionally in cats.
- It is characterized by a portion of forward blood leaking backward through the incompetent (insufficient) mitral valve while being pumped from left ventricle to the aorta (systemic circulation). This backward leakage of blood into the left atrium results in less blood being pumped out of the left ventricle and therefore decrease in stroke volume.
- Hemodynamic management should be directed to avoid bradycardia and avoid increasing afterload. Bradycardia could cause left atrial volume overload due to accumulation of the regurgitant volume. Increases in afterload could cause higher pressure gradients and impede forward systemic blood flow, resulting in more distension of the left atrium. Maintenance

of a slightly higher HR improves stroke volume by facilitating forward left ventricular blood flow.
- Anesthetic management is similar to dilated cardiomyopathy: avoid bradycardia or excessive decreases in contractility and avoid increased systemic vascular resistance (SVR). Avoid the use of alpha-2 agonist sedatives, which cause bradycardia and increased afterload and result in regurgitant fraction. Low doses of acepromazine, propofol, and isoflurane lower systemic resistance, thus improving left ventricular forward blood flow.

TRICUSPID REGURGITATION

- Tricuspid regurgitation is more commonly observed in small breed dogs.
- Swelling of the right ventricle or injury of the tricuspid valve results in leakage of the valve causing blood to leak back into the right atrium during ventricular contraction.
- Hemodynamic management should be directed at avoiding an increase in pulmonary vascular resistance and to improve forward pulmonary blood outflow.
- Anesthetic management should be aimed at maintaining right ventricular filling and avoiding pulmonary hypertension. Ventricular filling should be maintained with proper fluid administration; avoid intermittent positive-pressure ventilation (IPPV) or significant drug-induced vasodilation. IPPV with excessive airway pressure greatly compresses the vena cavae and decreases venous return. High doses of vasodilatory drugs (e.g. acepromazine, propofol, or isoflurane/sevoflurane) also lead to peripheral pooling of blood and decreases in venous return. Pulmonary hypertension can be minimized by avoiding hypoxemia and hypercapnia, since both conditions result in increased pulmonary vascular resistance and lead to pulmonary hypertension. Alpha-2 anesthetics such as dexmedetomidine and medetomidine tend to induce pulmonary hypertension and should be avoided.

PULMONIC STENOSIS

- Pulmonic stenosis occur in breeds such as Boston Terriers, Jack Russel Terriers,

Miniature Schnauzers, West Highland White Terriers, Bulldogs and Labrador Retrievers as a congenital disorder. Pulmonic stenosis rarely occurs in cats.

- It is a congenital condition with narrowing of the pulmonic valve due to thickening or fusion of the pulmonic leaflets. The stenotic sites can be valvular or perivalvular or within the pulmonary trees. The stenosis obstructs the blood flow from the right ventricle to the pulmonary artery; as a result a higher contractile force must be generated by the right ventricle to overcome the stenosis. With this compensatory increase in contractility, the right ventricle becomes hypertrophic and dilated with various degrees of cardiac murmurs and arrhythmia that can lead to right-sided congestive heart failure. The cardiac murmur can be easily heard or palpated through thoracic auscultation and palpation.

- The dog may require sedation or general anesthesia to perform a physical examination, radiography, or echocardiography to determine the severity of the stenosis. Echocardiography evaluates the blood velocity flow across the stenosis and the pressure gradients between the right ventricle and pulmonary artery. Balloon valvuloplasty may be performed in suitable candidates after a diagnosis of pulmonic stenosis.

- Because pulmonic stenosis increases the right ventricular work load and impairs left ventricular output by reducing forward flow, the hemodynamic goals of managing pulmonic stenosis are to maintain right ventricular contractibility, to provide a balance between maintaining right ventricular preload and avoiding excessive fluid overload, and to maintain left ventricular contractility. The HR should preferably be kept at the low normal range.

- The anesthetic goal is to reduce pulmonary vascular resistance (i.e. pulmonary hypertension) and SVR. IPPV, arterial hypoxemia and hypercapnia, acidosis, and hypothermia all may result in an increase in pulmonary vascular resistance.

AORTIC STENOSIS

- Occurs in large breed dogs and occasionally in cats.

- Aortic stenosis can occur above (supra-), below (sub-), or right at the aortic valve itself. Subaortic stenosis is the most prevalent form of aortic stenosis in dogs.

- Aortic stenosis impedes the left ventricular forward flow due to narrowing of the left ventricular outflow tract. The stenotic aortic valve also requires extra energy (therefore increases myocardial oxygen consumption) needed to overcome the resistance of the narrowing orifice. This disease process eventually leads to increased left ventricular pressure and left ventricular hypertrophic cardiomyopathy.

- Hemodynamic goal should be directed at maintaining adequate systemic blood pressure to maintain CO. Hypotension and bradycardia drastically affect hemodynamic stability and are poorly tolerated by the patient. Maintaining sinus rhythm and HR is vital in order to protect diastolic filling time. Inotropic support via dopamine/ dobutamine and fluid is needed despite the poor ventricular function. Premature ventricular contractions may appear frequently during the stress (i.e. increased myocardial oxygen consumption) and should be treated with lidocaine to optimize hemodynamic stability.

- Anesthetic management should be directed at maintaining blood pressure and CO and avoiding hypotension. Profound vasodilation associated with high doses of acepromazine, propofol, and isoflurane or sevoflurane should be avoided.

PATENT DUCTUS ARTERIOSUS (PDA)

- PDA is a vascular structure pathology that occurs at the proximal descending aorta and the roof of the main pulmonary artery. This vasculature is supposed to close spontaneously soon after birth, but ends up remaining open and allowing an extracardiac left-to-right shunt. PDA frequently occurs in younger dogs due to a congenital defect and requires anesthesia for either surgical or transcardiac catheter closure of the patent ductus.

- Pulmonary overcirculation and left heart volume overload are the two main hemodynamic impacts of the PDA. Overcirculation of the pulmonary trees results in decreased lung compliance and increased work in breathing.

- Because of the left-to-right shunt, pulmonary fluid volume overload results in an increase in flow returning to the left atrial and an increase in left ventricular end-diastolic pressures. Increased HR and cardiac contractility in the PDA patient is a neuroendocrine adaptation. An untreated PDA may result in left-sided heart enlargement and eventually left-sided congestive heart failure. The diastolic blood pressure in the aorta decreases owing to diastolic 'runoff' through the patent ductus and this causes a lower than normal diastolic pressure with a hyperkinetic pulse pressure.

- A continuous 'machinery' heart murmur is usually detected around the third intercostal space at the heart base with a stethoscope, and there is a palpable thrill at this site. Patients with a small PDA may not have a palpable thrill.

- Catheter treatment of PDA, either performing transarterial embolization with detachable or free coils or transvenously using a device called an Amplatz Canine Ductal Occluder under fluoroscopy, aims to stop the abnormal blood flow through the PDA. These procedures cause a blood clot to form in the abnormal ductus arteriosus that closes off the abnormal patent blood vessel.

- Anesthetic management of the PDA includes:
  - Dogs with evidence of pulmonary edema should be treated with furosemide for 24–48 hours before anesthesia induction.
  - In poorly developed puppies with PDA, preoperative fasting should be <6 hours in duration and intraoperative glucose may have to be supplemented.
  - A balanced electrolyte solution should be administered intraoperatively at a rate of 3–5 ml/kg/hour.

- Midazolam with an opioid (butorphanol, methandone, or hydromorphone) can be used as IM premedication. Anesthesia may be induced with propofol, alfaxalone, or etomidate. Preoxygenation prior to anesthetic induction is helpful.

- Routinely using anticholinergic agents should be avoided. However, if the HR is low and the blood pressure is also low, an anticholinergic agent should be administered to improve blood pressure

- Inhalant maintenance should be kept at a low concentration by supplementing additional midazolam and opioid during the procedure so that blood pressure is better maintained.

PERICARDIAL EFFUSION

- Pericardial effusion is characterized by accumulation of fluid inside the pericardium, which results in a cardiac tamponade associated with a lower fixed stroke volume and low CO.

- Pericardial effusion can be due to tumors (hemangiosarcoma or mesothelioma), idiopathic or secondary to congestive heart failure.

- Patients with pericardial effusion may require general anesthesia to perform pericardiocentesis or pericardiectomy.

- Hemodynamic management is directed to maintain HR in order to maintain CO.

PROTOCOLS TO MINIMIZE THE RISK AND MAXIMIZE THE CHANCES OF A GOOD ANESTHETIC OUTCOME IN PATIENTS WITH PRE-EXISTING CARDIAC DISEASE

- Obtain an accurate cardiac diagnosis. The primary and secondary effects of the cardiac dysfunction must be understood and treated appropriately.

- Anesthetic drugs that offset, rather than aggravate, the cardiovascular disease should be used.

- The adverse hemodynamic effects of the surgery or procedure requiring general anesthesia need to be understood.

- Appropriate drugs must be available to treat autonomic and cardiovascular dysfunction in order to preserve cardiac function.

- Adequate preoperative, intraoperative, and postoperative monitoring should be provided. ECG, pulse oximetry, capnography, and blood pressure monitoring are required.
- A thorough physical examination, including pulse quality and determination of HR and rhythm, is very important. Thoracic auscultation should be performed to assess arrhythmias, murmurs, crackles, wheezes, and pulse deficits.
- A preanesthetic work-up may include thoracic radiographs, ECG, blood pressure measurement, echocardiogram, and blood gas analysis.

ANESTHETIC MANAGEMENT AND PHARMACOLOGIC CONSIDERATIONS

- The pharmacologic considerations for various anesthetic agents/drugs are listed in *Table 10.4*.
- Preservation of CO is the key concept in safely managing patients with cardiac dysfunction, as they may not have adequate cardiac reserve. All general anesthetics decrease CO. The anesthetist's goal is to maintain vital tissue perfusion using the lowest possible doses despite these limitations.

- CO is a function of HR, preload, afterload, and myocardial contractility. HR under general anesthesia should be properly maintained within certain limits. A HR that is too slow or too fast is suboptimal.
- Preload and myocardial contractility must be maintained as close to normal as possible throughout the perioperative period.
- Drugs that increase afterload should be avoided in patients with most cardiac conditions.
- As with any other patient, those with heart disease that are otherwise in optimal shape prior to anesthesia have the best outcome. Improve ventricular function (to maintain tissue perfusion); treat existing arrhythmias; maintain effective circulating drug volume; correct anemia; and maintain proper tissue oxygenation.
- Acepromazine is an antiarrhythmic drug that has minimal effects on cardiac contractility, but does cause vasodilation. Vasodilation from alpha-receptor blockade on the vasculature results in decreased afterload, as well as decreased preload.
- Anticholinergics (e.g. atropine and glycopyrrolate) are used to treat bradyarrhythmias. They must be used

Table 10.4 Pharmacologic considerations for various anesthetic agents/drugs	
Anesthetic/drug	*Pharmacologic considerations*
Acepromazine	Vasodilation, decreases afterload, and affects preload
Anticholinergics (atropine, glycopyrrolate)	Iatrogenic tachycardia, increase myocardial oxygen consumption and cardiac arrhythmia
Alpha-2 adrenergic agonists	Decrease in heart rate, cardiac contractility and increase in afterload through peripheral vasoconstriction
Benzodiazepines	Minimal sedation with minimal cardiac depression
Opioids	Decrease heart rate, but do not depress cardiovascular function
Thiopentone, propofol, alfaxalone	Dose-dependent cardiac contractility reduction and vasodilation
Etomidate	Minimal changes in heart rate and blood pressure
Dissociatives	Indirectly supportive of cardiac function due to their stimulation of the sympathetic nervous system
Inhalants (isoflurane and sevoflurane)	Dose-dependent cardiac output reduction and vasodilation

with caution in cardiac patients, as an iatrogenically-increased HR leads to increased myocardial work and increased myocardial oxygen demand. This may be associated with decreased myocardial perfusion and arrhythmias.

- The use of alpha-2 agents (e.g. dexmedetomidine, medetomidine, or xylazine) is usually not recommended in cardiac patients. These drugs result in a decreased HR, contractility, and CO. The primary concern after administration of an alpha-2 agent is the large increase in afterload due to peripheral vasoconstriction, which increases SVR.
- BNZs, such as diazepam or midazolam, while possessing only mild sedative properties, have minimal cardiac effects and are a good choice in cardiac patients.
- Opioids can produce mild bradycardia by increasing vagal tone. This can be prevented by the concurrent administration, of anticholinergics. They are a good choice for most cardiac patients, as they do not decrease contractility (except meperidine). Meperidine and morphine release histamine, which can cause hypotension in some patients.
- Thiopentone, propofol, and, to a lesser degree, alfaxalone produce dose-dependent decreases in myocardial contractility, vasodilation, and compensatory increases in HR, arrhythmia formation, and hypotension.
- Etomidate is the drug of choice for patients with severe cardiac disease. It has minimal effects on HR and myocardial contractility, maintaining the initial level of CO. Propylene glycol, a vehicle of etomidate, may be associated with severe red cell shrinkage and may cause adrenocortical suppression in animals up to 1 week following administration. Etomidate, when used alone, without premedication, causes muscle twitching, and a muscle relaxant, such as diazepam (midazolam), administered IV prior to etomidate administration can help reduce this side-effect.
- Dissociative agents (e.g. ketamine and tiletamine) are indirectly supportive of cardiac function due to their stimulation of the sympathetic nervous system. They produce increases in HR, stroke volume, CO, and blood pressure.

When using larger doses, they inhibit myocardial contractility and can act as negative inotropes in patients lacking a sympathetic nervous system response. Use of appropriate doses of these drugs is helpful in dilated cardiomyopathy cases.
- Isoflurane and sevoflurane are superior to halothane in cardiac patients, except in those patients that cannot tolerate decreases in SVR. All inhalants cause dose-dependent CO reduction. Isoflurane and sevoflurane also induce dose-dependent reduction in SVR and peripheral pooling of blood, which reduces venous return. Caution should be taken when using high concentrations of these inhalants in tricuspid regurgitation and hypertrophic cardiomyopathy patients.
- Avoid tachycardia or bradycardia in cardiac patients.
- Monitor fluid administration carefully since the Frank–Starling law (which states volume loading the ventricle will improve cardiac contractility of the heart) may not apply. Diligence should be taken to balance adequate ventricular filling with fluids and excessive fluid administration. Reducing the crystalloid fluid rate to 3–5 ml/kg/hour may be necessary in some of these patients when under anesthesia.
- Avoid hypovolemia, blood loss, and decreased preload.
- Maintain contractility as much as possible, including the use of inotropes as appropriate.
- Preoxygenate the patient prior to anesthetic administration. This is because administering a high fraction of inspired oxygen for 3 minutes before induction of anesthesia will increase intrapulmonary oxygen reserves and delay the onset of hemoglobin desaturation with anesthetic-induced apnea.

EXAMPLES OF ANESTHETIC PROTOCOLS FOR DOGS WITH CARDIAC DYSFUNCTION

Premedication
- Midazolam or diazepam, 0.2–0.4 mg/kg IM.
- Opioid:
  - Butorphanol 0.2–0.4 mg/kg IM or
  - Buprenorphine 40–60 µg/kg, IM or

- Hydromorphone 0.05–0.1 mg/kg IM or
- Morphine 0.25–0.75 mg/kg IM.

Intravenous induction
- Propofol 4–6 mg/kg IV.
- Etomidate1–2 mg/kg IV.
- Alfaxalone 2–3 mg/kg IV.

Maintenance
Anesthesia is maintained with low concentrations of isoflurane or sevoflurane.

ANESTHETIC PROTOCOLS FOR CATS WITH CARDIAC DYSFUNCTION
- Similar anesthetic protocols to those listed above for dogs can be used.
- Ketamine (1–2 mg/kg IM) or tiletamine/zolazepam (1–2 mg/kg IM) can be added to midazolam and the opioid for premedication, but it should not be used in cats with hypertrophic cardiomyopathy or hyperthyroidism since increases in cardiac contractility arising from the ketamine/tiletamine could be detrimental.

Respiratory dysfunction

Specific respiratory disease-induced dysfunctions relating to anesthesia are listed in *Table 10.5*.

GENERAL CONSIDERATIONS
- General anesthesia compromises ventilation and gas exchange in all patients, but it is of particular concern in patients with respiratory disease because of their inability to compensate for these changes.
- Respiratory disease can be divided into extrapulmonary dysfunction and intrapulmonary dysfunction.
- Examples of extrapulmonary dysfunction include:
  - Diaphragmatic hernia.
  - Pneumothorax.
  - Hydrothorax.
  - Space-occupying lesions of the thorax.
  - Flail chest.
  - Anything that decreases chest wall expansion.
- Examples of intrapulmonary dysfunction include:
  - Pneumonia.
  - Pulmonary edema.

- Intrapulmonary hemorrhage (contusions).
- Atelectasis.
- Interstitial disease.
- Airway obstruction.
- Collapsing trachea.
- Laryngeal dysfunction.

ANESTHETIC MANAGEMENT AND PHARMACOLOGIC CONSIDERATIONS
- Extrapulmonary dysfunction should be corrected prior to anesthesia whenever possible. This may include the removal of any accumulated fluid via thoracocentesis.
- General anesthesia should be avoided in patients with pulmonary edema, pneumothorax, hemothorax, and pneumonia since gas exchange is significantly reduced and hypoxia is likely.
- Supplemental oxygen therapy should be available perioperatively.
- Patients with respiratory dysfunction should be carefully observed after sedation. Mild sedatives such as acepromazine, which produces minimal respiratory depression, are preferred. Low doses should be used, as a prolonged

Table 10.5 Respiratory disease-induced dysfunctions relating to anesthesia

Disease-induced abnormality	Consequences	Management
Difficulty in gas exchange	Hypoxia, hypercapnia	Provide 100%, oxygen Assisted or controlled ventilation
Reduced functional residual capacity	Unable to generate adequate tidal volume and lung capacity	Reduce space-occupying fluids, air, and mass
Airway obstruction	Hypoxemia, hypercapnia	Establish airway and maintain patency

recovery secondary to high doses of acepromazine is not desirable in these cases.

- Induction should be accomplished quickly with an injectable anesthetic agent so that the airway can be established and positive-pressure ventilation initiated, if necessary.
- The use of a laryngoscope and stylet is necessary to facilitate endotracheal intubation in brachycephalic breed dogs or patients with upper airway obstruction. (See Chapter 11 for more information.)
- Mask induction is often suboptimal in patients that cannot ventilate well.
- All opioids, including morphine, hydromorphone, and fentanyl, cause significant respiratory depression. Butorphanol and buprenorphine have less of a respiratory depressive effect.
- All IV induction agents, including thiopentone, propofol, etomidate, and alfaxalone, are significantly respiratory depressive. They all induce apnea and hypoventilation when administered rapidly as a large bolus. To avoid apnea, these induction agents should be titrated slowly using an IV catheter over a period of 60–90 seconds. For patients requiring immediate positive-pressure ventilation (e.g. in cases of diaphragmatic hernia), a more rapid bolus injection can be administered so that positive-pressure ventilation can be instituted immediately.
- Both isoflurane and sevoflurane have dose-dependent respiratory depressive effects.

Preparation for extrapulmonary dysfunctional patients

- Preoxygenate the patient before anesthetic induction.
- Remove any fluid, air, purulent material, or blood from the thoracic cavity via thoracocentesis before anesthetic induction.
- Rapidly induce anesthesia and follow with endotracheal intubation and positive-pressure ventilation using 100% oxygen.
- Position patients with a diaphragmatic hernia so as to avoid compression of the

functional lung lobes by herniated viscera. The cranial portion of the thorax should be higher than the abdomen in these patients.

- Anticipate sudden bradycardia when positioning the animal for surgery.

Preparation for intrapulmonary dysfunctional patients

- For patients with an upper airway obstruction, establish an airway by intubating with an endotracheal tube immediately after induction. Depending on the location of the obstruction, the endotracheal tube may well resolve the problem.
- Whenever possible, avoid general anesthesia in other types of intrapulmonary dysfunction.
- Monitor these patients closely and continuously for oxygenation immediately following surgery and until fully recovered.

EXAMPLES OF ANESTHETIC PROTOCOLS FOR DOGS AND CATS WITH RESPIRATORY DYSFUNCTION (E.G. BRACHYCEPHALIC OBSTRUCTIVE AIRWAY DISEASE)

Premedication

- Diazepam or midazolam (0.1–0.2 mg/kg IM or IV) or acepromazine (0.01 mg/kg IM or IV).
- Opioids (IM):
  - Butorphanol, if the procedure is not significantly painful.
  - Methadone may be useful for painful procedures with less potential for vomiting.
  - Hydromorphone or morphine for painful procedures.

Intravenous induction

- Always provide preoxygenation with either a face mask or flow-by method with enriched oxygen prior to anesthetic induction.
- Propofol or alfaxalone or ketamine (with midazolam).

Maintenance

Anesthesia is maintained with sevoflurane or isoflurane.

Central nervous system dysfunction

Specific central nervous system (CNS) disease-induced dysfunctions relating to anesthesia are listed in *Table 10.6*.

GENERAL CONSIDERATIONS

- All general anesthetics depress the CNS, which superimposes additional depression on top of an already diseased nervous system.
- Cerebral blood flow (CBF) is autoregulated by the body and influenced by systemic blood pressure, $PaCO_2$, and severe hypoxia, which are all affected by general anesthesia.
- Specific concerns for general anesthesia are most indicated when the patient has signs of increased intracranial pressure (ICP) due to brain trauma or space-occupying lesions, a history of seizures, or intracranial lesions.
- In patients with increased ICP, a history of seizures with suspected brain tumors, or intracranial lesions, hypoventilation should be avoided and hyperventilation provided to achieve the target range for $PaCO_2$ of 25–30 mmHg ($ETCO_2$ of 15–25 mmHg), which will decrease CO_2-driven increases in CBF and therefore lower ICP. For every 1 mmHg decrease in $PaCO_2$, there is approximately a 2% decrease in CBF.
- CBF is determined by cerebral perfusion pressure (blood pressure providing perfusion to the brain) and cerebral vascular resistance. Cerebral perfusion pressure is determined from mean arterial blood pressure (MAP), ICP, and central venous pressure. Cerebral perfusion pressure is usually the net difference between MAP and ICP. Under normal circumstances, MAP is between 60 and 100 mmHg and normal ICP is 5–15 mmHg, so the cerebral perfusion pressure ranges from 50 to 70 mmHg. Ischemic brain damage occurs if cerebral perfusion pressure is <50 mmHg for a sustained period of time. Therefore, it is important to maintain MAP and carefully manage ICP during the perioperative period.
- Hypoxia should be avoided because this also induces a high ICP.
- IV fluids should be used to support systemic circulation during general anesthesia, but overhydration, which increases central venous pressure and potentially lowers cerebral perfusion pressure, must be avoided.
- Bradycardia may be observed as a result of large increases in ICP. A breathing pattern, called Biot's respiration, may be seen in cases of increased intracranial pressure. Biot's respiration is characterized by a series of rapid, shallow inspirations followed by regular or irregular periods of apnea. Biot's respiration is caused by damage to the medulla oblongata due to trauma or by pressure on the medulla due to herniation.
- The use of anesthetics that might stimulate muscle rigidity or trigger seizures (i.e. ketamine or tiletamine) should be avoided. Dissociatives increase ICP and should be avoided in patients with CNS dysfunction.

Table 10.6 Central nervous system disease-induced dysfunctions relating to anesthesia

Disease-induced abnormality	Consequences	Management
Increase in intracranial pressure	Prolonged recovery Bradycardia	Controlled ventilation to reduce $PaCO_2$ Avoid hypoxemia and hypercapnia
Loss of mobility	Various neurologic signs	Caution when moving patients Standard anesthesia management
Impaired cerebral blood flow and loss of autoregulation	Various neurologic signs	Proper maintenance of blood pressure using fluids and inotropes
Convulsion	Increased oxygen consumption Loss of airway	Establish airway Provide oxygen Avoid using drugs that trigger seizures

- Anticonvulsants (e.g. diazepam or midazolam) should be available to treat seizures during the postoperative period. A patent IV catheter will facilitate this.

ANESTHETIC MANAGEMENT AND PHARMACOLOGIC CONSIDERATIONS

- Recent evidence suggests that acepromazine is not associated with decreased seizure threshold and does not promote seizure activity when used in epileptic patients. Therefore, acepromazine can be used judiciously as part of the premedication in patients with a history of seizures.
- Dexmedetomidine and medetomidine decrease ICP and are acceptable agents for use in neurologic patients at low doses.
- Diazepam and midazolam are helpful for muscle relaxation and seizure control in neurologic patients when used for premedication or postoperative seizure control.
- The use of opioids may be necessary for pain management. If assisted or controlled ventilation is not provided, high doses of potent opioids, such as fentanyl or hydromorphone, may lead to hypoventilation and indirectly increase ICP by increasing the $PaCO_2$.
- Propofol, alfaxalone, or etomidate are effective IV induction agents in cases with head injuries, as they decrease ICP.
- Ketamine or tiletamine should be avoided in neurologic patients given that they increase ICP and are associated with seizure activity.
- Inhalant anesthetic agents, such as isoflurane and sevoflurane, lead to increased ICP. Mild increases may be offset with slight hyperventilation of the patient.

EXAMPLES OF ANESTHETIC PROTOCOLS FOR DOGS WITH CNS DYSFUNCTION
Premedication

- Acepromazine 0.01–0.03 mg/kg IM or midazolam 0.2–0.4 mg/kg IM.
- Butorphanol 0.2–0.4 mg/kg IM, or hydromorphone 0.1–0.2 mg/kg IM, or methadone 0.2–0.4 mg/kg IM.

Induction

- Propofol 4–6 mg/kg IV.
- Alfaxalone 2–3 mg/kg IV.

Maintenance

- Anesthesia should be maintained with isoflurane or sevoflurane.
- Hyperventilation to maintain $PaCO_2$ at 25–30 mmHg ($ETCO_2$ of 15–25 mmHg) may be needed in patients with a suspected brain tumor or head trauma.

OTHER CONSIDERATIONS

- Be aware of head-down patient positioning, occlusion of jugular veins, or coughing, which all increase ICP.
- Fluid administration should be carefully monitored to prevent fluid overload.
- Be prepared for postoperative treatment of seizures.

Endocrine dysfunction

DIABETES MELLITUS

GENERAL CONSIDERATIONS

- An abnormal blood glucose level is the most common complication in these patients.
- Like any other patient, diabetic patients must be fasted prior to general anesthesia, but blood glucose needs to be closely monitored prior to anesthesia induction and every 30–60 minutes throughout the procedure and until the patient is fully recovered.
- Treatment is required if glucose levels deviate outside the normal range (3.7–7.4 mmol/l [67–134 mg/dl]).
- In general, a half insulin dose is administered to the fasted patient, with no insulin being provided if the blood glucose level is <11.1 mmol/l (200 mg/dl). Diabetic patients should be the earliest surgeries of the day to allow quick resumption of regular feeding and insulin schedule.

- If the blood glucose level is <3.3 mmol/l (67 mg/dl), supplemental fluids with dextrose (2.5–5%) should be administered during the procedure. Blood glucose should be monitored every 30 minutes.
- Ketoacidotic patients need to be stabilized prior to induction of general anesthesia. Excessively high blood glucose levels with a lack of insulin lead to a breakdown of body fat for energy, with resultant accumulation of ketones in the blood and urine. Severely affected patients also exhibit hyperglycemia (levels as high as 22.2–27.8 mmol/l [400–500 mg/dl] have been recorded), profound metabolic acidosis, and hyperketonemia. These patients require stabilization by correcting the dehydration, hyperglycemia, electrolyte abnormalities, acid–base imbalance, and hyperosmolarity before anesthesia.
- Insulins are divided into four types based on their duration of action: rapid-acting (lasts for 2–4 h), short-acting (or regular; lasts for 3–6 h), intermediate-acting (lasts for 12–18 h), and long-acting (lasts for 24 h).
- Caution should be taken when administering insulin to reduce blood glucose during anesthesia. Only the rapid-acting (Humalog, NovoLog) or short-acting (Humulin R, Novolin R) types of insulin should be administered immediately prior or during anesthesia. The intermediate-acting or long-acting types of insulin (Humulin U and Lantus) take more than 1 hour to reduce the blood glucose and will not be able to alleviate hyperglycemia during the anesthetic period; rather it will induce profound hypoglycemia hours later following administration.
- The short-acting types of insulin take more rapid action (within 30 minutes) to reduce blood glucose than the intermediate- and long-acting types of insulin.
- Profound and prolonged postoperative hypoglycemia has occurred following 2–3 doses of intraoperative administration of intermediate-acting types of insulin (Humulin N, Novolin N, Humulin L); this has resulted in patients requiring prolonged hypoglycemia management after anesthesia recovery.

ANESTHETIC MANAGEMENT AND PHARMACOLOGIC CONSIDERATIONS

- Anesthetic management is directed more toward preanesthetic preparation and maintaining euglycemia, normal electrolyte balance, and normal blood gasses.
- Alpha-2 agents, such as dexmedetomidine, medetomidine, or xylazine, promote insulin resistance and should be avoided in diabetic patients.
- Drugs with a long duration of action should be avoided to prevent a prolonged recovery. Rapid recovery allows the patient to resume a normal feeding schedule as soon as possible.

Hypothyroidism

GENERAL CONSIDERATIONS

- Most patients with mild-to-moderate hypothyroidism tolerate general anesthesia without complications.
- Body temperature should be monitored and every effort made to keep the patient at a normal body temperature.

ANESTHETIC MANAGEMENT AND PHARMACOLOGIC CONSIDERATIONS

- The use of acepromazine should be avoided as the drug has a long duration of action, causes vasodilation, and results in hypothermia.

Hyperthyroidism

GENERAL CONSIDERATIONS

- Dogs and cats should be rendered euthyroid prior to general anesthesia if at all possible.
- Many hyperthyroid cats have associated cardiac disease, in particular hypertrophic cardiomyopathy. These cases should be managed for hypertrophic cardiomyopathy, as discussed earlier.
- Drug protocols should be tailored to individual conditions.

ANESTHETIC MANAGEMENT AND CONSIDERATIONS

- Drugs that elevate HR (anticholinergics) or sympathetic tone (ketamine and tiletamine) should be avoided.
- Thiopentone has antithyroid activity, but may not be appropriate for cats in heart failure.

EXAMPLES OF ANESTHETIC PROTOCOLS FOR DOGS AND CATS WITH ENDOCRINE DISORDERS
Premedication

- Acepromazine 0.02–0.05 mg/ kg IM. (**Note:** Avoid high doses of acepromazine in cats with hypertrophic cardiomyopathy as it causes prolonged and profound peripheral vasodilation and hypotension.)

Urinary and renal dysfunction

GENERAL CONSIDERATIONS

- All anesthetic agents decrease renal blood flow and glomerular filtration rate (GFR). This in turn reduces the patient's ability to metabolize and excrete anesthetic drugs through the kidneys.
- Patients presenting with renal dysfunction may be well compensated or uncompensated.
- Compensated patients require little change in anesthetic protocol from those without renal disease, while uncompensated patients will require extensive intervention to normalize hydration, electrolyte balance, and acid–base status.
- General anesthesia increases sympathetic nervous system activity and stimulates the renin–angiotensin system, resulting in decreased renal blood flow. This response is exaggerated by hypovolemia, hypotension, hypoxemia, hypercapnia, or by agents that stimulate the sympathetic nervous system, such as ketamine or catecholamines. An animal with pre-existing renal disease may not be able to withstand these changes and renal failure may ensue.
- Renal disease can be subdivided into prerenal, renal, and postrenal disease and

- Midazolam 0.2–0.4 mg/kg with alfaxalone 1–2 mg/kg and one of the opioids works well for a reasonable sedation.
- Opioids:
  - Butorphanol 0.2 mg/kg or
  - Hydromorphone 0.1 mg/kg or
  - Methadone 0.5–1.0 mg/kg or
  - Buprenorphine 0.04–0.06 mg/kg.

Induction

- Chamber or face mask induction with isoflurane or sevoflurane or
- Propofol 6 mg/kg IV or
- Alfaxalone 2–3 mg/kg IV.

Maintenance

- Anesthesia can be maintained on isoflurane or sevoflurane.

anesthetic management should be tailored accordingly.
- Anesthesia and the stress associated with surgery causes release of aldosterone, vasopressin, renin, and catecholamines and decreases in GFR, renal blood flow, and urine production. This may prolong recovery from drugs that require renal excretion.
- Fluids should be administered to correct dehydration and promote diuretic excretion of wastes prior to anesthesia. Water intake should not be restricted.
- Azotemia (see also Chapter 2) is associated with potentiation of anesthetics. Azotemia may be associated with changes in the blood–brain barrier, increasing CNS drug activity. Lower doses are generally required for induction and maintenance of anesthesia in patients with renal disease.
- Patients with renal insufficiency, urethral obstruction, or a ruptured bladder may present with hyperkalemia and other electrolyte imbalances. Normal serum potassium concentrations for cats range from 4.2 to 5.9 mmol/l (4.2 to 5.9 mEq/l) (see also Chapter 2). Elevated serum potassium concentrations are associated with ECG changes. The P-R interval becomes prolonged when serum

potassium exceeds 8 mmol/l (8 mEq/l). Serum potassium concentrations >8.7 mmol/l (8.7 mEq/l) are associated with tall T-waves and small P waves. A serum potassium >9.8 mmol/l is associated with bradycardia or cardiac standstill, which is often followed by cardiac arrest. It is essential to monitor and correct plasma electrolyte imbalances prior to anesthesia. It is also important to monitor cardiac arrhythmias associated with these electrolyte imbalances and to treat them accordingly.

- Retention of metabolic byproducts by the kidney causes metabolic acidosis. This can be corrected with IV fluids. The administration of sodium bicarbonate may also be considered. Generally, rehydrating a patient is sufficient to return pH to normal over time. Sodium bicarbonate administration during anesthesia is only necessary if the pH is <7.2 or HCO_3 is <18 mmol/l (18 mEq/l).
- Patients with renal failure are frequently anemic. Anesthesia is associated with a decreased hemoglobin concentration, fluid administration causes hemodilution, and surgery is associated with blood loss. A PCV in the range of 0.27–0.3 l/l (27–30%) is desirable.
- The use of nephrotoxic antibiotics, which may worsen renal function, should be minimized.

ANESTHETIC CONSIDERATIONS OF HEMODIALYSIS AND HEMOPERFUSION CASES

Hemodialysis/hemoperfusion involves large volumes of a patient's anticoagulated blood being filtered through an adsorbent material (resins or columns of activated charcoal) in order to remove toxic substances and toxic waste from the blood. The clinical application of these treatments is to buy more time for dogs and cats that are suffering from acute renal damage (acute kidney injury, AKI) due to acute intoxication from ethylene glycol (antifreeze), NSAIDs (aspirin or acetaminophen), or sedative/antiseizure drugs (pentobarbital or phenobarbital). Occasionally, this can be applied to dogs infected with leptospirosis or with chronic renal diseases.

Clinically, the health status of dogs and cats undergoing hemodialysis/hemoperfusion can be largely classified into three categories: (1) overall healthy animals that are in the toxin-induced first- (initial pathologic renal changes with >25% decrease in GFR) or second-stage (ischemia, hypoxia, inflammation, and cellular injury of the kidney with >50% reduction in GFR) AKI due to toxic substance ingestion; (2) dogs and cats with third-stage AKI, which is characterized by azotemia or uremia or anuria/oliguria (urine output <0.5 ml/kg/hour, with >75% reduction in GFR or total loss of renal function) with electrolyte derangement (hyperkalemia) and severe metabolic acidosis; (3) dogs and cats with urinary outflow tract obstruction, where animals with stones in the ureter just prior to their subcutaneous ureteral bypass surgery can be stabilized by hemodialysis.

Patients in third-stage or end-stage AKI or with obstructed urinary tract outflow frequently come to the hemodialysis/hemoperfusion center with fluid overload. This is because initial fluid resuscitation frequently has a higher fluid rate administered to these animals, but the animals usually are unable to match this with increased urinary excretion because of the the injured kidneys. It has been documented in humans that such fluid overload is associated with poor survival rate. It is better to leave the fluid correction to hemodialysis. Fluids should be used conservatively for these categories of fluid-overloaded patients that are undergoing hemodialysis/hemoperfusion.

Hemodialysis/hemoperfusion patients need anesthesia for placing the hemodialysis catheter in the jugular vein and at times need an esophagostomy tube placement. There is a tendency to lean toward not correcting hyperkalemia in dogs and cats subjected to hemodialysis catheter placement prior to hemodialysis. The short anesthesia time (less than 30 minutes) is likely tolerated by these animals. The main concerns for treating hyperkalemic animals with sodium bicarbonate, insulin, and glucose to drive the potassium back into the intracellular space is that some urologists worry about rebound of potassium following a short dialysis treatment. This may mean that a previously dialyzed animal has to undergo hemodialysis sooner.

ANESTHETIC MANAGEMENT AND PHARMACOLOGIC CONSIDERATIONS
Premedication

- Acepromazine may be advantageous in renal patients due to the vasodilatory nature of the drug. Since acepromazine is a dopamine antagonist, it should not be used if dopamine administration is planned to improve renal blood flow.
- A study compared the effect of IV administration of acepromazine–butorphanol, diazepam–butorphanol, and diazepam–ketamine on GFR values in clinically healthy dogs. The results indicated that acepromazine–butorphanol provides the best sedative effects and was associated with GFR values identical to those in awake dogs. Furthermore, the systemic hypotension caused by acepromazine did not decrease the GFR in clinically normal dogs. Hypotension will be an issue in renal-compromised dogs and cats if high doses of acepromazine are used.
- Opioids can be used for renal patients and are helpful for pain management.
- Alpha-2 agents are generally avoided due to the associated decrease in CO, potential for bradycardia, and reduced renal blood flow (due to vasoconstriction).

Induction

- The choice of induction agent is not critical in patients with compensated renal disease.
- Patients that are severely depressed should have an anesthetic plan that maximizes CO and stability.
- In cats, ketamine is highly dependent on the kidney for excretion, so large doses of ketamine should not be administered to cats with renal disease.

Maintenance

- Maintenance on isoflurane or sevoflurane decreases GFR and it is important to maintain proper blood pressure to support renal perfusion pressure, thus minimizing the damage to remaining nephrons.

Other considerations

- Fluid administration:
  - Peripheral volume support through the use of 10–20 ml/kg/hour of

crystalloid isotonic fluids is essential. However, caution should be taken to watch out for fluid overload in AKI patients.
- Patients should not be hypovolemic prior to general anesthesia and any volume deficits should be corrected before induction.
- Urine output should be measured by aseptic catheterization of the bladder. Normal urine output is 1–2 ml/kg/hour.
- Dopamine therapy may be considered in debilitated patients (1–10 µg/kg/min). Low doses of dopamine will increase renal blood flow, GFR, and urine output. Higher doses will activate beta adrenoceptors, which may dilate renal arterial beds and increase CO.
- Adequate analgesia is very important since pain will cause catecholamine release, vasoconstriction, and decreased blood flow.
- NSAIDs should be avoided or used with caution.

EXAMPLES OF ANESTHETIC PROTOCOLS FOR DOGS AND CATS WITH URINARY AND RENAL DYSFUNCTION

COMPENSATED RENAL FAILURE

Premedication

- Acepromazine 0.01–0.02 mg/kg IM or midazolam 0.1–0.2 mg/kg IM.
- Opioids (IM):
  - Morphine 0.25–0.5 mg/kg or
  - Hydromorphone 0.05–0.1 mg/kg or
  - Butorphanol 0.2–0.4 mg/kg or
  - Buprenorphine 0.04–0.06 mg/kg.
  - Methadone 0.4–0.8 mg/kg.

Induction

- Propofol 3–5 mg/kg to effect or
- Alfaxalone 2–3 mg/kg IV.

Maintenance

General anesthesia can be maintained with isoflurane of sevoflurane.

Other considerations

- Blood pressure and fluid administration should be carefully monitored. Patients

should be well hydrated prior to premedication.
- The use of NSAIDs for pain management should be avoided or used with extreme caution.

UNCOMPENSATED RENAL FAILURE
- Patients should be rehydrated as completely as possible to decrease azotemia.
- Urine output should be monitored.

Gastrointestinal dysfunction

GENERAL CONSIDERATIONS
- Patients with gastrointestinal dysfunction requiring anesthesia may present for upper and lower gastrointestinal endoscopy, retrieval of foreign bodies, or treatment of gastric dilatation/volvulus (GDV).
- The use of NSAIDs should be avoided or used with caution.
- Dogs with GDV often have sinus tachycardia and require immediate decompression. The use of opioids, such as butorphanol or hydromorphone, is helpful to sedate these patients, providing immediate analgesia and suppressing tachycardia through activation of vagal tone.
- Postoperative arrhythmias are common in GDV patients and these may or may not respond to antiarrhythmic treatment. Cardiovascular monitoring of GDV patients, including ECG, during the perioperative period is critical for successful management of these cases.

ANESTHETIC MANAGEMENT AND PHARMACOLOGIC CONSIDERATIONS
- With the exception of opioids, routine protocols can be used for patients presenting for upper and lower gastrointestinal endoscopy.
- There is some debate about the use of opioids as a premedication in dogs and cats for upper gastrointestinal endoscopy. Full mu agonists may cause tightening of the pyloric sphincter in dogs, which increases the difficulty of gastroduodenoscopy. In a recent study, cats premedicated with hydromorphone, hydromorphone and glycopyrrolate, medetomidine, or butorphanol had no significant differences in difficulty or time required to pass the endoscope through the cardiac and pyloric sphincters.

- Managing cardiovascular and pulmonary functions perioperatively is just as important as the selection of the anesthetic protocol for successful anesthesia of GDV patients. Balanced electrolyte fluids should be administered as quickly as possible at a rate of 20–30 ml/kg to stabilize GDV patients.
- While administering balanced electrolyte fluids during the perioperative period it is important to monitor PCV and TP to prevent iatrogenic hemodilution.
- Monitoring arterial blood pressure, arterial blood gases, ECG, HR, and fluid administrations is key to managing GDV patients.

EXAMPLES OF ANESTHETIC PROTOCOLS FOR DOGS WITH GDV
Premedication
- An opioid, such as hydromorphone at 0.1 mg/kg IV.
- Orogastric tubing for decompression and simultaneous IV fluid administration.

Induction
- Induction with propofol, alfaxalone, or etomidate to effect for endotracheal intubation.

Maintenance
- General anesthesia should be maintained with isoflurane or sevoflurane.

Other considerations
- Additional opioids, such as fentanyl or hydromorphone, can be provided intra- and postoperatively for pain management.
- The use of a lidocaine–morphine CRI during the perioperative period is also useful to spare inhalant anesthetic concentration and provide pain management.

- Postoperative complications of GDV include cardiac arrhythmias, cardiovascular collapse, gastric necrosis, and sepsis. All efforts should be directed to supporting and maintaining cardiovascular function. Supportive analgesia is essential.

Cesarean section

GENERAL CONSIDERATIONS

- The goal of emergency or elective cesarean section is to produce lively, thriving puppies or kittens that are minimally affected by the anesthetic and perianesthetic drugs that have been administered and to prevent anesthesia-related problems in the bitch or queen.
- In cases of prolonged dystocia and fetal death *in utero*, the focus is on appropriate management of the bitch or queen. Appropriate analgesia should be instituted prior to surgery.
- There are two types of patients that present to the veterinarian for cesarean section: the stable patient presenting for elective surgery and the animal presenting for an emergency cesarean secondary to dystocia of variable duration.
- The emergency patient may well be exhausted, hypovolemic, hypotensive, hypo- or hyperthermic, and painful. Anesthetic management of these patients may include immediate supportive therapies including fluid and oxygen administration, sedative and analgesic drugs, general anesthesia, regional anesthesia, or any combination of these.
- Pregnant patients will have increased CO and increased intravascular volume.
- The functional residual capacity, or the amount of lung available to participate in gas exchange, will be reduced given the increased abdominal pressure against the diaphragm. Pregnant patients are, therefore, at risk for hypoventilation during surgery and ventilatory assistance may be required.
- Normal arterial CO_2 tensions are lower than in non-pregnant animals. Iatrogenic hyperventilation also puts pregnant patients at severe risk for hypocapnia, which decreases uterine blood flow. Consequently, ventilation of the pregnant patient must be supported appropriately.
- While the minimum alveolar concentration (MAC) of the administered inhalant anesthetic agent will be decreased, the large increase in CO may override any effect of decreased MAC.
- A pregnant patient may be at risk of increased gastric pressure predisposing to aspiration. Intubation should be accomplished quickly and the endotracheal tube cuff inflated (properly) in a timely fashion to protect the patient's airway.
- If a patient has been in labor for a long period of time, hypovolemia, acidosis, or other metabolic derangements, and exhaustion will all be considerations. Hypovolemia should be corrected prior to general anesthesia to maintain appropriate blood pressure. If time or viability of the fetuses is an issue, then a balanced isotonic crystalloid fluid can be administered rapidly at 10–30 ml/kg/hour prior to induction.
- The main goal of a cesarean section is to deliver live neonates, but anesthetic management should also be directed to improving the anesthetic care of the bitch/queen as well as producing vigorous neonates. While analgesia should not be neglected, opioid or dissociative analgesics will cross the placenta and affect fetuses.
- Anesthetic protocols that utilize just propofol induction and isoflurane or sevoflurane maintenance prior to retrieval of fetuses have been associated with decreased maternal and neonate mortality during cesarean section. Opioid and other analgesics can be supplemented to the bitch once the fetuses are removed.
- Any sedative or anesthetic drugs administered to the bitch will quickly cross the placenta and affect the fetus. Placental transfer of drugs depends

primarily on the ionization of the drug and the concentration of the drug in the bitch's blood stream.

ANESTHETIC MANAGEMENT AND PHARMACOLOGIC CONSIDERATIONS
Premedication
- Premedication (including the use of opioids) may not be suitable since these drugs can depress fetuses. Careful consideration should be taken before using any premedication in a cesarean section with known live fetuses.
- Preclipping the hair and scrubbing the surgical site will shorten exposure of fetuses to inhalant anesthetics (**Fig. 10.1**).
- Opioids used as preanesthetic drugs in cesarean sections have the advantage of providing analgesia to the bitch/queen and reversibility in the neonate if their effects compromise vigor at the time of birth. However, opioids will cross the placenta and affect the fetuses.
- Hydromorphone, morphine, oxymorphone, or fentanyl are suitable choices after removal of the fetuses.

- Anticholinergics may be administered if there is concern regarding a falling HR. Atropine will cross the placental barrier, while glycopyrrolate will not.
- An IV catheter should be placed soon after premedication or before induction if no premedication is used (**Fig. 10.1**).
- Bolus fluids can be administered to hypovolemic patients.

Induction
- Oxygen should be provided via a face mask (2–3 l/minute flow rate) for 5 minutes prior to and during injectable anesthetic induction.
- Injectable agents commonly used include thiopentone, alfaxalone, propofol (**Fig. 10.2**), or etomidate. The rapid redistribution of propofol provides an advantage in cesarean section anesthesia and has been associated with reduced risk to bitch/queen and neonate alike.
- A recent study indicates that similar good results may be provided by alfaxalone for canine cesarean section with a potential improvement in neonate vitality during the first 60 minutes after delivery.

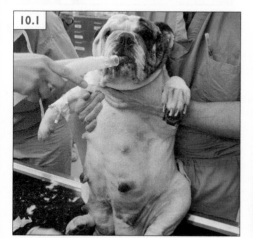

Fig. 10.1 Preparation for a cesarean section in a bitch includes preplacement of a catheter for intravenous induction, preclipping and prescrubbing the dog's surgical site, and preoxygenation prior to intravenous induction. Selection of several sizes of endotracheal tubes are also vital for rapid control of the dog's airway.

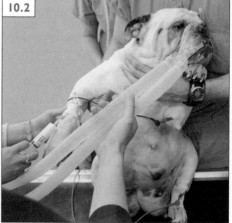

Fig. 10.2 Propofol can be used for intravenous induction and endotracheal intubation for rapid control of the airway. Note that the electrocardiogram is monitored and flow-by oxygen is provided during propofol induction in this dog.

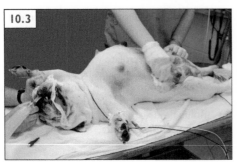

Fig. 10.3 Once the dog is anesthetized, further surgical scrubbing can be carried out before surgery. Inhalant anesthesia should be kept at the lightest plane possible.

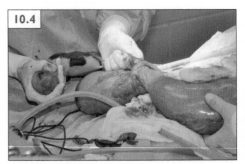

Fig. 10.4 Once the fetuses have been removed, the plane of anesthesia can be deepened and opioid analgesics provided intravenously for additional pain management.

- Face mask inductions may increase the risk of aspiration in pregnant patients.

Maintenance
- The use of an inhalant agent (isoflurane or sevoflurane) is preferred for maintenance (**Fig. 10.3**).

Other considerations
- Fluid therapy should be provided to maintain blood pressure. IV crystalloid fluids at a rate of 10 ml/kg/hour, or higher if blood pressure is not well maintained, is appropriate.
- Blood pressure should be monitored and managed carefully to support uterine blood flow.

EXAMPLES OF ANESTHETIC PROTOCOLS FOR CESAREAN SECTION IN DOGS
Premedication
- No premedication: opioids may be provided after the neonates are removed from the uterus:
  - Hydromorphone 0.05 mg/kg IV.
  - Fentanyl 0.002–0.005 mg/kg IV.

Induction
- Propofol 5 mg/kg IV to effect.
- Alfaxalone 2–3 mg/kg IV.

Maintenance
- Anesthesia should be maintained on isoflurane or sevoflurane.

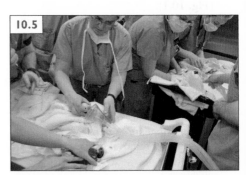

Fig. 10.5 A team should be assembled to assist in newborn care. The puppy's mucus and airway should be cleared with a suction bulb. Rubbing to stimulate spontaneous breathing, checking heart and respiratory rates, and providing exogenous heat and 100% oxygen are vital to the newborn.

Other considerations
- Fluid therapy: 10–20 ml/kg/hour LRS or Normosol-R (Plasma-Lyte A).
- Monitor blood pressure and hemoglobin saturation with oxygen.

RESUSCITATION OF NEONATES
- Rub neonates dry immediately post delivery (**Figs. 10.4, 10.5**).
- Listen for a heartbeat and watch for breathing efforts.
- Administer oxygen by mask and use one drop of doxapram under the tongue if not breathing (**Fig. 10.6**).

- A drop of naloxone and/or doxapram with a 22 gauge needle and syringe may be administered under the tongue if opioids were administered to the bitch/queen.
- If bradycardia (<180 beats per minute) occurs, a drop of atropine or epinephrine should be administered under the tongue.
- Keep the puppies or kittens as close to normal body temperature as possible (**Fig. 10.6**).
- After the bitch or queen has recovered from anesthesia, try to encourage nursing of the neonate as much as possible.

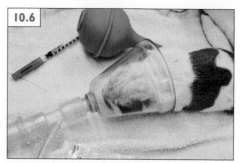

Fig. 10.6 Oxygen via a face mask and an exogenous heat source are vital in newborn care. A suction bulb can be used for removal of airway secretions.

Trauma

GENERAL CONSIDERATIONS

- Tissue injury caused by trauma can be largely classified into external and internal injuries. Patients may need to be anesthetized for treatment of injuries sustained in a number of ways, including motor vehicle injuries (blunt force trauma), falls, bite wounds, and burns. Motor vehicle injury scoring systems for trauma patients have been categorized over the years. The injured tissue categories are superficial soft-tissue, skeletal, or soft organ injury. The affected body regions are classified into head, neck, thorax, abdomen, pelvis, and extremities and the degree of injuries are subcategorized as minor, moderate, severe, severe and life-threatening, and fatal.
- External injuries include fracture and muscular trauma of the extremities and/or trunk (such as flail chest). Internal injuries include pulmonary contusion, traumatic myocarditis, hemo/pneumothorax, diaphragmatic hernia, rupture of spleen, liver, and/or bladder.
- Motor vehicle trauma patients may suffer hemorrhagic hypovolemic shock and/or cardiogenic shock. Hemorrhagic shock is due to severe blood loss and loss of intravascular volume. Cardiogenic shock may be due to restrictive movements of the heart associated with diaphragmatic hernia or severe cardiac arrhythmias due to traumatic myocarditis.

- The goals of handling these types of emergency trauma patients are: (1) to provide rapid stabilization and prevent shock induced decompensation; (2) to optimize oxygenated blood perfusion to the tissue; (3) to immediately alleviate pain and provide comfort; and (4) to medically prepare patients for surgical repair and management of the trauma.
- Managing cardiovascular and pulmonary function perioperatively is just as important as selection of the anesthetic protocol for successful anesthesia of trauma patients. Three factors determine oxygen delivery to tissue: arterial oxygen content, hemoglobin, and CO. Steps that optimize tissue oxygenation include providing 100% oxygen supplementation, maintaining a patent airway, support of ventilation, giving blood products and fluid replacement to increase oxygen delivery and improve circulating volume, and improvement of CO by alleviating any pleural space-occupying lesion (remove air or blood) and treatment of life-threatening arrhythmias.
- Cardiac arrhythmias may or may not be present within the first 24 hours of traumatic injuries. The arrhythmias commonly seen are ventricular premature contractions and ventricular tachycardia. Dogs sustaining significant injury should have more than one ECG performed to

detect cardiac arrhythmias. Studies have shown that a single ECG assessment may not detect some cardiac arrhythmias.

- Proper survey of the patient following injury is vital, especially in the thoracic region. Dogs are predisposed to myocardial injury when struck by motor vehicles more often than cats due to the shape of the thorax and the relative mobility of the heart within the thorax.

- HR, rhythm, pulse quality, respiratory patterns (shallow-fast versus deep-slow), heart and lung sounds, mucous membrane color, and CRT have to be thoroughly examined. Monitoring equipment, such as a pulse oximeter, ECG, and blood pressure monitor, is helpful in providing more objective assessments of cardiorespiratory function.

- Muffled heart or lung sounds, open-mouth breathing, and cyanosis are indicative of problems such as hemothorax, pneumothorax, or diaphragmatic hernia. Thoracocentesis may be performed anywhere from the 6th–10th intercostal space, with the needle or catheter introduced cranial to the rib. Radiographic diagnosis under general anesthesia should only be attempted once the animal is stabilized. Flail chest, rib fracture, and subcutaneous emphysema may be detected by careful palpation.

- Hypoxia and hypoventilation are common sequelae of thoracic trauma (see Chapter 12). Pain may prevent the animal from moving the thoracic muscles or rib cage properly. Providing 100% oxygen and analgesic agents tends to alleviate the animal's suffering and improve oxygenation. A shock dose of crystalloid fluid may have to be administered if the animal is hypotensive due to hypovolemia and acute blood loss (see Chapter 7).

- Dogs and cats with abdominal trauma may suffer rupture of the spleen or liver. Hemoabdomen may be present. Hypovolemic shock due to diminished venous return and lack of ventricular filling will result in low stroke volume and a compensatory high HR in the patient. This critical decrease in circulatory volume has to be rapidly restored with a shock dose (80–90 ml/kg in dogs and 60–70 ml/kg in cats) of crystalloid fluids. Alternatively, colloids may be given at 10–20 ml/kg over 20–30 minutes. Animals with blood loss >25% of their blood volume should be administered blood products (see Chapter 8).

- Dogs and cats suffering traumatic urinary system damage may have uroabdomen, uroretroperitoneum, direct renal parenchymal trauma, or urethral damage. Close monitoring of the animal's BUN, creatinine, and urine output are necessary. Abdominal ultrasound, radiography, or a contrast media study is required for a definitive diagnosis. Urine production should be 1–2 ml/kg/hour.

ANESTHETIC MANAGEMENT AND PHARMACOLOGIC CONSIDERATIONS
Premedication

- Opioids used as preanesthetic drugs in trauma patients have the advantage of providing analgesia, which provides immediate pain relief, plus a mild sedative effect.

- Hydromorphone, morphine, fentanyl, butorphanol, pethidine, or methadone are suitable choices for premedication.

- Anticholinergics may be administered if there is a concern of bradycardia.

- Bolus fluids should be administered to hypovolemic patients prior to anesthesia induction.

Induction

- Oxygen should be provided via face mask (2–3 liters/minute flow rate) for at least 5 minutes prior to and during injectable anesthetic induction.

- Constant ECG monitoring before, during, and after anesthesia induction is wise to detect any life-threatening cardiac arrhythmias and indicate appropriate treatment. Positive-pressure ventilation with 100% oxygen and repeated 2 mg/kg of lidocaine IV bolus injections (up to 6–8 mg/kg total) may be necessary to suppress some of these ventricular cardiac arrhythmias.

- Injectable induction agents such as propofol, alfaxalone, or etomidate are preferred. Given IV these agents are less likely to induce arrhythmias than

thiopentone or dissociatives (ketamine, tiletamine). Furthermore, these agents rapidly induce unconsciousness with muscle relaxation, allowing establishment of a patent airway via endotracheal intubation. All anesthetic agents should be administered 'to effect', utilizing the lowest dose possible.
- Face mask induction is not suitable for patients with thoracic trauma, especially with suspected pneumo/hemothorax or diaphragmatic hernia.

Maintenance
- The use of an inhalant agent (isoflurane or sevoflurane) is preferred for maintenance.

Other considerations
- Fluid therapy should be provided to maintain blood pressure. IV crystalloid fluids and fresh blood at a rate of 10 ml/kg/hour (or higher if blood pressure is not well maintained) are appropriate.
- Monitor blood pressure, PCV, and urine output (1–2 ml/kg/h) carefully to ensure adequate tissue perfusion with oxygen. PCV and TP (solids) should be maintained above 0.2 l/l (20%) and 40 g/l (4 g/dl), respectively.

EXAMPLES OF ANESTHETIC PROTOCOLS FOR TRAUMATIZED ORTHOPEDIC PATIENTS
Premedication
- Hydromorphone 0.1–0.2 mg/kg IM or IV.
- Acepromazine 0.01–0.02 mg/kg IM or IV.

- Preoxygenation (3 liters/minute via oxygen face mask).

Induction
- Propofol 5 mg/kg IV to effect.
- Could use a regional anesthesia technique, such as epidural or brachial plexus block with lidocaine or bupivacaine (1 mg/kg).
- CRI using either fentanyl (3–5 µg/kg/h) or morphine–lidocaine–ketamine at 1–2 ml/kg/hour starting soon after anesthesia induction and continuing for 24–48 hours after surgery.

Maintenance
- Isoflurane or sevoflurane.
- Provide additional hydromorphone of 0.05 or 0.1 mg/kg as supplemental analgesia if CRI is not used during the surgery to reduce the isoflurane concentration.

Other considerations
- ECG monitoring should be performed throughout the anesthesia process and starting from premedication in case of any prior cardiac arrhythmias.
- Measure intraoperative PCV and TP to ensure hydration status and oxygen carrying capacity.
- Fluid therapy: 10–20 ml/kg/hour LRS or Normosol-R (Plasma-Lyte A).
- Monitor blood pressure, ECG, oxygen hemoglobin saturation, and $ETCO_2$ concentration.
- Additional hydromorphone (0.05–0.1 mg/kg IV) or fentanyl (1–3 µg/kg/h CRI) can be given for postoperative pain management.

Further reading

Agarwal R, Porter MH, Obeid G (2013) Common medical illnesses that affect anesthesia and their anesthetic management. *Oral Maxillofac Surg Clin North Am* **25(3)**:407–38.

Bakti G, Fisch HU, Karlaganis G *et al.* (1987) Mechanisms of the excessive sedative response of cirrhotics to benzodiazepines: model experiments with triazolam. *Hepatol* **7**:629–38.

Donaldson LL, Leib MS, Boyd C *et al.* (1993) Effect of preanesthetic mediation on ease of endoscopic intubation of the duodenum in anesthetized dogs. *Am J Vet Res* **54**:1489–95.

Kolata RJ, Johnston DE (1975) Motor vehicle accidents in urban dogs: a study of 600 cases. *J Am Vet Med Assoc* **167**:938–41.

Rockar RA, Drobatz KS, Shofer FS (1992) Development of a scoring system for the veterinary trauma patient. *J Vet Emerg Crit Care* **4**:77–83.

Smith AA, Posner LP, Goldstein RE *et al.* (2004) Evaluation of the effects of premedication on gastroduodenoscopy in cats. *J Am Vet Med Assoc* **225**:540–4.

Snyder PS, Cooke KL, Murphy ST *et al.* (2001) Electrocardiographic findings in dogs with motor vehicle-related trauma. *J Am Anim Hosp Assoc* **37**:55–63.

Wong PL (1992) Anesthesia for gastric dilatation/volvulus. Anesthetic protocols for specific conditions. *Vet Clin North Am Small Anim Pract* **22**:471–4.

Airway management and ventilation

Ann B Weil and Jeff C Ko

Introduction

This chapter focuses on airway management under general anesthesia in dogs and cats. A discussion on how to set up the ventilator is also covered. More information on anesthetic equipment, anesthetic emergencies, normal endotracheal tube placement, and hypoventilation can be found in Chapters 1 and 21.

Managing the difficult airway

DIFFICULTY IN INTUBATION
- Inadequate depth of anesthesia:
  - If the plane of general anesthesia is too light, it increases the difficulty of intubation. It requires 30% more anesthetic depth than some surgeries to overcome airway reflexes.
  - When anticipating a difficult intubation, it is desirable to produce general anesthesia with an IV injectable agent instead of using inhalant mask induction. Injectable induction can be achieved rapidly with improved muscle relaxation, facilitating visualization of the airway.
  - A few drops of lidocaine applied to the larynx in cats can assist intubation if sufficient time (90–120 seconds) is allowed for the agent to work.
- Anatomic problems:
  - Cannot visualize the larynx. Laryngoscopes can be an invaluable aid to help visualize the airway, especially in brachycephalic breeds (**Figs. 11.1, 11.2**). Guide tubes and stylets may also be helpful (**Fig. 11.3**) for directing the endotracheal tube into place.
- Obstruction due to tumors (**Figs. 11.4, 11.5**), masses, or redundant soft tissues in the upper airway can make intubation difficult.
- If the airway cannot be controlled, spontaneous ventilation should be maintained and apnea avoided as much as possible to protect the patient.
- Whenever a difficult intubation is anticipated, administration for 5 minutes of 100% oxygen via a face mask (or a flow-by using a breathing circuit) immediately prior to anesthetic induction will help delay desaturation of the patient while the airway is being established.

LARYNGOSPASM
- A few drops of local anesthetic placed on the arytenoids can be very helpful.

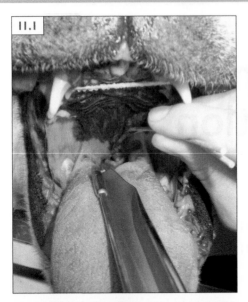

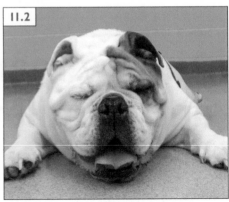

Figs. 11.1, 11.2 (**11.1**) The airway and laryngeal opening are better visualized with the aid of a laryngoscope and a light source. (**11.2**) This is particularly true for brachycephalic dogs with redundant tissues of the upper airway.

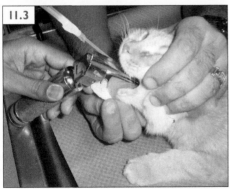

Fig. 11.3 A polypropylene stylet is being used coaxially with an endotracheal tube to intubate a cat. Note that the stylet is protruding out of the endotracheal tube. The protrusion of the stylet serves two purposes: (1) because the stylet has a smaller diameter, the view of the laryngeal opening is not blocked by the endotracheal tube; and (2) the stylet serves to guide the endotracheal tube into the trachea. Tracheal damage could occur if the stylet is too rigid, so metal stylets should not be used.

- Depth of anesthesia must be adequate.
- The use of a polypropylene stylet will help to guide the endotracheal tube (**Fig. 11.3**).
- A smaller endotracheal tube can be used to establish an airway and be later

replaced with an endotracheal tube of a larger diameter when the animal is well anesthetized and the airway is no longer spasming.

AIRWAY OCCLUSION AND CHANGING THE ENDOTRACHEAL TUBE

- Airway occlusion can occur with or without an endotracheal tube in the trachea. The latter situation may happen during recovery or soon after premedication, but before anesthetic induction, especially if the animal vomits.
- The airway must be immediately examined and a patent airway established when an obstruction occurs. General anesthesia is required to accomplish this.
- Endotracheal tube occlusion is identified by increased respiratory effort or an additional increase in airway pressure to ventilate the lungs.
- Endotracheal tube occlusion may occur because of:
  - A mucous plug or foreign body obstruction.
  - Overinflation of the endotracheal tube cuff leading to the cuff obstructing the distal opening.
  - Endotracheal tube being bent or collapsed.

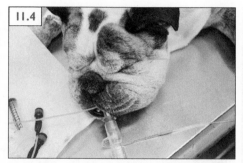

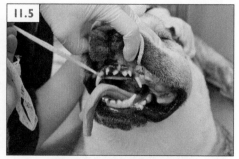

Figs. 11.4, 11.5 A 13-year-old Bulldog with an oral tumor. (**11.4**) This dog poses a great challenge for anesthesia for radiation therapy. Note the bulging of the cheek pouch due to tumor growth, which poses further challenges for endotracheal intubation in this brachycephalic dog. (**11.5**) The oral tumor has metastasized onto the hard palate, the laryngeal–pharyngeal area, and the maxilla, which not only causes airway obstruction, but also limits the ability of the jaws to be opened widely for visualization during endotracheal intubation. The use of a laryngoscope with a long blade and a guiding stylet (see **Fig. 11.3**) are necessary for better visualization of the airway for endotracheal intubation. A temporary tracheostomy is another option to establish an airway.

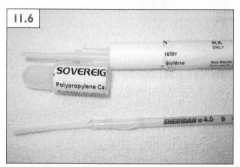

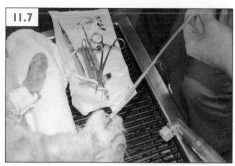

Figs. 11.6, 11.7 (**11.6**) A canine polypropylene urinary type of catheter can be used to facilitate the exchange of an endotracheal tube, especially when the animal is positioned in dorsal recumbency. (**11.7**) The stylet is inserted into the existing endotracheal tube while it is still in the trachea and left in place while the tube is removed. A functional endotracheal tube is reinserted over the stylet while it is still in the trachea.

- General anesthesia must be maintained while the airway is re-established; an injectable agent (e.g. propofol) is useful to accomplish this.
- A guide wire or tube may be used while changing the damaged or obstructed endotracheal tube, especially if the patient is positioned in dorsal recumbency and surgery is ongoing. Canine urinary polypropylene catheters (8 to 10 French) are useful as guide tubes (**Figs. 11.6, 11.7**).
- Use of a small amount of water-soluble sterile lubricant may be helpful to ease intubation; however, excessive amounts of lubricant may occlude the lumen of small diameter airways.

ORAL SURGERY
- An orally-placed endotracheal tube may be impractical for oral surgery. In this situation the airway can be established and maintained via pharyngotomy or tracheostomy to improve conditions for surgical access (**Fig. 11.8**).
- Pharyngotomy placement of an endotracheal tube can be accomplished while the animal is anesthetized by creating an opening on the side of the oral–pharyngeal area. An endotracheal tube is inserted into the oral cavity through the pharyngotomy site. The endotracheal tube in the trachea is extubated, the new endotracheal tube inserted into the trachea via the

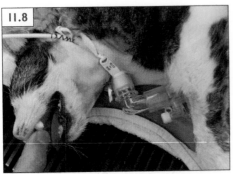

Fig. 11.8 Since the cat had dental binding of the jaws, oral–tracheal intubation was not possible. A tracheostomy was created in order to allow inhalant anesthesia to be performed for frequent dental works of this cat. Also note that an esophageal gastric tube (white tubing) was also placed to facilitate feeding of this cat.

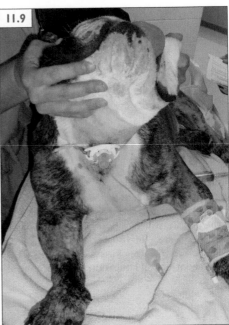

Fig. 11.9 A tracheostomy tube is being placed for recovery of a dog prone to airway obstruction problems.

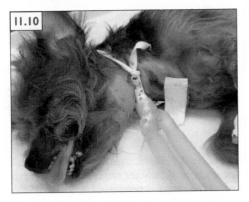

Fig. 11.10 A tracheostomy tube may be attached to the breathing circuit for anesthesia maintenance.

oral–pharyngeal site, and inhalant anesthesia is maintained with the pharyngotomy tube.
- For tracheostomy placement, a regular endotracheal tube may be placed through the tracheostomy site and secured to the patient for use with the anesthetic breathing circuit. A tracheostomy tube may also be used on recovery (**Fig. 11.9**). Conversely, a cuffed, tracheostomy tube may be attached to the breathing circuit during anesthesia (**Figs. 11.8, 11.10**).

PERIOPERATIVE OXYGEN ADMINISTRATION
- Preanesthetic oxygenation and denitrogenation is especially helpful for patients with:
  - Cardiac disease.
  - Respiratory disease.
  - Anticipated difficult intubation.
- Postanesthetic (i.e. during the early recovery period when the patient is extubated but still has some degree of unconsciousness) oxygen support is especially helpful for patients with:
  - Critical disease.
  - Lengthy anesthetic procedures.
  - Thoracotomy.
  - Pulmonary diagnostic procedures (e.g. an endotracheal wash or bronchial alveolar lavage).
- Oxygen administration methods:
  - Mask administration (**Fig. 11.11**). This method works well with doligocephalic breed dogs and cats, but does not work well with brachycephalic dogs or cats. This is because the rim of the face mask tends to cause corneal

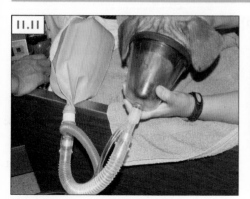

Fig. 11.11 Enriched oxygen can be administered through a face mask.

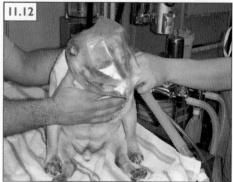

Fig. 11.12 A transparent plastic bag is an alternative way of providing enriched oxygen to brachycephalic dogs or dogs that will not tolerate a face mask.

damage to the eyes of brachycephalic animals.

- Oxygen hood or transparent plastic bag. Enriched oxygen can be administered with a transparent plastic bag that encloses the head (**Fig. 11.12**) or a commercially available hood. Transparent plastic bags for oxygenation are easy to obtain, economical, disposable, effective, and well-tolerated by the animal.
- Nasal insufflation can be used to increase the inspiratory fraction of oxygen to patients via a nasal catheter. A variable percentage of oxygen can be administered. Nasal insufflation is useful in the critical care setting and is helpful for postoperative patients requiring increased oxygen support. Typical oxygen flow rates of 1–7 liters/minute are used.
- Oxygen cage. A variable percentage of oxygen can be administered with humidification when using an oxygen cage.

EXTUBATION

- Patients should be extubated when pharyngeal reflexes have returned or they can swallow and protect the airway.
- Patients with difficult intubation characteristics (e.g. brachycephalic breeds, pharyngeal masses) should remain intubated as long as possible to avoid any airway occlusion due to residual muscle relaxation.

- Care should be taken to protect the endotracheal tube from being bitten by a recovering animal. Tubes can be chewed completely in half and remain lodged in the patient such that the remainder of the tube must be retrieved from the distal trachea. Sudden awakening can occur during recovery. Dogs that have received opioids can be startled by noises such as vacuum cleaners or the loud closing of a metal cage, resulting in very sudden, unanticipated arousal and damage to the endotracheal tube.
- Oxygen supplementation via a face mask should be available after extubation for difficult airway patients.
- Some patients may have to be reintubated after initial extubation if they cannot spontaneously ventilate or the airway is occluded. An injectable anesthetic agent (e.g. propofol) and a laryngoscope should be available to aid in reintubation. Inducing the animal back into a deeper plane of anesthesia allows the recovery process to start all over again.
- Dogs or cats receiving neuromuscular blockers (atracurium or pancuromium) without reversal should be monitored carefully (see also Chapter 6). A definitive and sustained head lift is an important sign that signifies the animal is strong enough to maintain spontaneous breathing and airway protection. Simply having a swallowing reflex does not mean it is safe to extubate these animals.

Ventilation (assisted or controlled)

INDICATIONS FOR USE

- Hypoventilation induced by anesthetic agents.
- Respiratory failure due to disease conditions.
- Thoracic surgery where the chest is open or a diaphragmatic hernia is present.
- Patients receiving neuromuscular blockade.
- Obese dogs and cats placed in dorsal recumbency and unable to breathe properly.

TYPES OF VENTILATION

- Intermittent positive-pressure ventilation (IPPV) may be as simple as the anesthetist occasionally squeezing the reservoir (or rebreathing) bag to assist ventilation.
- Ventilation may be controlled completely with a mechanical ventilator or with an anesthetist squeezing the reservoir bag at regular intervals.
- Side-effects of IPPV:
  - Has negative effects on cardiac output since the positive pressure in the thorax compresses the great vessels, including the vena cavae, and prevents venous return
  - Overventilation that reduces arterial blood CO_2 levels to <25 mmHg will drastically reduce cerebral blood flow. This, in turn, may cause delays in return of consciousness during recovery. Furthermore, lower arterial blood CO_2 tensions result in alkalemia.
  - Mechanical ventilation can induce lung trauma. There are several medical terms used to describe this in human anesthesia, including volutrauma (direct injury to alveoli from overdistension of the lung), barotrauma (injury resulting from high intrapulmonary air pressures), biotrauma (lung and distant organ injury resulting from the release of inflammatory mediators into the airspaces and into the systemic circulation), and atelectrauma (injury to alveoli resulting from the cyclic collapse and opening of atelectatic alveoli).

- Most lung trauma associated with mechanical ventilation is due to using excessively large tidal volumes and high peak inspiratory pressures (>35 cmH_2O). The best way to avoid mechanical ventilator-associated lung trauma is to use appropriate tidal volumes and permissive hypercapnia (see below).
- Underventilation may result in significant hypercapnea with associated respiratory acidosis and poor oxygenation due to inadequate lung expansion.

VENTILATOR SETTINGS

- Four settings are usually required to set up a mechanical ventilator. These are respiratory rate, tidal volume, peak inspiratory pressure (PIP), and inspiratory to expiratory (I:E) time ratio.
- Respiratory rates can be set between 8 and 14 breaths per minute, depending on the size of the animal and the chest compliance.
- A tidal volume of 10–20 ml/kg is useful for most small animals. Recent suggestions from human literature suggest using a tidal volume of approximately 9–10 ml/kg to allow for mild hypercapnea ($ETCO_2$ of 50–55 mmHg) and to avoid lung trauma. This is called permissive hypercapnea.
- Peak airway pressure, or PIP, should be between 12 and 20 cmH_2O for most anesthetized dogs and in cats. The PIP should not exceed 30 cmH_2O.
- The I:E ratio is the inspiratory time compared with the expiratory time and should be 1:2 or less (1:3 or 1:4). Many ventilators have a 'set' I:E ratio; in other words, the time spent in the inspiratory part of the cycle compared with the expiratory time has been programed by the manufacturer and cannot be changed.
- Occasionally, positive end expiratory pressure (PEEP) is used to increase oxygenation by keeping the airways opened in between breaths. PEEP is usually set between 0 and 2 cmH_2O for animals with healthy lungs. Settings >15–20 cmH_2O are dangerous because they impair venous return as well as induce barotrauma.

ASSESSING VENTILATORY EFFICIENCY

- Ventilation efficiency can be determined non-invasively by assessing $ETCO_2$ with a capnograph and SpO_2 with a pulse oximeter.
- Alternatively, an arterial blood gas sample can be used to assess the $PaCO_2$ and PaO_2.
- Effective ventilation should maintain arterial and $ETCO_2$ between 35 and 45 mmHg and SpO_2 of 99–100% or PaO_2 of 300–600 mmHg, if breathing 100% oxygen. Animals with significant pulmonary pathology may not be able to achieve this level of ventilation and oxygenation. (See Chapter 6 for more information on anesthesia monitoring.)
- To avoid oxygen toxicity, 100% oxygen should not be used for more than 18–24 hours. Long-term ventilator patients should be administered a sufficient oxygen percentage to keep the PaO_2 close to 90–100 mmHg. Variable air–oxygen mixture ratios aimed at yielding an inspiratory fraction of oxygen between 33% and 100% can be used to provide long-term ventilation to the patient.

TYPES OF VENTILATORS

- Ventilators can be largely classified as volume limited or pressure limited:
  - Volume-limited ventilators deliver a set volume to the patient regardless of airway pressure. The ventilator stops as soon as the preset volume is reached.
  - Pressure-limited ventilators deliver a tidal volume to the patient until a preset airway pressure is met. Therefore, the preset peak inspiratory pressure determines the ventilator's action, regardless of the tidal volume delivered.
- Most ventilators are time cycled.
- Ventilators can be driven (power source) by electricity or compressed gas, where compression of the bellows is accomplished by compressed gas (oxygen or medical air).
- Ventilators can be stand alone units attached to the rebreathing bag or part of the anesthesia machine.

- Ventilators can be further classified by the direction of bellows movement during the expiratory phase:
  - Bellows that push down to deliver a breath to the patient and ascend during expiration are classified as ascending bellows (see **Fig. 1.58**). Newer ventilators tend to have ascending bellows.
  - Bellows that extend up to deliver a breath to the patient and descend during expiration are classified as descending bellows (see **Fig. 1.57**). The bellow rising is powered by compressed gas or electricity. Bellow descent is caused by a weight attached to the bottom of the bellow.
- Ascending bellow ventilators provide several advantages over descending bellow ventilators. They do not draw air from the patient's airway during expiration because the bellow is lightweight and is gradually inflated during expiration.
- In contrast, descending bellows draw air out of the patient's airway during expiration as the weight on the bottom of the descending bellow descends with gravity. Since expiration is not passive, air is withdrawn from the patient's airway. This greatly increases the work of breathing to raise the bellows, so there is potential for pulmonary damage if a patient breathes spontaneously while on a descending bellow ventilator.

Engler ADS 1000 and 2000

The Engler ADS 1000 and 2000 anesthetic delivery system/positive-pressure ventilator is a ventilator without bellows (**Fig. 11.13**). Listed below are some key facts about this unique anesthesia machine:

- It is a pneumatic ventilator with a partial anesthesia machine design. It is a deviation from the basic anesthesia machine design with 'FROGS' components.
- It does not have a flowmeter, a reservoir bag, ventilator bellows, or a bellow housing.
- It acts like a non-rebreathing anesthetic delivery system and, as such, it does not have a CO_2 absorbent canister or one-way valves.

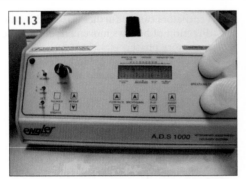
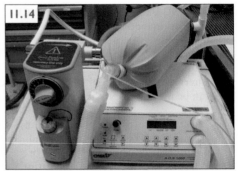

Figs. 11.13, 11.14 (11.13) An Engler ADS 1000 anesthetic delivery system/positive-pressure ventilator. **(11.14)** The ADS 1000 requires a vaporizer (in this case a sevoflurane vaporizer) to function as an anesthesia machine. A breathing hose is connected to the delivery system and then connected to the patient (a reservoir bag is used here for illustration).

- It does require a precision vaporizer (**Fig. 11.14**), a breathing hose, an oxygen supply of 50 psi (equipped with a laboratory animal model uses only 5 psi for animals <1 kg with the Engler ADS 2000 model), and a scavenging system to function as an anesthetic delivery system.
- It has a microprocessor that controls the oxygen flow rate, respiratory rate, and PIP based on the patient's body weight (1–68 kg [2.2–150 lb]) as entered by the operator using the key pad of the device. Some consider this system easy to use and reliable for providing anesthesia via positive ventilation to the animal.
- Most anesthetic machines deliver a continuous oxygen flow to the vaporizer, but the Engler ADS1000 (and 2000 model) delivers intermittent bursts of oxygen at a high flow rate (between 2 and 60 liters/minute) through the vaporizer, which inflates the patient's lungs via pneumatic positive pressure.
- It is not known whether this high intermittent oxygen flow rate passing through the vaporizer has damaging effects on the internal structures of the anesthetic vaporizer. There are some concerns that vaporizers used with the Engler ADS models have a 'shorter useable life span' than when used with a traditional anesthesia machine. However, this shorter useable life span still lasts for years.
- Similar to a non-rebreathing circuit, the exhaled CO_2 is washed out with the anesthetic waste gas through exhalation and enters the scavenging system connected to the machine.
- Basically, the ADS 1000 and ADS 2000 function the same way. The practitioner needs to use $ETCO_2$ or blood gas $PaCO_2$ values to fine tune the settings (respiratory rate and PIP) to make the $ETCO_2$ of the ventilator patient fall between the normal range (35–45 mmHg). The ADS 2000 allows the preset breathing parameters to be more flexibly altered by the operator than those of the ADS 1000 model.

Further reading

Ambros B, Carrozzo MV, Jones T (2018) Desaturation times between dogs preoxygenated via face mask or flow-by technique before induction of anesthesia. *Vet Anaesth Analg* **45(4)**:452–8.

Dorsch JA, Dorsch SE (1999) *Understanding Anesthesia Equipment*, 4th edn. Wilkins and Wilkins, Baltimore, pp. 75–269.

Hartsfield SM (2007) Airway management and ventilation. In: *Lumb and Jones' Veterinary Anesthesia and Analgesia*, 4th edn. Blackwell Publishing, Ames, pp. 495–531.

CHAPTER 12

Anesthetic considerations for patients requiring upper airway surgery and patients requiring thoracic surgery

Jennifer C Hess

Introduction

This chapter will discuss preoperative, intra-operative, and postoperative concerns for patients undergoing airway and thoracic surgery. It will also consider patient preparation and pre- and postoperative analgesia, with options of regional or local techniques to lower the requirement of inhalant agents or total dose of opioids.

Patient preparation

Patient preparation includes:
- Preserving the drive to ventilate after anesthesia, minimizing the likelihood of emesis, and ensuring patient comfort for a safe recovery.
- Assessing the preoxygenation status and planning for the necessary items for emergency airway treatment.

- For airway surgery patients, consider preparing for tracheotomy.
- A low-stress presurgical environment can help. Availability of oxygen supplementation, either through nasal supplementation or through cooled oxygen cages, is desirable. Airway and brachycephalic patients become

overheated more easily than other patients.

- For thoracic surgery patients, prepare for thoracic tube placement or replacement of a surgically placed chest tube as they can become dislodged or clogged. For thoracic surgery, emergency interventions may require the removal of air or fluid from the thoracic cavity in the perianesthetic period.
- An endotracheal tube (ETT) is NOT complete protection against liquid entering the trachea. It is an airtight seal against gas leaving the trachea, but the cuff can fail when sufficient liquid from flushing or regurgitation gathers around it (see Chapter 6).
- The author suggests extreme care if one chooses to infuse liquids into the stomach or esophagus as a treatment for regurgitation. If the lower esophageal sphincter is weak enough to allow regurgitation once, it may recur. Although esophageal injury is devastating, aspiration pneumonia is more quickly fatal.

Premedication

- Consider the use of an antiemetic in a single prophylactic dose, such as maropitant citrate and or ondansetron prior to pure mu opioid agonists (MOAs). The airway surgery patient may benefit greatly from interventions to prevent emesis because the airway may lack a protective ETT at certain points. The ETT may be removed and reinserted during surgery, and this can stimulate emesis.
- All patients can experience passive regurgitation, but brachycephalic dogs are especially prone. Older, gestational, or obese dogs are more likely to regurgitate and aspirate.
- Surgical procedures, such as tie-back or laryngeal implant, can make dogs susceptible to aspiration immediately after the procedure because the patients gain airway diameter at the expense of tracheal protection.
- No proven technique exists to prevent all regurgitation, but consider the patient risk and the use of continuous infusion of prokinetics, such as cisapride or metoclopramide, in the brachycephalic patient or gastrointestinal motility compromised patient.
- Continually review the evolving literature as well as the controversies over fasting times. Thoracic surgery patients are likely to have a consistently protected airway but are often subject to prolonged anesthetic times owing to the complex nature of working inside a cavity with moving viscera.
- MOAs provide the strongest analgesia while simultaneously suppressing the innate drive to ventilate by suppressing the hypercapnic ventilatory response centrally in the medulla, as well as the hypoxic ventilatory response in the carotid bodies. Kappa opioids such as butorphanol do not have this effect. Partial MOAs such as buprenorphine have a much weaker or no effect at normal doses on ventilatory drive.

Anxiolysis and sedation (also see Chapter 3)

- For one patient, a medication may provide anxiolysis and for another it may not, or only at a higher dose. In anesthesia practice, the benzodiazepines (BNZs) and the phenothiazine tranquilizer acepromazine are two common medication used for anxiolysis in the perioperative period.
- The concerns with airway patients is that elevated levels of anxiety or panic may lead to more respiratory distress, therefore these medications are administered to help patients be amenable to evaluation or treatment before anesthesia and arouse smoothly after anesthesia.
- The competing concern is maintaining a patient's awareness and compensatory mechanisms and to do so, avoid profound sedation. Too much anxiety or too much sedation is undesirable. It is the 'Goldilock Principle' of anesthesia.

- BNZs help sedate and augment the actions of opioids and inhalant anesthetic agents. Acepromazine is controversial as to whether it masks the patient's true state of anxiety or whether it helps. In this author's opinion it can be helpful in patients with airway problems, brachycephalic dogs, sighthounds, and others. There is a wide safety margin and a slow onset. Hypotension is avoided by using low doses, allowing 30 minutes before redosing, and using care in combination with inhaled anesthetics.
- The alpha-2 adrenergic agonist dexmedetomidine can provide profound but rousable sedation and analgesia to healthy patients. Patients with airway or thoracic disease should be sedated with this medication when there is no other option and for as short a duration as possible; for example, to control an emergency because there is a reliable reversal agent (atipamezole). CRI at low doses may augment opioid analgesia. Overall, the cardiac side-effects of increased afterload are well-tolerated in healthy patients only. Minimal case study series suggests its safe use in the hypertrophic obstructive cardiomyopathy subset of hypertrophic cardiomyopathy (HCM) cats.
- Trazodone provides longer-term anti-anxiety and mild sedation. It can be used in collapsing trachea medical management, so may be encountered in the emergency stent placement patient. The doses of other medications should be lowered and a short-acting induction agent, such as propofol or alfaxalone, used to effect. Trazodone is a useful treatment for postsurgical confinement anxiety. Trazodone is most effective when administered consistently for a week or two before surgery rather than as a large bolus dose. There is no reversal agent and it is often used in combination with behavioral medications such as fluoxetine in dogs, so question the owner regarding other medications administered daily. While there is no specific reversal for trazodone sedation, there is an antihistamine, cyproheptadine, that can reverse the serotonin effects. Combining multiple serotonin-acting pharmaceuticals can lead to serotonin syndrome, so use care in combining trazodone, selective serotonin reuptake inhibitors, and the medications used for general anesthesia.

MEDICATION INTERACTIONS

- There is a dearth of literature on multiple medication interactions in veterinary patients undergoing general anesthesia.
- Monitoring the patient and using short-acting anesthetic medications with appropriate reversal or antidotes available is the safest course of action. Often, patients with airway or thoracic problems do not have 'reserve' and are living on the edge of health, are acclimated to their problems when fully awake and aware, and the addition of medications may potentially remove a margin of safety. Therefore, monitoring and making changes consecutively instead of simultaneously, while being able to intubate and control ventilation or perform emergency interventions (tracheotomy or remove fluid or air from the chest) in an efficient manner, is advisable. This requires planning, visualizing anatomical landmarks, and making checklists.

Monitoring (see also Chapter 6)

- Oxygenation is monitored using a pulse oximeter and by blood samples analyzed by a co-oximeter (benchtop). The requirements for a pulse oximeter are a minimal peripheral pulse and a heart rate within the settings of the machine's algorithm. Pulse oximetry (S_pO_2) is a surrogate for blood oximetry (SaO_2), the gold standard. Newer pulse oximeters measure different wavelengths of light to assess multiple hemoglobin types. When the pulse oximeter fails to read, assess patients for heart rate changes or falling oxygenation before attributing the failure to monitor error.
- Ventilation is measured by assessing the blood levels of CO_2 through a minimum of end-tidal capnography

and ideally correlated to arterial blood gas (ABG) sampling in the airway or thoracic surgical patient. $ETCO_2$ (less reliable than $SaCO_2$) can be measured non-invasively by a direct mainstream capnograph or by a sidestream sampling line conveying the sample to the monitor. The mainstream is more accurate. The sidestream loses accuracy in higher oxygen flows and smaller patients, when the sample is diluted with incoming fresh gas flow. This author has observed 20 mmHg underestimations of $ETCO_2$ in small patients on non-rebreathing circuits when compared with ABG measurement. The second problem is that $ETCO_2$ monitoring approximates the blood levels of CO_2 when there is no impairment of the lungs. In patients with thoracic disease there may be an impairment of lung function or blood circulation to the lungs. An ABG sample can be correlated with an $ETCO_2$ after induction and repeated when changes are made to ventilation or if the patient is unstable. Ventilation should be adjusted in response to ABG results over $ETCO_2$.

Induction (see also Chapter 4)

- Short-acting, quick onset medications are preferred. One should be prepared to intubate or treat an emergency when administering the premedication or induction. One regimen the author finds useful for this is fentanyl IV followed by alfaxalone IV, with immediate intubation and manual ventilation.
- Anesthetic depth for intubation is one of the deepest levels of anesthesia and pushes the physiologic limits of the patients. In the airway or thoracic diseased patient, this is a critical time for expert intervention. Short-acting, easily titratable agents, such as propofol, alfaxalone, or etomidate, are the first choice. Alfaxalone is a newer induction agent that may have better cardiovascular stability. It is a better choice for patients with a known allergy to egg or soy, or a known negative reaction to propofol. Various reports of 'twitching' or rough recoveries have been anecdotally reported with both medications. Etomidate and a BNZ/dissociative combination are also used with care. Etomidate administered after a BNZ is unique in its cardiac stability; however, it also can induce emesis.
- Propofol is commonly used and the main concern is apnea and rare propofol 'reactions' including reddening of the pinna, erythematous facial features, and stiff arms to paddling at the extreme. It can cause short-lived, temporary and reversible cardiac depression in a dose-dependent manner. Propofol is metabolized by the plasma and is the best choice for patients with hepatic comorbidities. Propofol reaction has an anecdotal treatment of diphenhydramine and steroids or epinephrine. Severe reactions including facial swelling should be treated as an anaphylactic reaction and epinephrine administered. IgE testing can be used at 4–6 weeks post reaction to confirm an allergy. Patients at risk of anaphylaxis during anesthesia should be pretreated with diphenhydramine (2 mg/kg q6 h for 1–2 days) and epinephrine should be available. Prior exposure to intralipid solutions (parenteral feeding) and dermatologic sensitivities have been associated with propofol anaphylaxis.
- A BNZ/dissociative combination, such as midazolam or diazepam plus ketamine, is a safe option in dogs, but less so in cats because of the prevalence of asymptomatic HCM.

Analgesia options

- Pain levels vary with the procedure and the clinician. There is always both visceral and somatic pain in airway surgery and thoracic surgery. The pain level can be roughly monitored by increases in heart rate, blood pressure, or respiratory rate. Because veterinary patients have compelling reasons to hide pain, analgesia should be planned based on the procedure as well as pain assessments. Suppressing ventilation should be avoided after the end of anesthesia by using NSAIDs where safe and/or low doses of MOAs or kappa opioids. During recovery, patients should not be struggling because this may dislodge sutures, chest tubes, or nasal oxygen and could create an oxygen debt.

- For airway surgery, methadone, butorphanol, or buprenorphine may provide sufficient analgesia, along with the use of topical lidocaine or other local anesthetic on the surfaces being surgically revised. Butorphanol CRI has been used, giving a single dose initially (0.1–0.2 mg/kg) with the remaining dose (0.1–0.3 mg/kg) over 1 hour or several hours. Variable sedation may result and all CRIs need to be reduced in dosage over time to maintain the same plasma concentration.

- Regional and local anesthesia and analgesia for thoracic surgery provides a way to reduce the minimum alveolar concentration of an inhalant anesthetic and minimize the need for opioid CRI. This attenuates cardiac depression and better maintains perfusion. It can reduce or eliminate the heart rate and respiratory rate depression from potent opioid infusions. Regional anesthesia (see also Chapter 23) blocks the regional transmission of the nociceptors' chemical information to the spinal cord, hindering the forward transmission of pain to the spinal cord and brain. During thoracic surgery, non-inhaled anesthesia and analgesia are important to maintain a stable plane of anesthesia.

- Neuraxial anesthesia can be a 'single shot' epidural injection of morphine plus saline and will provide thoracic analgesia to patients receiving thoracotomies. The total dose of morphine (0.1 mg/kg) is lower than the morphine equivalent dose of many opioids given parenterally. Morphine is contained within the epidural and thecal space, reaching the cerebrospinal fluid in the brain in 10 minutes after lumbosacral injection and binding to the substantia gelatinosa

in the spinal cord. Morphine travels to the blood and is removed, with plasma levels lower than parenteral administration. Local anesthetics administered into the lumbosacral space are not suitable for epidurals for thoracic pain. Local anesthetic can be used to block a specific region by inserting an epidural catheter in the L–S space and using fluroscopic guidance to reach the level of the dermatome to be blocked. This is an uncommon veterinary practice. Epidural catheters can be used to dose morphine repeatedly and can help patients with severe pain from thoracotomies. When using an epidural catheter, clean practices (gloves, antiseptics) will avoid infections, and clear labeling of the epidural port will prevent IV medications being administered administered accidentally and will prevent complications. Conscious patients can have epidurals administered after surgery while still sedate by using a lidocaine block of the skin above the L–S site.

- Intercostal (IC) block is an often misunderstood and overlooked block that provides analgesia for lateral thoracotomy. The IC space is a potential space that feels similar to the epidural space with a lack of resistance to injection. The IC space is located caudal to the rib near its insertion on the spinous process and is often described as 'walking off the caudal border of the rib with a needle'. The location can be verified with a negative aspiration for air (thoracic cavity entrance). This analgesic blockade can also be applied using a nerve stimulator and insulated needle. Blocking three IC spaces cranial and caudal to incision is recommended.

- Intrapleural regional analgesia is the application of bupivacaine or lidocaine through the chest tube. This analgesia assists in postoperative pain management of lateral thoracotomy or sternotomy. Another newer option is to administer a thoracic paravertebral block that places the local anesthetic near the spinal nerves as they emerge from the intervertebral foramen.

- Chest tube placement and troubleshooting are useful for the anesthetic care of patients recovering from thoracotomies. Tubes are often placed by the surgeon at the end of the procedure, and might be dislodged during recovery or transfer. Common errors with the chest tubes center around the three-way stopcock. The arrow on the stop cock indicates the off position, unlike gas or plumbing lines where the arrow indicates flow. Accidental injections of air intrathoracically should be removed. Loosening of a 'Christmas tree' adapter is another problem. To test if a chest tube is patent, a small volume of saline may be injected and then the tube can be milked. A negative aspiration from the chest tube is interpreted as being negative for aspiration of fluid or air. If the patient is in respiratory distress, check the tube placement or replace the tube, or intervene short term with a butterfly catheter set to remove air while the chest tube is replaced. Gently rotating the patient may improve ventilation or improve the function of the chest tube.

OPIOID ANALGESIA

- Opioids are a key component of any multimodal analgesic protocol. The problem is that they tend to depress respiration. This effect may be reduced if opioids are used at lower doses in combination with regional anesthesia and analgesia as described above.
- Fentanyl, along with remifentanil, alfentanil, and sufentanil, are short- or ultrashort-acting opioids with little or no organ metabolism. They can be used to manage intense surgical stimulation (higher doses) and postoperative pain (lower doses). Ventilation must be controlled through manual or mechanical IPPV to counteract the opioid-induced reduced response to hypercapnia and hypoxia. Methadone is a unique opioid because it has NMDA antagonism, a property shared with ketamine, and usually does not produce nausea. It is perceived to be not as sedating as other opioids, which may help the respiratory compromised patient. It is often used in brachycephalic dogs undergoing airway surgery.

- Butorphanol is useful for airway surgery analgesia, especially as a CRI (see above). For some patients, it is sedating without the same effects on vagal tone and heart rate and has none of the respiratory depression caused by MOAs. This can be beneficial because both airway and thoracic disease cases often have increased vagal tone. There is a risk of sedation in those patients on whom it has a profound effect and unlike MOAs, these effects are not easily antagonized. The antitussive effect and antiemetic effects of butorphanol are beneficial.
- Hydromorphone is a MOA that provides excellent analgesia of longer duration than the fentanyl class. Redosing and CRI during surgery may cause a prolonged extubation time. Morphine causes the most histamine release, nausea, and vomiting of the MOAs mentioned, so parenteral use is less desirable. Morphine is excellent in the epidural space, superior to fentanyl. Fentanyl is lipophilic and tends to leave the epidural/thecal area quickly so that an epidural injection achieves almost the same plasma level as a parenteral injection quickly. (See previous chapters for details.)

POSTOPERATIVE ANALGESIA

- This author recommends analgesia with methadone single injection, which can be repeated, butorphanol with a priming dose and a CRI, or lower doses of stronger opioids. Ketamine CRI can be used for postoperative pain management and oral NMDA antagonists might prove helpful as they add analgesia and do not depress ventilation.
- Lidocaine CRI may provide analgesia and lower opioid CRI requirements. Lidocaine is currently thought to have anti-inflammatory as well as analgesic properties.
- Epidural catheters can be used to redose epidural morphine and will last approximately 3 days. A single shot epidural of morphine (described above) may lower dose requirements of other analgesics and so assist postoperative recovery.

Emergencies (see also Chapter 21)

- Emergency medications for airway surgery patients can include dexamethasone sodium phosphate, furosemide, and epinephrine. Epinephrine has potent and immediate bronchodilation. Dexamethasone may decrease swelling in the airway and furosemide has protective effects against bronchospasm. Atropine, a choice for severe bradycardia, also has mild bronchodilator effects. Other injectable bronchodilators include terbutaline and aminophylline. The latter has more drug to drug interactions. These are mentioned to suggest maximizing the respiratory system reserve in those patients who may have problems in other, upper anatomic spaces.

- Emergency access to the airway is the most important skill to have at hand when working with masses in the retropharyngeal region or brachycephalic syndrome. Intervention with a tracheotomy is a simple surgical procedure. Other options include using a large bore needle between the tracheal rings as a short-term solution. The most critical patient can be the collapsing trachea or malfunctioning stent patient. If it is a more distal collapse, it is not possible to access the trachea below the obstruction. Intubation is still worth performing and then IPPV might be able to supply some oxygen past the obstruction as a short-term solution. This can create time to create a surgical or endoscopic intervention.

- An anti-inflammatory dose of steroid, epinephrine and furosemide may be helpful. Furosemide has protective action in bronchospasm/bronchoconstriction. Doxapram as an emergency treatment for failure to respire has fallen out of favor because it increases oxygen consumption; it has shown favorable outcomes in dogs oversedated with acepromazine in one study. Laryngospasm can be treated by a few drops of lidocaine on the arytenoids or deepening the plane of anesthesia while providing oxygen. Using excess pressure to pass the obstruction should be avoided; instead use a smaller tube, a small amount of lubrication, and patient positioning. This will avoid rupture, injury, or inflammation of the larynx.

- Laryngeal paralysis surgical interventions usually begin with a distressed patient on presentation. Understanding the individual anatomy will help an anesthetist prepare for the case. Some patients have paralyzed and flaccid arytenoids. Some patients are paralyzed and have arytenoids that are fixed medially. Damage can be unilateral or bilateral. The most concerning are the bilateral paralyzed and fixed medial arytenoids, as this is an obstructed airway. Oxygen supplementation can be given before and during induction, including a separate small oxygen cannula that can be placed close to the slit of an opening of the arytenoids. The use of a long polypropylene stylet with an ETT smaller than expected is useful for a guided intubation. The other option is to have a small ureteroscope or bronchoscope upon which the ETT is threaded, and use this to navigate the obstruction. Again, tracheotomy is an option for the challenging case.

- Both laryngeal tie-back (arytenoid lateralization) and laryngeal implants may involve removing and replacing the ETT, usually with the same or smaller size. Preparation includes laryngoscopes, polypropylene stylets, and emergency medications. Another problem can be that the arytenoids can be inadvertently sutured to the ETT. The surgical site must be reopened and the sutures removed. Replace with a new, clean unpunctured ETT.

- Emergencies after surgery include airway obstruction that presents as stertorous breathing or panic. Examples include ear flushes and total ear canal ablations. After making a quick assessment, administer the medications discussed above. Check if it is possible to retract or reduce the swelling. Inducing the patient again and reintubating the patient may be necessary. The patient may need IPPV under sedation until the medications can reduce the swelling. Gentle extension of the neck, gentle massage of the lymph nodes, and alternating cold/warm compresses may encourage circulation in the swollen but otherwise stable patient.

- Brachycephalic syndrome and corrective surgery presents difficult airway challenges: regurgitation under anesthesia, aspiration of gastrointestinal contents, and increased vagal tone causing bradycardia. As discussed above, a careful choice of analgesics is needed to avoid vomiting, with either pretreatment with antiemetics or choosing an analgesic less likely to cause nausea. Preoxygenation and a cool, low-stress environment will help. The surface area to body mass ratio makes these breeds more difficult to cool. It may be necessary to administer acepromazine or dexmedetomidine in recovery to calm the patient. Stress in these patients is inadvisable because that will increase oxygen consumption in a patient that struggles to meet its oxygen demand at rest.

- Brachycephalics may have a high PCV/hematocrit (0.55–0.60 l/l [55–60%]). Intravenous fluids can help in the pre-, intra-, and postoperative periods. Careful monitoring of heart rate may reveal bradycardia, but treating it with an anticholinergic may increase the thickness of airway secretions, which is undesirable. A bronchodilator should be considered to recruit lower airways.

- Brachycephalic airway surgery may incur more hemorrhage with soft palate reduction using a scalpel instead of a laser. Laryngeal saccule resection and nares resection are also more likely to hemorrhage with scalpel use. Laser scalpels cause less hemorrhage, but requires protective eyewear and ETT protection. If the tube is inadvertently cut by the laser, discontinue the oxygen immediately to prevent a fire. Use injectable anesthetics to reintubate. When the procedure ends some patients seem painful and need immediate analgesia. Some will retain the ETT for an extended time while meeting other benchmarks of recovery, such as becoming sternal or standing. Careful monitoring will prevent chewing of the tube; worst case, swallowing the tube will require endoscopy and, rarely, bronchoscopy. Because having a hypoplastic trachea is a component of brachycephalic syndrome, preparation for intubation should include multiple small sizes of ETTs. Use an appropriately-sized laryngoscope so that the larynx may be visualized. Intubation may be aided by the use of a wire stylet to better control the ETT, or the use of a long polypropylene tom cat catheter as a guide for the ETT. Also, a tongue depressor can be used to retract a long soft palate dorsally when performing intubation.

- High-pressure, low-volume cuffed ETTs allow for a wider airway than do low-pressure, high-volume ETTs and this can be important because a small ETT can become more readily clogged with mucus, causing an iatrogenic airway obstruction. Careful monitoring of the capnograph can show formation of a mucus plug by a change in exhalation portion and a sharp upward slope ('shark fin').

Thoracic surgery

- Thoracotomy causes severe pain. There will be impairment of circulation of the blood in the lungs and there will be ventilation–perfusion (V/Q) mismatch depending on what is needed to alter, remove, or biopsy the contents of the thoracic cavity. Changes in peak inspiratory pressure (PIP) will be needed when the thorax is opened to room air. Efficient communication between the surgical and anesthesia team helps, although one can often feel the difference during manual IPPV. ABG monitoring is critical for thoracotomy. Controlling ventilation by manual or mechanical IPPV is required. Patients cannot spontaneously ventilate with an open thorax. The blood pressure may vacillate as pressure is placed on the major vessels.

- Both lateral and median sternotomy incisions cause pain. Analgesia options include morphine epidurals, IC or thoracic paravertebral blocks. CRIs of fentanyl or similar medications provide analgesia or partial IV anesthesia. Ketamine CRI is possible but it can increase oxygen consumption and make it harder to work around the heart as ketamine increases systolic function and heart rate.
- Chest tubes are often placed by the surgery team. Common problems include dislodgment or the blockage and air or fluid will not drain. The chest tube may need to be replaced if conservative measures fail to restore patency. Gently rotating the patient slowly and aspirating the chest tube may help the patient ventilate and oxygenate. Time can help atelectatic lungs inflate. Other complications from this type of surgery include pneumothorax from improper handling of chest tube, re-expansion pulmonary edema, and kinking or blockage of the chest tube. Closely monitor the patient for signs of respiratory distress, such as increased respiratory rate or a drop in pulse oximeter values below normal.

Pleural space disease

- These cases require patient preparation to be able to remove the air via the chest tube and CRI to maintain stable anesthesia. Inhalants may be less reliable in patients with lung injury because of changes in intrathoracic pressures and blood circulation. These changes affect uptake and distribution of inhalant anesthetics. The CRI may become partial or total IV anesthesia to facilitate the surgery.
- Hemothorax is a pleural space disease with an effusion that has a PCV/hematocrit of 0.25 l/l (25%) or greater. There are many causes and stabilization for anesthesia usually does not involve aggressive thoracentesis, and removing too much fluid may destabilize the patient. Sufficient fluid is removed to allow ventilation. Often the presentation for surgery is to determine or correct the cause of hemothorax. The general principles of treating an unstable patient are to be followed: continuous monitoring as much as tolerated, quick induction with short-acting medications, and quick intubation and control of ventilation. $ETCO_2$ should be measured but ventilation and oxygenation should be assessed with ABG samples from an arterial catheter (dorsal pedal artery of dogs and cats is recommended). Serial blood gases, with notations of the $ETCO_2$ at the time the sample was taken, should be used for monitoring and controlling ventilation for the patient with pleural space disease. Patients who present are usually higher risk anesthesia candidates. If the hemothorax is not the result of a coagulation disorder, an epidural, IC, or paravertebral block may help smooth the anesthesia. If a coagulation disorder is suspected, local or regional anesthesia is contraindicated.
- Chylothorax is a pleural space disease caused by a thoracic duct leak that results from either comorbidities or trauma. When the patient presents for a thoracotomy, the same recommendations apply for a quick induction and control of ventilation through manual or automatic IPPV. The electrolyte concentrations should be monitored in real-time If it is a traumatic chylothorax or hemothorax, monitor the cardiac rhythm closely as trauma to the chest may result in dysrhythmias and anesthetic medications, including inhalant agents, can increase the likelihood of dysrhythmias. Any disease or injury of the chest may cause changes in vagal tone, which may result in a bradyarrhythmia.
- Pneumothorax can present as mild, moderate, or severe disease. In patients with insignificant amounts of air and a sealed leak, gentle IPPV at low pressures may suffice or may worsen the injury. As more air enters the area around the lung, the same PIP will result in less chest

excursion unless the extrapulmonary air can be emptied. This can change the feel of manual IPPV to a 'stiff' feel and the SPO_2 will decrease. Moderate or severe cases need periodic removal of any air that accumulates in the pleural space.

- Patients who underwent trauma may have undiagnosed pneumothorax. When managing the difficult oxygenation and ventilation in a case that was stable before IPPV, this should be considered as a rule-out. Spontaneous pneumothorax can be caused by injuries remote from presentation, such as a migrating porcupine quill or other foreign body. When pneumothorax is known and managed actively, the anesthetic outcome can be good.

- Chylothorax and hemothorax patients benefit from striving to use the minimum amount of PIP to achieve normal or close to normal levels of CO_2. The concern driving this notation is the possibility of re-expansion pulmonary edema (RPE). RPE is poorly described in veterinary species. It is always a risk with chest tubes and chest 'taps', but in the human medical literature it is a less than 1% occurrence. When it does occurs, RPE has a 20% mortality. Treatment is mainly supportive, with one case report of putting drained fluid back into the chest as a treatment, although this is not compelling evidence. Whether draining air or fluid, if the situation gets worse, radiographs are warranted to monitor RPE. Of note is that vascular permeability plays a role, so patients who have copious amounts of protein in the fluid drained from the thorax are more likely to have a problem such as RPE, but overall it is a rare condition. The current trend is to remove fluid slowly and the minimal amount needed to allow normal oxygenation and ventilation.

- Space-occupying thoracic lesion surgery challenges the anesthetist to control ventilation in the face of rapidly changing V/Q mismatch, large changes in blood pressure and perfusion, and the risk of catastrophic hemorrhage. Sometimes, the procedure can be short and free of complications. In cats whole blood should be typed and cross matched prior to anesthesia if possible; in dogs without a previous history of transfusion, typing is helpful but not necessary, therefore securing access to whole blood or pRBCs quickly is a measure of safety for the patient. As major vessels are compressed and released there will be many changes in the ABG, $ETCO_2$, blood pressure, and SPO2, so vigilant and frequent monitoring may be labor intensive and require constant supervision by the anesthetist for periods of time.

- Lung lobe torsion is a rare condition that can happen in any species. It may be associated with neoplasia and is always a clinical emergency. It may present in systemic inflammatory response syndrome or sepsis. Preoperative and intraoperative blood chemistry and counts should be checked carefully and frequently. An arterial catheter should be placed as monitoring the blood pressure invasively is indicated in these critical cases. (See also the recommendations for thoracotomies including analgesia and serial ABG monitoring above.) Lung lobe resection can involve bullectomy, pneumonectomy, lobectomy, or a wedge resection. The blood pressure and SPO_2 may fluctuate greatly during removal of the lung or portion of the lung as hemostasis is achieved. This usually resolves when the patient is sternal and able to inflate the remaining lung tissue. The patient may need time in the oxygen cage for any atelectasis of the healthy lung lobes to resolve.

- These surgeries can be done while ventilating without any special equipment and using an inhalant anesthetic agent. However, there will be exposure of personnel to the inhalant agent if this is the method employed. The patient may require an IV anesthetic to maintain a stable plane of anesthesia. This can be the induction agent in a CRI, a CRI of remifentanil, or a CRI of fentanyl and midazolam, for example.

- One lung ventilation is a technique used for lung lobe partial or complete resections. Methods include equipment such as endobronchial tubes (double lumen tubes preferred; single lumen tubes rarely used) and endobronchial blockers. Endobronchial blockers induce lung collapse distal to the bronchus. One practical aspect is that if these techniques are not commonly used, employing them will introduce the risk factor of inexperience. Often, lung resections are done without special equipment.

- High-frequency ventilation (HFV), which uses special equipment and keeps the motion of the lungs at a minimum, may be helpful for RPE and other thoracic diseases and surgical interventions in the thorax. The ventilator used may be cost prohibitive currently, but affordable equipment in the future. This technique is based on the physiology of panting dogs and includes tidal volumes that are less than the volume of dead space while ventilating the patient. This minimizes parenchymal movement. HFV includes high-frequency jet ventilation, high-frequency positive-pressure ventilation, and high-frequency oscillatory ventilation. Ventilating patients without parenchymal excursions would be extremely helpful for surgeons because visibility would be increased and this could reduce the risks of tumor removal, but it is not widely practiced in veterinary anesthesia. Anesthetizing patients for diagnostic and irradiation treatment of space-occupying lesions in the thorax may benefit from HPV.

- Diaphragmatic hernia patients or patients undergoing repair procedures share the same concerns as thoracotomy patients with regard to pulse oximetry, oxygen saturation, and CO_2 levels. They also shares the rare potential for RPE described above. Often there is an atelectatic lung lobe, and if the situation is chronic, a patient who may have compensated before surgery may have trouble intra- and postoperatively. Recovery in an oxygen cage with enough time for the body to compensate for the intrathoracic, intra-abdominal, and anatomic changes is helpful.

- Pericardiectomy patients should be stabilized prior to surgery by removal of enough fluid from the pericardial sac so that the patient can tolerate the cardiovascular challenges of general anesthesia. The same general thoracotomy rules apply of analgesia, opioid, or local/regional anesthesia. Usually a chest tube will be placed and local anesthetics may be administered through the chest tube for comfort. These patients are different from lung lobectomy as they are often as stable or more stable after the pericardiectomy. If they appear unstable, check for excess air or hemorrhage in the thorax.

- For heart-base mass removal and patent ductus arteriosus (PDA) repair the risk of needing a transfusion is elevated by the location. Whole blood or pRBCs should be readily available. The surgeon will need good visualization and the only option is to hyperventilate and hold inspiration so there is no movement during the procedure. This is another potential application for HFV ventilation.

- PDA surgical occlusion is often reserved for the patients with a large shunt. The PDA has the same risks as the heart-base removal but has more drastic changes in the circulation as the blood begins to take a path that leads to better oxygenation as the ductus is occluded. The perilous part is the risk of hemorrhage if the suture cuts through the ductus instead of merely occluding it. If this should happen, it may be useful to lower the blood pressure immediately, either by short-term increase in inhalant anesthetic agent or by administration of nitroprusside.

ACID–BASE ABNORMALITIES

- The acid–base status of most of the patients described will be normal or acidemic as a result of inefficient ventilation from lung or airway impairment. The exception is that the patient may be normal or alkalemic because of a respiratory alkalosis from panting or air escaping between the arytenoids in the patient with laryngeal disease.

- Correct this by adjusting the ventilation as described using ABG over the $ETCO_2$. Providing sodium bicarbonate IV is only beneficial for patients who have the ability to ventilate enough to exhale the CO_2 generated by the dissociation of sodium bicarbonate. If there is no other abnormality, the safest course of action for the patient is to maintain normal blood volume, stabilize perfusion, and provide a balanced crystalloid fluid at a rate that is tolerated by the patient's illness.

Further reading

Campoy L, Reade MR (2013) (eds) *Small Animal Regional Anesthesia and Analgesia*. Wiley-Blackwell, Ames.

Galmén K, Harbut P, Freedman J *et al.* (2017) The use of high-frequency ventilation during general anaesthesia: an update *F1000Research* **6(F1000 Faculty Rev):**756.

Hartsfield SM (2007) Airway management and ventilation. In: *Lumb and Jones' Veterinary Anesthesia and Analgesia*, 4th edn. Blackwell Publishing, Ames, pp. 495–531.

Hasan P, Williams J (2012) Basic opioid pharmacology: an update. *Br J Pain* **6(1):**11–16.

Lerche P, Aarnes TK, Covey-Crump G *et al.* (2016) *Handbook of Small Animal Regional Anesthesia Techniques*. Wiley-Blackwell, Ames.

Patinson KPS (2008) Opioids and the control of respiration. *Br J Anaesth* **100(6):**747–58.

Pypendop B (2009) Jet ventilation. In: *Small Animal Critical Care Medicine*. (eds) D Silverstein, K Hopper) Saunders Elsevier, St. Louis, pp. 910–11.

CHAPTER 13

Anesthetic considerations for upper and lower gastrointestinal endoscopic procedures

Ann B Weil

Introduction

Endoscopy is the process of looking inside the body by inserting a rigid or flexible tube and examining an image of the interior of an organ or cavity. An additional instrument may be inserted to biopsy an organ or to retrieve foreign objects. Although most endoscopic procedures are considered to be minimally invasive, most animals will require general anesthesia. Some of the potential complications of the endoscopic procedure may be related to general anesthesia, and some endoscopic procedures may benefit from special anesthetic considerations. A thorough understanding of the physiologic changes produced by the various endoscopic procedures is necessary to properly support the anesthetized patient. Some endoscopic procedures will require the use of insufflation gas to improve visualization, which has a physiologic impact on the patient. Patient positioning may also affect the cardiovascular and respiratory systems. Minimally invasive procedures under general anesthesia need the same monitoring care as any other anesthetized patient.

GENERAL CONSIDERATIONS

- Although preoperative fasting prior to general anesthesia is somewhat controversial, patients undergoing upper and lower gastrointestinal (GI) endoscopic procedures will benefit from such fasting. It is difficult to visualize the interior of the stomach and GI tract if there is a lot of fluid and ingesta present. Preoperative fasting of the patient will help reduce the incidence of aspiration of gastric contents. It is customary for adult patients to have food withheld for 12 hours prior to general anesthesia. Pediatric patients should have a shorter fasting period than adults, depending on age and size. Water should be available up to 1 hour prior to anesthesia.

- Baseline data include a CBC, chemistry panel with electrolytes, and a urinalysis (see Chapter 2). Other tests may include thoracic and abdominal radiographs, computed tomography (CT) imaging, ECG (see Chapter 22), echocardiogram, and/or blood gas analysis depending on the patient's physical condition, body systems affected, and anticipated procedure.
- Drug choices should be made on an individual basis. Careful consideration should be made to the use of preanesthetic agent sedatives (see Chapter 3) and analgesics, as the use of these drugs will reduce the amount of injectable and inhalant anesthetics needed, thus improving the cardiovascular performance of the patient. Sample protocols are included at the end of this chapter and specific drug concerns are discussed in each section.
- Monitoring (see Chapter 6) patients undergoing minimally invasive procedures is of paramount importance because they are undergoing general anesthesia. Blood pressure measurement, capnography, and pulse oximetry as well as ECG should be used to assess patient welfare during the procedure. An IV catheter should be placed for drug administration and fluid therapy during the procedure. Mean arterial pressure should be maintained above 60 mm Hg in dogs and cats. $ETCO_2$ should be between 35 and 45 mm Hg and SpO_2 >95%.
- Crystalloid fluids (see Chapter 7) should be administered IV as inhalant anesthetics will impose vasodilation and reduced contractility, thus reducing cardiac output. Fluids are generally administered at the rate of 5 ml/kg/hour unless the patient is hypoproteinemic or has cardiac disease or renal considerations. Patients that are dehydrated before the procedure should have volume deficits corrected prior to anesthesia. Colloids may be useful in some patients.

Pharyngeal/oral examination

- Many patients will require profound sedation or general anesthesia in order to accomplish a thorough pharyngeal or oral examination. Keep in mind that many of these patients may have a pharyngeal mass that could occlude the airway. It is wise to be prepared for a difficult intubation should that become necessary.
- Preoxygenation for 5 minutes will help prevent the patient from desaturating should intubation prove difficult. This author prefers to avoid drugs that cause vomiting or regurgitation for this type of examination, so butorphanol or methadone may be the opioid of choice. Note that an oral examination is not the same as an examination for laryngeal function.

Upper gastrointestinal endoscopy

- Drugs that potentiate vomiting should be avoided in cases of esophageal or gastric foreign bodies. If the patient has experienced prolonged vomiting, the animal should be carefully examined for dehydration and/or electrolyte disturbances. Volume depletion and electrolyte imbalance should be corrected prior to general anesthesia. The animal may be sedated with a mild tranquilizer such as acepromazine if it is not dehydrated.
- Acepromazine has the added advantage of an antiemetic effect. A benzodiazepine such as midazolam or diazepam may be a useful sedative if the patient is debilitated. Full mu opioid agonists (MOAs) such as morphine, oxymorphone, or hydromorphone may promote vomiting when administered IM. Methadone may be an alternative MOA that is less likely to promote vomiting.
- Maropitant may be useful as a premedication to decrease the incidence of vomiting and provide additional analgesia for the procedure. Kappa agonist opioids such as butorphanol are less likely to

promote vomiting. The animal should be induced with an injectable anesthetic and intubated quickly in order to avoid aspiration. Propofol, alfaxalone, ketamine, or etomidate (see Chapter 4) may be used for this purpose, depending on the rest of the animal's condition. The patient may be maintained on inhalants after intubation. An appropriately inflated endotracheal tube cuff should be maintained at all times to avoid inadvertent aspiration of fluid during the procedure.

- Balanced, isotonic crystalloid fluids (such as Normosol-R [Plasma-Lyte A] or lactated Ringer's solution [LRS]), administered at 5 ml/kg/ hour, should be used for patients with normal oncotic pressure and plasma proteins. Hypoproteinemic patients may benefit from colloid administration. Plasma or VetStarch can be used to assist in maintaining sufficient oncotic pressure. VetStarch can be used at a rate of 2–5 ml/kg/hour along with crystalloid fluid administration during the procedure. Care must be taken to avoid fluid overload.

- Insufflation of the stomach with air must be carefully monitored to avoid overinflation and attendant cardiovascular and respiratory compromise. Pulse oximetry, blood pressure measuring, and capnometry are very helpful to monitor anesthesia in these patients. Frequently, respiration must be supported with intermittent positive-pressure ventilation if abdominal pressure is increased. The size of the stomach should be continuously monitored during gastroscopy in order to prevent excessive insufflation.

- Care must be taken to avoid aspiration of gastric contents. The endotracheal tube cuff should be properly inflated on intubation and maintained throughout the procedure. The cuff should not be deflated until the patient is extubated, ensuring that the patient can swallow and protect the airway.

- Nearly every drug will alter intestinal motility. Sphincter function is of particular concern when performing upper GI endoscopy in order to examine the upper duodenum. The esophagus, stomach, and upper duodenum can be visualized and biopsied if warranted. The cardiac and pyloric sphincters can impede endoscopy. Comparison of premedication with atropine, glycopyrrolate, morphine, meperidine, acepromazine, and saline prior to general anesthesia for gastroduodenoscopy in dogs resulted in more difficulty entering the pyloric sphincter when a combination of morphine and atropine was used. This has led to the suggestion that all full MOAs should be avoided when duodenoscopy is performed. The use of atropine in dogs as a premedication does not facilitate duodenal intubation and may inhibit it. Alpha-2 agonists such as dexmedetomidine or medetomidine do not hinder passage of the endoscope through the pylorus in dogs, although vomiting may be an issue in some patients.

- More recent work has evaluated the effects of various premedications (see Chapter 3) on ease of duodenoscopy in the cat. The results suggest that hydromorphone (a full MOA), glycopyrrolate (anticholinergic), medetomidine (alpha-2 agonist), or butorphanol (agonist antagonist opioid) are all satisfactory for use as a premedication prior to gastroduodenoscopy in the cat.

- Experienced clinicians may not have any difficulty passing the endoscope into the duodenum, despite the anesthetic protocol used. Butorphanol may be used without difficulty and has the additional benefit of not inducing as much vomiting as a full MOA when used as a premedication. Its short duration is helpful in avoiding excessive postanesthetic sedation.

LOWER GASTROINTESTINAL ENDOSCOPY

- Colonoscopy is often performed in patients with signs of large bowel or rectal disease. In order to adequately visualize the colonic mucosa, the bowel is prepared for the procedure with

234 CHAPTER 13 Anesthetic considerations for GI endoscopic procedures

food withdrawal, administration of a GI lavage solution (e.g., GoLYTELY, Braintree Laboratories), and a series of enemas. This preparation can cause dehydration in some patients. Careful evaluation should be performed to ensure adequate hydration prior to general anesthesia. Volume deficits should be corrected prior to general anesthesia with IV administration of crystalloid fluids.

• Complications associated with colonoscopy are reported to be relatively rare in dogs, with minor and major complications developing in 30 out of 355 procedures (8.5%). Minor complications were most frequently associated with vomiting of GoLYTELY. Anesthetic complications such as bradycardia, which resolved after the anesthetic episode, were also reported under minor complications. Major complications may also be associated with general anesthesia. Aspiration of vomited GoLYTELY was responsible for mortality of one patient in the study and has been reported in humans. Many different anesthetic plans can be used appropriately for this procedure.

SAMPLE ANESTHETIC PROTOCOLS
Pharyngeal examination
1 Preoxygenation with 100% oxygen via face mask if patient permits.
2 Premedication with dexmedetomidine (0.005 mg/kg) + butorphanol (0.2 mg/kg) IV or IM.
3 Induction with propofol (4–6 mg/kg) IV to effect if sedation not enough to complete examination (catheter placement recommended).
4 Intubation with oxygen administration.

5 Maintenance with sevoflurane or isoflurane if needed.
6 Normosol-R (Plasma-Lyte A) (5 ml/kg/h) if inhalant anesthetic used.

Upper GI endoscopy
1 Premedication with acepromazine (0.01–0.02 mg/kg) + butorphanol (0.2–0.4 mg/kg) IV or IM.
2 Place IV catheter.
3 Induction with propofol (6 mg/kg IV) to effect or alfaxalone (2 mg/kg IV) to effect.
4 Maintenance with isoflurane or sevoflurane.
5 Normosol-R (Plasma-Lyte A) (5 ml/kg/h) if patient has normal serum proteins.
6 Normosol-R (Plasma-Lyte A) (2.5 ml/kg/h) + VetStarch (2.5 ml/kg/h) if hypoproteinemic.

Colonoscopy
1 Premedication with maropitant (1 mg/kg IV or SC) 30 minutes prior to other drugs.
2 Midazolam (0.2 mg/kg) + hydromorphone (0.1 mg/kg) IM.
3 Place IV catheter (if not already in place).
4 Induction with propofol (6 mg/kg IV to effect) or alfaxalone (2 mg/kg IV to effect).
5 Maintenance with isoflurane or sevoflurane.
6 Normosol-R (Plasma-Lyte A) (5 ml/kg/h) if patient has normal serum proteins.
7 Normosol-R (Plasma-Lyte A) (2.5 ml/kg/h) + VetStarch (2.5 ml/kg/h) if hypoproteinemic.
8 Hydromorphone (0.05 mg/kg IV) if additional analgesia needed.

Further reading

Weil AB (2009) Anesthesia for endoscopy in small animals. *Vet Clin North Am Small Anim Pract* **39**:839–48.

CHAPTER 14

Anesthetic considerations for minimally invasive surgical procedures

Ann B Weil

(Refer to Chapter 13 for a basic overview of endoscopy.)

Laryngoscopy/tracheoscopy

- Diagnosis of laryngeal paralysis relies on evaluating arytenoid activity under a light plane of anesthesia. Many patients undergoing this diagnostic procedure will have signs of obstructive upper airway disease. They are dyspneic and easily stressed. Thoracic radiographs should be added to the minimum database if the images can be obtained without excessive stress to the patient.
- Evaluation of laryngeal function is most frequently done under a light plane of general anesthesia, but there are many clinical opinions as to the optimal anesthetic plan and a variety of injectable anesthetics have been used. All sedative drugs and deeper planes of anesthesia tend to diminish arytenoid function with much individual variation, therefore this author prefers to utilize

only a short-acting injectable anesthetic without premedication with sedative drugs.
- The perfect technique of general anesthesia for laryngeal function evaluation has yet to be established, as the depth of anesthesia must be sufficient enough to open the jaw and protect the examiner and equipment, yet still maintain arytenoid cartilage movement for evaluation. False-positive examinations can occur with most sedatives and anesthetic combinations.
- Preoxygenation of the patient via oxygen mask or flow-by oxygen (**Fig. 14.1**) with the breathing circuit is very helpful. Two to three liters per minute of oxygen should be given for 5 minutes immediately prior to drug administration. This allows increased

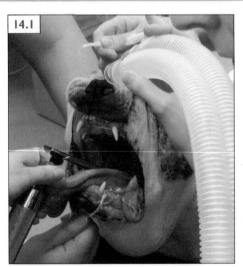

14.1

Fig. 14.1 A Bulldog's airway is being examined to assess its laryngeal function. Preoxygenation (not shown) and continuous oxygen with flow-by method is being provided during the examination process.

time for examination of the airway before the patient desaturates.

- A variety of injectable anesthetic protocols have been evaluated. One study showed that arytenoid motion at recovery was significantly greater with thiopental compared with propofol alone, acepromazine with thiopental or propofol, and ketamine and diazepam. This is comparable to what has been shown in people, where propofol has been reported to have a more detrimental effect on vocal cord motion than thiopental. A more recent study compared alfaxalone with propofol or thiopental. The results of this study showed that all three agents could be successfully used for laryngeal function evaluation. Propofol may have the advantage of a shorter examination time.

- Comorbidities of the patient may dictate the final selection of anesthetic agent, as well as the conditions under which the examiner is accustomed to performing the evaluation. It is helpful for an assistant to announce inspiration by the patient while evaluating arytenoid abduction. Propofol may be administered at 6 mg/kg IV to effect or alfaxalone at 2 mg/kg

to effect. Administration of supplemental oxygen during the examination is useful, as is pulse oximetry to monitor oxygen saturation. Doxapram (2–5 mg/kg IV) may be used at the end of the examination to stimulate more vigorous respiratory movements and eliminate false positives.

- General anesthesia is used for tracheoscopy and bronchoscopy in animals in order to minimize laryngospasm and coughing and protect the endoscope. Tracheoscopy/bronchoscopy is performed without an endotracheal tube in very small patients or via the endotracheal tube in patients with sufficient tracheal diameter (size 7 or 8 endotracheal tube). Inhalant anesthesia can be used to maintain the patient during bronchoscopy if the patient is large enough for an endotracheal tube, using a special T-shaped adapter to accommodate the scope as well as administer oxygen and anesthetic gas. There should be sufficient room inside the endotracheal tube for exhalation of gases without resistance.

- Injectable anesthetics can be used to maintain anesthesia in patients with small tracheal diameter, while oxygen is administered through the scope or via a catheter placed beside the scope if there is sufficient room. A variety of injectable protocols may be used, depending on the patient's condition. In general, a protocol that has minimal cardiovascular effects and allows rapid recovery, is preferable, as many patients undergoing bronchoscopy have significant respiratory impairment. Short-acting opioids such as fentanyl or butorphanol can be used for premedication. Butorphanol is a potent cough suppressant. Acepromazine has little respiratory depression and is useful at low doses to calm patients with upper respiratory disease. Propofol has little accumulative effect and can be administered in intermittent boluses or via CRI to maintain anesthesia. The use of anticholinergics to 'dry up' small airways is no longer recommended. Oxygen supplementation post tracheoscopy or bronchoscopy is important to support patients through the recovery period until airway reflexes are normal.

- Oxygen saturation should be monitored via pulse oximetry throughout the procedure, with the goal of maintaining saturation above 95%. Mean arterial blood pressure should be >60 mmHg. Balanced, isotonic crystalloid fluids should be administered with inhalant anesthesia and propofol CRI of moderate duration.

Rhinoscopy

- Rhinoscopy is a procedure that often requires a surgical plane of general anesthesia. A full mu agonist opioid, such as hydromorphone, morphine, methadone, fentanyl, or oxymorphone, can be administered as part of the premedication plan in addition to a tranquilizer/sedative such as acepromazine or dexmedetomidine. Short-acting, potent opioids, such as fentanyl or remifentanil, can be bolused IV prior to biopsy to prevent excessively high vaporizer settings.
- Regional anesthetic techniques, such as infraorbital blocks (see Chapter 23) with lidocaine, mepivacaine, or bupivacaine, will also improve patient comfort. Postprocedure bleeding can be minimized if the patient is well sedated after biopsies are taken, as excessive head shaking and activity can lead to continued bleeding and increased irritation of the area.
- The endotracheal tube cuff should be properly inflated (see Chapter 1) prior to rhinoscopy and the procedure halted anytime there is a concern about the cuff. The patient should be extubated with the cuff partially inflated to assist in clearing blood from the airway if it has not been packed prior to beginning the procedure.

Laparoscopy

- Laparoscopic non-invasive surgery (see **Fig. 6.34**) has become common as more procedures are attempted in a non-invasive fashion. Healthy patients may present for elective procedures such as ovariectomy or animals with significant disease may present for procedures such as liver biopsy. In order to perform this type of surgery, a pneumoperitoneum is established to allow room to place the trocar and cannula assemblies safely and improve visualization for the procedure. CO_2 is most frequently chosen as the insufflation gas for laparoscopy. The use of medical air has increased potential for air embolism and increased potential to support combustion if electrocautery is used. CO_2 is able to diffuse across the peritoneal cavity and enter the blood stream, where it stimulates the sympathetic nervous system to release endogenous catecholamines. Higher levels of arterial CO_2 tend to increase heart rate, blood pressure, and cardiac output. Excessively high levels of CO_2 will lead to narcosis, arrhythmia, acidemia, and myocardial depression. Nitrous oxide does not alter the patient's acid–base status.
- Regardless of the type of gas used, insufflation of gas increases intra-abdominal pressure (IAP) in the patient, with the potential to cause respiratory impairment. Tidal volume usually decreases, with resultant hypoventilation. Functional residual capacity and lung compliance decrease during general anesthesia and the increase in IAP from gas insufflation causes cranial displacement of the diaphragm. All of these factors contribute to the need for increased ventilation support for the anesthetized patient undergoing laparoscopy. Depression of ventilation increases with increasing IAP, and IAP <20 mmHg is recommended.
- Increased IAP also leads to decreased venous return and a reduction in cardiac output. Tissue blood flow may be compromised with increased IAP, as elevated IAPs are associated with

decreased hepatic blood flow and oliguria. Anesthetic conditions for the patient will be improved by using the least amount of IAP necessary to complete the procedure.

- Changes in body position have the potential to adversely affect the anesthetized patient, especially when coupled with abdominal insufflation. Inhalant anesthetics alter the baroreflex, leading to a depressed reflex control of circulation in response to changes in body posture. Head-down tilt of a dorsally recumbent patient (Trendelenburg position) allows better exposure of caudal organs in the operative field. Reverse Trendelenburg position (head up and dorsally recumbent) is used when improved exposure of cranial organs is desired. The head-down tilt position has more effect on respiratory and cardiovascular mechanics, leading to decreases in minute ventilation and cardiac output, amongst other effects. Mean arterial pressure may increase. The head-up tilt position will also affect cardiovascular mechanics, leading to reflex vasoconstriction and increased heart rate and arterial blood pressure in dogs.

- Excellent monitoring of the anesthetized patient undergoing laparoscopy is essential. IAP results in hypoventilation, so the use of a mechanical ventilator is helpful to provide pulmonary support, as normocapnia should be a monitoring goal. If CO_2 is the insufflation gas used, absorption of CO_2 across the peritoneal membrane will lead to higher $PaCO_2$, regardless of the respiratory status of the patient.

- $ETCO_2$ monitoring and pulse oximetry (see Chapter 6) will provide continuous monitoring of the respiratory system. Invasive blood pressure monitoring is warranted in more critical patients undergoing laparoscopy, while non-invasive methods (Doppler or oscillometric cuff-based monitors) can be used in healthy patients undergoing elective laparoscopic procedures. Arterial catheter placement will allow easier sampling for blood gas analysis if CO_2 is the insufflation gas. Abdominal insufflation must be monitored and the Rule of 15s is a good general guideline: no more than 15 mmHg IAP or 15 degrees of tilt.

- While general anesthesia is most frequently used for laparoscopic procedures in small animals, it is important to consider the increased stress to the patient of abdominal insufflation and tilted body posture. These effects are aggravated by general anesthesia.

- Complications of laparoscopy include hemorrhage, pneumothorax, gas embolism, or puncture of an organ with placement of the Veress needle. Splenic enlargement will occur if thiopental (still available internationally) was used as the induction agent, increasing the likelihood of inadvertent puncture of this organ. Serial PCV determinations and TP measurements can help assess the need for blood replacement products.

- Packed RBCs and plasma, or whole blood transfusion (see Chapter 8), should be considered if the PCV falls below 0.2 l/l (20%) and the TP below 40 g/l (4 g/dl). Pneumothorax created by high peak inspiratory pressure during mechanical ventilation or by migration of CO_2 may require placement of a chest tube. Despite the relative safety of CO_2 as an insufflation gas, fatal embolism has been reported in people and animals. If embolism is suspected, insufflation should be immediately discontinued and cardiac massage started.

- Anesthetic plans for laparoscopic procedures depend on the individual patient. Young and healthy patients for elective procedures will have little restriction on drug choices. Diseased patients may require anesthesia care that suits their disease state. Regardless, animals undergoing laparoscopic procedures require careful monitoring. Hypotension is managed with reducing the anesthetic dose, fluid therapy, and sympathomimetic drug administration. The analgesic needs of the patient must be considered, despite it being considered a minimally invasive procedure. Intraoperative and postoperative analgesic needs can be met with parenterally administered opioids. Lidocaine patch application at the port sites can be used to provide regional analgesia without systemic effects.

Sample anesthetic protocols

LARYNGEAL EXAMINATION
1 Assure volume status of the patient is normal.
2 Preoxygenate with 100% oxygen via face mask.
3 Propofol (4–6 mg/kg IV to effect), maintaining as light a plane of anesthesia as possible.
4 Continued administration of 100% oxygen.
5 Doxapram IV if increased respiratory effort needed to complete examination.
6 Intubation if possible after examination.

RHINOSCOPY
1 Premedication with dexmedetomidine (0.005 mg/kg) + methadone (0.3 mg/kg) IM.
2 Preoxygenate with 100% oxygen via face mask for 5 minutes.
3 Induce with propofol or alfaxalone.
4 Maintain with isoflurane or sevoflurane in oxygen.
5 Normosol-R or Plasma-Lyte A® (5 ml/kg/h).

6 Fentanyl (5 µg/kg IV bolus) if additional analgesia necessary.
7 Infraorbital nerve block.
8 Carprofen (2.2 mg/kg SC).

LAPAROSCOPIC GASTROPEXY
1 Maropitant (1 mg/kg SC) 30 minutes prior to premedication with opioid.
2 Premedication with dexmedetomidine (0.005 mg/kg) + hydromorphone (0.1 mg/kg) IM.
3 Preoxygenate with 100% oxygen via face mask for 5 minutes.
4 Induce with propofol or alfaxalone.
5 Maintain isoflurane or sevoflurane in oxygen.
6 Normosol-R or Plasma-Lyte A® (5 ml/kg/h).
7 Fentanyl (5 µg/kg IV bolus) if additional analgesia necessary (5 µg/kg/h CRI if desired or additional boluses of hydromorphone may be used instead).
8 Carprofen (2.2 mg/kg SC).

Further reading

Mama K, de Rezende ML (2015) Anesthesia management of dogs and cats for laparoscopy. In: *Small Animal Laparoscopy and Thoracoscopy*. (eds BA Fransson, PD Mayhew) John Wiley & Sons, Hoboken, pp. 73–80.

Radkey DI, Hardie RJ, Smith LJ (2018) Comparison of the effects of alfaxalone and propofol with acepromazine, butorphanol, and/or doxapram on laryngeal motion and quality of examination in dogs. *Vet Anaesth Analg* **45(3)**:241–9.

Weil AB (2009) Anesthesia for endoscopy in small animals. *Vet Clin North Am Small Anim Pract* **39**:839–48.

Anesthetic considerations for neurologic patients

Stefania C Grasso

Introduction

Animals with neurologic problems are often anesthetized for diagnostic procedures such as brain or spine magnetic resonance imaging (MRI), computed tomography (CT) scan, cerebrospinal fluid (CSF) (**Fig. 15.1**) collection, and nerve/muscle biopsy, or for surgical procedures including thoracolumbar and cervical intervertebral disc disease (IVDD) and brain tumor resection (**Fig. 15.2**). Less common procedures performed include atlantoaxial instability correction, ventriculoperitoneal shunt placement, vertebral distraction and fusion for Wobbler disease, and vertebral fracture repair.

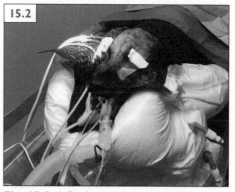

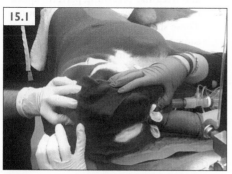

Fig. 15.1 Cerebrospinal fluid sampling at the level of the cisterna magna. Pulse oximetry and capnography should be closely monitored during the procedure to quickly detect airway obstruction due to the position of the neck.

Fig. 15.2 A Barbet in the operating room prepared for a transfrontal craniotomy to remove a right forebrain mass. Inflatable cushions are used to properly position the head and ensure immobility during the surgery. The eyes are kept closed with clean gauzes and tape to protect them from penetration of surgical debris and blood.

Brain diseases

GENERAL CONSIDERATIONS

- General anesthesia carries higher risks in patients with a suspected space-occupying lesion, head trauma, and seizures, due to the possibility of increased intracranial pressure (ICP).
- Understanding cerebral blood flow autoregulation is necessary to appreciate the impact of general anesthesia on neurologic patients.
- Cerebral blood flow is dependent on cerebral perfusion pressure (CPP) and cerebral vascular resistance. CPP is the net difference between mean arterial blood pressure (MAP) and ICP, and maintaining MAP within 70–80 mmHg will ensure a CPP >70 mmHg, considering that normal ICP is 10–15 mmHg. Cerebral vascular resistances are affected by changes in blood flow, changes in cerebral metabolism, and chemical factors such as oxygen and CO_2 levels. Physiologically, blood flow is constant despite changes in MAP when in the autoregulation range (60–160 mmHg). Outside this range, the CPP will change linearly to the MAP; if the MAP falls to <60 mmHg, the CPP will decrease.
- The Monroe–Kellie doctrine states that the skull is a rigid box in which different compartments (blood, CSF, cerebral tissue) exist in dynamic balance. The ICP will rise when the volume of one compartment increases without a concomitant decrease in another one:
  - Increased blood: hemorrhage due to trauma, cerebral vasodilation due to hypoxemia and hypercapnia, seizures, hyperthermia, anesthetics, and hypotension.
  - Increased CSF: congenital hydrocephalus, obstruction of the CSF outflow (congenital or acquired).
  - Increased cerebral tissue: tumor (e.g. meningioma/glioma), cerebral edema/contusion.
- The main anesthetic goal is to prevent the increase of ICP.

- General anesthetics depress the central nervous system (CNS) and this can aggravate the depression already present.
- Factors that increase the ICP and that need to be avoided are:
  - Vomiting.
  - Coughing.
  - Obstruction of the venous return through the jugular veins (struggling, jugular blood sampling, high intrathoracic positive pressure).
  - Hypoxia.
  - Hypercapnia/hypoventilation.
  - Hypotension.
  - Fluids overload.
- Ventilation needs to be supported in order to avoid hypercapnia, which leads to cerebral vasodilation and increased ICP. $PaCO_2$ should be maintained at 35–40 mmHg and therefore $ETCO_2$ at 30–35 mmHg. $PaCO_2$ <30–35 mmHg is associated with vasoconstriction and risk of ischemic damage.
- The head should be kept elevated with a maximum 30° angle at all times after anesthetic induction in order to facilitate venous drainage of the head.
- Treatment of pain after head trauma or during surgical procedures is paramount.
- Increased ICP leads to a strong sympathetic response clinically manifested as the Cushing's triad: systemic hypertension, reflex bradycardia, and irregular breathing pattern/apnea (Cheyne–Stokes or Biot's respiration). These signs may not be present all at the same time when there is compression on the brainstem. Furthermore, the Cushing's reflex might not be present despite documented herniation on imaging. Imaging is the most sensitive method to clinically confirm brain herniation.

ANESTHETIC MANAGEMENT AND PHARMACOLOGIC CONSIDERATIONS

- Preanesthetic assessment should focus on:
  - Level of consciousness.
  - Neurologic evaluation, especially pupil size.

- Ventilation and oxygenation.
- Minimum blood database: hematocrit, total solids, blood glucose, and electrolyte levels. Further blood parameters should be assessed based on the signalment and anamnesis of the animal.
- Diagnostic imaging: chest radiographs and abdominal ultrasound should be considered, especially in trauma or suspected space-occupying lesion cases.
- Signs of increased ICP should be excluded before induction of anesthesia and, if present, the animal should be stabilized first. Therefore, ECG and arterial blood pressure readings should be obtained before induction.
- The effects on the CNS of different anesthetics as well as recommendations for their use are listed in *Table 15.1*.
- Sedatives/analgesics may have more profound effects even at low doses if the mentation status of the patient is altered. The premedication drugs and doses are chosen based on the level of consciousness of the patient and may not always be required.
- Ideal pain management should include short-acting opioids such as fentanyl/remifentanil as CRI, due to the easier dose titration and rapid elimination if neurologic assessment is required.
- Intubation is performed when the anesthetic plan is appropriate to avoid coughing. Lidocaine 2% at 1 mg/kg can be administered IV slowly 1 minute before induction to decrease the stimulation of the intubation.
- Face mask anesthetic induction with inhalants should be avoided, as struggle and stress can increase ICP.
- The animal needs to be mechanically or manually hyperventilated to maintain $ETCO_2$ around 30–35 mmHg. The hyperventilation offsets the mild increase of ICP caused by inhalant anesthetics. High inspiratory peak pressure (>20 cmH_2O) as well as high positive end-expiratory pressure (>5 cmH_2O) should not be used as the increase in intrathoracic pressure raises the central venous pressure and ICP.

- Hypoxemia leads to cerebral vasodilation, therefore oxygenation should be closely monitored from induction to recovery using pulse oximetry or arterial gas analysis. If needed, oxygen can be provided after extubation via face mask or oxygen cage. Nasal cannulas may be used; however, they can cause sneezing, which increases ICP.
- The essentials for anesthetic monitoring are ECG, arterial blood pressure, pulse oximetry, and capnography. An arterial line can be used in most critical cases to closely monitor the blood pressure and obtain arterial blood samples for gas analysis (PaO_2, $PaCO_2$).
- Administration of isotonic crystalloid fluids (Plasma-Lyte A®, LRS) at 5 ml/kg/hour is usually appropriate for well-hydrated animals with no ongoing blood loss. In the past, fluid restriction was contemplated to prevent cerebral edema formation; however, this practice is no longer recommended. Patients with signs of dehydration should receive IV fluids before undergoing general anesthesia. If hypotension occurs, artificial colloids or hypertonic saline can be titrated until the blood pressure is restored.

ADDITIONAL CONSIDERATIONS FOR PATIENTS WITH HEAD TRAUMA
- Assessment of the airway patency.
- Presence of mandibular/maxillary fractures, which can complicate intubation.
- Fluid resuscitation: hypertonic saline 7.5% (1–4 ml/kg) or colloids are preferred over large volumes of crystalloids.
- Presence of pulmonary contusions/pneumothorax.
- Presence of abdominal trauma.
- Supported ventilation during general anesthesia should aim for eucapnia ($PaCO_2$ = 40 mmHg) as lower values can aggravate the ischemic neuronal damage.
- Use of high doses of corticosteroids is contraindicated.
- Use of dextrose-supplemented IV fluids should be avoided since hyperglycemia may already be present and is correlated with the severity of the trauma.

Table 15.1 Pros and cons of common anesthetic drugs and recommendations for their use

Anesthetic agent/drug	Pros	Cons	Recommendations
Acepromazine	Reduction of seizure threshold controversial Duration dose dependent	High doses have long duration	Use with caution Low doses (0.01–0.02 mg/kg IM/IV) are not contraindicated
Alpha-2 agonists	Dexmedetomidine and medetomidine decrease ICP at low doses	Moderate to profound CNS depression Hypertension and bradycardia mimic the Cushing's reflex	Use with caution Usually the sedation induced by these agents is not needed in depressed animals Low doses (0.5–2 µg/kg IV) or use of a CRI are not contraindicated
Benzodiazepines	Reduction in $CMRO_2$, minimal changes in CBF Muscle relaxation Minimal impact on the respiratory and cardiovascular system Good sedation in combination with opioids Seizure control	Contraindicated when signs of hepatic encephalopathy are present Can cause excitement in some patients	Drugs of choice for premedication
Opioids	No direct effects on ICP Kappa-agonists cause minimal respiratory and cardiovascular depression	Hydromorphone and morphine cause vomiting Mu-agonists are more likely to cause bradycardia and hypoventilation	Hydromorphone/morphine: contraindicated as premedication for brain pathology Butorphanol: opioid of choice for diagnostic procedures Short-acting mu agonists (fentanyl, remifentanil) when painful procedures
Barbiturates, propofol, alfaxalone	Decrease ICP, CBF, and $CMRO_2$ Muscle relaxation Short duration	Respiratory depression Arterial vasodilation	Induction agents of choice Doses can be decreased if combined with a benzodiazepine Propofol and alfaxalone CRI can be used for maintenance of anesthesia
Etomidate	No impact on cardiac output	Cerebral hypoxia Ischemic injury Likely coughing at induction	Contraindicated
Dissociatives	Does not cause apnea	Increase CBF and $CMRO_2$ Associated with seizure activity	Contraindicated
Inhalants	Rapidly eliminated Dose-related effects and easily titratable Sevoflurane causes faster recovery	Respiratory depression Hypotension Enflurane causes seizures	Halothane and nitrous oxide contraindicated Desflurane not suitable (more effect on ICP than others) Use ≤1 MAC

CBF, cerebral blood flow; $CMRO_2$, cerebral metabolic rate; CNS, central nervous system; CRI, constant rate infusion; ICP, intracranial pressure; MAC, minimum alveolar concentration.

POTENTIAL COMPLICATIONS

- Increased ICP:
  - Causes of progressive or sudden bradycardia with/without hypertension or vice versa during anesthesia should be investigated immediately, and if increased ICP is suspected, treatment should be started promptly (**Fig. 15.3**).

Changes in breathing pattern may be more difficult to assess as the ventilation of the animal is controlled during anesthesia.
- Signs of Cushing's reflex can appear during recovery and the animal can manifest difficulty breathing after extubation.

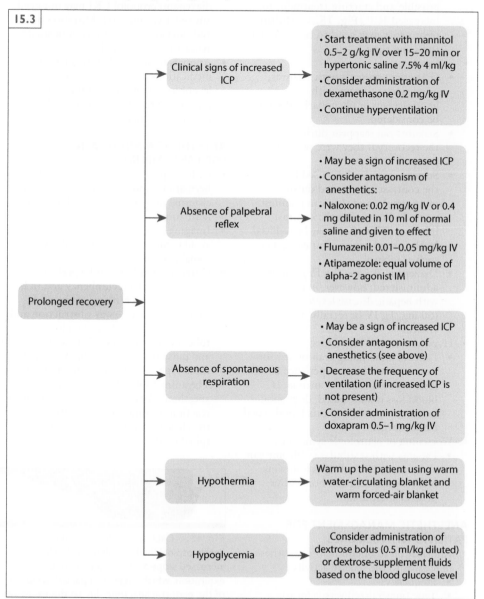

Fig. 15.3 Flow chart for management of prolonged recovery in animals with cerebral space-occupying lesions or head trauma. ICP, intracranial pressure.

- Prolonged recovery:
  - If a space-occupying lesion or head trauma is present, extubation can be delayed as much as 30–60 minutes from the end of the inhalant anesthetic. Recommendations to speed up the recovery include reversal of anesthetic drugs whenever possible and starting treatment for increased ICP (**Fig. 15.3**). Multiple treatments may need to be started at the same time.
- Seizures:
  - If a patient presents with seizures, prophylactic therapy with levetiracetam or phenobarbital should be considered.
  - Seizures can reappear during the recovery if they were present preoperatively.
  - Seizures can also be caused by the contrast agents used during myelography and they can manifest up to 24 hours after the contrast injection. This effect may be reduced by the use of newer contrast agents such as iohexol.
  - Diazepam (0.5 mg/kg IV) can be administered; however, in patients with hepatic disease levetiracetam (60 mg/kg IV or rectally) is a better choice.
- Hypotension and blood loss:
  - Patients undergoing craniotomy for tumor removal may experience blood loss, hypotension, and anemia. If blood loss is anticipated, dogs should be cross matched and cats blood typed before surgery.
- Worsening of neurologic symptoms:
  - Patients with vestibular syndrome can show worse clinical signs following recovery up to 24–48 hours after general anesthesia.

ANESTHETIC MANAGEMENT FOR PATIENTS WITH SEIZURES

- Information to obtain before anesthesia in regards to the seizure activity:
  - Frequency.
  - Type (generalized versus focal).
  - Chronological progression.
  - Treatment with anticonvulsants (if any).
  - Previous diagnostic imaging findings (if any).
- Anesthetic and pharmacologic considerations are similar to patients with a brain tumor or head trauma discussed above.
- Patients presented in status epilepticus on diazepam/propofol CRI may not need any sedative and careful titration of IV and inhalant agents is recommended to avoid anesthetic overdose.
- Animals treated with anticonvulsant medications (e.g. phenobarbital, levetiracetam, potassium bromide) should receive their regular dose until the perioperative period.

ANESTHETIC MANAGEMENT FOR CSF SAMPLING

- CSF sampling is contraindicated if herniation is present. Both lumbar and cisternal sampling carries risk of brain herniation.
- Imaging is suggested prior to sampling to avoid complications from kinking of the spinal column.
- Cisternal sampling can be performed in lateral or sternal recumbency and in both cases it requires kinking of the neck, which can cause airway obstruction and hypoxemia if a reinforced endotracheal tube is not used (**Fig. 15.1**). Capnography and pulse oximetry can quickly detect these types of complications (**Fig. 15.4**).
- The animal should be at an adequate anesthetic depth to avoid any movement/reactions leading to complications due to the close proximity of the needle to the spinal cord.

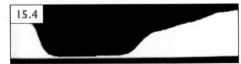

Fig. 15.4 Capnogram during cisternal cerebrospinal fluid sampling. Note the increased slope at the beginning of the expiration, which suggests a partial occlusion of the endotracheal tube due to the excessive kinking of the neck.

EXAMPLES OF ANESTHETIC PROTOCOLS FOR DOGS AND CATS

- Premedication:
  - Butorphanol (0.1–0.2 mg/kg IM/IV).
  - Midazolam/diazepam (0.1–0.2 mg/kg IM/IV) (care with hepatic disease).
  - Fentanyl (2–5 µg/kg IV followed by CRI [2–10 µg/kg/h]) or methadone (0.1–0.2 mg/kg IV/IM) for painful procedures.
- Induction:
  - Propofol (1–6 mg/kg IV).
  - Alfaxalone (0.5–3 mg/kg IV).
  - Propofol or alfaxalone with a benzodiazepine.
- Maintenance:
  - Isoflurane.
- Sevoflurane.
- Propofol CRI (0.1–0.5 mg/kg/min) (not recommended for cats due to prolonged recovery) or alfaxalone CRI (0.06–0.1 mg/kg/min).
- Adjunctive therapies:
  - Dexmedetomidine (0.5–1 µg/kg IV with/without CRI [0.5–1 µg/kg/h]) can be used for premedication or in the postoperative period to provide sedation and analgesia.
  - Low-dose acepromazine (0.005–0.01 mg/kg IV) can be used in the postoperative period in animals that shows circling, vocalization, and confusion.

Spinal and vertebral diseases

ANESTHETIC MANAGEMENT FOR THORACOLUMBAR AND CERVICAL SPINAL DISEASE

- Pain:
  - Multimodal approach should be used.
  - A combination of opioids and lidocaine or/and ketamine CRI is suggested; ketamine and lidocaine provide neuroprotection and allow reduction of the inhalants requirements.
  - NSAIDs can be used if corticosteroids have not been administered.
  - Preservative-free morphine (0.1 mg/kg) can be applied directly onto the spinal cord before surgical closure in thoracolumbar surgery. Alternatively, collagen devices can be soaked into the analgesic and left on the spinal cord.
  - Lidocaine patch 5% can be applied around the surgical incision to decrease postoperative local hyperalgesia.
  - Gabapentin can be given pre- and postsurgically.
  - Muscle relaxants such as diazepam or methacarbamol can be considered.
- Positioning:
  - Thoracolumbar surgery: sandbags/inflatable cushions used for proper positioning and excessive pressure from the surgeon on the chest can decrease the thoracic compliance and induce hypoventilation.
  - Cervical surgery: requires excessive extension of the neck and attention needs to be paid to position the head at the same level of the body (**Fig. 15.5**).

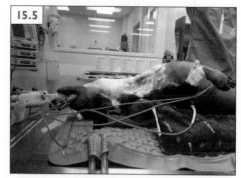

Fig. 15.5 A Dachshund in the anesthetic induction room being surgically prepared for a cervical ventral slot. Note the marked extension of the neck and the multiple lines on the fluid pump as well as the syringe pump to administer different analgesics during the procedure.

- Capnography is a useful tool to detect the need for assisted ventilation, which should be started when $ETCO_2$ is 45–50 mmHg.
- Monitoring:
  - Standard anesthetic monitoring is recommended. Invasive blood pressure monitoring is preferred whenever possible with cervical procedures due to the higher risk of hemorrhage.
- Complications:
  - Blood loss due to accidental laceration of the venous sinuses. Changes in arterial blood pressure, heart rate, mucous membranes color, and hematocrit/total solid value should be closely monitored.
  - Bradycardia caused by parasympathetic stimulation following retraction of the vagal trunk during cervical surgery.
  - Alteration of the breathing pattern due to retraction of the trachea during cervical surgery. Use of a reinforced endotracheal tube is recommended.
  - Bradycardia has been reported in Dachshunds during spinal imaging; anecdotally, hypertension has also been noted during thoracolumbar imaging/surgery in this breed. It is important to prevent hypothermia and opioids should be titrated in order not to aggravate the bradycardia.
  - Regurgitation is reported with higher incidence in patients with cervical disease. The esophagus should be suctioned and a flush with bicarbonate should be considered.

ANESTHETIC MANAGEMENT FOR PATIENTS WITH ATLANTOAXIAL INSTABILITY

- Atlantoaxial instability can impair respiratory function.
- Careful handling of the neck is required, especially after induction and during intubation, when normal muscle tone is lost during general anesthesia.
- Struggling to place an IV catheter or when providing preoxygenation should be avoided.
- During intubation the neck should be supported and kept parallel to the ground.
- Benzodiazepines should be avoided as they can cause excessive muscle relaxation.

EXAMPLES OF ANESTHETIC PROTOCOLS FOR DOGS AND CATS

- Premedication:
  - Acepromazine (0.01–0.02 mg/kg IV/IM)
  - Opioids:
    - Butorphanol (0.1–0.2 mg/kg IV/IM).
    - Hydromorphone (0.05–0.1 mg/kg IV/IM).
    - Fentanyl (2–5 µg/kg IV).
    - Methadone(0.2–0.4mg/kgIV/IM).
- Induction:
  - Propofol or alfaxalone.
- Maintenance:
  - Isoflurane or sevoflurane.
- Other considerations:
  - Dexmedetomidine CRI can be used as part of a multimodal approach to pain with opioid/lidocaine/ketamine CRI.
  - Avoid hydromorphone when vomiting is not desirable.

Neuromuscular diseases

GENERAL CONSIDERATIONS

- The presence of megaesophagus and dysphagia predispose these animals to increased risk of aspiration of gastric contents.
- Respiratory muscle weakness can lead to hypoxemia and hypoventilation.
- The thermoregulation ability may be impaired and predisposes to hypothermia/hyperthermia.

ANESTHETIC MANAGEMENT AND PHARMACOLOGIC CONSIDERATIONS

- Benzodiazepines and alpha-2 agonists may worsen the muscle weakness and should be avoided or used with caution. Agents causing vomiting and nausea (hydromorphone, morphine) should be avoided.
- The use of antiemetics and prokinetic agents (maropitant, metoclopramide) should be considered in the perioperative period.

- The goal at induction is to obtain rapid control of the airway. Use of induction agents that have a quick onset and provide good muscle relaxation, such as propofol or alfaxalone, is recommended. The animal should be intubated in sternal recumbency, keeping the head elevated until the endotracheal tube cuff has been inflated.
- Ventilation should be assisted manually or mechanically and the efficacy of gas exchanges should be assessed using pulse oximetry, blood gas analysis, and capnography.
- Suction should be available at induction and recovery. If megaesophagus is present, the esophagus and stomach should be suctioned after induction.

- Patients with laryngeal paralysis should be kept in a quiet environment to avoid any respiratory distress and a low dose of acepromazine can be given to decrease anxiety.
- Extubation should be delayed until the animal is able to protect its airways.
- Patients affected by myasthenia gravis treated with anticholinesterases should receive their regular dose on the day of the anesthesia unless the use of a neuromuscular blocker is anticipated.

EXAMPLES OF ANESTHETIC PROTOCOLS FOR DOGS AND CATS

See under Brain diseases, Examples of anesthetic protocols for dogs and cats, above.

Further reading

Armitage-Chan EA, Wetmore LA, Chan DL (2006) Anesthetic management of the head trauma patient. *J Vet Emerg Crit Care* **17**:5–14.

Ko J (2013) *Small Animal Anesthesia and Pain Management*, 1st edn. Manson Publishing, London.

Leece E (2015) Neurological disease. In: *BSAVA Manual of Canine and Feline Anaesthesia and Analgesia*, 3rd edn. (eds T Duke-Novakovski, M de Vries, C Seymour). British Small Animal Veterinary Association, Gloucester, pp. 392–408.

Otto KA (2015) Physiology, pathophysiology, and anesthetic management of patients with neurologic disease. In: *Veterinary Anesthesia and Analgesia: The 5th Edition of Lumb & Jones*. (eds KA Grimm, LA Lamont, WJ Tranquilli, SA Greene, SA) Wiley Blackwell, Ames, pp. 559–83.

Wendt-Hornickle E (2015) Neurologic disease. In: *Canine and Feline Anesthesia and Co-existing Disease*, 1st edn. (eds LBC Snyder LBC, R Johnson) Wiley Blackwell, Ames, pp. 71–81.

Anesthetic considerations for ophthalmic surgeries

Tokiko Kushiro-Banker

Overview

Commonly performed ophthalmic procedures in dogs and cats include:

- For corneal disease: keratectomy, conjunctival graft, parotid duct transposition.
- For cataract: phacoemulcification, intracapsular cataract extraction.
- For cherry eye: pocket technique.
- For eyelid disease: entropion correction.
- For glaucoma: cyclophotocoagulation, intravitreal injection.
- For retinal disease: trans-scleral retinopexy.
- For multiple conditions: evisceration and prosthesis, enucleation.

The anesthetic effects on intraocular pressure (IOP) and tear production are important concerns in many cases. Intraocular procedures are unique, often requiring the use of neuromuscular agents for globe positioning as well as consideration of pupil size. Cataract patients are often diabetic and careful perioperative planning and close monitoring are critical.

General considerations

- The cornea possesses a substantial amount of sensory innervation. A pain management plan is particularly important for corneal surgeries.
- Some drugs may cause miosis or mydriasis. These properties should be considered for intraocular surgeries and glaucoma patients.
  - Atropine: marked mydriasis (glycopyrrolate has no effects on pupil size).

- Opioids: the effects vary depending on species and individuals. In general, miosis and mydriasis are commonly seen in dogs and cats, respectively. The degree of miosis/mydriasis is more prominent with mu receptor opioid agonists than with kappa opioid agonists.
- Ketamine: mydriasis is often seen in cats. In dogs, a slight increase in pupil diameter may be observed for a short period.
- Careful handling of patients is important as some may have fragile ophthalmic tissues or protruded globes, especially in brachycephalic patients. Additional attention should be paid when applying a mask for preoxygenation.
- Eye signs (e.g. palpebral reflex, blinking, globe position) and jaw tone are often unavailable for assessment of anesthesia depth. Anal tone is a useful alternative method in addition to physiologic values (e.g. heart rate, blood pressure, respiratory rate and patterns.)

Sedation protocols for ophthalmic examinations and/or minor procedures

- Sedation may be required to perform an ophthalmic examination in uncooperative patients or ones with severe pain. Also, some minor procedures (e.g. tarsorrhaphy, intravitreal injection) may be completed under sedation rather than general anesthesia. However, one should be aware that sedation often cause third eyelid elevation and medioventral rotation of the globe.

SEDATION PROTOCOL EXAMPLES
(Refer to Chapters 3 and 9 for additional information.)

- Dexmedetomidine (5–7 µg/kg) IM + butorphanol (0.2–0.4 mg/kg) IM, or hydromorphone (0.05–0.1 mg/kg) IM or methadone (0.2–0.4 mg/kg) IM (dogs and cats):
  - Possible proemetic effect due to dexmedetomidine and hydromorphone:
    - Avoid if increase in IOP must be prevented OR
    - Administer maropitant (1 mg/kg SC) 1 hour prior to sedation.
  - Butorphanol for minor pain, hydromorphone or methadone for moderate to severe pain.
  - Good for agitated animals, patients in pain, or minor procedures.
  - Add 0.5–1.0 mg/kg IM (dogs) or 3–7 mg/kg IM (cats) of ketamine for fractious animals.
  - Dexmedetomidine can be antagonized with atipamezole IM.
- Acepromazine (0.01–0.03 mg/kg) + butorphanol (0.2–0.4 mg/kg), hydromorphone (0.05–0.1 mg/kg) or methadone (0.2–0.4 mg/kg) IM (dogs):
  - Possible proemetic effect with hydromorphone; maropitant (1 mg/kg SC) 1 hour prior to sedation can prevent vomiting.
  - Sedation may last for several hours.
- Butorphanol (0.2–0.4 mg/kg) or hydromorphone (0.05–0.1 mg/kg) IV or IM, then propofol (2–3 mg/kg to effect slow IV) (dogs, cats):
  - Good for animals with cardiac/hepatic/renal diseases.
  - Short duration (5–15 minutes); propofol (1 mg/kg IV) will give an additional 3–5 minutes for each injection.
  - Provide oxygen, prepare for intubation just in case of severe respiratory depression.
- Alfaxalone (2–4 mg/kg) + butorphanol (0.2–0.4 mg/kg), hydromorphone (0.05–0.1 mg/kg) or methadone (0.2–0.4 mg/kg) IM (cats):
  - Good for agitated cats with cardiac/hepatic/renal diseases.
  - Recovery may be rough in some patients (e.g. transient opisthotonos, paddling).
  - Moderate duration: 30–60 minutes.

SEDATIVES AND ELECTRORETINOGRAPHY
- Alpha-2 adrenoceptor agonists (e.g. dexmedetomidine) affect electroretinography (ERG) responses, but have been accepted for clinical use.
- Inhalant anesthetics significantly decrease ERG responses.
- Ketamine may affect the ERG minimally.

Intraocular pressure

- In patients with deep corneal ulcers, glaucoma, trauma, or any concerns of possibly increased IOP, care must be taken to prevent increasing IOP to avoid worsening the condition (e.g. rupture of the globe). The common factors of increasing IOP are listed below.
  - Pressure on the globe.
  - Coughing.
  - Vomiting.
  - Excitation.
  - Intubation.
  - Trendelenburg (head-down) position.
  - Increase in central venous pressure (e.g. holding jugular vein off).
  - Hypercapnea.

- Ketamine.
- Etomidate (if myoclonus occurs).
- Avoiding certain medications with proemetic property (e.g. dexmedetomidine, hydromorphone) or possible excitatory effect (e.g. benzodiazepines) and refraining from intubating lightly anesthetized animals are important in such patients. Emesis/vomiting due to opioids can be prevented by maropitant (1 mg/kg SC) 1 hour prior to opioid injection.
- Recovery should be quiet and smooth without excitation. Analgesics and/ or sedatives may be given if indicated. Cataract surgery patients should be treated similarly, as postoperative glaucoma is not uncommon.

Tear production

- Sedation and general anesthesia can decrease tear production significantly and this may persist for up to 24 hours post anesthesia, especially in patients who have received longer than 2 hours anesthesia.

Ophthalmic lubricant should be applied on the unaffected eye to prevent any corneal damage during the perianesthesia period (do not apply lubricant on the surgical eye).

Airway management

- Ophthalmic procedures often require patients to be in a dorsal position with their neck flexed. Use of a regular endotracheal tube may cause airway obstruction due to kinking. A spiral embedded (reinforced, guarded, spiral) tube should be used to prevent this occurring (**Fig. 16.1**; see also Chapter 1).

OCULOCARDIAC REFLEX
- Although its incidence is very low, traction of extraocular muscles or pressure on the globe can evoke oculocardiac reflex. Bradycardia is the most common symptom, but sinus arrest or ventricular fibrillation can be caused in very severe cases. In such cases, any stimulation to the globe or surrounding tissues should be stopped immediately and antimuscarinic agent (atropine or glycopyrrolate) given if indicated (only atropine should be used for emergency conditions).

PAIN MANAGEMENT
- The sensory systems for the eyes are extensively developed and many ophthalmic procedures cause severe pain,

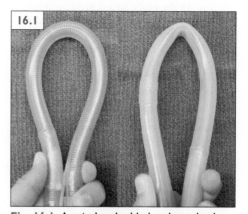

Fig. 16.1 A spiral embedded endotracheal tube (left) and a regular silicone endotracheal tube (right). A spiral embedded tube does not cause kinking even when flexed significantly.

thus appropriate analgesia should be applied:
- Retrobulbar block (see Chapter 23). Most useful regional anesthesia technique in small animals:
  - Loss of sensation to the entire globe and ocular muscle (cause central positioning of the globe).
  - For enucleation.
- Topical anesthesia. 0.5% proparacaine, quick onset (<15 seconds) and short duration (5–10 minutes).
- Infiltration block of eyelids: bupivacaine.
- Perineural injection/splash block for enucleation: bupivacaine.
- Systemic analgesia:
  - Opioid: intermittent administration or fentanyl infusion.
    - Possible miosis/mydriasis.
    - Possible proemetic property: morphine, hydromorphone. Methadone is unlikely to cause vomit, whereas oxymorphone/ hydromorphone is more likely to do so. Administration of maropitant (1 mg/kg SC) 1 hour before opioid administration can prevent vomit/emesis.
    - Lidocaine infusion (25–50 µg/ kg/min).
    - Ketamine infusion (10 µg/ kg/min) (in cases without IOP concerns).
- An auriculopalpebral nerve block provides only akinesia (loss of motor function) on the upper eyelid; no analgesia is produced.

Globe position

- Many intraocular surgeries and corneal surgeries require the eye globe to be in the central position. As general anesthesia causes medioventral rotation of the eye, especially in dogs, a neuromuscular blocking agent (NMBA) is used for central positioning of the eye. Commonly used NMBAs and reversal agents (acetylcholinesterase inhibitors) are summarized in *Table 16.1* (see also Chapter 6). Although a retrobulbar block can fix the globe to a central position, this method should not be used except for enucleation, due to several possible adverse effects (e.g. increase in IOP, hemorrhage; see Chapter 23).
- The initial dose is administered shortly before the beginning of surgery.
- One-half of the initial dose may be used as repetitive doses.
- Neuromuscular function should be monitored by using a nerve stimulator to determine the necessity of a repetitive dose and a reversal agent (see Chapter 6).
- Use of a NMBA must be followed by appropriate ventilatory care as respiratory muscles become paralyzed as well as ocular muscles.
- NMBAs do not provide any analgesic effects. Skeletal muscle paralysis makes anesthesia depth assessment difficult. Careful monitoring of physiologic data (e.g. heart rate, blood pressure) and appropriate pain management must be performed to avoid a patient suffering.
- A reversal agent should be administered if the train-of-four (TOF) ratio is <0.7 or the patient is unable to breath spontaneously with an adequate tidal volume.
- Common reversal agents are edrophonium (0.5 mg/kg IV) and neostigmine (0.04 mg/kg IV); atropine (0.01–0.02 mg/kg IV) must be administered 5 minutes prior to neostigmine.

Table 16.1 Commonly used neuromuscular blocking agents (NMBAs) in dogs and cats

NMBA	IV dose (mg/kg)	Onset (min)	Duration (min)	CRI rate (µg/kg/min)
Atracurium	0.2	3–5	20–30	3–8
Vecuronium	0.1	4–8	25	1–1.7
Rocuronium	0.4	1–2	30–40	3.3
Pancuronium	0.06	2–3	40–110	–

DIABETIC PATIENTS

- Many patients with cataract have diabetes mellitus as a coexisting disease, either regulated or recently diagnosed. If possible, only well-regulated patients should be anesthetized. These patients require well-planned preparations and close monitoring. Ketoacidotic patients must be stabilized prior to anesthesia.
- Recent full blood works (see Chapter 2) should be available to assess the patient's status, especially electrolyte balance and hydration status.
- Insulin (*Table 16.2*; see also Chapter 10) should be continued as usual until the night before.
- Fasting period should be similar to a non-diabetic patients. However, it is recommended to check the patient overnight. In unregulated patients, periodic blood glucose (BG) monitoring should be performed and a dextrose-containing IV fluid or corn syrup (e.g. Karo Syrup®) PO administered as needed.
- Surgery should be scheduled as the first case in the morning to avoid hypoglycemia due to delayed resumption of normal feeding (see Chapter 10).
- On the morning of surgery (at least a couple of hours prior to anesthesia induction), BG should be remeasured.

If BG is >8.33 mmol/l (150 mg/dl), an intermediate-acting insulin (takes about 2 hours to reduce blood glucose; see also Chapter 10) at half the patient's usual morning dose should be administered. (The timing of this administration should be at least a couple of hours prior to anesthetic induction. See Chapter 10.) If BG is <8.33 mmol/l (150 mg/dl), the morning dose of insulin may be skipped and dextrose-containing fluid may be given IV as needed.

- BG should be checked at the time of induction and repeated every 30 minutes (every 60 minutes if very stable).
- During anesthesia, the range of BG may be maintained between 8.33 and 13.9 mmol/l (150 and 250 mg/dl.) If BG is >13.9–16.6 mmol/l (250–300 mg/dl) during anesthesia, rapid-acting insulin should be given IV or IM. Thirty to 50% of the patient's usual dose is typically a good starting dose. Otherwise, 0.1 unit/kg could be administered.
- Rapid-acting insulin may be infused at the rate of 0.038 unit/kg/hour if preferred. The rate should be adjusted depending on BG level.
- If BG become <5.5–6.9 mmol/l (100–125 mg/dl), dextrose should be added in fluid (1–5%) as needed.

Table 16.2 Classification of insulin preparations commonly used in veterinary medicine

Insulin preparation	Species	Route	Onset (hours)	Peak (hours)	Duration (hours)	Product name/s
Short-acting (or regular)	Dogs, Cats	IV	Immediate	0.5–2	1–4	Humulin-R®, Novolin-R®
		IM	0.5	1–4	3–8	
		SC	0.5	1–4	4–10	
Intermediate-acting						
NPH (isophane), lente	Dogs	SC	0.5–2	2–10	4–24	Humulin-N®, Novolin-N®
	Cats	SC	0.5–2	2–8	4–12	
Porcine insulin zinc	Dogs	SC	0.5–2	1–10	10–24	Vetsulin®
	Cats	SC	0.5–2	2–6	8–24	
Long-acting						
PZI	Dogs	SC	0.5–8	4–14	6–28	Prozinc®
	Cats	SC	0.5–8	5–7	6–28	
Glargine		SC	4–18	None	>24	Lantus®

NPH, neutral protamine hagedorn; PZI, protamine zinc insulin.

- BG should also be measured during recovery. Hypoglycemia prolongs anesthesia recovery. Once the patient recovers fully from anesthesia, its normal feeding/insulin regimen should be resumed.

Commonly used ophthalmic drugs and possible systemic adverse effects

- Carbonic anhydrase inhibitor (e.g. acetazolamide): metabolic acidosis, hypovolemia/dehydration.
- Parasympathomimetic (muscarinic) (e.g. pilocarpine): bradycardia, hypotension, bronchospasm.
- Non-selective beta-blockers (e.g. timolol): bradycardia, bronchoconstriction, hypotension.
- Osmotic diuretics (e.g. mannitol): initial increase in cardiac preload, hypovolemia/dehydration, hypokalemic hypochloremic alkalosis.
- Phenylephrine: hypertension (vasoconstriction) with bradycardia (baroreceptor reflex).
- Epinephrine: tachycardia, ventricular dysrhythmias, hypertension.

EXAMPLES OF ANESTHETIC PROTOCOLS FOR DOGS FOR NON-INTRAOCULAR PROCEDURES

- Premedication:
  - Maropitant (1 mg/kg SC) 1 hour prior to the rest of the premedications (not necessary if methadone is used as an opioid, rather than hydromorphone or oxymorphone).
  - Acepromazine (0.01–0.03 mg/kg) or dexmetomidine (3–7 µg/kg) IM.
  - Opioid:
    - Hydromorphone or oxymorphone (0.05–0.1 mg/kg IM).
    - Methadone (0.2–0.4 mg/kg IM).
- Induction:
  - Propofol (4–6 mg/kg to effect IV).
  - Alfaxalone (2–3 mg/kg to effect IV).
- Maintenance:
  - Isoflurane or sevoflurane.
  - Propofol (0.1–0.5 mg/kg/min IV).
- Pain management:

- Opioid:
  - Intermittent injection of:
    - Hydromorphone or oxymorphone (0.05 mg/kg IV q1–2 h).
    - Methadone (0.1–0.2 mg/kg IV q1–2 h).
    - Fentanyl (1–5 µg/kg IV q20–30 min).
  - Fentanyl (0.1–0.7 µg/kg/min IV).
- Lidocaine (25–50 µg/kg/min IV).

EXAMPLES OF ANESTHETIC PROTOCOLS FOR DIABETIC DOGS FOR INTRAOCULAR SURGERIES

- Premedication:
  - Acepromazine (0.01–0.03 mg/kg or dexmetomidine 3–7 µg/kg IM.
  - Opioid:
    - Buprenorphine (0.01–0.02 mg/kg IM).
- Induction:
  - Propofol (4–6 mg/kg to effect IV).
  - Alfaxalone (2–3 mg/kg to effect IV).
- Maintenance:
  - Isoflurane or sevoflurane.
  - Propofol (0.1–0.5 mg/kg/min IV).
- Pain management:
  - Buprenorphine (0.005–0.01 mg/kg IV).
  - Lidocaine (25–50 µg/kg/min IV).

EXAMPLES OF ANESTHETIC PROTOCOLS FOR CATS FOR OPHTHALMIC PROCEDURES

- Dexmedetomidine may be preferred to acepromazine in most cases as the latter provides only mild sedation in cats.
- Alfaxalone dose in cats is 2–5 mg/kg to effect IV.
- Otherwise similar to dogs.

Further reading

Gross ME, Pablo LS (2015) Ophthalmic patients. In: *Veterinary Anesthesia and Analgesia: The 5th Edition of Lumb & Jones.* (eds KA Grimm, LA Lamont, WJ Tranquilli, SA Greene, SA) Wiley Blackwell, Ames, pp. 963–82.

Lerch P (2015) Ophthalmic disease. In: *Canine and Feline Anesthesia and Co-Existing Disease.* (eds LBC Snyder, RA Johnson) Wiley Blackwell, Ames, pp. 179–86.

Nanji KC, Roberto SA, Morley MG *et al.* (2018) Preventing adverse events in cataract surgery: Recommendations from a Massachusetts Expert Panel. *Anesth Analg* **126(5)**:1537.

Thompson S (2007) Ophthalmic surgery. In: *BSAVA Manual of Canine and Feline Anaesthesia and Analgesia*, 2nd edn. (eds C Seymour, T Duke-Novakovski) British Small Animal Veterinary Association, Gloucester, pp. 183–93.

CHAPTER 17

Anesthesia and sedation for radiography, ultrasound, CT, and MRI patients

Jeff C Ko

Introduction

There is an increasing need for using various modes of diagnostic imaging to obtain further detailed images in dogs and cats. The most commonly used of these diagnostic imaging modes are radiography, ultrasound, computed axial tomography (CT), and magnetic resonance imaging (MRI). Some of these diagnostic imaging modes require absolute immobilization for the patient to remain still for a long period of time (MRI, ultrasound-guided biopsy, and possibly some of the slow CT), while others only need a short duration of immobilization (radiography, 64-slice and higher slice CT). For ultrasound, most of the imaging can tolerate slight movements of these patients without sacrificing a lot of detail and quality of the images. In addition to these motion-still demands, each patient has a unique disease state that needs to be considered when selecting a sedative or anesthetic protocol. This chapter describes sedative and anesthetic protocols for using with each of these diagnostic imaging modes.

Clinical considerations for selecting sedation or general anesthesia for radiographic-related procedures

- Several criteria related to the patient's age and concurrent diseases can be used to determine whether the patient should undergo sedation or general anesthesia for radiography, ultrasound, or CT.
- Aged patients with cardiac, liver, or kidney dysfunctions likely will not tolerate well the use of high doses of heavy sedation or repeated injectable drugs to maintain a long duration of sedation.
- Patients with a compromised airway (e.g. profound signs of the brachycephalic syndrome) would be more suitable for

general anesthesia with a secured patent airway (endotracheal intubation) to provide assisted or controlled ventilation with 100% oxygen using inhalant anesthetics.

- The same goes for patients with severe obesity (due to compromisation of the ability to breathe) and patients with abdominal or thoracic space-occupying lesions, including patients with ascites, diaphragmatic hernia, pleural effusion, and pneumothorax. These patients may have distinct clinical signs of respiratory difficulty, including increased respiratory rates, flared nostrils, restrictive breathing pattern with a short and shallow breath, abdominal labored breathing pattern, dyspnea, and refusal to lie down. Using general anesthesia will likely assist or control the breathing in these patients.

- Patients with skeletal muscle compromise, including thoracic wall injury or intracranial trauma, neuropathies, or high risk of gastrointestinal regurgitations, should be subjected to general anesthesia instead of using heavy sedation. These patients are better managed with endotracheal intubation for airway security with access to provide immediate assisted or control ventilation.

- If imaging requires the use of controlled ventilation to minimize cranial abdomen and lung motion artifact or the use of positive end-expiratory pressure to minimize lung atelectasis, then general anesthesia is preferred to sedation.

- Other than the above situations, calmed patients will tolerate well with just gentle physical restraint and mild sedation. Nervous animals require chemical restraint with either moderate or heavy sedation to complete the radiographic diagnostic procedures.

CASES SUITABLE FOR RADIOGRAPHY, ULTRASOUND, AND CT PROCEDURES USING SEDATION

- Radiography, ultrasound, and CT cases suitable for sedation are described as follows:
  - Healthy dogs and cats may be subjected to radiographic procedures to evaluate their skeletal muscular configurations under sedation.

- Ultrasound procedures with or without needle biopsy can be performed under reasonable sedation instead of using general anesthesia.

- A lot of institutes are using 64-slice CT scanners that are capable of complete radiographic images from snout to tail of a dog within minutes. Some research institutions have even more advanced scanners that are 256, 320, or 640 slices. The 320-slice CT scanner covers 16 cm of imaging area in one rotation. The newest 640-slice scanner provides adult human whole body images from head to toe in 1 minute. With the new and powerful CT scanners having such a stunning speed, using sedation seems to offer significant advantages over anesthetizing every animal with traditional general anesthesia. More and more teaching institutions and private practices are using sedation to achieve these diagnostic purposes.

SAFETY KEYS TO CONSIDER WHEN USING SEDATION FOR RADIOGRAPHY, ULTRASOUND, CT, AND MRI PROCEDURES

- Important safety keys to remember when sedating patients for these procedures include:
  - The animal should have an IV catheter in place. Should sedation fail, the catheter will offer a rapid way to provide additional sedative or convert the sedation into general anesthesia.
  - 100% oxygen should be delivered whenever possible via face mask or through insufflation during the sedation (**Fig. 17.1**).
  - Sedated animals should be monitored for vital signs to ensure their safety, and action taken if abnormalities occur. Pulse rate, respiratory rate, hemoglobin oxygen saturation, body temperature, and blood pressure (if possible) should be monitored as with general anesthesia and recorded accordingly.

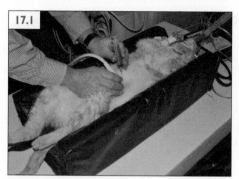

Fig. 17.1 A cat is sedated with an intramuscular injection of midazolam (0.4 mg/kg), alfaxalone (2 mg/kg), and butorphanol (0.2 mg/kg) for ultrasound-guided liver biopsy. Note that 100% oxygen is provided via a face mask for insufflation and a Doppler is used to monitor the blood pressure and pulse rate of the cat.

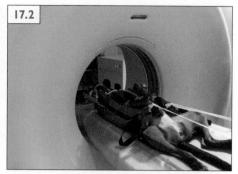

Fig. 17.2 A dog was sedated with midazolam (0.2 mg/kg)–dexmedetomidine (3 μg/kg)–butorphanol (0.2 mg/kg), and alfaxalone (1 mg/kg) IM for CT of the head and thorax. An IV catheter was placed and anesthesia maintained with alfaxalone intermittent boluses.

- Owners should be informed that there is a possibility that the sedation may be converted to a general anesthesia if considered necessary.
- An endotracheal tube and laryngoscope with a blade should always be ready to provide an airway; also access to an Ambu bag or breathing circuit to ventilate with enriched oxygen.

SEDATIVE PROTOCOLS FOR RADIOGRAPHY, ULTRASOUND, CT, AND MRI PROCEDURES
(See *Table 17.1*)
- The sedatives can be administered either IV, IM (or SC), or a combination of both routes, pending on the animal's temperament and health status. IV administration requires an IV catheter (ideally) so that repeated injection can be easily achieved. When using IV injection of some sedatives (e.g. alpha-2 agonists), caution should be taken since they impact significantly on the cardiovascular system immediately compared with IM or SC.
- Sedation may be induced with an IM injection to start with (**Fig. 17.2**). When the animal is sedated, an IV catheter can be easily placed and maintenance of sedation/anesthesia sustained with intermittent boluses of alfaxalone

(0.25–1 mg/kg) or propofol (0.5–1 mg/kg). Repeated IV bolus injections can be used for maintenance of sedation for up to 1–2 hours using alfaxalone or propofol. These short-acting IV agents are quickly metabolized and recovery is usually smooth and rapid.
- It is important to monitor respiratory function and oxygenation when using intermittent boluses of IV anesthetic agents, because they can induce general anesthesia if higher doses are administered. As a result, apnea and profound respiratory depression can occur. Endotracheal intubation and a means of providing ventilation should be readily available when using this method of sedation.
- For overall healthy dogs and cats, medetomidine/dexmedetomidine together with an opioid (butorphanol, morphine, hydromorphone, methadone, or pethidine) can be used. These drugs may be administered IV or IM (*Table 17.1*).
- IM use of alfaxalone provides a significant advantage over propofol, which does not have any effect when administered other than by the IV route (*Table 17.2*).
- The advantage of using alfaxalone with midazolam is that both sedation and

Table 17.1 Sedation protocols for radiographic, CT, and ultrasound procedures in dogs and cats

Drug combination, dose, and routes** of administration	Duration of action	Side-effects and comments
Dexmedetomidine (0.005–0.015 mg/kg) (medetomidine [0.01–0.03 mg/kg]) + an opioid* ± alfaxalone (0.5–1 mg/kg)	20–40 minutes	Use in patients without cardiovascular dysfunction
Dexmedetomidine (0.005–0.015 mg/kg) (medetomidine [0.01–0.03 mg/kg]) + opioid* + midazolam (0.2–0.4 mg/kg) or diazepam (0.2–0.4 mg/kg) ± alfaxalone (0.5–1 mg/kg)	25–50 minutes	Use in patients without cardiovascular dysfunction
Midazolam (0.4 mg/kg) or diazepam (0.4 mg/kg) + an opioid*	10–20 minutes	Sedation is less reliable, and some patients may have paradoxical excitement
Midazolam (0.4 mg/kg) or diazepam (0.4 mg/kg) + acepromazine (0.005–0.01 mg/kg) + an opioid*	20–30 minutes	Sedation is better than midazolam (or diazepam) with the opioid combination; however, hypotension likely to occur due to acepromazine
Midazolam (0.4 mg/kg) or diazepam (0.4 mg/kg) + alfaxalone (0.5–2 mg/kg) + an opioid*	15–20 minutes	Sedation is better than midazolam (or diazepam) with opioid Blood pressure is better maintained than midazolam + acepromazine + opioid Suitable for using in cardiovascular dysfunctional patients Recovery is rapid and smooth

** IV with the low dose and IM with the high dose.

* Opioids: butorphanol (0.2–0.3 mg/kg), morphine (0.15–0.25 mg/kg), hydromorphone (0.05–0.1 mg/kg), methadone (0.2–0.5 mg/kg), or pethidine (3–5 mg/kg).

muscle relaxation can be enhanced. If a painful procedure is to be introduced, lidocaine infiltration or use of an opioid should be considered. When alfaxalone is used with midazolam, medetomidine/dexmedetomidine, and butorphanol (or any other opioids), the sedation, muscle relaxation, and analgesia are all greatly enhanced (*Table 17.2*).

- Alfaxalone provides an additional advantage of being used IM in combination with midazolam and any of the opioids in dogs and cats. Alfaxalone at 1–2 mg/kg can be combined with midazolam (0.2–0.4 mg/kg) and butorphanol (0.2–0.4 mg/kg) or methadone (0.4–0.6 mg/kg) in the same syringe as a single IM injection.

Sedation quality is reasonable and cardiorespiratory function is relatively well maintained (**Fig. 17.1**). Recovery from this combination is rapid and smooth. In order to maintain proper oxygenation, enriched oxygen insufflation should be provided during the radiographic procedures via face mask or flow-by with a breathing circuit.

- In hyper, aggressive, or extremely nervous cats and dogs, a small dose of dexmedetomidine/medetomidine can be added to enhance the alfaxalone–midazolam–butorphanol (or any other opioids)-induced sedation (**Fig. 17.2**). This small amount of alpha-2 agonist usually does not compromise the cardiovascular function of the animals (*Table 17.2*).

Table 17.2 Intramuscular injection of alfaxalone in cats and dogs. Butorphanol can be replaced with any other opioid (morphine [0.25 mg/kg], methadone [0.3–0.5 mg/kg], or hydromorphone [0.1 mg/kg])

Health status	Drug combination	Dosage of drug	Degree of sedation	Onset and duration of sedation	Suitable procedures
Healthy patients	Dexmedetomidine (medetomidine) Butorphanol	5 μg/kg (10 μg/kg) 0.2 mg/kg	Mild to moderate	8–10 min 10–20 min	Ultrasound, radiography, CT
	Alfaxalone Dexmedetomidine (medetomidine)	1–2 mg/kg 5 μg/kg (10 μg/kg)	Mild to moderate	8–10 min 10–25 min	Ultrasound, radiography, CT
	Alfaxalone Dexmedetomidine (medetomidine) Butorphanol	1–2 mg/kg 10–15 μg/kg (20–30 μg/kg) 0.2–0.4 mg/kg	Moderate to profound	5–8 min 25–40 min	Ultrasound, radiography, needle biopsy, CT, MRI
	Alfaxalone Midazolam Dexmedetomidine (medetomidine) Butorphanol	1–2 mg/kg 0.2–0.4 mg/kg 10–15 μg/kg (20–30 μg/kg) 0.2–0.4 mg/kg	Moderate to profound	5–7 min 35–40 min	Ultrasound, radiography, CT, MRI, biopsy or other minor invasive procedures
Sick patients	Alfaxalone Midazolam	2 mg/kg 0.4 mg/kg	Mild	10–12 min 20 min	Ultrasound, radiography
	Alfaxalone Midazolam Dexmedetomidine (medetomidine)	2 mg/kg 0.4 mg/kg 2–3 μg/kg (4–8 μg/kg)	Moderate	8-10 min 20-30 min	Ultrasound, radiography, biopsy, CT
	Alfaxalone Midazolam Butorphanol	2 mg/kg 0.4 mg/kg 0.2–0.4 mg/kg	Moderate to profound	8–10 min 20–30 min	Ultrasound, radiography, biopsy, CT, MRI
	Alfaxalone Midazolam Butorphanol Dexmedetomidine (medetomidine)	2 mg/kg 0.4 mg/kg 0.2–0.4 mg/kg 3–5 μg/kg (6–10 μg/kg)	Moderate to profound	5–10 min 25–35 min	Ultrasound, radiography, CT, MRI, biopsy or other minor invasive procedures

Further reading

Arlachov Y, Ganatra RH (2012) Sedation/ anaesthesia in paediatric radiology. *Br J Radiol* **85(1019)**:e1018–31.

Derbent A, Oran I, Parildar M *et al.* (2005) Adverse effects of anesthesia in interventional radiology. *Diagn Interv Radiol* **11**:109–12.

Deutsch J, Jolliffe C, Archer E et al. (2017) Intramuscular injection of alfaxalone in combination with butorphanol for sedation in cats. *Vet Anaesth Analg* **44(4)**:794–802.

Khenissi L, Nikolayenkova-Topie O, Broussaud S (2017) Comparison of intramuscular alfaxalone and ketamine combined with dexmedetomidine and butorphanol for castration in cats. *J Feline Med Surg* **19(8)**:791–7.

Anesthetic considerations for orthopedic surgical patients

Bonnie L Hay Kraus

Introduction

Patients requiring surgical orthopedic procedures usually suffer from developmental or traumatic abnormities. In dogs, the common developmental orthopedic diseases requiring surgery include: osteochondritis dissecans of the shoulder, elbow and stifle, and hock; elbow dysplasia; elbow incongruity; patellar luxation; avascular necrosis of the femoral head; and hip dysplasia (femoral head/neck excision, triple pelvic osteotomy, total hip replacement). Cranial cruciate disease is the most common cause of hindlimb lameness in dogs and typically presents in middle age, although it can occur at any age. Ligament rupture is the result of degeneration from a combination of factors, including age, obesity, poor physical condition, genetics, conformation, and breed predilection. Traumatic fractures are most commonly the result of motor vehicle accidents; the most common fractures requiring surgical intervention are of the femur, pelvis, radius/ulna, tibia, and humerus. In cats, trauma is the most common reason for surgical orthopedic intervention, with 70–87% of fractures occurring in the hindlimb, most often the femur.

Preoperative evaluation

- The preanesthetic work-up should begin with a complete and thorough physical examination to identify potential health concerns. Overall health, species, breed, temperament, and body condition score are all important factors that may affect the anesthetic plan. The preanesthetic laboratory and diagnostic database depends on the status of the patient.

- Patients with developmental orthopedic surgical disease are typically young and healthy. A minimum laboratory database (see Chapter 2) for these patients should include a PCV, TP, blood glucose, and Azostix (reagent strip for blood urea nitrogen).
- Otherwise healthy patients >5–7 years of age are at a higher risk for subclinical disease (~30%) and should have a CBC and serum biochemical analysis.
- Once trauma patients are stabilized with respect to airway, breathing, circulation (see Chapter 20), and level of consciousness, a more extensive work-up is required, including: CBC, biochemical profile, serum electrolytes, urinalysis, thoracic and abdominal radiographs, and ECG. Blood gas analysis and clotting profiles may be required in critically injured patients.
- Thoracic and abdominal radiographs should be evaluated for signs of trauma including pneumothorax, lung contusions, rib fractures, diaphragmatic hernia, intracavity effusion, and urinary bladder integrity. Trauma patients may experience significant hemorrhage, especially if they have incurred a femur or pelvic fracture. It is important to recheck the PCV/TS 12–24 hours post trauma. Ideally, the PCV should be >0.2 l/l (20%) and TP >35 g/l (3.5 g/dl) prior to anesthesia/surgery. Even if the ECG is normal on presentation, the patient should be re-evaluated prior to anesthesia for the development of ventricular premature contractions 2–5 days post trauma due to traumatic myocarditis. Trauma patients should be stabilized with appropriate supportive care as much as possible prior to anesthesia and surgery.

- The Centers for Disease Control and Prevention (in the USA) provide guidelines for the prevention of surgical site infections (SSI) in humans. These include recommendations to identify and treat remote infections prior to elective surgeries and to only remove hair immediately prior to surgery. Elective veterinary orthopedic patients that have skin infection (pyoderma) should be identified and treated prior to elective surgery. However, they should not have their hair clipped the day/night before surgery to identify skin infection as it is associated with a significantly higher risk of SSI. The surgical area may be clipped under premedication if tolerated by the patient in order to identify skin infection and avoid unnecessary risk and owner expense of cancellation of the surgical procedure after anesthetic induction.

Sedation protocols for radiographic examination (*Table 18.1* and see Chapter 17)

- Sedation for radiographic examination in otherwise healthy dogs and cats may be accomplished with a combination of dexmedetomidine–butorphanol. In dogs, 5.0 μg/kg of dexmedetomidine and 0.3 mg/kg of butorphanol is mixed in the same syringe and half of the volume administered IV.
- Dogs generally become laterally recumbent within 1–2 minutes, otherwise the remainder of the dose is administered. Adequate sedation may take longer (5–10 minutes) with IM administration and the entire dose should be administered. It is important to allow adequate time for the drug combination to take effect; stimulated patients will require additional or higher doses. Patients sedated with this protocol will have a decreased heart rate (HR) and normal/high normal blood pressure; generally, the higher the dose

Table 18.1 Sedation protocols for radiographic examination

	Dexmedetomidine	Butorphanol
Dogs	2.5–5.0 μg/kg IV	0.15–0.3 mg/kg IV
	5–10 μg/kg IM	0.3 mg/kg IM
Cats	5.0–7.5 μg/kg IV	0.15–0.3 mg/kg IV
	10–15 μg/kg IM	0.3 mg/kg IM

of dexmedetomidine, the lower the HR. Most patients become mildly hypoxemic and therefore, should be monitored with a pulse oximeter and provided flow-by oxygen supplementation (50–100 ml/kg/min) via face mask. Reversal of the dexmedetomidine can be achieved at any time with the same volume of atipamezole administered IM. Partial reversal can be achieved by administering one-quarter to one-half the volume of atipamezole, or the patient may be left to fully recover on its own within 1–2 hours. Patients not receiving reversal should be monitored for hypoxemia and hypothermia and supported with oxygen and external heat supplementation as needed.
- Some feline patients may be difficult to handle or fractious, especially when painful, and a full cardiorespiratory

evaluation may not be possible. Occult forms of feline cardiac disease such as hypertrophic cardiomyopathy may not be detectable on physical examination alone. In these situations, an alternative protocol consisting of alfaxalone (2.0 mg/kg) and either butorphanol (0.2–0.3 mg/kg) or methadone (0.2 –0.5 mg/kg) IM may be considered. Lateral recumbency is achieved within 10 minutes for butorphanol but may be quicker with higher doses of methadone. Cats typically recover within ~45 minutes. This protocol has been found to have minimal effect on echocardiographic parameters in healthy cats and, although it is not reversible, it provides a smooth and fairly short recovery time and does not cause vomiting.

Anesthesia/analgesia protocols for dogs (see also Chapter 24)

- Pre-emptive and multimodal analgesia are basic tenets of good perioperative pain management. When devising an analgesic plan for surgical orthopedic patients, it is helpful to use a pre-emptive pain scale to classify both the severity and the type(s) of pain the patient may be expected to experience based on the pathophysiology of the disease and the planned surgical procedure. The pre-emptive scoring system uses a simple descriptive scale to assign a degree of pain based on the procedure performed and the amount of tissue trauma involved (i.e. no pain, mild pain, moderate pain, or severe pain). The classification of types of pain includes somatic, visceral, neuropathic, inflammatory, and acute or chronic/maladaptive pain.
- Orthopedic pain is widely accepted as moderate to severe (76%) in human patients. Somatic pain generally arises from damage to bones, joints, muscle, and skin. Orthopedic surgical pain can generally be classified as moderate to severe, acute somatic pain. However, trauma patients may also experience visceral and/or neuropathic pain from concurrent injuries and some veterinary orthopedic patients may be experiencing chronic or

maladaptive pain syndromes based on the duration of lameness. Multimodal pain management uses a variety of analgesic drugs and techniques in order to affect multiple levels of the pain pathway. Different drugs exert their effects at different steps or levels of the pain pathway (**Fig. 18.1**). This classification helps to target sites along the pain pathway and to choose drugs most effective for treating those types of pain.
- These strategies assist in pre-emptive/intraoperative/postoperative analgesia planning. The limitations are that such a plan is not tailored to the individual and is not useful in assessing response to therapy. Therefore, monitoring and regular assessment using a validated pain scoring system is needed to evaluate the effectiveness of the original analgesic plan and to allow modification according to the individual patient's needs.
- Opioids (*Table 18.2*) should form the basis of analgesic protocols for orthopedic patients and, since orthopedic pain is typically categorized as moderate to severe, a mu agonist opioid is indicated. Hydromorphone and morphine are associated with a 50–100% incidence

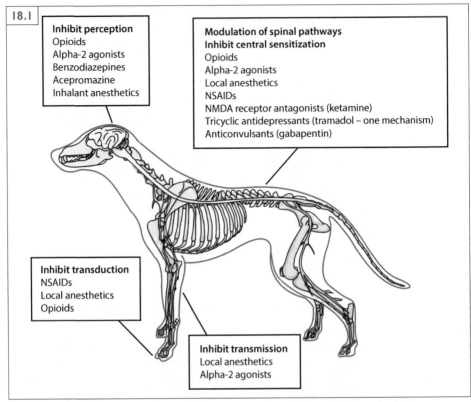

18.1

Inhibit perception
Opioids
Alpha-2 agonists
Benzodiazepines
Acepromazine
Inhalant anesthetics

Modulation of spinal pathways
Inhibit central sensitization
Opioids
Alpha-2 agonists
Local anesthetics
NSAIDs
NMDA receptor antagonists (ketamine)
Tricyclic antidepressants (tramadol – one mechanism)
Anticonvulsants (gabapentin)

Inhibit transduction
NSAIDs
Local anesthetics
Opioids

Inhibit transmission
Local anesthetics
Alpha-2 agonists

Fig. 18.1 The Pain Pathway and site(s) of action of common classes of drugs used to treat pain in veterinary patients.

Table 18.2 Opioid choices for orthopedic procedures in dogs and cats

Drug	Dose range*	Duration of action	Specific attributes
Hydromorphone	0.1–0.2 mg/kg IM, IV	2–4 hours	Causes vomiting, signs of nausea Panting, vocalization in dogs Associated with hyperthermia in cats
Morphine	0.5–1.0 mg/kg IM, IV	4–6 hours	Causes vomiting, signs of nausea Histamine release with rapid IV administration
Methadone	0.2–1.0 mg/kg IM, IV	2–4 hours	Does not cause vomiting Vocalization in dogs Mydriasis, euphoria in cats
Fentanyl	2–10 µg/kg IV	<30 minutes	Does not cause vomiting, may cause nausea Not associated with histamine release Used IV for induction/CRI

* In general, the lower end of the dose range is used for cats.

of vomiting depending on dose, route of administration, and concomitant administration of acepromazine.

- Perioperative vomiting has been associated with the development of postoperative aspiration pneumonia. Maropitant is a neurokinin-1 antagonist that prevents vomiting and signs of nausea associated with opioids when administered at a dose of 1.0 mg/kg SC at least 1 hour prior to opioid administration. It may also reduce inhalant requirements and has been shown to provide a faster return to feeding postoperatively. IV administration has recently been added to the label and allows a faster onset of action.

- Hydromorphone or morphine are administered IM, along with acepromazine or dexmedetomidine, in ASA I–I1 maropitant–pretreated orthopedic canine patients. Methadone is more expensive, but does not cause vomiting and can be used in patients not pretreated with maropitant. Fentanyl is administered IV and the short duration of action requires continued administration with a CRI.
- The choice of sedative/tranquilizer and dosing (*Table 18.3* and see Chapter 3) depends on patient history, signalment, temperament, physical status, length of procedure, and desired side-effect profile preferred by the anesthetist. Most healthy patients will benefit from acepromazine or dexmedetomidine added to an opioid analgesic to ease the stress of handling and IV catheter placement, and reduce the dose of induction and inhalant required. Dexmedetomidine is a more potent sedative, has adjunct analgesic properties, and is reversible; however, it significantly decreases cardiac output and has a short duration of action. If used as a premedication for procedures lasting longer than 1 hour, sedation with a microdose of dexmedetomidine (1.0 µg/kg IV) or

acepromazine (5.0 µg/kg IV) should be considered prior to discontinuing the inhalant to provide a smooth transition to wakefulness. Acepromazine has less effect on cardiac output than dexmedetomidine but can contribute to vasodilation and hypotension. It also lacks analgesic properties and is not reversible. It has a longer duration of action (4–6 hours depending on dose) and is likely to provide sedative effects through the recovery period. Although benzodiazepines cause minimal cardiovascular depression, they provide the least reliable sedation and are reserved for very young (<3 months), advanced geriatric, and critically ill patients.

INDUCTION

- Healthy patients may be induced with any of the currently available agents. The dose of induction agent is decreased in proportion to the level of sedation provided by the premedication protocol.
- Suggested agents/combinations include:
  - Propofol (2–4 mg/kg).
  - Alfaxalone (0.5–2.0 mg/kg).
  - Propofol (2.0 mg/kg) + ketamine (2.0 mg/kg).
  - Ketamine (5.0 mg/kg) + midazolam (0.25 mg/kg).
- Induction adjuncts may be administered to lower the dose of propofol and/or provide a loading dose for intraoperative analgesic CRI:
  - Lidocaine (2.0 mg/kg IV slowly over 2 minutes prior to induction), followed

Table 18.3 Sedative and tranquilizer choices for orthopedic procedures in dogs and cats

Drug	Dose range	Duration of action	Specific attributes
Acepromazine	0.005–0.05 mg/kg	4–6 hours	Not reversible Hypotension due to alpha-1 antagonism Provides sedation through recovery
Dexmedetomidine	2–10 µg/kg	~60–90 minutes depending on dose	Reversible Significant (40%) decrease in cardiac output Provides adjunct analgesia May need additional sedation for recovery
Midazolam	0.1–0.5 mg/kg	~2 hours	Reversible (flumazenil) Minimal cardiovascular depression May cause paradoxical excitement in healthy adult patients

by ketamine (0.5 mg/kg IV) if not included in the induction protocol.
- Midazolam (0.2–0.4 mg/kg) administered after 1.0 mg/kg of propofol has been shown to decrease the induction dose of propofol.
- The occurrence and severity of hypoventilation, apnea, and hypotension is directly related to the dose and rate of induction agent administered. Administering alfaxalone at a rate of 0.5 mg/kg/min and propofol at a rate of 1.0 mg/kg/min has been shown to reduce the induction doses of both drugs and decrease the incidence of postinduction apnea. All patients will benefit from preoxygenation with 50–100 ml/kg/ minute for 3–5 minutes prior to induction to delay the onset of hypoxemia during induction and intubation.
- Trauma or critically ill patients may be induced with fentanyl (5.0–10.0 µg/kg, slowly over ~2 minutes) followed by midazolam (0.2 mg/kg) IV. Adjunct agents such as lidocaine or ketamine may also be used in these patients to lower induction doses and provide loading doses for intraoperative CRI. These patients should be preoxygenated and monitored with pulse oximetry and ECG during induction.

INTRAOPERATIVE ANALGESIA
Choices for intraoperative analgesia include CRI or loco-regional anesthesia/analgesia (*Table 18.4*).

Intraoperative CRI
- The following drug combinations can be used: morphine–lidocaine–ketamine (MLK), hydromorphone–lidocaine– ketamine (HLK) fentanyl–lidocaine– ketamine (FLK).

- MLK should be infused at a rate of 5 ml/kg/hour for the first hour; thereafter it may be reduced to 2.5 ml/ kg/hour. These restrictive IV fluid administration rates are intended for euhydrated, stable, healthy patients. Goal-directed fluid therapy with additional crystalloid and/or colloid fluids should be tailored to patient needs according to hydration status and intraoperative considerations such as hypotension and/ or blood loss. It is recommended, but not imperative, to use an IV fluid pump for accurate infusion and to avoid inadvertent bolus administration. Hydromorphone (10 mg/ml) may be used as a substitute opioid: addition of 0.2 ml (2 mg) gives an infusion dose of 0.02 mg/kg/hour (this is a total dose of 0.05 mg/kg over 4 hours).
- MLK can greatly reduce the MAC of inhalants (up to ~48%), therefore it is imperative that anesthetic depth is monitored and the inhalant gas reduced. It is common for dogs undergoing major orthopedic surgery (e.g. tibial plateau leveling osteotomy [TPLO], tibial tuberosity advancement [TTA], triple pelvic osteotomy, fracture repair) to be maintained on a vaporizer setting of 1% isoflurane (ET_{ISO} ~0.7–0.8%). Individual patients may require additional opioids; these are patients that continue to have HR and blood pressure responses to surgical stimulation and need to be maintained on >1.5% isoflurane. These patients typically respond favorably to an intraoperative IV dose of hydromorphone 0.05 mg/kg. $ETCO_2$ monitoring is recommended to identify patients with significant respiratory depression ($ETCO_2$ >58 mmHg). Loading doses should be administered prior to CRI in order to

Table 18.4 Intraoperative constant rate infusion of morphine–lidocaine–ketamine in dogs*

Drug (concentration)	Volume to add (mg)	Infusion dose 1st hour	2nd hour and after
Morphine (10 mg/ml)	3.0 ml (30 mg)	0.3 mg/kg/hour	0.15 mg/kg/hour
Lidocaine (20 mg/ml)	15 ml (300 mg)	50 µg/kg/minute (3 mg/kg/hour)	25 µg/kg/minute (1.5 mg/kg/hour)
Ketamine (100 mg/ml)	1.2 ml (120 mg)	20 µg/kg/minute (1.2 mg/kg/hour)	10 µg/kg/minute (0.6 mg/kg/hour)

* Morphine, Lidocaine, Ketamine (MLK) Constant Rate Infusion (CRI) – Iowa State University College of Veterinary Medicine. Modification of original recipe by Dr. W. Muir. Add to 500 ml bag of crystalloid fluids.

more quickly achieve adequate plasma levels (see above).

- Fentanyl may also be substituted as the opioid in the multimodal analgesic CRI when the desire is to have more control/titration of the opioid dosage and retain the multimodal, neuroprotective, and/or anti-inflammatory effects of lidocaine and ketamine. Fentanyl is administered via a syringe pump and the LK is added to the IV crystalloid fluids (see above). The intraoperative dose of fentanyl is 5.0–10.0 µg/kg/hour, but doses as high as 20–40 µg/kg/hour may be used in painful multitrauma patients or critical patients in need of significant inhalant sparing to maintain cardiovascular stability. $ETCO_2$ monitoring is recommended to identify patients with significant respiratory depression ($ETCO_2$ >58 mmHg). Patients at higher doses may require intermittent positive-pressure ventilation despite titration of inhalant. Bradycardia is a common side-effect with all mu agonist opioids, especially fentanyl (HR <60 large/medium dog, HR <70–80 small dogs) and should be treated with an anticholinergic (glycopyrrolate [0.005 mg/kg] or atropine [0.02 mg/kg] IV) if there is a significant effect on blood pressure (MAP <60 mmHg).

- Dexmedetomidine (0.5–1.5 µg/kg/h intraoperatively, 0.5–2.0 µg/kg/h postoperatively) provides adjunct analgesia and synergism with opioid analgesics. It is helpful in decreasing the stress response to surgery/anesthesia, as an adjunct analgesic in stable trauma patients, and in patients with high anxiety/aggression. It provides significant MAC reduction of inhalants so attention to vaporizer setting and monitoring of $ETCO_2$ is necessary, in addition to expression of urinary bladder prior to recovery.

- NSAIDs are also effective in treating orthopedic pain. Injectable or oral NSAIDs may be administered prior to anesthesia/surgery or injectable NSAIDs may be administered at recovery (for doses and routes see Chapter 24). Although there are minimal hematologic or renal side-effects in healthy, euhydrated patients, prostaglandin blockade under conditions of hypotension (which can occur in ~40% of anesthetized small animal patients) may negatively affect renal hemodynamics.

- A new class of non-COX inhibiting NSAID (grapiprant) has been approved by the Food and Drug Administration (FDA) Center for Veterinary Medicine (in the USA) for treatment of osteoarthritis in dogs. Grapiprant (Galliprant®) is a prostaglandin E2 EP4 receptor antagonist. The EP4 receptor is the primary mediator of the PGE2-elicited inflammation and sensitization of sensory neurons. The specificity of EP4 receptor antagonism rather than blocking prostaglandin synthesis should result in a better safety and side-effect profile than the currently available COX-1-/COX-2-inhibiting NSAIDs. The dose of Galliprant (grapiprant tablets) is 2 mg/kg once daily. This drug is approved for use in dogs only.

LOCO-REGIONAL ANESTHESIA/ANALGESIA

- Loco-regional anesthesia/analgesia techniques are effective and relatively inexpensive modalities that should be considered as part of the multimodal analgesic plan for orthopedic patients. In general, the block that provides anesthesia/analgesia most specific to the surgical site should be implemented. The brachial plexus block may be used for forelimb surgeries from the mid-humerus and distally (see also Chapter 23). A radius/ulna/median/musculocutaneous (RUMM) block may be used for procedures of the carpus and paw. For the hindlimb, a lumbosacral (LS) epidural or femoral/sciatic nerve (FSNB) block are options depending on the surgical procedure and postoperative care profile desired. The LS epidural may be utilized for procedures involving the pelvis and hindlimb (see also Chapter 23). Preservative-free morphine alone or in combination with bupivacaine is the most commonly used drug for LS epidural.

- Opioids modulate pain signals at the level of the spinal cord whereas local anesthetics have the ability to completely block the nociceptive pathway. In addition to motor and sensory nerves, local anesthetics also block autonomic nerves and may increase the risk of intraoperative hypotension. Epidural morphine can cause postoperative urine retention due to increased urinary sphincter tone and detrusor muscle relaxation; therefore, it is important to empty the urinary bladder prior to recovery from anesthesia and to monitor urinary bladder size and urine output postoperatively.

- The FSNB can be utilized for procedures involving the stifle (i.e. mid-femur and distally). The addition of dexmedetomidine to bupivacaine extends the duration of action of the FSNB to up to 6–24 (median 14) hours. Recent studies have found no significant difference in pain scores between MLK CRI, FSNB, and LS epidural, so all are reasonable choices for surgical procedures of the stifle in canine patients. Intra-articular administration of local anesthetics has been associated with chondrolysis in multiple species *in vivo* and *in vitro* and therefore is not recommended.

Femoral/sciatic nerve block

- FSNB techniques are a practical alternative to epidural techniques. These blocks produce less urine retention and reduce opioid consumption in the 24 hours after surgery. As with LS epidurals, performing these blocks is of intermediate technical difficulty but they are comparatively less invasive. There is a good success rate once the technique is mastered and a low risk of complications. However, this technique does require good anatomic knowledge in order to increase success and minimize complications.

- The sciatic nerve block can be used alone for procedures of the foot and hock, but the femoral block needs to be included if the procedure involves the tibia or stifle. Examples of diagnoses/surgical procedures where a FSNB can be used include: tibial fracture repair, stifle arthroscopy, patellar luxation, cruciate ligament repair (TPLO or TTA), surgery of foot and tarsus.

- Standardized patient positioning is an important aspect of the procedure and helps to ensure a successful block and potentially decrease complications. It is important to verify that the needle is not located in the nerve or a vessel prior to injection of the local anesthetic. Before injecting, the clinician should ALWAYS aspirate for blood. It is also important to verify that the needle is not placed intraneurally. When using the electrolocation technique, it is recommended that the current of the nerve stimulator is decreased to 0.2 mA, eliminating motor stimulation; then increased again to 0.4 mA to re-establish the twitch (see also Chapter 23). As the local anesthetic is injected, the twitch response should cease as the nerve is displaced away from the needle; this is called the 'Raj Test'. Encountering resistance during injection may also signal an intraneural injection and the needle should be repositioned before continuing injection. Bupivacaine (*Table 18.5*) is highly cardiotoxic if inadvertently injected IV; therefore, the patient should be monitored for signs of toxicity, such as tachycardia, hypotension, cardiac arrhythmias, muscle twitching, or seizures, during and after the block.

- Femoral nerve block (**Fig. 18.2**). The femoral nerve arises from ventral branches of the L4, L5, and L6 spinal nerves and courses through the iliopsoas muscle, then exits the muscle and continues across the femoral triangle. The femoral triangle

Table 18.5 Femoral/sciatic nerve block	
Femoral/sciatic nerve block drugs	*Dose: mix in same syringe, administer half dose at each site*
Bupivacaine	1.0–1.5 mg/kg
Dexmedetomidine	0.1 µg/kg

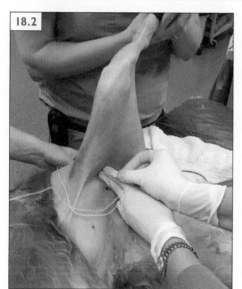

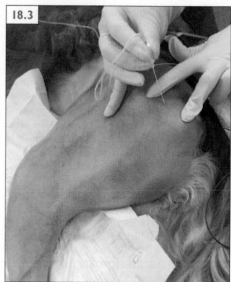

Fig. 18.2 Femoral nerve block using electrolocation.

Fig. 18.3 Sciatic nerve block using electrolocation.

is delineated by the pectineus muscle caudally, the sartorius muscle cranially, and the iliopsoas proximally. The femoral nerve is located cranial to the femoral artery and vein and directly medial to the caudal belly of the sartorius muscle. The patient is placed in lateral recumbency with the limb to be blocked positioned uppermost, abducted 90°, and extended caudally (**Fig. 18.2**). The inguinal area should be clipped and prepared. A 22 gauge, 50 mm insulated needle should be used with the peripheral nerve stimulator. The stimulating needle is inserted cranial to the femoral artery, caudal to the sartorius muscle within the femoral triangle, and advanced towards the iliopsoas muscle at a 20–30° angle with the nerve stimulator set at 1 mA. When the needle is within range of the femoral nerve, contraction of the quadriceps muscle and stifle extension will be observed. The current is decreased gradually to 0.4 mA, until the the same response can be elicited. Reposition the needle if necessary. In medium-sized breed dogs, the femoral nerve is fairly superficial (~0.5–1 cm under the skin), so deep needle insertions should be avoided. Contraction of the sartorius muscle should not be considered an acceptable endpoint;

the needle should be advanced further or repositioned.
- Sciatic nerve block. The sciatic nerve is formed by ventral branches of the L6, L7, and S1 spinal nerves. It exits the pelvis through the greater sciatic notch and descends between the greater trochanter and ischiatic tuberosity. It also gives off muscular branches supplying caudal thigh muscles. The patient should be placed in lateral recumbency with the limb to be blocked uppermost in a natural position (**Fig. 18.3**). The area between the greater trochanter and the ischiatic tuberosity should be clipped and prepared. Identify the greater trochanter and the ischiatic tuberosity and draw a line between these two points. The needle is placed at a point between the cranial and middle thirds (**Fig. 18.3**). The stimulating needle (22 gauge, 50 mm) is inserted at a 45° angle off skin with the nerve stimulator initially set at 1 mA. A positive contraction response is dorsiflexion or plantar extension of the foot. The current is decreased gradually to 0.4 mA (threshold current) until the same response can be elicited, repositioning the needle if necessary. Contraction of the biceps femoris muscle

should not be considered an acceptable endpoint. This response can be due to direct muscle stimulation and not sciatic nerve stimulation. This usually indicates the needle is too superficial. Contractions of the semimembranosus or semitendinosus muscles without foot movement are also NOT an acceptable endpoint. The needle is located too far caudally and the muscular branches of the sciatic nerve are being stimulated. Injections here will miss the main sciatic nerve and result in block failure.

- Complications of femoral nerve block include puncturing of the femoral artery, vein, or nerve itself. Complications of the sciatic nerve block include nerve injury resulting in temporary or permanent foot knuckling. Local anesthetic should not be injected when resistance is encountered during injection. Use of higher doses of dexmedetomidine may result in more systemic absorption and typical side-effects of this drug (vasoconstriction and bradycardia).

- Ultrasound (US)-guided peripheral nerve blocks (PNB)s are gaining popularity in the specialty of veterinary anesthesia/analgesia. US allows visualization of the needle, peripheral nerves and vessels, muscles and fascial plane. US-guided PNB are beyond the scope of this text and the reader is referred to other resources.

Anesthesia/analgesia protocols for cats (see also Chapter 24)

- Of the mu agonists mentioned above, methadone may have the most favorable behavioral profile in cats. Cats will typically become friendly, playful, and euphoric with dilated pupils. Methadone usually does not result in significant sedation when used alone unless the patient is geriatric or ill, and it should be administered with dexmedetomidine or alfaxalone for additional sedation.

- Buprenorphine may be used in cats undergoing an orthopedic procedure associated with mild to moderate pain; however, there are several limitations. Buprenorphine is a partial mu agonist and so does not have the full analgesic effect of a pure mu agonist. It also has an analgesic ceiling where administration of additional drug does not result in more significant analgesia effects. These attributes, along with its comparatively long onset of action of 45–60 minutes, make it a less desirable pre-emptive and intraoperative analgesic unless combined with a loco-regional anesthesia/analgesia technique and/or intraoperative CRI. The new long-acting formulation of buprenorphine (Simbadol™) is FDA approved (in the USA) for single dose administration SC per 24 hours in cats. Side-effects include euphoria, hyperactivity, and hyperthermia.

- Cats typically do not experience sedation with opioids alone; the addition of dexmedetomidine (5–15 µg/kg) provides good sedation, muscle relaxation, and adjunct analgesia. Ketamine (2–5 mg/kg) or tiletamine/zolazepam (Telazol®, 2–3 mg/kg) can be added to premedication for additional restraint/analgesia if the patient is painful or fractious. Alfaxalone (2.0 mg/kg IM) can be substituted for dexmedetomidine (and ketamine/Telazol) in cats where fewer cardiovascular effects are desired. Dexmedetomidine, when administered alone (20–25 µg/kg) is associated with a high incidence of vomiting. The addition of butorphanol (0.1–0.2 mg/kg) prevents vomiting and decreases the severity of signs of nausea; however, butorphanol provides only mild analgesia with a short duration of action (~30–90 minutes). Maropitant (1.0 mg/kg SC) significantly decreases the incidence of vomiting but not signs of nausea in cats; however, cats object robustly to SC administration. Oral administration (8 mg/kg PO) 2–18 hours prior to premedication significantly decreases, but does not prevent, vomiting and signs of nausea in cats administered dexmedetomidine and morphine.

- Depending on the dose and patient response to premedication drugs, cats may be able to be intubated. If needed, the induction protocols listed above for dogs may also be used in cats. An exception is lidocaine, which is not recommended for routine use IV in cats because cats are more susceptible to local anesthetic toxicity.

INTRAOPERATIVE ANALGESIA, INCLUDING NSAIDS

- Intraoperative CRIs will differ slightly in feline orthopedic patients since lidocaine CRI is not recommended. Dexmedetomidine (0.5–2.0 µg/kg/h) +/– ketamine (10–20 µg/kg/min, 0.6–1.2 mg/kg/h) can be used after loading doses in premedication or induction.
- Meloxicam is approved for a single postoperative dose in cats. Robenacoxib is available in both injectable and oral formulations for 3 days of perioperative administration. Safety and efficacy studies are underway for the new grapiprant EP4 antagonist in cats.
- All the loco-regional anesthesia/ analgesia techniques mentioned

above for canine orthopedic patients may also be applied in cats. Careful attention to local anesthetic dosing and diligent aspiration to avoid inadvertent blood vessel penetration prior to local anesthetic injection is imperative.

MONITORING

- Standard monitoring should include anesthetic depth, adequate oxygenation, ventilation, circulation, and body temperature with appropriate interventions taken when indicated (see Chapter 6). In addition to subjective, vigilant monitoring by the anesthetist, use of ECG, non-invasive blood pressure, pulse oximetry, capnography, and thermometer are indicated. Invasive blood pressure monitoring and blood gas analysis are indicated in trauma patients or patients with moderate to severe systemic illness (ASA III or more).

Complications

- As with all canine and feline patients undergoing anesthesia, orthopedic patients should be monitored for the following common anesthetic complications: hypoventilation, hypoxemia, hypotension, cardiac arrhythmias, hypothermia, and hyperthermia. The anesthetist should anticipate and have a plan for identification and intervention for anesthetic complications. Intraoperative hemorrhage is also a concern in trauma patients or in the uncommon event of the popliteal artery being severed during TPLO surgery for cranial cruciate ligament deficiency. The patient's starting total blood volume should be calculated, along with increments of 10%, 20%, and 30% losses. Blood loss can be quantitated by evaluating blood soaked gauze sponges (5–15 ml/ 4 × 4 gauze), weighing the sponges (1 g = 1 ml blood) and measuring a PCV on the suction fluid, and using the equation:

$$\text{ml of blood in suction} = PCV \text{ fluid}/PCV$$
of the patient × volume of fluid in the suction canister

In patients starting surgery with a normal PCV/TS, total blood volume (TBV) losses should be replaced as follows:

- 10–15% TBV loss: replace with 3–4 times the volume lost with crystalloid.
- 15–25% TBV loss requires the addition of colloid fluids (colloids, albumin, or plasma). Of these, colloids (Hetastarch) is the most economical and readily available. Colloids are administered as a bolus of 2–5 ml/kg and/or 2.0 ml/kg/ hour up to 20–50 ml/kg/day.
- >25–30% TBV loss requires oxygen carrying capacity replacement in the form of pRBCs or whole blood replacement.
- Trauma patients with a PCV <20% should receive pRBCs or whole blood prior to anesthesia and surgery, in order to maintain oxygen delivery to tissues.
- Dogs undergoing orthopedic surgery, especially those weighing >40 kg (88 lb) are at high risk for gastroesophageal reflux (GER). A high percentage of GER is 'silent' in that, unless esophageal

pH is monitored, it goes unnoticed. If GER fluid is noticed from the mouth or nostrils, the esophagus should be suctioned and lavaged with warm water and 5–10 ml of sodium bicarbonate should be diluted in an equal volume of water and infused into the lower esophagus. This will increase the pH of the lower esophagus for ~4 hours. It is important to check the ET cuff for any leaks prior to suction and lavage of the lower esophagus.

Postoperative considerations

- Appropriate analgesia and nursing care are important factors in the postoperative care of orthopedic patients. Pain evaluation/assessment should be performed regularly, preferably by the same individual, and the analgesic plan adjusted as indicated. The patient's level of sedation should be assessed after the expected onset of action of administered analgesic drug(s) or if the patient is maintained on CRI(s) in the postoperative period. Overly sedated patients are at risk for hypoventilation/hypoxemia and significant risk for aspiration if they regurgitate and cannot protect their airway with appropriate reflexes. Attention to urinary bladder function and care is another consideration. Dexmedetomidine will increase urine production and opioids, especially when administered epidurally, can lead to urinary retention. Urinary bladder distension stimulates the sympathetic nervous system, causing discomfort, vocalization, and restlessness and leading to confusion with the patient's surgical pain. The urinary bladder should be palpated and expressed prior to discontinuation of inhalant gas. Thereafter, bladder size should be assessed every 6 hours, especially if the patient is on a dexmedetomidine CRI, and treated appropriately with sling walk, manual expression, or intermittent catheterization. Partial/full opioid reversal is rarely needed for urinary retention associated with morphine epidural.

Case examples

CASE 1

- A 5-year-old spayed female Labrador Retriever presented for cranial cruciate repair. Weight, 35 kg (77 lb); body condition score (BCS), 7/9; temperament

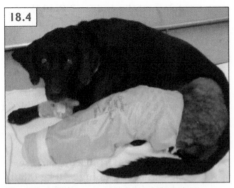

nice but slightly nervous; CBC and serum biochemistry within normal limits, heart and lungs auscult within normal limits (**Fig. 18.4**).

- Maropitant (1.0 mg/kg SC) 1 hour prior to opioid administration.
- Other options to avoid vomiting and signs of nausea include: (1) maropitant (1.0 mg/kg SC) the evening prior to anesthesia/surgery; (2) maropitant + acepromazine (0.005–0.01 mg/kg SC) 30 minutes prior to opioid administration; (3) maropitant (1.0 mg/kg IV) ~5 minutes prior to opioid administration; (4) substitute methadone for hydromorphone or morphine.
- Premedication. Hydromorphone (0.1–0.2 mg/kg) + acepromazine (0.005–0.01 mg/kg) both IM.
- Induction. Propofol (2 mg/kg) + ketamine (2 mg/kg) mixed in the same syringe; administer half the dose slowly

Fig. 18.4 Five-year-old spayed, female Labrador Retriever presented for cranial cruciate repair.

over 30–60 seconds; administer at a rate of 1.0 mg/kg/min until intubation can be accomplished.
- Intra-/postoperative analgesia. F/S nerve block with bupivacaine (1.5 mg/kg) + dexmedetomidine (0.1 µg/kg); dose split between the two nerve block sites; provides local anesthesia/analgesia for 4–10 hours.
- Other options for intra-/postoperative analgesia. LS epidural: bupivacaine alone will provide ~2.5–6 hours anesthesia/analgesia; morphine (preservative-free 0.1 mg/kg) +/– bupivacaine (0.2 ml/kg, 0.5%) up to 12–18 hours of analgesia.
- Other options for intraoperative analgesia. MLK or HLK CRI.
- Postoperative analgesia options. (1) intermittent opioid administration +/– NSAID; (2) CRI – continue MLK or HLK postoperatively +/– NSAID; (3) FSNB or LS epidural (supplemental opioid according to pain evaluation) for evening and overnight; if using FSNB or LS epidural, it is important to monitor patients regularly with a pain scoring system and adjust or add appropriate analgesic treatment in the form of additional opioids, NSAID, or CRI if deemed necessary.

CASE 2
- A 10-month-old castrated male, domestic medium hair cat with a fracture of the tarsus due to having a door closed on it. Weight, 5 kg (11 lb); BCS, 4/5; temperament nice but very active (**Fig. 18.5**).

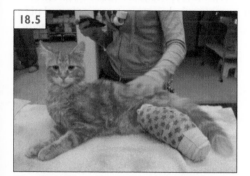

Fig. 18.5 Ten-month-old castrated male, domestic medium hair cat with a fracture of the tarsus due to having a door closed on it.

- Premedication. Dexmedetomidine (10 µg/kg) + methadone (0.5 mg/kg) IM.
- Additional options for premedication. (1) Add ketamine (2 mg/kg) IM if additional restraint or total injectable anesthesia for induction or loading dose for intraoperative CRI is desired; avoid in cats with hypertrophic cardiomyopathy; (2) substitute alfaxalone (2 mg/kg IM) for dexmedetomidine if fewer cardiovascular effects are desired in an older patient, patients with moderate comorbidities, or suspected or confirmed cardiovascular disease.
- Induction. Intubation may be possible with the premedication protocol. If not, options include: (1) propofol (2 mg/kg) + ketamine (2 mg/kg) IV mixed in the same syringe; administer half the dose slowly over 30–60 seconds; continue at the same rate until intubation can be accomplished; (2) alfaxalone (2 mg/kg IV).
- Intra-/postoperative analgesia. Intermittent injection of methadone (0.2–0.5 mg/kg IV) and F/S nerve block with bupivacaine (1.5 mg/kg) + dexmedetomidine (0.1 µg/kg); dose is split between the two nerve block sites; provides local anesthesia/analgesia for 4–10 hours.
- Other options for intra-/postoperative analgesia. LS epidural: bupivacaine alone will provide ~2.5–6 hours anesthesia/analgesia; morphine (preservative-free 0.1 mg/kg) +/– bupivacaine (0.2 ml/kg, 0.5%) up to 12–18 hours of analgesia.
- Other options for intraoperative analgesia in addition to intermittent injection of methadone. Dexmedetomidine (1–2 µg/kg/h) +/– ketamine (10–20 µg/kg/min, 0.6–1.2 mg/kg/h) CRI.
- Postoperative analgesia options. (1) Intermittent opioid administration (methadone or buprenorphine) +/– NSAID; both buprenorphine and methadone can be given by oral transmucosal administration postoperatively; (2) CRI – continue dexmedetomidine +/– ketamine (decrease to 1–2 µg/kg/min) CRI postoperatively

+/– NSAID. (3) FSNB or LS epidural (supplemental opioid according to pain evaluation) for evening and overnight; if using FSNB or LS epidural, it is important to monitor patients regularly with a pain scoring system and adjust or add appropriate analgesic treatment in the form of additional opioids, NSAID, or CRI if deemed necessary.

Further reading

Bigby SE, Beths T, Bauquier S *et al.* (2017) Effect of rate of administration of propofol and alfaxalone on induction dose requirement and occurrence of apnea in dogs. *Vet Anaesth Analg* **44**:1267–75.

Boscan P, Pypendop BH, Siao KT *et al.* (2010) Fluid balance, glomerular filtration rate and urine output in dogs anesthetized for an orthopedic surgical procedure. *Am J Vet Res* **71(5)**:501–7.

Campoy L, Reed M (2012) The thoracic limb. In: *Small Animal Regional Anesthesia and Analgesia.* (eds L Campoy, M Read) Wiley Blackwell, Ames, pp. 141–66.

Campoy L, Mahler S (2012) The pelvic limb. In: *Small Animal Regional Anesthesia and Analgesia.* (eds L Campoy, M Read) Wiley Blackwell, Ames, pp. 199–226.

Hay Kraus BL (2013) Efficacy of maropitant in preventing vomiting in dogs premedicated with hydromorphone. *Vet Anaesth Analg* **40(1)**:28–34.

Kogan DA, Johnson LR, Sturgess BK *et al.* (2008) Etiology and clinical outcome in dogs with aspiration pneumonia: 88 cases (2004–2006). *J Am Vet Med Assoc* **233**:1748–55.

Lamata C, Loughton V, Jones M *et al.* (2012) The risk of passive regurgitation during general anaesthesia in a population of referred dogs in the UK. *Vet Anaesth Analg* **39(3)**:266–74.

Leppänen MK, McKusick BC, Granholm MM *et al.* (2006) Clinical efficacy and safety of dexmedetomidine and buprenorphine, butorphanol or diazepam for canine hip radiography. *J Small Anim Pract* **47(11)**:663–9.

Ovbey DH, Wilson DV, Bednarski RM *et al.* (2014) Prevalence and risk factors for canine post-anesthetic aspiration pneumonia (1999–2009): a multicenter study. *Vet Anaesth Analg* **41**:127–36.

Ramsey D, Fleck T, Berg T *et al.* (2014) Cerenia prevents perioperative nausea and vomiting and improves recovery in dogs undergoing routine surgery. *Intern J Appl Res Vet Med* **12(3)**:228–37.

Ribas T, Bublot I, Junot S *et al.* (2015) Effects of intramuscular sedation with alfaxalone and butorphanol on echocardiographic measurements in healthy cats. *J Feline Med Surg* **17(6)**:530–6.

Tart KM, Babski DM, Lee JA (2010) Potential risks, prognostic indicators, and diagnostic and treatment modalities affecting survival in dogs with presumptive aspiration pneumonia: 125 cases (2005–2008). *J Vet Emerg Crit Care* **20**:319–29.

Wilson DV, Evans AT (2007) The effect of topical treatment on esophageal pH during acid reflux in dogs. *Vet Anaesth Analg* **34**:339–43.

Anesthetic considerations for dental and oral–facial surgeries

Jeff C Ko

Introduction

Dentistry is among one of the most performed procedures in the veterinary practice. Dental patients range from overall healthy, young animals for dental prophylaxis to aged animals with concurrent diseases for multiple dental work-up and extractions. The overall death rate associated with anesthesia in dogs is estimated at between 0.11% and 0.43%. This rate increases as the animal's age increases.

A recent retrospective study compared 100 overall healthy geriatric (>10–11 years old) with another 100 dogs with cardiac dysfunctions but without congestive heart failure undergoing dental procedures in a university teaching hospital. The results showed that cardiac arrhythmias were uncommon and the anesthetic-induced complication rates were similar, regardless of whether the dogs had cardiac disease or not. The take-home message from this study is that dogs with heart disease pose no more significant anesthetic risk of complication when subjected to routine dental procedures than non-cardiac disease geriatric dogs, provided the anesthesia is carried out by trained personnel and with carefully monitoring. However, the three most observed complications in non-cardiac disease geriatric dogs were hypotension (49%), bradycardia (35–36%), and hypoventilation (21–24%).

For details of dental patients with concurrent diseases, consult the relevant chapters in this book. This chapter will only cover the most commonly encountered issues as well as describing anesthetic considerations and protocols for dentistry and oral surgeries in dogs and cats.

Anesthetic considerations for dental and oral–facial surgical procedures

- Physical examination and blood work is needed to identify potential systemic dysfunction or dehydration. For young and healthy animals, basic blood work (see Chapter 2), such as PCV, TP, BUN, and blood glucose, are sufficient. For geriatric patients with concurrent specific diseases, a CBC, serum chemistry, and urine analysis may be necessary prior to dental procedure. Some clinicians consider such testing troublesome and use this as an excuse to promote performing dental procedures on awake animals without the use of general anesthesia. This concept is incorrect and owners should be educated to allow their pet's dental procedure to be performed properly under general anesthesia.

- Hospital visit-related and/or physical examination-related anxiety is a common problem in dogs and cats. It is a frequently encountered challenge for owners taking their pets to the hospital for dental prophylaxis. Trazodone and gabapentin have been used in dogs and cats prior to transportation and a hospital visit to reduce the animal's anxiety.
  - Trazodone is a human antidepressant that acts as a serotonin antagonist/reuptake inhibitor. It is also an alpha-1 adrenergic receptor antagonist. It has been used at a dose of 5–10 mg/kg PO 2 hours prior to transportation or hospital visit to reduce anxiety in dogs and cats.
  - The cardiorespiratory effects of trazodone (5.0–7.5 mg/kg PO) are comparable to acepromazine (0.01–0.03 mg/kg IM) in healthy dogs undergoing propofol induction and isoflurane for maintenance. Both drugs induce hypotension in dogs. When animals receive trazodone prior to anesthesia, hypotension should be anticipated and managed accordingly.
  - Gabapentin is a human antiseizure drug. It has also has been used to treat chronic pain in dogs and cats. Gabapentin (20 mg/kg PO) 1 hour prior to the visit has been

used to reduce anxiety in cats for transportation-related and hospital visit-related anxiety. The cardiorespiratory effect of gabapentin administered prior to anesthesia induction is unknown, but it is likely to have minimal effect.
  - Recently, it has been shown that a combination of trazodone (5 mg/kg) with gabapentin (10 mg/kg) PO at 2 hours prior to the hospital visit induced a greater degree of anxiolytic/tranquilizing effect than either drug used alone in dogs and cats.

- General anesthesia is required for dental cleaning.
  - The 2013 American Animal Hospital Association Dental Care Guidelines for Dogs and Cats, which were endorsed by the American Veterinary Dental College, considered dental cleaning without general anesthesia to be unacceptable.
  - Anesthesiologists would absolutely agree that general anesthesia provides the necessary immobilization and masseter muscle relaxation to allow proper dental work (include intraoral radiography, gum probing, removal of dental tartar, and polishing) to be performed without causing the animal distress.

- Endotracheal intubation is needed to maintain a patent airway.
  - Oral-tracheal intubation is necessary to maintain a patent airway and prevent any potential aspiration of water, saliva, blood, or dental materials.
  - To prevent potential microaspiration, the endotracheal tube (ETT) should be lubricated with a water-soluble lubricant, especially the cuff portion (see Chapter 1).

- Pharyngotomy (at times, tracheostomy) may be necessary for oral surgery.
  - Various maxillofacial, mandibular, or maxillary fractures can occur and will need surgical repair. Because of the difficulty in accessing some of these fracture sites, surgery may require a

pharyngotomy (tracheostomy) to allow the surgeon to have maximum space to work on the fracture.

- Dental occlusion is another procedure that will require general anesthesia or profound sedation to guide mandibular realignment with complex fractures. Pharyngotomy is one of the options when the ETT is in the way during precise alignment of the upper and lower arcades.
- An alternative to pharyngotomy is repeated intubation and extubation during the dental occlusion. This should only be performed in otherwise healthy dogs. This technique carries a high risk when applied to patients with cardiorespiratory dysfunction because of potential hypoxia. This technique also does not work well in brachycephalic breeds because of the difficulty of airway accessing. Obese patients requiring intermittent positive ventilation are also not suitable for repeated intubation and extubation.
- Security of the ETT is important to prevent the tube disconnecting or dislodging.
  - Both dental and oral surgical procedures require frequent repositioning of the animal's head. This may result in dislodging or disconnection of the ETT. Accidental extubation with the tube within the oral cavity followed by inadvertently reinserting the ETT into the esophagus commonly occurs. It is therefore important to properly secure the tube to prevent this situation happening.
- Avoid tracheal trauma.
  - When repositioning the animal's head or body for the dental procedure, it is vital to disconnect the ETT from the breathing circuit to avoid potential tracheal torque or rupture.
  - Avoid excessive ETT cuff inflation. The cuff should be measured with a pressure manometer (see Chapter 1) and the cuff pressure maintained within 20–25 cmH$_2$O of water during the anesthetic procedure.

- Avoid airway obstruction.
  - Airway obstruction due to airway secretions, mucus plug, blood, or dental-related debris can occur. The position of the head for dental or oral surgery could also result in kinking of the ETT. Therefore, selecting a flexible but kink-resistant type of tube (e.g. a reinforced silicone tube) is important.
  - It is vital to monitor the patent's airway patency via capnography (see Chapter 6) or breathing bag excursion.
  - Dental and oral surgical gauze pads must be counted before and after the procedure to ensure none are left inside the oral cavity or upper airway.
- Proper eye lubrication is vital during the dental or oral surgery.
  - During the dental and oral surgical procedure, excessive water, blood, or other types of fluid are likely to contaminate the globes and cause severe irritation to the eyes of the anesthetized patient. Eye ointment should be applied liberally to the eye for protection and this will need to be repeated several times during the course of the procedure to prevent dryness of the eyes.
- Prevention of hypothermia.
  - Dental polishing frequently results in patients becoming wet. Heat loss from wet hair is far more rapid and profound than from dry hair. Avoiding excessive watering of the patient's body and hair helps to avoid cutaneous heat loss.
  - Drugs such as acepromazine and inhalants are potent vasodilators and tend to cause cutaneous heat loss.
  - Unnecessary use of a high oxygen flow rate also promotes heat loss from the airway.
  - External heat, such as water heating blanket, rice socks (see Chapter 31), or forced hot air warmer, should be provided to prevent hypothermia. At times, long-haired animals may develop hyperthermia due to their inability to vent heat. Monitoring body temperature is vital in detecting hypo- and hyperthermia.

- Avoid excessive long duration of anesthesia.
  - A lot of dental procedures may take hours to complete due to their complexity. Frequently, extra dental works are undertaken after the practitioner has had a chance to examine the tooth and obtain dental radiographs.
  - A long duration of anesthesia places an extra burden on geriatric and diabetic patients. Hypothermia associated with a long duration of anesthesia occurs because of prolonged inhibition of the thermoregulatory center, extensive heat loss from just being under general anesthesia, inhalant-induced vasodilation, and cold oxygen exposure through the airway. All these factors, together with an inability to warm up the hypothermic patient effectively, will greatly prolong the recovery further.
- Consider dealing with the diabetic patient (see Chapter 10) as the first case in the morning so that prolonged fasting and a delayed return to regular feeding time do not occur.
  - Blood glucose should be checked perioperatively to ensure the level falls within the normal range. A half dose of an ultra-short acting insulin can be given as part of the premedication protocol and the blood glucose checked every 20–30 minutes until the dog resumes feeding.
- Taking care of perioperative pain management using the multimodal analgesic technique.
  - Premedication with an opioid together with intraoperative local anesthetic blockage (see Chapter 23) and using NSAIDs is a typical multimodal analgesic technique that can be applied to dental and oral surgical patients.
- Anticipate common anesthetic problems that could occur.
  - Hypotension, hypoxia, hypothermia, hypoventilation, and cardiac arrhythmias all can occur with dental and oral surgical patients.
- Tachycardia, bradycardia, and ventricular premature contractions commonly occur during the procedures. Tachycardia could be related to pain. Bradycardia could be due to hypothermia or high vagal tone manipulation. Ventricular premature contractions could be related to the high sympathetic tone due to the pain and stress of the patient.
- The three most commonly occurring anesthetic complications are hypotension (49%), bradycardia (35–36%), and hypoventilation (21–24%).
- Hypotension should be treated with fluids (both colloid and crystalloid fluids), reducing the anesthetic depth by turning down the inhalant and supplementing with an opioid and/or using a local anesthetic technique to take care of the pain, and considering using inotropes if all these corrective procedures are undertaken without success (see Chapter 6).
- Bradycardia should be treated with anticholinergic agents if it is associated with hypotension (see Chapter 6).
- Hypoventilated animals should receive either assisted or controlled artificial ventilation.
- Avoid the use of a spring-loaded mouth gag to maximally open the mouth.
  - Several studies have shown that the use of a spring-loaded mouth gag when maximally opened is likely to compress the maxillary arteries of cats because of their anatomic location in this species.
  - Another study has shown that the use of smaller mouth gags was associated with fewer alterations of maxillary artery blood flow. Therefore, when performing a dental procedure with the mouth opened maximally, using a smaller mouth gag is suggested instead of a wide spring-loaded mouth gag.

Pain management for in-hospital and as take-home medication

- Using local anesthetic (lidocaine or bupivacaine, or a mixture of both) with infraorbital (for maxillary tooth extraction analgesia) and mental (for mandibular tooth extraction analgesia) blocks is usually helpful for pain relief during dental or oral–facial surgeries (see Chapter 23).
- A recently available bupivacaine liposome injection suspension (Nocita®) can be used to infiltrate the tooth extraction

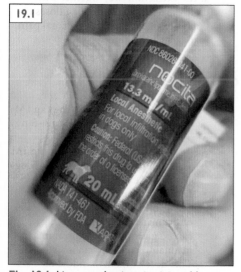

Fig. 19.1 Liposome bupivacaine injectable suspension. Note the white suspension solution.

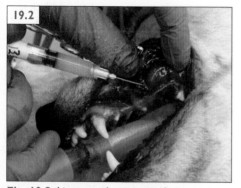

Fig. 19.2 Liposome bupivacaine being infiltrated at the maxillary molar extraction site. Note the bulging of the mucosal area.

(**Fig. 19.1**) or oral–facial surgical site for pain relief for up to 3 days when the surgical procedure is being closed. The infiltration should cover the various layers of muscle, mucosa, and skin (**Fig. 19.2**). Bupivacaine liposome injection suspension starts to act in approximately 30 minutes. Immediate pain relief should be considered if the bupivacaine injection suspension is infiltrated immediately prior to anesthesia recovery of the animal. Alternatively, regular bupivacaine should be administered prior to surgery. This is timed to fill the interval between the regular bupivacaine and the bupivacaine liposome injection suspension.

- It is debatable whether the liposome bupivacaine injection suspension can be used for regional dental or oral–facial regional blocks. The concern is that if it lasts for 3 days, the motor function of the facial nerves (including the lingual never) might be paralyzed for such a duration with a potential adverse outcome.
- If there is no specific contraindication, NSAIDs such as robenacoxib (2 mg/kg PO or 1 mg/kg SC) can be administered in cats for up to 3 days. Carprofen (2.2 mg/kg PO, SC q12h, or 4.4 mg/kg PO, SC q24h) can be used in dogs for 3 days.
- If an opioid is needed, buprenorphine OTM is a good way to provide a long duration of analgesia. The author's preference is to use buprenorphine (Simabdol™ 1.8 mg/ml). This high concentration of buprenorphine overcomes the large volume required for administration to large-sized animals. It can be used in dogs and cats.
- For buprenorphine the dosages are: dogs: 80–120 µg/kg OTM; cats: 80–160 µg/kg OTM. This lasts approximately 12–24 hours with a single application and can be repeated once daily for 3 days.
- Dogs are more sensitive to buprenorphine than cats and may appear to be more sedate if a high dose is used. The sedation usually occurs between 20 and 30 minutes after OTM application and

lasts approximately 1–2 hours. During the sedation, the dog can be aroused.

- Tramadol is a weaker opioid than buprenorphine but can be used because of its convenient oral administration.
- The tramadol dose for dogs and cats is approximately 5–10 mg/kg q12h. Sedation may be prominent in dogs and less in cats. Tramadol tablets are bitter tasting and cats dislike them intensely. Administration may be difficult and the use of piller likely necessary.
- Recent studies have questioned the analgesic efficacy of tramadol in dogs. Pharmacokinetic studies indicate that tramadol is likely to be more effective in cats than in dogs. This is because tramadol's analgesic effect relies on its two metabolites, the O-desmethyltramadol (M1) and N,O-didesmethyltramadol (M5), to work on the opioid receptor. There is minimal measurable M1 and a low detectable M5 plasma concentrations in dogs. In contrast, there is a relatively high detectable M1 plasma concentrations in cats. Therefore, the use of tramadol in dogs for managing dental pain deserves reconsideration and is likely to be falling out of regular consideration. Therefore, this author's recommendation is that a long-acting local anesthetic filtration at the extraction site, together with daily NSAID and a couple of doses of buprenorphine, is the ideal dental pain management at home.

Recommendations for dental and oral–facial surgeries

PREMEDICATION

- Premedication prior to the procedure will facilitate animal handling and IV catheterization.
- Neuroleptic analgesic combinations work well in both dogs and cats for these procedures. (See also neuroleptic–analgesic combinations in Chapter 3.)
- For ASA I–II patients, the author's choices are
  - Acepromazine (0.01–0.03 mg/kg IM) or azaperone (0.2–0.4 mg/kg IM).
  - Medetomidine (10–20 µg/kg IM) or dexmedetomidine (5–10 µg/kg IM) combined with one of the following opioids:
    - Butorphanol (0.2–0.4 mg/kg IM).
    - Buprenorphine (40–80 µg/kg IM).
    - Hydromorphone (0.01–0.02 mg/kg IM).
    - Methadone (0.5–1.0 mg/kg IM).
    - Morphine (0.25–1 mg/kg IM).
  - The author also use two sedatives to induce a more profound sedation as part of the sparing effect to reduce the total dose of each sedative use. The following are examples:
    - Acepromazine (0.01 mg/kg IM) with midazolam (0.2–0.4 mg/kg IM).
    - Acepromazine (0.01 mg/kg IM) with dexmedetomidine (3–5 µg/kg IM).
    - Midazolam (0.2–0.4 mg/kg IM) with dexmedetomidine (3–5 µg/kg IM).
- In addition to these premedicants, a dose of medetomidine (10 µg/kg) or dexmedetomidine (8 µg/kg) can be given IM once the animal is maintained on inhalant anesthesia. This dose of medetomidine or dexmedetomidine serves two purposes:
  - It reduces the maintenance inhalant anesthetic concentration.
  - It counteracts the vasodilation induced by the inhalant, so that blood pressure is better maintained.
- For ASA III–IV patients, the author's choices are:
  - Midazolam (0.2–0.4 mg/kg IM) combined with one of the following opioids:
    - Butorphanol (0.2–0.4 mg/kg IM).
    - Buprenorphine (30–60 µg/kg IM).
    - Hydromorphone (0.05–0.1 mg/kg IM).
    - Methadone (0.25–0.5 mg/kg IM).
    - Morphine (0.25–0.3 mg/kg IM).

- In cardiac or geriatric ASA III–IV patients, when the animal's temperament requires a little more profound sedation, alfaxalone (0.5–1 mg/kg IM) can be added to the above midazolam–opioid combination to further enhance the sedation. The drawback of adding alfaxalone as part of the IM combination is that the injection volume is large in large-sized dogs because a 1% formulation of alfaxalone is currently only available.

INTRAVENOUS INDUCTION
- Propofol (2–6 mg/kg).
- Alfaxalone (2–4 mg/kg).
- Etomidate (1–2 mg/kg).

INHALANT ANESTHETICS
- Isoflurane to effect.
- Sevoflurane to effect.

FLUID ADMINISTRATION
- 3–5 ml/kg/hour of crystalloid fluids.

- If hypotension occurs, follow the hypotension treatment guideline (see Chapter 6).
- A combination of colloid (3 ml/kg/h) and crystalloid (3 ml/kg/h) fluids can be coadministered.

PAIN MANAGEMENT
- Prior to dental extraction, a regional dental block can be used with lidocaine or bupivacaine.
- During wound closure, use liposome bupivacaine injectable suspension for local infiltration.
- Give a dose of buprenorphine (see previously mentioned dosages). Buprenorphine can be taken home (120 µg/kg OTM daily for 3 days). (Note: The take-home opioid should follow the local veterinary narcotic regulation for allowing pet owners to access such controlled substances.)
- Administer an injectable NSAID and follow with 3 days of take-home NSAID.

Further reading

Carter JE, Motsinger-Reif AA, Krug WV et al. (2017) The effect of heart disease on anesthetic complications during routine dental procedures in dogs. *J Am Anim Hosp Assoc* **53(4):**206–13.

Martin-Flores M, Scrivani PV, Loew E et al. (2014) Maximal and submaximal mouth opening with mouth gags in cats: implications for maxillary artery blood flow. *Vet J* **200:**60–4.

Stevens BJ, Frantz EM, Orlando JM et al. (2016) Efficacy of a single dose of trazodone hydrochloride given to cats prior to veterinary visits to reduce signs of transport- and examination-related anxiety. *J Am Vet Med Assoc* **249(2):** 202–7.

Stiles J, Weil AB, Packer RA et al. (2012) Post-anesthetic cortical blindness in cats: twenty cases. *Vet J* **193:**367–73.

Analgesia and sedation of emergency/intensive care unit patients

Elizabeth J Thomovsky and Aimee C Brooks

Introduction

This chapter briefly introduces the most common groupings of emergency and intensive care unit (ICU) cases with the aim of recommending analgesic and sedation protocols as well as discussing possible long-term ICU-related complications in these patients.

Basic triage of emergency cases

- Airway and breathing. Ensure that the patient is able to breathe without extreme effort. Consider using an oxygen cage, flow-by oxygen, nasal oxygen, or intubation (**Figs. 20.1–20.4**) (see Chapter 11).
- Circulation. Ensure that all cardiovascular parameters are normalized; ideal parameters and monitoring techniques are outlined in *Table 20.1*.
  - Administer repeated boluses of 20–30 ml/kg of IV crystalloid fluids up to a total of 90 ml/kg in dogs or 60 ml/kg in cats to stabilize hypovolemic patients (see Chapter 7).
  - If needed, colloids are given in boluses of 5–10 ml/kg IV up to 20 ml/kg (see Chapter 7).

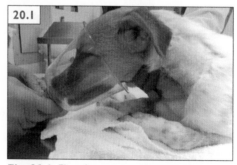

Fig. 20.1 Flow-by oxygen administration using a mask. This is a minimally invasive way to administer oxygen while handling a patient. Movement of the head away from the oxygen, oxygen mixing with room air, and stress induced by the mask limits the efficacy.

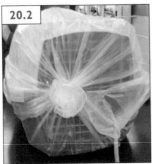

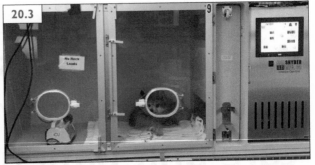

Figs. 20.2, 20.3 Oxygen chambers. These are advantageous because they allow for administration of oxygen without handling the animal. However, all enclosures run the risk of having increased temperature and humidity within the chamber. They also do not allow for ease of patient handling and require that the animal be removed from oxygen prior to receiving treatments. Placing a cat or dog carrier into a plastic garbage bag (**20.2**) and filling the bag with oxygen creates a make-shift oxygen cage. Cutting a hole at the caudal end of the bag is important to allow carbon dioxide and excessive heat to exit the cage. Alternatively, a commercial oxygen cage that regulates the oxygen level and actively scavenges carbon dioxide while controlling temperature (**20.3**) can be used. A third alternative is to place the animal's head into an oxygen hood (not pictured).

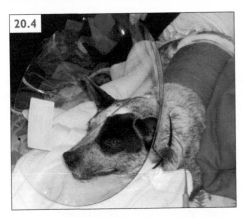

Fig. 20.4 Nasal oxygen cannula. This route of oxygen administration is more invasive than a chamber or flow-by but is advantageous because it allows continuous handling/treating of an animal while it is getting oxygen. The patients do not suffer from increased heat and humidity since they are not within an enclosure while they receive oxygen.

- Use blood products, vasopressors, and/or positive inotropic drugs to maintain blood pressure and tissue perfusion if fluid therapy is not effective or is contraindicated (see Chapter 6).
- If possible, gain IV access and obtain blood for blood work such as PCV/TP, glucose, lactate, electrolytes, and acid–base.
  - Other point of care monitoring (e.g. non-invasive blood pressure, SpO$_2$, ECG, ultrasound) is considered depending on the patient's presentation (*Table 20.1*).
- Further diagnostics (CBC, serum chemistry, coagulation times (see Chapter 2), radiographs) are obtained once the patient is stabilized.
- Mild sedation (as outlined in the sections below) may be needed to facilitate initial diagnostics.

Table 20.1 Suggested monitoring techniques for triage and subsequent ICU monitoring (see Chapter 6 for more details)

Parameter	Methodology	Goals
Tissue perfusion	Doppler indirect blood pressure. Readings may approximate mean arterial blood pressure when 90 mmHg or below Oscillometric indirect blood pressure Direct (invasive) blood pressure via arterial catheter	Maintain systolic blood pressure >90 mmHg or mean arterial blood pressure >60 mmHg
	Lactate measurements	<0.22 mmol/l (2 mg/dl) or a 50% reduction from presenting value within 3 hours
	Serial physical examination	
	Pulse quality	Subjectively strong, easy to palpate
	Mucous membrane color	Pink color
	Capillary refill time	<2 seconds
	Extremity temperature	Ears and paws feel warm to the touch
Oxygenation/ ventilation	Pulse oximetry	Maintain SpO_2 above 94%
	Arterial blood gas	Maintain PaO_2 >80 mmHg
	Respiratory rate/effort and auscultation findings	Not tachypneic (respiration rate <60 bpm); no labored breathing; lung sounds audible but not increased
Heart rate/ arrhythmias	Heart rate monitoring (auscultation or via ECG, arterial line, or SpO_2 plethysmograph)	Heart rate should be 60–140 bpm in dogs or 180–200 bpm in cats
	ECG continuous monitoring	Identify and treat any specific arrhythmias noted
Urine production	Urine output quantification via catheter or weighing of bedding	Urination during resuscitation indicates perfusion to the kidneys If urinary catheter in place, urine output after resuscitation should be at least 0.5 ml/kg/hour
	Serial monitoring of patient weight	Increases of more than 10% of body weight from presentation could indicate fluid retention Weight loss more than 10% from presenting body weight might indicate fluid deficiency or excessive fluid losses (e.g. polyuria, drains, diarrhea)
	Serial palpation or ultrasound of bladder size if not urinating	Bladder should be enlarging with urine over time; small bladder with no urine production after fluid therapy presents a concern for appropriate kidney function
	Serial renal values/electrolytes	BUN, creatinine, and potassium should not become higher on serial rechecks after fluid therapy
Body temperature	Serial rectal temperatures	Maintain normothermia (37.2–39.2°C [99–102.5°F])
Electrolytes/ acid–base	Serial blood gas and electrolyte monitoring	Normalization of electrolytes and acid–base parameters with fluid therapy and supplementation of potassium and other electrolytes as indicated
Hemoglobin/ hematocrit	Monitor serial hemoglobin or hematocrit	Transfuse red blood cell products if anemia with clinical signs (weakness, tachycardia)
	Co-oximetry (if underlying disease indicates)	Identify methemoglobin (acetaminophen intoxication) or carboxyhemoglobin (smoke inhalation)

Specific emergency/intensive care unit conditions

SKIN/INTEGUMENT/MUSCULOSKELETAL

Common examples include traumatic wounds, bite wounds, and burns with or without concurrent fractures. After following the rules of basic triage (above), address the wounds:

- Cover the wound with a clean, dry dressing (e.g. gauze, non-adherent pad) during triage.
- Stop any bleeding with a tourniquet, hemostats, application of pressure bandaging, and/or application of hemostatic agents.
  - If bleeding is excessive, this is done during basic triage to help stabilize cardiovascular parameters.
  - Tourniquets should be released for 5 min for every 30 min of application to preserve distal tissue and nerve viability.
- After the patient is stabilized, pursue appropriate wound care including lavage and debridement of the wounds. (See *Further reading* for specifics on wound care.)
- Since wounds are inherently painful, analgesics must be used during triage/wound care. Opioids and/or local anesthetics are the best options for these patients (see Chapters 23 and 24):
  - NSAIDs are not used acutely, especially in patients presenting with shock or with concerns about perfusion to the heart, kidney, and/or gastrointestinal (GI) tract.
  - Once an animal is fully resuscitated (typically 6–24 hours post trauma), NSAIDs may be used.
- If sedation is required for wound care, there are two options:
  - If the patient is cardiovascularly stable, sedation with either acepromazine or dexmedetomidine in combination with an opioid analgesic is recommended (see Chapters 9 and 24).
    - Generally a full mu agonist such as hydromorphone or methadone is preferable to butorphanol/buprenorphine.
    - Full mu agonists have a longer duration of analgesic effect, provide small amounts of sedation, and can be fully reversed with naloxone.

- Buprenorphine is difficult to reverse and takes up to 30 minutes to provide an analgesic effect.
- If the patient is too painful to effect wound care with sedation, general anesthesia is suggested (see Chapters 5 and 9).
- If the patient is not cardiovascularly stable, use a full mu opioid analgesic and benzodiazepine combination (see Chapter 9).
  - Both of these drugs can be reversed.
  - Benzodiazepines have fewer negative cardiovascular effects than acepromazine and dexmedetomidine.
  - Regularly dose opioids and/or use a CRI of a short-acting opioid such as fentanyl during wound care to prevent pain. Local analgesia/anesthesia can be used during wound care.
- Radiographs are taken to better characterize the extent of injury.
  - Pursue radiographs AFTER the patient is stabilized.
  - Cover wounds for radiography and perform definitive wound treatment after radiography.
  - Sedation for radiographs ranges from opioid analgesics to general anesthesia (see above and Chapter 17).
    - Tranquilizers such as acepromazine or dexmedetomidine can facilitate proper radiographic positioning without inducing further pain or distress.
    - General anesthesia is required for radiography if it is too painful or difficult to position the patient with only sedation.
    - Do not tranquilize or anesthetize an animal until it is cardiovascularly stable.
- Fracture external coaptation with a splint, cast, or bandage is performed under heavy sedation with analgesia or general anesthesia.
  - Bandages and/or splints are used acutely until definitive surgical repair (if indicated) is pursued.
  - See *Further reading* for details on fracture repair and external coaptation.

- Longer-term care in the ICU:
  - Chronic IV fluid therapy is given for maintenance and ongoing losses. When calculating and providing for ongoing losses, be sure to account for drainage from wounds both in bandages and collected in wound drains.
  - Opioids are used to control pain until the wound is closed surgically or has healed.
    - Consider CRI of an opioid such as fentanyl (see Chapter 24).
    - NSAIDs are excellent for longer-term use in stable ICU patients.

- Local anesthetics can be used for multiple days to spare the patient from opioids and/or NSAIDs (see Chapter 23).
- Chronic use of pain medications in ICU patients can lead to ileus and decreased appetite (*Tables 20.2, 20.3*).
  - Ileus typically occurs after 1–3 days with an opioid CRI or sooner with a CRI including ketamine and/or lidocaine.
  - Regular reassessment and weaning of pain medications is important.

Table 20.2 Pros and cons of long-term analgesia and sedation in the intensive care unit

Intervention	Advantages	Disadvantages
Intermittent or CRI opioid use more than 2–3 days	Fewest renal side-effects Good in hypotensive patients Provides mild sedation and relief of anxiety Reversal agents available for full mu agonists (e.g. hydromorphone, methadone)	Induces ileus Constipation possible Regurgitation possible Excessive sedation Anorexia Occasionally results in urinary retention
Constant rate infusion opioid +/– lidocaine +/– ketamine longer than 24 hours	Improved analgesia versus opioids alone Lowers opioid dose to reduce opioid side-effects More profound sedation than opioid alone (specifically ketamine CRI) Lidocaine may help with concurrent ventricular arrhythmias (e.g. post gastrointestinal surgery)	Very uncommon for animals to eat when on a CRI of opioids, lidocaine, and ketamine Greater chance of ileus after 24 h than opioid alone Greater risk of regurgitation than opioid alone after 24 h Urinary retention and constipation risks similar to receiving opioid alone

CRI, constant rate infusion.

Table 20.3 Recommendations to avoid complications of long-term analgesia and sedation in the intensive care unit

If long-term analgesia or sedation is needed (e.g. postoperative septic peritonitis, polytrauma) given intermittently or via constant rate infusions:

Anticipate ileus and take steps to avoid this expected side-effect:

- Titrate doses of opioids, ketamine, and lidocaine to the lowest possible doses that still achieve analgesia or sedation
- Start prokinetic agents (metoclopramide 1–2 mg/kg/d) or erythromycin 1 mg/kg IV or PO prior to signs of ileus as long as not contraindicated by the type of surgery
- Start antiemetic such as maropitant (1 mg/kg IV or SC) or ondansetron (0.1 mg/kg IV)
- Consider placing nasogastric (NG) tube and suctioning fluid from stomach q12–24 h to provide gastric decompression and improve patient comfort; possibly decreases regurgitation and/or nausea resulting from a distended stomach
- Start enteral nutrition via NG or other feeding tube as soon as reasonable after surgery to stimulate gut motility. Typically, small amounts (e.g. 25% of an animal's daily energy requirement given over 24 h as a constant rate infusion) will stimulate enterocyte health and gut motility with a low risk of regurgitation
- If possible, attempt to have patient stand or move for short periods of time several times a day to stimulate gut motility
- Consider alternative analgesic options to reduce or avoid systemic drugs, such as local wound soaker catheters or epidural catheters for animals who will likely require high-dose analgesia for >24–48h

- Nutrition is important to provide amino acids for wound healing.
  - When routinely withholding food to facilitate sedation for daily wound care, it can be difficult to provide enough nutrition.
  - Long-term opioid use decreases appetite and creates ileus, leading to inappetence and anorexia.
  - Many animals require a temporary feeding tube, such as a nasogastric or nasoesophageal tube, or even an esophagostomy tube to administer enough nutrition. (See *Further reading* for information on placing feeding tubes.)
  - Start feeding animals immediately after sedation/anesthesia for wound care and withhold food for as short a period of time as possible prior to repeated sedation/anesthesia events.
  - If tolerated, bolus feeding via a feeding tube rather than CRI may promote more complete provision of nutrition per day.
  - Coordinate the need for food with the need for sedation for bandage changes and wound care to allow both things to occur.

NEUROLOGIC EMERGENCIES

The most common neurologic emergencies include head trauma, seizures, or spinal cord disease.

- Basic triage of these patients is the same as indicated above. This should be performed regardless of the neurologic status and prior to or concurrent with specific treatment of the neurologic disease.
- Seizure management is the next priority.
  - Animals having active seizures are first given diazepam (0.5 mg/kg IV or 1–2 mg/kg per rectum) or midazolam (0.5 mg/kg IV, IM, or intranasal).
  - Long-term antiepileptic treatment, such as levetiracetam (20 mg/kg IV or PO q8 h) or phenobarbital (loading dose 16–20 mg/kg IV or PO followed by 2.5–3 mg/kg PO q12 h), is commenced immediately after the

diazepam or midazolam therapy. This reduces the risk of further seizures occurring when the short-acting benzodiazepines wear off in ~20 minutes.

- Concerns for an increase in intracranial pressure must be addressed.
  - Clinical signs include a decline in mental status or abnormalities in cranial nerves such as anisocoria, absent gag, lack of pupillary light responses, or lack of physiologic nystagmus.
  - Some animals display the Cushing's reflex (bradycardia with hypertension with marked elevation in intracranial pressure).
  - Treatment includes mannitol 0.5–1 g/kg IV over 20–30 minutes or hypertonic saline (4 ml/kg) as a bolus.
  - Do not give mannitol unless the patient is cardiovascularly stable. Hypertonic saline will transiently increase intravascular volume and can be used in unstable patients with increased intracranial pressure.
- Longer-term care in the ICU:
  - Sedation may be required for the neurologic patient that is anxious or in danger of injuring itself. Examples include the dog with intervertebral disk disease that is restless or moving in its cage or spinal trauma/fracture cases that will not rest comfortably. Many dogs that have had seizures are anxious.
    - Sedation includes anxiolytics such as acepromazine or trazodone +/– pain medications (see Chapter 9).
    - Avoid NSAIDs acutely when there is concern about decreased perfusion to the brain, kidneys, or GI tract.
    - Long term, dogs may become less responsive to sedative drugs (especially acepromazine) and require increasing drug dosages.
      - Beware of continually adding drugs or increasing drug dosages in animals that are not responsive to sedatives.

At some point, the animal could become dysphoric, which in turn can cause anxiety.
- Too much sedation can decrease nutritional intake. If the need for sedation outweighs the importance of oral food intake, a feeding tube should be used.
- Pain management is indicated long term for neurologic conditions including spinal cord fracture and intervertebral disk disease.
  - These cases should be managed acutely with opioids and NSAIDs (once cardiovascular stability has been achieved) (see Chapter 24).
  - Longer-term pain medications include opioid-derivatives such as tramadol or acetaminophen with codeine (in dogs only) and NSAIDs. Gabapentin can also be used for neuropathic pain (see Chapter 26).
  - Oral opioids used long term for pain often cause less appetite suppression than injectable opioids.
  - When opioids are used chronically (see *Tables 20.2, 20.3*), ileus can occur. This leads to decreased appetite or constipation. Since most dogs and cats do not receive full mu agonist drugs long term, this side-effect is less common in animals than humans.

RESPIRATORY EMERGENCIES

Common presentations include pleural space disease (effusions, pneumothorax), upper or lower airway conditions, and parenchymal lung disease (e.g. pneumonia, edema).
- Oxygen should be provided to all patients in respiratory distress.
  - Initially if tolerated, provide oxygen by mask. Holding the tubing in front of the nose is less effective in raising inhaled FiO_2 (see **Figs. 20.2, 20.4**).
  - For long-term ICU care, use nasal cannulas, oxygen cages, or oxygen hoods/tents to provide oxygen (see **Figs. 20.2–20.4**).
    - It is ideal to monitor the temperature, humidity, and oxygen levels within any oxygen cage/space.
    - Heat and humidity commonly increase within oxygen enclosures and create patient discomfort and stress.
  - Serially monitor the patient's oxygen level via SpO_2 or arterial blood gas to determine effectiveness of the oxygen supplementation.
    - Visual clues such as cyanosis are only apparent in non-anemic patients at severe levels of hypoxemia (SpO_2 <75%).
    - Monitor the animal's breathing to identify respiratory patterns that might lead to exhaustion including increased respiratory effort.
  - Patients requiring >60% FiO_2 for longer than 12–24 hours are at risk of oxygen toxicity.
  - Offer mechanical ventilation if available when there is prolonged increased respiratory effort or hypoxemia (PaO_2 <60 mmHg or SpO_2 <90%) despite oxygen supplementation (**Fig. 20.5**).

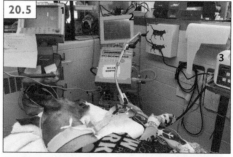

Fig. 20.5 Patient on a mechanical ventilator. The dog has a tracheostomy tube in place, which is in turn attached to the ventilator tubing. Note that ventilator patients receive continual monitoring including end-tidal carbon dioxide, pulse oximetry, and invasive blood pressure. They also receive multiple injectable medications to provide for sedation/analgesia via syringe pumps. (1) invasive blood pressure; (2) ventilation parameters; (3) enteral nutrition.

- Avoid stress in all respiratory distress patients
  - Dyspnea can induce panic and increase the effort of breathing.
    - Mild to moderate sedation in patients with respiratory distress can reduce panic, allow animals to take more effective breaths through compromised airways, and facilitate medical procedures.
    - It is unlikely that a strong respiratory drive will be overridden by appropriate doses of opioids for sedation and/or pain.
    - If an animal is nearing respiratory exhaustion or hypoxemia is not relieved with oxygen therapy, intubation may be necessary +/- positive pressure ventilation (see below).
- **Upper airway emergencies** include brachycephalic airway disease and laryngeal paralysis.
  - Animals with mild to moderate difficulty moving air can be managed with oxygen, external cooling if hyperthermic, and sedation.
    - Butorphanol (0.2–0.4 mg/kg) +/- acepromazine (0.01–0.05 mg/kg with a maximum of 3 mg) IV or IM are commonly used to relax animals with upper airway obstructions.
    - Use a pure mu opioid in place of butorphanol if the cause of the upper airway obstruction is painful (e.g. bite wounds).
- Patients may require repeated dosing with sedative drugs to relieve stress and prevent further airway crises over time.
  - Butorphanol can be administered as a CRI (0.1–0.4 mg/kg/h).
  - Trazodone is given PO to reduce anxiety long term, starting at 2–5 mg/kg q8–12 h and can be titrated up to 20 mg/kg/day. Rarely, high doses of trazodone can lead to serotonin syndrome. This occurs only if the animal is concurrently receiving high doses of drugs that elevate serotonin levels (e.g. tramadol or selective serotonin reuptake inhibitors such as fluoxetine).
- Intubate animals with severe upper airway obstruction.
  - Give intravenous propofol to effect to facilitate intubation.
  - A propofol CRI is used short term to maintain intubation while pursuing further diagnostics.
  - Perform an emergency tracheostomy if oral intubation is not possible (**Fig. 20.6**) (see Chapter 11 and *Further reading*).

20.6

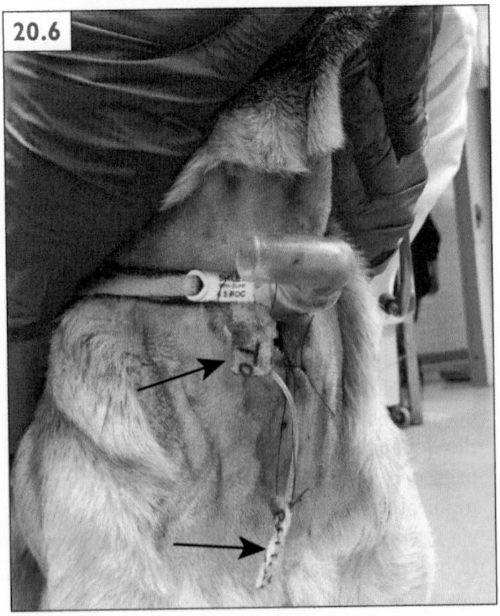

Fig. 20.6 Patient with a tracheostomy tube to relieve an upper airway obstruction. Note that there is a right-angle adaptor on the end of the tracheostomy tube in the patient, which helps to allow the animal to breath normally even when resting with the neck on the ground or the bedding. There are also two tape tags attached to sutures placed in the cartilage rings proximal and distal to the tracheostomy site (arrows), which allow the tracheostomy tube to be replaced. (The animal in **Fig. 20.5** also has a tracheostomy tube attached to the ventilator tubing.) Tracheostomy tubes easily accumulate secretions (as shown) and frequent care is necessary to maintain a patent airway.

– Perform anesthetic monitoring while the animal is heavily sedated/intubated (see Chapter 6).
– Drugs needed to maintain intubation often compromise ventilation. The patient may require assisted ventilation by hand (Ambu bag, anesthesia bag) or mechanical ventilation (see Chapter 11 and *Further reading*).
- If **pleural space disease** (i.e. pneumothorax or pleural effusion) is suspected based on physical examination (heart and lung sounds are muffled along with an inspiratory dyspnea) and history (i.e. trauma cases), emergency thoracocentesis can be life-saving (see *Further reading* for instructions on performing thoracocentesis) (**Fig. 20.7**).
  - Point-of-care ultrasound or radiographs help to detect effusion and guide thoracocentesis but are not necessary prior to thoracocentesis when there is a high level of clinical suspicion.
  - Repeated drainage of fluid or air indicates the necessity for a chest tube.
    – Typically, heavy sedation or preferably brief general anesthesia is used to place chest tubes.
    – Be aware that giving positive-pressure breaths under general anesthesia will rapidly worsen a pneumothorax. Perform thoracocentesis immediately prior to induction of general anesthesia. Collect all supplies for chest tube placement prior to induction of anesthesia.

- Longer-term care in the ICU for all respiratory patients:
  - Oxygen is often required for several days depending on the reason for the respiratory distress.
  - Ongoing or repeated sedation may be needed to reduce stress until definitive therapy is achieved.
  - Sedation protocols used for animals with upper respiratory disease (see above) can be utilized in any respiratory patient.

CARDIOVASCULAR EMERGENCIES

The most common presenting cardiovascular emergencies in small animal patients are right- or left-sided heart failure, pericardial effusions, and arrhythmias.
- With the possible exception of pericardial effusion, IV fluids are contraindicated for patients in heart failure.
- Low stress handling, provision of oxygen, and a single dose of furosemide (1–2 mg/kg IV or IM) is indicated if there is a high level of suspicion for left-sided congestive heart failure in a respiratory distressed animal.
- Mild sedation for animals in respiratory distress (see below) may facilitate diagnostics and handling.
- For patients in severe distress, the animal should be intubated and ventilated.
- In right-sided heart failure, if pleural and pericardial fluid accumulations compromise breathing, a therapeutic tap is indicated
- In cases of pericardial effusion, pericardiocentesis can be painful.

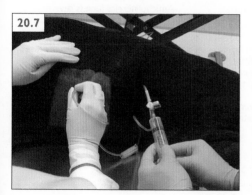

20.7

Fig. 20.7 Thoracocentesis is performed in dogs and cats cranial to the rib (to avoid the neurovascular bundle) in the 7th–9th rib space. A closed collection system (shown here) including a needle or catheter, extension set, 3-way stopcock, and syringe prevents movement of air into the chest and reduces the risk of contamination of the pleural space or the diagnostic sample (if fluid) during the procedure.

- Sedation with butorphanol (0.2–0.4 mg/kg IV or IM) and local anesthetic at the site of the tap is used to facilitate pericardiocentesis.
- In severely compromised animals, local block alone is often enough.
- Avoid sedative/anesthetic drugs that may exacerbate common causes of heart disease (*Table 20.4*). Benzodiazepines and opioids are generally good choices for sedation of most cardiac patients as they have the least effect on cardiac parameters and can be reversed if necessary (see Chapter 3).
- For heavier sedation in patients that need brief procedures, low doses of propofol, etomidate, or alfaxalone can be titrated in addition to benzodiazepines/opioids, but ventilation, oxygenation, and blood pressure should be closely monitored (see Chapter 4).
- General anesthesia should be avoided in patients in heart failure if possible.

For patients with stable underlying heart disease requiring anesthesia, anesthetic plans should be tailored to the underlying disease process and appropriate monitoring and supportive medications (e.g. positive inotropes) should be available (*Table 20.4*, see Chapter 6).
- Longer-term care in the ICU:
- Oxygen therapy.
- Continuous ECG monitoring for detection and treatment of significant arrhythmias (see Chapter 6 and *Further reading* for specifics of arrhythmia treatments).
- Long-term sedation (see above) to avoid stress.
- Monitoring of electrolytes (especially potassium) and renal values at least daily if patients are on diuretic therapy.
  - Supplement electrolytes as needed orally or in IV fluids.
  - If IV fluids are needed to maintain hydration, supplement electrolytes

Table 20.4 Considerations for sedative drugs with specific cardiac diseases (see Chapter 10)

Cardiovascular disease	Physiology	Drugs to restrict/avoid
Mitral valve endocardiosis	Most common cause of congestive heart failure in medium to small breed dogs Regurgitation of blood through a leaky mitral valve during systole increases left atrial volume/pressure and can lead to hydrostatic overload and pulmonary edema As long as the patient is not already hypotensive, drugs that decrease afterload (e.g. acepromazine) may help reduce regurgitant jet volume	Dexmedetomidine: increased afterload and bradycardia Anticholinergics (unless severe bradycardia): increased myocardial oxygen demand, arrhythmias High doses of inhaled anesthetics; use a balanced approach to general anesthesia to reduce inhalants as much as possible
Dilated cardiomyopathy (DCM)	Common in large/giant breed dogs and occasionally in cats Reduced cardiac contractility results in decreased cardiac output Tachycardia and bradycardia are detrimental Mitral regurgitation often occurs secondary to DCM	High doses of inhaled anesthetics; use a balanced approach to general anesthesia to reduce inhalants Dexmedetomidine: decreased contractility, bradycardia, and increased afterload Anticholinergics (unless severe bradycardia): increased myocardial oxygen demand, arrhythmias
Hypertrophic cardiomyopathy	Common, especially in hyperthyroid cats Increased stiffness of the ventricular wall reduces ventricular filling in diastole Avoid increases in contractility, tachycardia, and vasodilation Decreased afterload may worsen systolic anterior motion of the mitral valve	Ketamine/Telazol/xylazine: increased contractility and tachycardia Acepromazine: vasodilation/decreased afterload Anticholinergics (unless severe bradycardia): increased myocardial oxygen demand, arrhythmias, tachycardia High doses of inhaled anesthetics; use a balanced approach to general anesthesia to reduce inhalants as much as possible

or provide IV drugs, use the smallest possible volumes of low sodium (5% dextrose in water, 0.45% sodium chloride) fluids to avoid volume overload.

- Placement of short-term feeding tubes (nasoesophageal or nasogastric) can maintain hydration and provide electrolytes and nutrition more safely than IV fluids in patients not eating and drinking voluntarily.

METABOLIC DISORDERS

Metabolic disorders include electrolyte disturbances, severe acidosis/alkalosis, and hypoglycemia.

- It is common for animals with metabolic disturbances to need some form of sedation/anesthesia within hours of arrival to facilitate instrumentation (e.g. urinary catheterization, central venous catheter placement, dialysis catheters).
- It is important to normalize metabolic abnormalities in these patients prior to sedation/anesthesia to avoid catastrophic complications including cardiac arrest.
- Metabolic abnormalities may exacerbate anesthetic complications such as arrhythmias and hypotension and should be identified and addressed promptly (**Fig. 20.8**) prior to or during sedation/anesthesia.

Electrolyte disturbances

- **Hyperkalemia** is common secondary to acute kidney injury, post renal obstruction, or hypoadrenocorticism (Addison's disease).
  - Hyperkalemia raises the resting membrane potential of a cell leading to an inability to depolarize.
  - The primary life-threatening sequela is cardiac dysfunction: bradycardia, arrhythmias, and hypotension. Classic ECG changes (tall, tented T waves, increased P-R interval, loss of P waves, and widening of the QRS complex [see Chapter 22]) may be noted.
  - Hyperkalemia should be treated if the potassium level is >8 mmol/l (mEq/l) or at lower levels if animals are clinically affected (*Table 20.5*).
- **Hypokalemia** most commonly occurs secondary to high-volume urinary diuresis or therapy with medications such as furosemide.
  - Hypokalemia causes muscular weakness, decreased ability to concentrate urine (which further exacerbates potassium loss), arrhythmias, and metabolic acidosis.
  - Supplementation is usually with KCl, although potassium phosphates can be used if phosphorus supplementation is also desired, as in diabetic ketoacidosis (DKA) therapy (see *Further reading*).

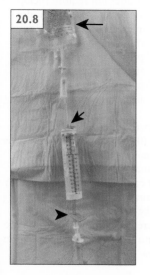

Fig. 20.8 A burette can be filled with up to 150 ml of fluids from the upper bag (arrow). Various medication additives are injected directly into the burette from the top ports (short arrow); when the concentration of additives is changed or when the burette is empty, the burette/line to patient is emptied, new additives added, and the burette filled to the desired volume from the upper bag. The new fluid is run through the line before reconnection to the patient. The burette is labeled (yellow sticker) to indicate the current additive concentration in the burette. The arrowhead designates a clamp that is closed to ensure the contents of the burette are properly mixed before administration to the patient. The clamp is opened when the contents of the burette are being given to an animal.

Table 20.5 Therapeutics for treatment of hyperkalemia

Drug	Mechanism of action	Dose
IV fluid therapy	Dilutes potassium and increases urinary potassium excretion through improved glomerular filtration rate Any isotonic crystalloid is effective, including 0.9% NaCl	See IV fluids in basic triage section as well as acute kidney injury section
10% calcium gluconate	Transiently restores cellular electrical gradients to allow for continued cellular (cardiac myocyte) depolarization Does not lower serum potassium levels	0.5–1.5 ml/kg IV slowly over 5–10 minutes with ECG monitoring Duration of effect ~20 minutes
Regular (short-acting) insulin + dextrose	Translocates potassium into the intracellular space	0.25–0.5 U/kg with a 1 ml/kg bolus of 25% dextrose To avoid hypoglycemia, subsequent fluid therapy should contain dextrose supplementation for the next 4 hours
Sodium bicarbonate	Translocates potassium intracellularly in exchange for H^+ ions Reserved for severely acidemic patients (pH <7.0)	1–2 mmol (mEq)/kg IV slowly over 15 minutes Rebound alkalosis and elevations in $PaCO_2$ can occur
Terbutaline	Stimulates Na/K/ATPase pump to translocate potassium intracellularly	0.01 mg/kg IV slowly

Table 20.6 Recommended potassium supplementation rates

Serum potassium level (mmol [mEq]/l)	Recommended supplementation (mmol [mEq]/kg/h)
<2.0	0.5 or greater (with monitoring)
2.1–2.5	0.4–0.5
2.6–3.0	0.3–0.4
3.1–3.5	0.2
3.6–5.0	None or 0.1

- A sliding scale is often used to determine supplementation rates based on potassium deficits (*Table 20.6*).
- Rates >0.5 mmol (mEq)/kg/h should only be administered with careful ECG monitoring to avoid arrhythmias.
- Concentrations >80 mmol/l (mEq/l) should not be given peripherally to avoid phlebitis.

- **Hypercalcemia** can cause polyuria/polydipsia, weakness, GI upset, seizures/tremors, or even death secondary to arrhythmias or seizure activity.

Over time, hypercalcemia can lead to renal failure by organ mineralization.

- Organ mineralization is hastened by concurrent high phosphorus levels, especially when the calcium/phosphorus product is >600 mg/l (60 mg/dl).
- Definitive therapy requires treatment of the underlying cause.
- Acute therapy is outlined in *Table 20.7.*
- **Hypocalcemia** does not require therapy if the decrease is mild and the patient does not exhibit clinical signs. Clinical signs (occurring with severe hypocalcemia) include facial pruritus, tremors/seizures, behavioral changes (agitation/excitation), pyrexia, weakness, polyuria/polydipsia, or even myocardial failure and respiratory arrest.
- Emergency treatment: 10% calcium gluconate (0.5–1.5 ml/kg IV slowly over 10–15 minutes while monitoring ECG.
- 10% Calcium gluconate contains 9.3 mg of calcium/ml. If continued IV supplementation is needed, a CRI of 1–3 mg/kg/hour of calcium can be administered. Use 0.9% NaCl to dilute the calcium so as to avoid precipitation in IV lines.

Table 20.7 Therapeutics for treatment of hypercalcemia

Drug	Mechanism of action	Dose
IV fluid therapy	Dilutes the calcium concentration Increases calcium excretion through the kidney 0.9% NaCl is the fluid of choice; the high sodium content increases renal calciuresis	See IV fluids in basic triage section as well as acute kidney injury section
Furosemide	Enhanced urinary calcium wasting	2 mg/kg q8–12 h or 2 mg/kg bolus followed by 0.5 mg/kg/hour CRI Do not allow patients to become dehydrated during this therapy
Glucocorticoids	Reduce bone resorption, decrease intestinal uptake, increase renal excretion of calcium	1 mg/kg prednisone equivalent per day May confound later diagnostics for underlying cause (e.g. lymphoma) if unknown
Bisphosphonates (e.g. pamidronate)	Decrease osteoclast activity	Dose dependent on exact drug used Renal failure is a side-effect
Calcitonin	Decreases activity and function of osteoclasts	4–8 U/kg SC q12–24 h

- Long-term, oral supplementation with calcium carbonate (Tums®) at 25–50 mg/kg/day.
- **Hypernatremia/hyponatremia**. Gains or losses of free water lead to changes in sodium concentration (see *Further reading*).
  - While severe sodium derangements cause clinical signs regardless of timing, clinical signs typically depend more on how rapidly the sodium levels have changed rather than actual sodium concentrations.
  - The majority of complications come from overly-rapid correction of sodium levels (see *Further reading* for more details).

Severe acid–base disorders
- Severe acid–base disorders compromise anesthesia and sedation by compromising cardiac output, blood pressure, and oxygen delivery by hemoglobin.
- Acid–base disorders may predispose to arrhythmias, seizures, neurologic depression, and muscle weakness.
- Sedation and anesthesia can result in acid–base abnormalities if tissue perfusion or ventilation is affected by drugs.
- Definitive treatment is always focused on resolution of the underlying disease process resulting in the acid–base disturbance; rarely, treatment may focus on the acid–base condition itself (e.g. administration of bicarbonate) if the underlying problem is not easily resolved (see *Further reading*).
- Respiratory acidosis is caused by hypoventilation. Ventilation can be improved by increasing the rate or tidal volume of breaths given while under general anesthesia or removing the underlying cause (e.g. reverse drugs causing respiratory depression).
- Respiratory alkalosis is caused by hyperventilation. The underlying cause of the hyperventilation (e.g. hyperthermia, pain, hypoxemia, CNS disease, drugs) should be removed/treated.
- Metabolic acidosis is secondary to bicarbonate loss or excessive organic acids in the body (e.g. hypoperfuson/hyperlactatemia, DKA, renal failure, or toxins such as ethylene glycol). Mainstays of treatment include IV fluid therapy but might include bicarbonate (see *Further reading*).
- Metabolic alkalosis results from GI losses (e.g. vomiting from an upper GI obstruction) or use of bicarbonate or diuretics. Treatment includes IV fluid therapy and treatment of the underlying cause.

Hypoglycemia
- Hypoglycemia causes neurologic signs such as dullness, weakness, and seizure activity. Severe, prolonged hypoglycemia can contribute to cardiovascular dysfunction, bradycardia, and signs of shock.
  - To avoid iatrogenic hypoglycemia, animals with diabetes mellitus who are fasted for general anesthesia are commonly given half their normal insulin dose on the morning of anesthesia.
  - Consider reduced fasting times (3–4 hours) and prophylactic dextrose supplementation in juvenile toy-breed dogs prior to anesthesia.
  - If hypoglycemia (blood glucose <3.7 mmol/l [67 mg/dl]) is noted, administer 0.5–1 ml/kg of 25% dextrose as an IV bolus.
  - After the bolus or in patients at high risk for hypoglycemia, supplementation of IV fluids with 2.5–5% dextrose is warranted.
  - Encourage small, frequent meals once the patient is able to eat.

RENAL DISEASES
Common examples of renal diseases in emergency cases and in the ICU include acute kidney injury, chronic kidney disease, and medullary washout occurring from diseases such as DKA and after relieving urinary obstructions.

Kidney injury and failure
- These cases can present through the emergency room as relatively stable animals with clinical signs related to anorexia, vomiting, and malaise.
- Many ICU patients develop renal injury or failure as a consequence of being critically ill and/or while being treated for their illness.
- Diagnosis is based on elevations in BUN, creatinine, phosphorus, and possibly potassium seen on blood work, together with isosthenuria (i.e. urine specific gravity 1.008–1.012). In some cases, the urine specific gravity is not isosthenuric but significantly lower than one would expect with prerenal azotemia.

- If patients are able to produce urine, treatment is initiated with IV fluids at rates calculated to replace the dehydration noted on the physical examination plus additional fluids to create diuresis.
  - Monitoring of electrolytes daily is important to avoid complications such as hypokalemia and to ensure that elevated electrolytes (i.e. hyperphosphatemia) are normalizing.
  - Placement of a urinary catheter to quantify the urine production is useful to ensure the animal's urine production is not exceeding the administered fluid volume (**Fig. 20.9**).
- If patients are unable to produce urine at the expected amounts (i.e. at least 0.5 ml/kg/h), management is more complex.
  - A urinary catheter must be placed to quantify urine production.

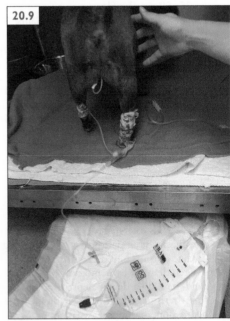

20.9

Fig. 20.9 A female dog with an indwelling Foley urinary catheter and a closed urinary collection system. The catheter is sutured to the body wall as well as secured to the left hind limb to prevent accidental removal by the patient. The patient is also wearing an e-collar (not shown).

- The amount of fluids given is matched to the amount of urine produced to avoid fluid overload.
- Close monitoring of electrolyte levels (especially potassium) is critical to avoid life-threatening electrolyte imbalances when the potassium levels increase above 7 mmol/l (mEq/l).
- Drug therapy for kidney injury/failure:
  - Gastric protectants (e.g. histamine blockers such as famotidine or hydrogen ion pump blockers such as pantoprazole) are given routinely. Gastric protectants improve uremia and reduce gastric ulcer formation.
  - Antiemetics (e.g. maropitant) may be given for nausea.
  - Antihypertensives (e.g. amlodipine) are given to control hypertension concurrent with the renal disease.
  - Pain management is not typical in renal injury/failure unless the patient is receiving analgesia for another problem (e.g. a postoperative patient with concurrent renal disease).
    - Opioids are the drug of choice for pain in renal failure patients. Full mu agonists such as fentanyl, hydromorphone, and methadone are good choices (see Chapter 3).
    - DO NOT use NSAIDs in renal injury/failure patients as they will worsen the renal injury.
    - Additional sedation/analgesia, such as a lidocaine and/or ketamine CRI, will further depress appetite/worsen nausea in animals already nauseous and anorexic from their renal disease.
    - Be aware that if drugs are renally excreted (e.g. ketamine), they will have a longer half-life in renal failure patients. Reduced doses can be considered (e.g. 25% less than published doses).
- Select sedative drugs that have the least chance of reducing blood flow to the kidneys and causing further renal tubular damage.
  - Mixing an opioid with a benzodiazepine such as diazepam or midazolam is the best combination (see Chapter 9).

- Typically, the authors use diazepam (or midazolam) at 0.2 mg/kg with a full mu agonist opioid.
- If further sedation is needed, small doses of an alpha-2 agonist (e.g. dexmedetomidine), which should preserve renal blood flow, can be given to effect (see Chapter 9).
- Exercise caution with sedative drugs such as acepromazine that will vasodilate indiscriminately, thus reducing renal perfusion and filtration.
- If general anesthesia is required, care must be taken to minimize reductions in renal blood flow (see Chapter 10).

Medullary washout
- Medullary washout occurs when the gradient of urea and sodium that normally exists in the renal medulla is lost. This commonly occurs secondary to severe polyuria post urinary obstruction or due to osmotic diuresis as in DKA.
- Medullary washout leads to an inability to concentrate the urine and production of large amounts of dilute urine.
- The greatest concern is development of new/worsening dehydration if IV fluid therapy is not adequate to keep up with urinary losses. This situation can lead to prerenal azotemia.
- Quantifying and replacing ongoing urine volume loss is important. Ideally, a urinary catheter should be placed and urine collected and quantified.
  - Once the patient is well hydrated and any prerenal azotemia has resolved, the urine volume is replaced with the same volume of IV fluids.
  - If a urinary catheter cannot be placed, urine output is roughly estimated by weighing bedding or litter boxes and/or attempting to catch and measure voided urine.
  - Weigh the patient at least 2–3 times daily.
    - Rapid changes in daily weight represent body water gained or lost, not body mass.
    - Remember 1 liter of water weighs 1 kg.

- Medullary washout will improve over days to weeks if the kidney is able to re-establish the gradient
  - To determine if medullary washout has improved, reduce fluid administration by 10–25% for 4–6 hours to observe the urine production during that time.
    - If the urine production drops to match the reduced fluid administration, the medullary gradient has been re-established. Continue to wean down the IV fluid amount every 4–6 hours until the desired fluid rate is obtained (often maintenance fluid rates).
    - If urine production remains unchanged or otherwise significantly exceeds the IV fluids given during the 4–6 hour period, increase the IV fluids to match the urine produced for another 12–24 hours. Then reduce the IV fluids again and observe the urine production.
      - If urine production matches the new IV fluid amount, continue to wean off the fluids every 4–6 hours.
      - If the urine production continues to exceed the fluid given, rematch the fluids to the urine and wait an additional 12–24 hours before trying to wean the fluids again.
  - Drug administration in medullary washout:
    - Animals with medullary washout may have azotemia due to prerenal causes (excessive fluid loss through the kidney). However, kidney function is normal.

- No specific medications are given for medullary washout.
- If nausea or increased gastric acidity is suspected secondary to the presence of azotemia, antiemetics such as maropitant, histamine blockers such as famotidine, or hydrogen pump inhibitors such as pantoprazole can be used.
- Sedation drugs are normally metabolized and excreted with medullary washout. Therefore, theoretically there are no limitations to the use of sedative drugs.
  - The authors often use combinations of full mu agonist opioids and benzodiazepines if the animals are extremely compromised due to their underlying disease (see above under Kidney injury and failure).
  - If the animals are minimally metabolically compromised (e.g. dog with a urethral obstruction and no changes on blood work), then normal sedation combinations can be used (see Chapter 9).
- The long-term ability of the kidneys to metabolize drugs should be unchanged in medullary washout, so there are theoretically no limitations on the analgesic or sedation drugs used long term in the ICU. NSAIDs should be avoided until any azotemia present on blood work has been corrected in the event that azotemia is due to pre-existing renal disease. NSAIDs should not be used in animals with renal disease.

Further reading

Balsa IM, Culp WT (2015) Wound care. *Vet Clin North Am Small Anim Prac* **45**:1049–65.

DeFrancesco TC (2013) Management of cardiac emergencies in small animals. *Vet Clin North Am Small Anim Prac* **43**:817–42.

Dibartola SP (2006) *Fluid, Electrolyte, and Acid–Base Disorders*, 4th edn. Elsevier Saunders, St. Louis.

Han E (2004) Esophageal and gastric feeding tubes in ICU patients. *Clin Tech Small Anim Prac* **19**:22–31.

Holahan M, Abood S, Hauptman J et al. (2010) Intermittent and continuous enteral nutrition in critically ill dogs: a prospective randomized trial. *J Vet Intern Med* **24**:520–6.

Hopper K, Powell LL (2013) Basics of mechanical ventilation for dogs and cats. *Vet Clin North Am Small Anim Prac* **43**:955–69.

Huang A, Scott-Moncrieff JC (2011) Canine diabetic ketoacidosis. *NAVC Clinician's Brief* **April**:68–70

Swaim SF, Renberg WC, Shike KM (2011) *Small Animal Bandaging, Casting, and Splinting Techniques.* Wiley-Blackwell, Ames.

Tseng LW, Waddel LS (2000) Approach to the patient in respiratory distress. *Clin Tech Small Anim Prac* **15**:53–62.

Waddell MS, Michel KE (1998) Critical care nutrition: routes of feeding. *Clin Tech Small Anim Prac* **13**: 197–203.

Ware WA (2007) *Cardiovascular Disease in Small Animal Medicine.* Manson Publishing, London.

Anesthetic emergencies and cardiopulmonary resuscitation

Ann B Weil and Jeff C Ko

Introduction

Despite careful attention when monitoring the anesthetized patient, emergencies related to general anesthesia can and do occur. Most anesthetic emergencies can be divided into two groups:

- Unexpected crises that develop in normal, healthy patients presented for elective surgeries. These are often related to the anesthetic machine and equipment errors and may be prevented with careful management.
- Events that develop as a result of the drugs given to produce general anesthesia. The side-effects of these drugs can be life-threatening.

This chapter reviews the most common life-threatening emergencies associated with anesthesia and their treatment.

Respiratory complications that result in anesthetic emergencies

APNEA

- Apnea (**Fig. 21.1**) is most often induced by IV induction agents.
- Apnea can occur with any agent, including thiopentone, propofol, alfaxalone, etomidate, or ketamine.
- It is most likely to occur when large doses of the drug are administered in a rapid bolus.
- Propofol, etomidate, or alfaxalone should be administered slowly and

'to effect', minimizing the potential for apnea (see also Chapter 4). Thiopentone can cause some stage II excitement at subanesthetic dosing.

- Transient apnea is not usually a major concern if the patient can be intubated and ventilated.
- Apnea is a significant clinical concern when the airway cannot be controlled, intubated, and ventilated (see also Chapter 11).

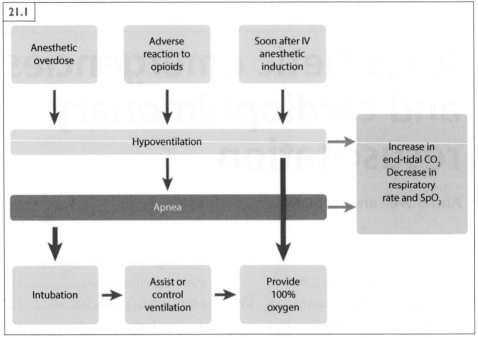

Fig. 21.1 Diagrammatic representation of the relationship between anesthetic-induced hypoventilation and apnea.

HYPOVENTILATION

- Every anesthetized patient hypoventilates as a result of CNS depression of the respiratory system imposed by the anesthetic drug (**Fig. 21.1**). The medullary respiratory center may not respond to higher levels of CO_2 with increased ventilation.
- Hypoventilation is an insidious problem, as most veterinarians and technicians assume that an adequate respiratory rate and respiratory efforts equate to adequate alveolar ventilation and gas exchange.
- The amount of gas exchanged with each breath (tidal volume) has two components: dead space gas and alveolar ventilation.
- Dead space gas is the air that is in the conducting airways and is not available for gas exchange. It remains relatively constant and is the first gas in and out of the mouth or nasal passages, trachea, and other conducting units of the respiratory tree.

- Under general anesthesia, tidal volume decreases and dead space gas remains the same, so alveolar ventilation must decrease.
- Hypoventilation can be confirmed by observing $ETCO_2$ values >45 mmHg and less frequent respiratory efforts (either rate, tidal volume, or both).
- Capnometers are useful monitors for the diagnosis of hypoventilation (see also Chapter 6).
- Mechanical ventilators may be used to prevent or treat hypoventilation during general anesthesia (see also Chapter 11).
- Assisting ventilation by occasional squeezing of the reservoir bag (sighing) may help prevent hypoventilation and atelectasis.
- Hypercarbia may also result from anesthetic equipment malfunction (see Chapter 6).

LOSS OF AIRWAY

- Loss of airway is a condition that has resulted in the deaths of many otherwise healthy patients and is a primary reason for anesthetic emergencies in all species. Loss of control of the airway, especially when unrecognized by the anesthetist, leads to problems due to the CNS depression and respiratory depression imposed by general anesthetics. Some examples of conditions that can lead to patient mortality include:

- Inadvertent extubation and placement of the endotracheal tube (ETT) into the esophagus.
- ETT occlusion by mucus plugs or blood.
- Kinking of the ETT.
- Overinflation of the ETT cuff.
- ETT is too short.
- ETT is too long, resulting in one-lung ventilation from improper tube placement.
- See Chapter 11 (Airway management and ventilation) for further information.

HYPOXEMIA

- Hypoxemia is a common complication of general anesthesia. The five major causes of hypoxemia or low arterial oxygen tensions (PaO_2) include:
  - Low inspired oxygen concentration most commonly occurs with equipment failures and errors. For example, the oxygen flow meter is inadvertently turned off or an ETT becomes kinked or obstructed. A common manifestation of this occurrence is the patient who appears to be 'waking up' or is mistaken to be at a lighter plane of anesthesia. Hypoxia will cause a ventilatory drive when PaO_2 levels are <50–60 mmHg and the gasping behavior of the severely hypoxic patient can mimic arousal.
  - Hypoventilation, especially when FiO_2 (inspiratory fraction of oxygen) = 21% (room air). Oxygen supplementation should be considered in patients undergoing injectable anesthetics (e.g. IM Telazol® or ketamine in cats). Hypoxia secondary to hypoventilation while breathing room air can lead to prolonged recovery and adverse

consequences such as blindness when cerebral blood flow and oxygen delivery are compromised during a general anesthesia.
- Barriers to diffusion of respiratory gases result from problems such as pneumothorax or pulmonary edema. Oxygen is usually affected first, since CO_2 is about 20 times more soluble than oxygen. Pulmonary edema, pleural effusion, and pneumothorax should be corrected as much as possible prior to general anesthesia. Occasionally, occult conditions will manifest during the course of general anesthesia and must be handled during the procedure.
- Ventilation–perfusion (V/Q) mismatch occurs in small animal patients, but with less frequency than in large animals. V/Q mismatch can be seen with embolic events.
- A right-to-left cardiac shunt (e.g. reversed PDA or tetralogy of Fallot) can occur.
- Patient oxygenation can be monitored via pulse oximetry or blood gas analysis. Pulse oximetry is more frequently used as it is economical, non-invasive, continuous, and easy to apply to the patient.
- The administration of positive end expiratory pressure (PEEP) (see Chapter 11) can be helpful in the hypoxemic patient, as it increases alveolar participation in gas exchange and may recruit collapsed alveoli.
- Desaturation events or low SpO_2 occur with the following situations:
  - Apnea.
  - Severe hypoxia.
  - Inadvertent bronchial intubation.
  - Embolic events.
  - Pulmonary edema.
  - Pleural effusion.
  - Hypoventilation if not breathing 100% oxygen.
  - Anaphylaxis.
  - Bronchospasm.
  - Low cardiac output.

LARYNGOSPASM

- See Chapter 11.

Cardiovascular complications that result in anesthetic emergencies

BRADYCARDIA (FIG. 21.2)
- General heart rate guidelines under inhalant anesthesia:
  - Large dogs: approximately 60 beats per minute (bpm).
  - Small dogs and cats: 80–90 bpm.
  - Puppies and kittens will need to maintain a higher heart rate than an adult animal.
  - Blood pressure monitoring can be a useful to guide therapy. If the heart rate is borderline low with good blood pressure, additional intervention may not be necessary.
- Many of the drugs used as adjuncts to anesthesia increase vagal tone (e.g. opioids, alpha-2 agonists).
- Many surgical treatments can stimulate vagal tone as well (e.g. airway surgery, ocular surgery, bladder surgery).
- Cardiac output is the product of stroke volume and heart rate. If the heart rate becomes critically low, output will suffer, especially under the conditions of general anesthesia, as stroke volume is already reduced by the anesthetic agents.
- If the heart rate is already faster then normal, increasing the heart rate drastically will not increase the patient's cardiac output and will compromise myocardial oxygenation.
- Anticholinergic drugs such as atropine or glycopyrrolate are appropriate therapy for bradycardia of vagal origin:
  - They can be administered IV or IM.
  - They are often administered IV in critical situations.
  - They may be administered IM for prevention of bradycardia when opioids are used.
- Heart rate under general anesthesia should be higher than if the patient was not anesthetized, as anesthetic drugs depress contractility and decrease venous return in addition to their effects on heart rate.
- Anticholinergic therapy with alpha-2 agents (e.g. medetomidine or dexmedetomidine) is controversial. Reversal of the alpha-2 agonist with an alpha-2 antagonist, such as atipamezole, may be used if the bradycardia from these drugs is severe. A partial dose of atipamezole may be administered to increase heart rate while preserving some alpha-2 analgesia.
- Some bradycardia is not due to parasympathetic activity and will not respond to anticholinergic therapy (e.g. excessive inhalant anesthetic depth, hypothermia).

HYPOTENSION
- Key concepts:
  - Low blood pressure can become an anesthetic emergency when tissue perfusion is compromised.
  - Tissue perfusion is a balance between cardiac output, organ blood flow, and peripheral vessel tone.
  - MAP is the best estimate of tissue perfusion pressure in a clinical situation.
  - A MAP of 60 mmHg should provide sufficient blood flow to the vital organs, such as the brain, heart, and kidneys.
- Inhalant anesthetic agents cause hypotension by two basic mechanisms:
  - Vasodilation (especially isoflurane and sevoflurane).

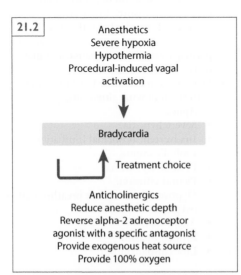

Fig. 21.2 Causes of bradycardia and its treatment.

- Cardiac output reduction by decreasing contractility.
- If the patient has a MAP <60 mmHg, therapy should be initiated. This therapy can consist of decreasing anesthetic depth, improving peripheral fluid volume, increasing cardiac output, or use of vasopressors.
- Decreasing anesthetic depth:
  - Decrease the vaporizer setting to the lowest necessary to provide general anesthesia. The addition of sedative/analgesics such as opioids or alpha-2 agonists may provide analgesia and allow lower vaporizer settings through a MAC-sparing effect.
- Adequate peripheral fluid volume:
  - Patients anesthetized with inhalants need fluid support regardless of any surgical blood loss or insensible fluid losses.
  - Venous return is the primary determinant of cardiac output in a healthy patient (Frank–Starling Law of the heart); an anesthetized, vasodilated patient will have greatly diminished venous return without fluid support. The patient will also be experiencing decreased contractility as a result of inhalant administration.
- Anesthesia fluid rates are usually between 5 and 10 ml/kg/hour with a balanced, isotonic crystalloid solution in a healthy patient with normal cardiac function. This rate can be maintained in an anesthetized patient for 3–4 hours and then reduced.
  - Occult hemoconcentration is a very common finding in patients presented for anesthesia, especially if they have been hospitalized. It is not necessary to withhold water prior to anesthesia, but many hospitalized patients may be too stressed to drink well.
  - Induction with propofol can cause profound vasodilation and hypotension. When encountering patients with a higher than expected heart rate, one of the first things to check is the volume status of the patient to determine if the high heart rate is a compensation for hypovolemia. A fluid challenge of

5–10 ml/kg can be very helpful in reducing the heart rate to a normal value.
- Hypoproteinemic patients (albumin <20 g/l [2.0 g/dl] or TP <40 g/l [4.0 g/dl]) benefit from colloid administration (e.g. VetStarch™ or plasma), while anesthetized. Crystalloid administration may need to be reduced to avoid further dilution of plasma protein, but the patient's volume needs must still be met.
- Central venous pressure monitoring via jugular catheterization is the gold standard, but careful attention to breath sounds and auscultation for crackles will be helpful as well.
- Sometimes, careful peripheral volume support and control of anesthetic level is not sufficient to correct a hypotension problem. A logical next step is to increase cardiac output if possible. Usually this is achieved by catecholamine administration. Some of the more commonly used sympathomimetic drugs for this purpose include dobutamine, dopamine, and ephedrine (see Chapter 6).

HEMORRHAGE

- Hemorrhage affects delivery of oxygen to tissues when blood volume losses are high. In general, a PCV of 0.2 l/l (20%) and a TP >35 g/l (3.5 g/dl) in the anesthetized patient is desirable. If a patient's blood loss is >20 ml/kg, or if the blood loss is not measurable but the PCV and TP are lower than the above values, some sort of oxygen-carrying solution is required.

CARDIAC ARRHYTHMIAS (SEE ALSO CHAPTER 22)
Definition

- Arrhythmias are defined as an abnormality in heart rhythm and/or rate in the site of origin of the cardiac impulse, or as a disturbance in the normal conductance of the cardiac impulse.
- Arrhythmias become anesthetic emergencies when they interfere with cardiac output to an extent that they decrease tissue perfusion.

Types of arrhythmia (*Table 21.1*)

- **Bradyarrhythmias (slower than normal rates)**. Should initially be treated with an anticholinergic drug (e.g. atropine or glycopyrrolate). Atropine (0.04 mg/kg IV) should be used if the heart rate is falling rapidly and severely. Glycopyrrolate is frequently used as a preanesthetic medication to stabilize the heart rate due to its longer duration of action than atropine (see Chapter 3).
- **Ventricular arrhythmias**. If ventricular arrhythmias (ventricular premature contractions [VPCs]) are discovered during anesthesia, several criteria can be used to determine how disruptive the arrhythmia is likely to be. In general, arrhythmias may be more of a problem during anesthesia if they are multifocal, if VPCs are >12/minute, or if they are associated with pulse deficits
- It is important to differentiate VPCs from ventricular escape beats. The two conditions have different therapeutic managements.
- When VPCs are detected during anesthesia, consideration must be given to what may be causing them and if they can be corrected during the anesthetic period.

Causes of arrhythmias (*Table 21.1*)

- Iatrogenic:
  - Caused by a drug administered as part of the anesthetic protocol.
  - Commonly used anesthetics and adjunctive drugs that can cause arrhythmias include thiopentone, propofol, xylazine, medetomidine/ dexmedetomidine, and anticholinergics. However, any drug may cause an arrhythmia in a sensitive individual.
- Metabolic and electrolyte disturbances:
  - Metabolic acidosis.
  - Hypokalemia.
  - Hyperkalemia. (**Note:** Hyperkalemia will cause bradycardia.)
  - Calcium disturbances.
- Hypercarbia:
  - High levels of CO_2 stimulate the sympathetic nervous system and can cause rhythm disturbances, as well as have a direct depressant effect on the myocardium.
- Hypoxia.
- Sympathetic stimulation or pain:
  - Paradoxically, the plane of anesthesia may need to be deepened and/or the addition of analgesic drug therapy may be warranted.
- High parasympathetic tone (vagal tone):
  - Manipulation of airway, bladder, or globe of the eye may cause a sudden decrease in heart rate.
  - Brachycephalic breeds tend to have higher vagal tone.
- Primary cardiac disease, such as:
  - Cardiomyopathy.
  - Primary rhythm disturbances.
- Hypothermia:
  - Usually causes bradycardia.

Investigating arrhythmias

- Blood gas and electrolyte analysis can be very useful when looking for the source of the problem.

Table 21.1 Arrhythmias: causes, types, and treatments

Causes	Types	Treatments
• Iatrogenic • Metabolic • Hypercarbia • Hypoxia • High sympathetic tone (pain) • High vagal tone • Primary cardiac diseases • Hypothermia • Hyperthermia	• Rate (tachycardia, bradycardia) • Rhythm (regular or irregular) • Site of origin (atrial, supraventricular, and ventricular) • Disturbance in the normal conductance of the cardiac impulse (single or multifocal)	• Treat primary causes first • For bradyarrhythmias use atropine (0.04 mg/kg IV) or reverse with atipamezole if it is induced by medetomidine or dexmedetomidine • For ventricular premature contractions (multifocal with pulse deficit) use lidocaine (2 mg/kg IV) • For ventricular escape beats use atropine

- Once an arrhythmia has been detected, blood pressure monitoring is very helpful. If the patient is able to maintain an acceptable MAP under anesthesia even though it has an arrhythmia, this is a good indication that the anesthesia can continue.
- Failure to maintain an adequate MAP is an indication that anesthesia should be terminated as quickly as possible.

- If a procedure requires general anesthesia despite significant ventricular arrhythmia, a test dose of lidocaine (2 mg/kg IV) can be given. If the patient responds to lidocaine therapy, a lidocaine CRI (50 µg/kg/min) can be started.

Other complications that result in anesthetic emergencies

HYPOTHERMIA
- Extremes in body temperature can cause considerable problems in anesthetized patients. Most patients will lose body heat as a result of general anesthesia. Heat loss is caused by:
  - Inhalants. These cause vasodilation, which promotes heat loss in the patient.
  - High oxygen flow rates, which will increase body cooling because compressed gas is very cold and dry.
  - Hair removal and surgical preparation solutions.
  - An open body cavity.
- Body temperature should be kept as near normal as possible for most anesthetized patients.
- The effects of hypothermia are:
  - It causes a significant stress response in the postoperative period (sevenfold increase in catecholamines).
  - It results in impaired coagulation.
  - It results in impaired tissue perfusion and delayed wound healing.
  - Temperature affects the MAC of inhaled anesthetics, which is a measure of potency, so the colder the patient, the less anesthetic will be required.
  - It causes a bradycardia that is unresponsive to anticholinergics.
- Steps should be taken to reduce the amount of body heat lost by anesthetized patients. Forced air warmers, circulating water heating pads, and fluid warmers are some of the devices that are very useful.

HYPERTHERMIA
- High body temperature can be seen in anesthetized patients and in the postoperative period.

- Hyperthermia can be a concern with heavy coated animals and animals that are panting.
- Inadvertent overheating with warming devices in a heavy coated animal during general anesthesia is a frequent cause of intraoperative hyperthermia.
- It is also a concern with metabolic and genetic hyperthermic syndromes (malignant hyperthermia). Triggers include all inhalant anesthetics and succinylcholine. Greyhounds may have more hyperthermic problems.
- The ability to monitor body temperature can be very helpful in identifying these problems in the early stages. Capnography will also register the increased CO_2 levels seen when muscle metabolism is high, which can be one of the first signs of malignant hyperthermia.
- Treatment of hyperthermia involves:
  - Early identification of the problem.
  - Rapid body cooling.
  - Heating pads turned off or removed.
  - Cold water baths.
  - Cold water enemas.
  - Ice packing (protect skin from direct contact).
  - Dantrolene therapy if malignant hyperthermia suspected.
  - Stopping the cooling process at 40°C (104°F).

Postanesthetic hyperthermia in cats
- More and more cats are seen with a high postoperative temperature.
- The temperature increase comes several hours after the end of the anesthetic and occurs with a variety of anesthetic protocols.

- Hydromorphone is strongly associated with hyperthermia in cats following anesthesia.
- Treatment has consisted of:

- Opioid reversal.
- NSAIDs.
- Acepromazine.
- Direct body cooling.

Cardiopulmonary resuscitation

IDENTIFICATION OF ARREST VIA CHECKING OF VITAL SIGNS
- Can you hear a heartbeat?
- Can you feel a pulse?
- Is the animal breathing?
- What is the mucous membrane color?

ACTION TO BE TAKEN
- If the signs of cardiopulmonary arrest are present, immediate action must be taken (see **Fig. 21.3** for a procedural flow chart).
- The longer the time between identification of the arrest and cardiopulmonary resuscitation (CPR), the less likely there will be successful resolution of the problem. Animals that have experienced an anesthetic mishap or accident and who are basically healthy are much more likely to be successfully resuscitated than animals that arrest with a lot of underlying disease problems.
- CPR can be divided into four steps: airway, breathing, circulation/compressions, and drugs (*Table 21.2*).

First step (airway)
- Is the animal intubated?
- Is the airway controlled?
- If the patient is under general anesthesia, is the patient correctly intubated and the tube unobstructed?
- If the patient is under general anesthesia, the inhalant anesthetic should be immediately terminated and the breathing circuit flushed with 100% oxygen to rapidly clear the residual anesthetic.

Second step (breathing)
- Previous recommendations for veterinary patients were to provide a ventilation rate of 20–24 breaths per minute.
- Newer guidelines suggest a lower rate of ventilation (8–12 breaths per minute) to avoid decreases in myocardial (due to positive-pressure ventilation-related reduction of venous return to the heart) and cerebral (due to lower arterial CO_2 resulting in cerebral vasoconstriction) perfusion.
- Ventilate the patient with 100% oxygen.

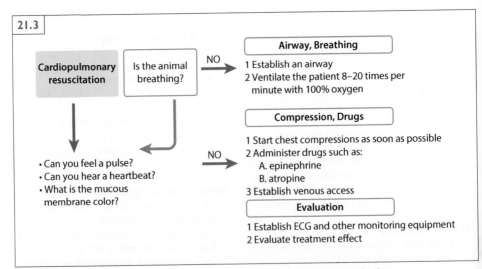

Fig. 21.3 Procedural flow chart for performing cardiopulmonary resuscitation.

Table 21.2 Cardiopulmonary resuscitation sequence (ABCD), drugs, and dosages

Airway	Validation of airway patency	
Endotracheal intubation with: • Endotracheal tube • Laryngoscope • Suction of blood or fluid	Correct endotracheal tube placement by: • Visualization of tube in the airway • Proper chest or anesthetic reservoir bag excursion • Palpation of endotracheal tube in the trachea • Use of capnography	

Breathing	Breathing	Sequence
Use an anesthetic machine with a breathing circuit or Ambu bag	Initially 2 breaths, 1–2 seconds in duration, with 100% oxygen	After establishment of a patent airway
	Evaluate spontaneous ventilation	If yes, observe the animal; if no, check for pulse and rhythm and consider reversal agents for drugs that may cause apnea
	No spontaneous ventilation	Give 10–12 breaths/minute with peak inspiratory pressure ≤20 cmH$_2$O

Circulation/compressions	Frequency	Sequence
Chest compression	80–100/minute with a 1:1 compression:relaxation ratio	Chest compressions should be initiated first and continued with no pauses during administration of endotracheal intubation, ventilatory breaths, placement of IV catheters, ECG assessment, palpation of pulses, or administration of drugs

Drug	Dose and route	Indication and details
Atropine	0.04 mg/kg IV 0.08–0.1 mg/kg IT*	Bradycardia. Can repeat every 3–5 minutes for a maximum of 3 doses
Atipamezole	0.1–0.2 mg/kg IV	Bradycardia induced by alpha-2 agonists; alpha-2 drug antagonist
Calcium gluconate (10% = 100 mg/ml)	0.5–1.5 ml/kg IV slowly	Hyperkalemia and documented ionized hypocalcemia. Do not give via IT route
Epinephrine	0.01 mg/kg IV 0.03–0.1 mg/kg IT*	Increases rate and force of cardiac contractions, increases peripheral vasocontractions. Repeat every 3–5 minutes
Lidocaine	2–4 mg/kg IV 4–6 mg/kg IT*	Ventricular tachycardia, ventricular premature contractions. Repeat every 3–5 minutes
Magnesium sulfate	0.15–0.3 mmol(mEq)/kg IV slowly over 10 minutes	Treatment of refractory ventricular arrhythmias including ventricular fibrillation and life-threatening mutilfocal ventricular tachycardia
Naloxone	0.02–0.04 mg/kg IV 0.04–0.06 mg/kg IT*	Opioid antagonist
Sodium bicarbonate	0.5–1 mmol(mEq)/kg IV	Metabolic acidosis
Vasopressin	0.2–0.8 U/kg IV 0.4–1.0 U/kg IT*	Increases peripheral, coronary, and renal vasoconstriction, but less than epinephrine
External defibrillation; shock energy	2–5 joules/kg: 50 joules for small dogs and cats; 100 joules for medium-sized dogs; 200 joules for large dogs	Asystole, ventricular fibrillations
Internal defibrillation; shock energy	0.2–0.5 joules/kg	Open chest is necessary for this procedure

* Medications administered intracheally (IT) should be diluted in 3–5 ml of sterile water.

- Make sure the vaporizer has been turned off.
- Does the chest expand easily? If not, check that the ETT is not obstructed or the patient does not have a chest full of blood (hemothorax) or air (pneumothorax).

Third step (circulation/compressions)

- Chest compressions should be commenced very quickly. The patient should be positioned in lateral recumbency with the back towards the person doing the compressions in order to prevent the animal from sliding around on the table (**Fig. 21.4**).
- The chest wall should be allowed to recoil completely after being compressed to approximately 30% of its diameter, with no pauses during administration of ventilator breaths or other necessary tasks (IV catheter placement, ECG assessment, or administration of medications).
- Forward flow of blood is the goal of chest compressions.
- There are two theories:
  - The cardiac theory utilizes direct compressions of the heart to provide forward flow.
  - The thoracic pump theory hypothesizes that changes in intrathoracic pressure created by cardiac compressions are responsible for forward flow.
- The larger the animal, the more difficult it is to do effective compressions.
- The current recommendation for chest compression is that there should be 80–100 compressions per minute, with a 1:1 compression to relaxation ratio.

Fourth step (drugs)

- Deciding what drugs to use to treat cardiac arrhythmia relies on an accurate ECG identification (**Fig. 21.5**).
- Epinephrine (1:10,000) should be administered as soon as the arrest is identified.
- Several dosing regimes are available (0.05–0.1 mg/kg), but in a crisis it can be difficult to take the time to look up the weight of the animal and calculate a dose.
- Alternatively, administer 0.5–1.0 ml to a small dog or cat, 2 ml to a medium size dog, and 3 ml to a large dog.
- Epinephrine should be given IV. If venous access is not available, a double dose can be administered down the ETT and washed in with several milliliters of water or saline.
- If a slow heartbeat is identified prior to the arrest, atropine should be given (0.04 mg/kg IV).
- Cardiac compression is necessary during bradycardia in order to deliver the IV emergency drugs to the heart through the compression-propelled forward blood flow.
- The following drugs are used for CPR:
  - Epinephrine: 0.01 mg/kg IV or 0.03–0.1 mg/kg IT.
  - Vasopressin: 0.2–0.8 U/kg IV or 0.4–1.0 U/kg IT.
  - Atropine: 0.04 mg/kg IV or 0.08 mg/kg IT with saline.
  - Lidocaine: 2–4 mg/kg IV.
  - Sodium bicarbonate: 0.5 mmol(mEq)/kg IV.

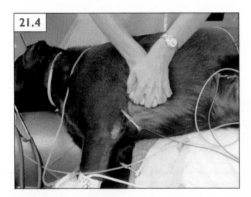

21.4

Fig. 21.4 The person performing cardiac compression should stand against the back of the animal to prevent the animal sliding away from the center of the compression. The compression is likely to be most effective with the heel of the palm against the animal's chest directly above the heart.

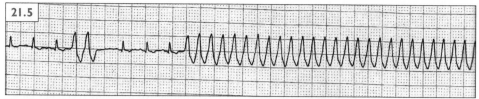

Fig. 21.5 An impending cardiac arrest with some irregular heartbeats before the heart went to ventricular tachycardia.

DEFIBRILLATION

- Ventricular fibrillation (**Fig. 21.6**) should be identified and the patient defibrillated as early as possible using a defibrillator (**Fig. 21.7**). With the patient in right or left lateral recumbency, one paddle is placed on the sternal side of the chest wall and the other paddle on the upper side of the chest wall; gel is applied to both paddles (**Fig. 21.8**).

- How much energy should be used? 50 joules for small dogs and cats; 100 joules for medium-sized dogs; and 200 joules for large dogs. (**Note:** One joule is defined as the amount of work or energy exerted when a force of 1 Newton is applied over a displacement of 1 meter. One joule is the equivalent energy of 1 watt of power radiated or dissipated for 1 second.)

- One shock should be administered rather than the three successive shocks previously recommended, with chest compressions resumed immediately for 2 minutes before reassessing the cardiac rhythm and administering any additional shocks.

- The energy may be doubled if the first shock is not effective in converting the fibrillation of the heart.

- When the defibrillator is discharged, a warning of 'clear' must be announced to stop contact with the patient (and anything connected to the patient) and protect personnel from being shocked.

SOME CONSIDERATIONS REGARDING CARDIOPULMONARY RESUSCITATION

- One person alone cannot do successful CPR.

- Venous access should be established as soon as possible, but not before airway management, ventilation, and chest compressions.

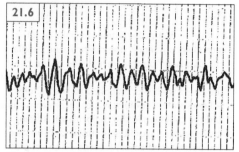

Fig. 21.6 A defibrillator is needed when ventricular fibrillation is identified on the electrocardiogram.

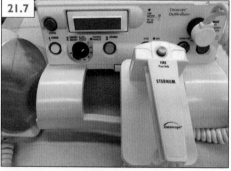

Fig. 21.7 A defibrillator is required for defibrillation. Two external paddles are shown, one to be used on the sternum (marked sternum) and the other on the apex (the metal side facing) of the animal. The metal portion of the paddle comes in contact with the animal and the conduction gel should be applied to the metal portion. Note the power button (green color) and the energy selection dial (5–360 joules) on the defibrillator. The fire button used to discharge the energy is located on the paddles. When firing the electrical shock to the patient, both buttons must be pressed simultaneously.

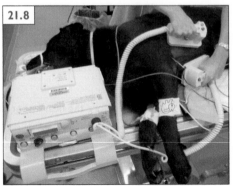

Fig. 21.8 With the patient in right or left lateral recumbency, one defibrillator paddle can be placed on the sternal side of the chest wall and the other paddle on the upper side of the chest wall. Gel is applied to the paddles. All personnel should stay clear from the animal and the table while the defibrillator is being discharged to avoid being shocked. Note the fire button (red color) located on the top of each paddle.

- A 'shock dose' of crystalloids (90 ml/kg/h for dogs and 45 ml/kg/h for cats) is only recommended if the patient was hypovolemic before cardiopulmonary arrest. In the euvolemic arrested patient, the recommended dose (based on a 2008 publication) is a 20 ml/kg bolus for dogs and a 10 ml/kg bolus for cats using crystalloid fluids. Excessive IV fluids during CPR to euvolemic patients decreases coronary perfusion pressure.

- The ABC (airway/breathing/compressions) protocol of CPR has been followed for many years, but CPR success rates remain low. Controversy exists over the best way to perform CPR and the subject will remain open to debate until outcomes are dramatically changed by the way it is performed. There is some evidence to show that cardiac compressions should be done first, rather than airway establishment.

- The patient must constantly be assessed during the procedure. Helpful monitoring equipment includes ECG, capnography, blood pressure monitors, and pulse oximetry.

- Remember that a capnometer may not be useful for assessing intubation in an arrested patient, as circulation is required to present CO_2 to the lung. The presence of $ETCO_2$ is an indication of effective cardiac compressions.

- Most patients will require some form of supportive care following arrest, depending on the severity of the arrest and the success of the resuscitation.

Further reading

Dorsch JA, Dorsch SE (1999) *Understanding Anesthesia Equipment*, 4th edn. Wilkins and Wilkins, Baltimore, pp. 75–269.

Fletcher DJ, Boller M (2013) Updates in small animal cardiopulmonary resuscitation. *Vet Clin North Am Small Anim Pract* **43(4):**971–87.

Greene SA (2007) *Veterinary Anesthesia and Pain Management Secrets*. Hanley and Belfus, Philadelphia.

Long B, Koyfman A (2017) Emergency medicine myths: epinephrine in cardiac arrest. *J Emerg Med* **52(6):**809–14.

Mitchell SL (2000) Tracheal rupture in cats: 16 cases (1993–1998). *J Am Vet Med Assoc* **216:**1592–5.

Muir WW (1998) Acute therapy of anesthetic emergencies. *Comp Cont Educ Pract Vet* **20:**10–13.

Plunkett SJ, McMichael M (2008) Cardiopulmonary resuscitation in small animal medicine: an update. *J Vet Intern Med* **22:**9–25.

Posner LP (2007) Postoperative hyperthermia in cats: an update. *Proceedings of the North American Veterinary Conference*, Orlando.

Vissers G, Soar J, Monsieurs KG (2017) Ventilation rate in adults with a tracheal tube during cardiopulmonary resuscitation: A systematic review. *Resuscitation* **119:**5–12.

Weil AB (2005) Anesthetic emergencies. *J Nat Vet Tech Am* **Spring:**42–8.

CHAPTER 22

Perioperative cardiac arrhythmias and treatments

Jeff C Ko

Introduction

Cardiac arrhythmias commonly occur in anesthetized patients during the perioperative period. Electrocardiography (ECG) provides a quick diagnosis of cardiac arrhythmias and should be part of the routine monitoring of the anesthetized patient. Unrecognized cardiac arrhythmias may develop into more serious types of arrhythmia, leading to hemodynamic instability, including a reduction in cardiac output and blood pressure, and eventually resulting in cardiac arrest. It is therefore important to detect cardiac arrhythmias early and take appropriate treatment actions before a serious cardiac event occurs. This chapter is not intended to be a comprehensive discussion of all cardiac arrhythmias. It describes briefly ECG formation, conduction pathways, types of cardiac arrhythmia, and commonly seen cardiac arrhythmias perioperatively, and discusses the treatment of arrhythmias while the patient is under general anesthesia.

Normal cardiac conduction pathways

- Often, perioperative cardiac arrhythmias do not require immediate treatment. However, close monitoring of these arrhythmias is essential. Once hemodynamic instability occurs, immediate treatment can be instituted, and the abnormality of the cardiac arrhythmia quickly identified and followed up. It is therefore important to understand the normal cardiac conduction pathways and recognize the types of cardiac arrhythmia in order to better approach the treatment decision.
- The normal heart (sinus) rate is determined by a natural cardiac pacemaker, called the sinoatrial (SA) node, located in the upper posterior wall of the right atrium (**Fig. 22.1**). The SA node has an intrinsic firing rate of 60–100 bpm. Under normal conditions, the electrical activity of the heart is associated with the mechanical activity of the heart (*Table 22.1*).

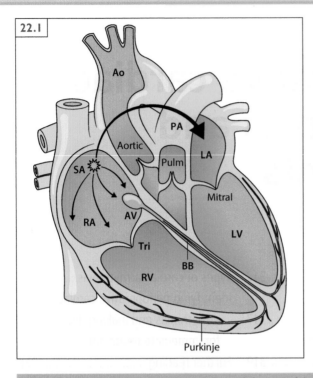

22.1

Fig. 22.1 Normal electrical conduction pathway of the heart. The electrical signal is conducted from the sinoatrial (SA) node to the atrioventricular (AV) node and then from the AV node to the ventricles along the pathway of the bundle of His, the right and left bundle branches (BB), and finally the Purkinje fibers in the myocardium of the ventricular wall. The electrical signal also spreads from the SA node to the left atrium (LA), as shown with the large black arrow. Ao, aorta; Aortic, aortic valve; LV, left ventricle; Mitral, mitral valve; PA, pulmonary artery; Pulm, pulmonary valve; RA, right atrium; RV, right ventricle; Tri, tricuspid valve. The green color represents the electrical signal conduction network.

Table 22.1 The electrical and mechanical myocardial events of the heart

Pulse origin and anatomic location	Electrical activity	Mechanical activity	Event
Sinoatrial (SA) node. Located within the upper posterior wall of the right atrium	Origin of the P wave Initiates the electrical impulse for cardiac electrical activity	Initiation of atrial contraction	The pacemaker of the heart
SA node electrical activity then spreads from the right atrium to the left atrium	P wave formation	Following SA node initiation, it triggers depolarization and passes through the myocardial cells of the atria This depolarization of the atria resulted in atrial contractions	Depolarization and contraction of both atria
Atrioventricular (AV) node is located on the bottom of the right atrium, just above the right ventricle	Atrial impulse continues to travel from the atria to the AV node	When the impulse goes through the AV node, there is a slight delay in response, which allows complete contraction of the atria and empties the atrial blood to fill the ventricles	Moves the blood from atria to ventricles
The impulse travels from the AV node to the ventricles through the bundle of His and the Purkinje fibers in the wall of ventricular myocardium	QRS formation	Ventricular contractions due to depolarization of the ventricular myocardium	Moves the blood from the ventricles to the aorta and pulmonary arteries
Cardiac cycle completion	T wave, impulse recovery with repolarization	No mechanical response to the repolarization	Strictly an electrical event without any mechanical response

The normal cardiac conduction pathway originates in the SA node and then spreads from the right atrium to the left atrium, which results in atrial contractions and subsequently moving of blood from the atrium to the ventricle. The impulse recorded for such action potential is the 'P' wave on the ECG.

- After the 'P' wave, the atrial impulse continues to travel from the atrium to the atrioventricular (AV) node, which is located on the bottom of the right atrium, just above the right ventricle. The AV node is a gatekeeper for electrical impulses between the atria and the ventricles. It has an intrinsic firing rate of 40–60 bpm. When the impulse passes through the AV node, there is a slight delay in response. This delay allows complete contraction of the atrium and empties the atrial blood to fill the ventricle.
- The impulse then travels onward from the AV node to the ventricle along the pathway of the bundle of His, the right and left bundle branches, and finally the Purkinje fibers in the myocardium of the ventricular wall. This electrical conduction is recorded on the ECG as a 'QRS' complex and results in ventricular contraction, which moves the blood from the ventricle to the aorta and pulmonary arteries. The cells in the ventricle have an intrinsic firing rate of 20–40 bpm.
- After the QRS complex, the cardiac cycle is completed with impulse recovery (repolarization) and this is recorded as a 'T' wave on the ECG.
- Any abnormality in the aforementioned electrical impulse formation results in a cardiac arrhythmia. There are many different ways of classifying cardiac arrhythmias. In general, ECG provides electrical information about the heart rate, rhythm, and origin of the complexes. Under general anesthesia, the ECG is usually evaluated by examining the heart rate and rhythm on the monitor screen, or on a print out of an ECG strip from the monitor if the origin of a cardiac complex is to be examined.

Causes of perioperative cardiac arrhythmias

- Perioperative cardiac arrhythmias can be largely classified as patient triggered, procedural triggered, and anesthetic agent triggered.
- Patient triggered cardiac arrhythmias arise mostly from the following conditions:
  - Excitation or extreme stress associated with high sympathetic tone. The types of cardiac arrhythmia are mostly associated with tachycardia and ventricular premature contractions (VPCs).
  - Debilitating diseases (e.g. gastric dilatation/volvulus [GDV], myocardial contusion, emaciation-associated hypothermia, malignant hyperthermia, renal dysfunction, or urinary tract outflow obstruction) associated with electrolyte or acid–base imbalance. The types of cardiac arrhythmia are mostly associated with severe bradycardia, atrial or junctional VPCs, paroxysmal supraventricular tachycardia, atrial standstill, and sinus arrest.
- Cardiac disease-associated cardiac arrhythmias. The types of cardiac arrhythmia can vary, but some obvious ones are sick sinus syndrome, sinus arrest, severe bradycardia, or excessive tachycardia with diverse types of atrial or ventricular conduction disturbances.
- Activation of parasympathetic tone-associated cardiac arrhythmias, mainly severe bradycardia, first-, second-, and third-degree heart block, pronounced sinus arrhythmia, wandering pace makers, ventricular escape beats, or even sudden cardiac arrest.
- Procedural-triggered cardiac arrhythmias are mostly associated with the following conditions:
  - Interventional cardiac procedures, including pace maker placement and balloon valvuloplasty.

- Surgical procedures of the thorax that involve the pericardium, heart valves, and myocardium.
- Surgical procedures related to any large blood vessel and GDV.
- Upper airway or bladder/urethral surgeries.
- Anesthetic agent-triggered cardiac arrhythmias are mostly associated with the following conditions:
  - Propofol may induce tachycardia or bradycardia. Alfaxalone on the other hand, induces a faster heart rate soon after induction.
  - Ketamine and tiletamine/zolazepam are known to induce tachycardia and VPCs.
  - Opioids are known to induce various degrees of bradycardia, heart blocks, sinus arrhythmias, or even sinus arrest.
  - Alpha-2 agonists, such as xylazine, medetomidine, and dexmedetomidine, are known to induce bradycardia, second-degree heart block, sinus arrest, and ventricular escape beats.

- Inhalant anesthetic agents, such isoflurane or sevoflurane, might not directly induce cardiac arrhythmia but can facilitate other types of cardiac arrhythmia by lowering the blood pressure or reducing cardiac output or coronary blood flow.
- Atropine and glycopyrrolate can induce both bradycardia (see Chapter 3) and tachycardia.
- Dopamine and dobutamine are likely to induce tachycardia.
- Ephedrine may induce reflex bradycardia following significant increase in blood pressure, secondary heart block, sinus tachycardia, or VPCs.
- Epinephrine and norepinephrine may induce tachycardia and reflex bradycardia.
- Reversal of neuromuscular block agents using neostigmine and edrophonium (less likely than neostigmine) may also trigger severe bradycardia.

Types of cardiac arrhythmias

The types of cardiac arrhythmia can be classified by their rate, rhythm, and impulse formation. Each of these cardiac arrhythmias can occur alone or in combination with other types of cardiac arrhythmia.

CARDIAC ARRHYTHMIAS DUE TO AN ABNORMAL HEART RATE

- Heart rate can be within the normal acceptable physiologic range, slow (bradycardia, **Fig. 22.2**) or fast (tachycardia), under general anesthesia or under sedation.
- Dogs and cats have different criteria for bradycardia and tachycardia under general

anesthesia/sedation. For dogs, a heart rate <60 bpm is considered as bradycardia. For cats, a heart rate <80–100 bpm is considered bradycardia. It is challenging to define what bradycardia is since giant and toy breed dogs tend to have different criteria. Also, some athletic dogs tend to have a lower heart rate than non-athletic dogs. One alternative is to use 20% lower than the awake baseline rate as a definition for bradycardia. Because cardiac output is a product of heart rate and stroke volume, and blood pressure is a product of cardiac output and systemic vascular resistance, if the heart rate decreases or increases to a

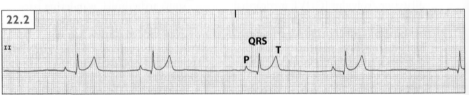

Fig. 22.2 Bradycardia. All the ECG complexes' morphology (P-QRS-T) are there, except the heart rate is slow.

certain threshold and the stroke volume cannot compensate such a change, it will cause cardiac output to fall and blood pressure to drop.

- In dogs, a heart rate faster than 180 bpm (giant breeds) or 200 bpm (toy breeds), and in cats a heart rate faster than 220 bpm, are considered as tachycardia.

Reasons for abnormal heart rates

- Bradycardia may be due to the high vagal reflexes (high parasympathetic activation) of the animal. Brachycephalic breed dogs are likely to have a higher vagal activity than dolichocephalic breed dogs. Manipulation of the upper airway (bronchial, pharyngeal, laryngeal), esophageal mucosa, tracking of the eye orbit (craniocardiac reflex), mechanical stimulation of abdominal viscera, especially the urinary bladder (abdominocardiac reflex), may trigger vagal activity-induced bradycardia.
- Anesthetics can induce bradycardia. Opioids such as fentanyl, morphine, and hydromorphone likely induce bradycardia. Alpha-2 agonists such as xylazine, medetomidine, and dexmedetomidine also induce bradycardia. Propofol and, less likely, alfaxalone may occasionally induce bradycardia. Low doses of anticholinergic agents (atropine and glycopyrrolate) can induce bradycardia before they increase heart rate. High concentrations of isoflurane and sevoflurane also can result in bradycardia.
- Electrolyte imbalance, such as hyperkalemia, low calcium, or severe acidosis, may trigger bradycardia; however, hypokalemia and hypomagnesemia patients may develop tachycardia.
- Mild hypoxia and/or hypercarbia may trigger tachycardia due to reflex sympathetic stimulation. Profound bradycardia will occur in cases of severe hypoxia, hypotension, tension pneumothorax, or pulmonary embolus.
- Diseases of the sinus node such as sick sinus syndrome. Others such as sinus arrest or cardiac tamponade also cause bradycardia.

- Bradycardia may occur with hypothermia or when reversing a neuromuscular blocker (e.g. atracurium, pancuronum) with neostigmine or edrophonium.
- Tachycardia may be due to pain, anesthetic drugs, or hyperthermia. Anesthetics such as ketamine and tiletamine/zolazepam are capable of inducing tachycardia. Long-haired animals with a poor ability to ventilate, overheating with warming devices, or infection can induce tachycardia. Tachycardia may also be an early sign of cardiac failure, with compensatory reflex to improve blood pressure. Acute hemorrhaging can also trigger reflex tachycardia to improve blood pressure.
- Propofol and alfaxalone also can induce transient tachycardia instead of bradycardia.
- Inotropic agents such as dopamine and dobutamine can cause tachycardia when using doses higher than 10–15 µg/kg/minute.
- Tachycardia may also be due to other cardiac arrhythmias such as supraventricular tachycardia (atrial or junctional) or ventricular tachycardia (see below).
- Episodes of tachycardia begin and end abruptly. This is called paroxysmal tachycardia.

CARDIAC ARRHYTHMIAS DUE TO ABNORMAL RHYTHMS

- Abnormal rhythms can be largely classified by their origin from sinus, atria, or ventricles.
- Sinus origin includes:
  - Sinus rhythm: the heart's normal regular rhythm.
  - Sinus arrhythmia: arrhythmia originating from the sinus but varying with respiration.
  - Sinus bradycardia: heart rate slower than sinus rhythm.
  - Sinus arrest: absence of SA node impulse activity.
  - Sinus tachycardia: heart rate faster than sinus rhythm.
  - Wandering pacemaker: sinus arrhythmia with different P wave shapes due to different pacemaker originated location.

- Atrial origin includes:
  - Atrial standstill.
  - Atrial premature complexes: an ectopic beat originates from the atrium and appears earlier than the normal P wave from the SA node. It is followed by a normal QRS complex because the impulse is transmitted by the same conduction pathway as the P wave from the atria.
  - Atrial tachycardia: if it is multifocal, then it is a fast run of wandering pacemaker.
  - Atrial flutter: a series of rapid firing from a single atrial focus. Usually called 'saw tooth' shape.
  - Atrial fibrillation: multiple irregular atrial activities without clear P waves.
  - Paroxysmal atrial tachycardia or paroxysmal supraventricular tachycardia: the tachycardia may originate from the atrium or a supraventricular focus with the QRS complex looking like of sinus origin.
- Atrioventricular junctional origin includes:
  - AV junctional premature beat: an ectopic focus in the AV junction fires before the normal SA node impulse. This abnormal premature impulse can conduct retrogradely to the atria and form an inverted P wave, or it can conduct along the normal pathway to the ventricle and form a normal QRS complex.
  - Supraventricular tachycardia (SVT) is a cardiac arrhythmia due to repetitive premature depolarizations of the supraventricular ectopic focus. The rate of depolarization varies widely in dogs; it can be as low as 150 bpm and as high as 300 bpm. Most of the R-R intervals are very regular (**Fig. 22.3**) with the QRS complexes typical of supraventricular complexes being narrow and upright (lead II).
  - Some dogs may have long runs of SVT, whereas others can have very short runs of SVT.
  - SVT is rarely seen under general anesthesia, likely due to reduction of sympathetic tone. Animals with SVT should not be anesthetized until any underlying disease has been treated.
- Ventricular origin includes:
  - Asystole.
  - VPCs: impulses originate from ventricles and occur earlier than the normal QRS complexes. VPCs may be single, multiple, in runs, or coupled with normal sinus rhythms. They also can be unifocal or multifocal (see also Chapter 10).
  - Ventricular tachycardia: more than 5–6 VPCs in a run
  - Ventricular flutter.
  - Ventricular fibrillation.
  - Idioventricular rhythm: when the pacemaker at the SA or AV nodes is either too slow or fails to trigger heartbeats, the ventricular myocardium itself becomes the pacemaker and starts to fire on its own to prevent the heart going into cardiac arrest. These are called escape beats. When there are multiple escape beats, it is called idioventricular rhythm, with the impulse signals transmitted between ventricular cardiomyocytes instead of by the normal conduction system, thus forming a series of wide and bizarre

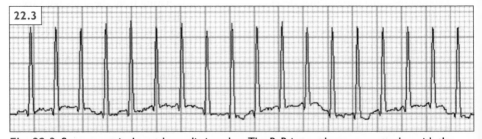

Fig. 22.3 Surpraventricular tachycardia in a dog. The R-R intervals are very regular with the QRS complexes typical of supraventricular complexes, being narrow and upright (lead II).

QRS rhythms. The rate is usually 20–40 bpm. If the rate is higher than 40 bpm, it is called accelerated idioventricular rhythm.

CARDIAC ARRHYTHMIAS DUE TO IMPULSE CONDUCTION ABNORMALITY

- A normal impulse conduction pathway initiates from the SA node to the AV node. It then goes in a ventricular direction to the bundle of His and then to the right and left bundle branches, and finally reaches the Purkinje fibers. Any impulse conduction deviating from this pathway results in an abnormal conduction and can be classified as follows:
- AV block:
  - First-degree: the P-R interval is prolonged, but the duration is consistent with each complex.
  - Second-degree: the P-R interval is progressively increased from one cycle to the next until no QRS complex occurs (Wenckebach phenomenon, **Fig. 22.4**). This is also called a Mobitz type I block.
  - Another type of second-degree AV block is called Mobitz type II, in which the P-R interval is fixed but the P waves stand alone without QRSTs following after that.
  - Third-degree (**Fig. 22.5**): no association between P waves and QRS complexes. A complete block occurs and none of the atrial impulses penetrate to the ventricles. When the heart rate becomes too slow, other secondary pacemakers may fire and ventricular escape beats may be seen.
- Bundle branch block (BBB):
  - BBB occurs when there is a delay or blockage along the left (LBBB, **Fig. 22.6**) or right (RBBB) bundle branch of His electrical impulse pathway.
  - When a BBB occurs, the heart is pumped less efficiently.
  - There is no specific treatment for the BBB itself under general anesthesia. The patient should be treated for any underlying heart diseases that caused the BBB before general anesthesia takes place.

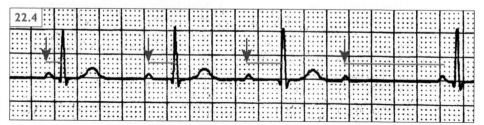

Fig. 22.4 Second-degree heart block with Wenckebach phenomenon (Mobitz type I), the P-R interval (the red line) is progressively increased from one cycle to the next until no QRS complex occurs. The P wave is indicated by the blue arrow.

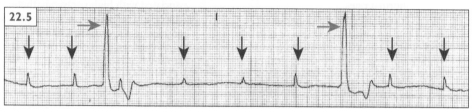

Fig. 22.5 Third-degree heart block with complete block occurring. Only P waves can be seen (blue arrows) with no atrial impulses penetrating to the ventricles (no QRS complexes). When the heart rate becomes too slow, other secondary pacemakers (ectopic foci) may fire on their own. If the foci originate from the atrioventricular junction or ventricle, they are termed junctional or ventricular escape beats. Two junctional ventricular escape beats (red arrows) are seen here.

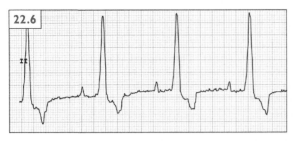

22.6

Fig. 22.6 Bundle branch block (BBB) occurs when there is a delay or blockage along the left or right bundle branch of His electrical impulse pathway. A left BBB is seen here.

Identifying perioperative cardiac arrhythmias and making decisions for immediate treatment

- An easy way to identify whether there is a perioperative cardiac arrhythmia is to follow the steps stated here when evaluating an ECG using a limb lead II on the monitor screen or from a printout (preferred method) (see Chapter 6).
  - Rate: a quick glance at the ECG monitor/strip will identify if the heart rate is fast or slow, and if the R-R intervals are regular or irregular.
  - Rhythm:
    - If R-R intervals are regular, it is likely a sinus rhythm.
    - If R-R intervals are irregular, then follow the next steps.
  - ECG morphology:
    - Identify if every P is followed by a QRST complex.
    - Identify if every QRST complex is preceded with a P wave.
    - Identify if all the QRST complexes look identical in size and shape.
    - If the ectopic (other than normal pacemaker) beat originates close to the SA node, the ECG complex looks only slightly different from normal ones.
- Most cardiac arrhythmias (*Table 22.2*) occur under general anesthesia or sedation and require only close monitoring without immediate treatment. However, if the arrhythmia threatens the hemodynamic stability (i.e. causes the MAP to decrease below 60 mmHg or systolic blood pressure to decrease below 80 mmHg), then it requires immediate treatment.
- The goal of treating cardiac arrhythmias under this condition is:
  - To control the heart rate and let it remain within a relatively normal range.
  - To restore normal cardiac rhythm if possible.
  - To optimize the conditions that minimize the cause of the arrhythmia.
  - To allow the corrected heart rate and rhythm to restore hemodynamic stability (i.e. maintain MAP of at least 60 mmHg).

COMMONLY OCCURRING CARDIAC ARRHYTHMIAS, CAUSES, AND TREATMENT PERIOPERATIVELY

The following cardiac arrhythmias require immediate treatment.

- Sinus bradycardia, sinus arrhythmia, first-, second-, or third-degree AV block (**Fig. 22.5**). Sinus arrhythmia is an arrhythmia induced by respiration with an irregular rhythm. The heart rate increases during inspiration and decreases during expiration.
- Severe wandering pacemaker may be seen and occasionally should be treated. This is characterized by irregular rhythm with various shapes of P waves:
  - These arrhythmias are frequently associated with high parasympathetic activity and, when severe, occur with a conduction abnormality characterized by a disruption along the conduction pathway from the SA node to the AV node; this results in one or more P waves not being followed by a QRS-T complex.
- Atrial and junctional or ventricular escape beats:
  - An escape beat is when an ectopic focus fires on its own due to a prolonged pause in the SA node pacing activity (**Fig. 22.5**).

Table 22.2 Cardiac arrhythmia under general anesthesia and its treatments

Arrhythmia	Rate (bpm)	Rhythm	Treatment	Reason/comment
Respiratory sinus arrhythmia	60–100	Regular irregular	None	Usually associated with higher vagal tone; heart rate is faster during inspiration and slower during expiration
Sinus bradycardia	<60 in dogs and <80 in cats	Regular	Anticholinergics or dopamine/dobutamine	High vagal tone, drug-induced (opioids and alpha-2 sedatives); slow rate likely decreases cardiac output
Sinus tachycardia	>180 in dogs and >200 in cats	Regular	Treat underlying problems (for example pain, fever, hypotension)	Increased myocardial oxygen consumption and reduced cardiac output
Atrial flutter	250–350	Regular or irregular	Esmolol (a beta1 receptor blocker used to control rapid heartbeats with fast onset and short duration of action) at 0.05 mg/kg IV	No P waves, 'saw tooth' pattern
Atrial fibrillation	350–400	Irregular	Esmolol at 0.05 mg/kg IV	No P waves, P-R interval not measurable
Supraventricular tachycardia (SVT)	>150	Regular	In most situations SVT may stop quickly and no treatment is needed; if it persists and affects blood pressure, try to use vagal maneuvers to stimulate the vagus nerve, or give an opioid to increase vagal tone Esmolol at 0.05 mg/kg IV	Fast rate resulting in decreased cardiac output
Ventricular premature contraction (VPC)	Variable, but can be normal	Irregular	Treat underlying problems if affecting blood pressure If multiple VPCs, give 2 mg/kg lidocaine 1–2 min apart with maximum of 8 mg/kg IV	Early beats, wide and bizarre shapes
Ventricular tachycardia	100–250	Regular	Give 2 mg/kg lidocaine at 1–2 min apart with maximum of 8 mg/kg, IV; if pulseless, use defibrillation	Wide, regular, fast rate, without P waves
Ventricular fibrillation	Rapid	Chaotic without pattern	Defibrillate, turn off anesthetic vaporizer and increase oxygen flow rate and control ventilation, perform cardiac compression	Impending death
Asystole	No activity	Flat line	Give epinephrine (0.01–0.1 mg/kg IV), defibrillate, turn off anesthetic vaporizer and increase oxygen flow rate and control ventilation, perform cardiac compression	Impending death

- If the ectopic focus is originates from the atrium, it is called an atrial escape beat. If it originates from the AV junction or ventricle, it is called a junctional or ventricular escape beat.

- Atrial and junctional or ventricular escape beats are due to:
  - Higher parasympathetic activity associated with brachycephalic breeds; also some athletic dogs may trigger such a response.

- Anesthetics such as alpha-2 agonists (xylazine, medetomidine, dexmedetomidine) and opioids induce high parasympathetic activity and lead to these arrhythmias.
  - Types of arrhythmia induced by electrolyte imbalance, diseases, or other drugs are mentioned earlier in this chapter.
- The arrhythmias can be either prevented or treated with atropine (0.02–0.04 mg/kg IV or IM) or glycopyrrolate (0.01–0.02 mg/kg IV or IM) if they are specifically related to the reasons mentioned here. Atropine at low doses may actually result in bradycardia or AV block itself before it increases the heart rate.

- VPCs may occur in several different forms:
  - Occasional single (**Fig. 22.7**) or two VPCs.
  - Rapid succession of three or more VPCs in a run.
  - Bigeminy (**Fig. 22.8**) or trigeminy VPCs (sinus rhythm sandwiched between every other VPC or every two VPCs in a fixed ratio).
  - A trigeminy (**Fig. 22.9**) is a type of cardiac arrhythmia characterized by the occurrence of three heartbeats in a repeating pattern. This pattern can be either two normal beats coupled to a VPC, or two VPC coupled to a normal beat.
  - Unifocal (from a single focus) or multifocal (from different ectopic foci) VPCs.

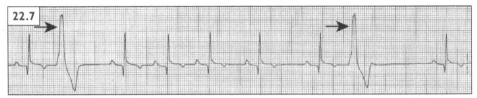

Fig. 22.7 Ventricular premature contractions (VPCs) may occur with several different forms. This is a single VPC.

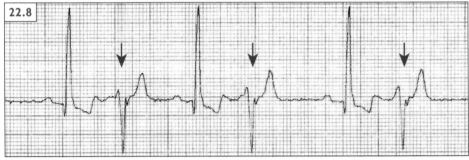

Fig. 22.8 Bigeminy VPCs with a normal sinus beat sandwiched between every other VPC in a fixed ratio.

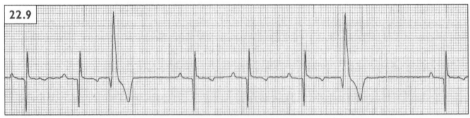

Fig. 22.9 A trigeminy can be either two normal beats coupled to a VPC (shown here), or two VPCs coupled to a normal beat. This trigeminy is formed with the first three beats.

- Most VPCs under general anesthesia may be triggered by several causes:
  - Increased catecholamine release triggered by the pain, distress, or excitement.
  - Hypoxia, hypercapnia, electrolyte imbalance, or acidosis.
  - Myocardial contusion following thoracic trauma.
  - Perioperative period of GDV.
  - Certain anesthetics such as thiopental, halothane, ketamine, or tiletamine/zolazepam may precipitate the occurrence of VPCs.
- Depending on the severity of the VPCs, occurrence of occasional one or two contractions does not require any treatment. A run of VPCs or multifocal VPCs affects cardiac output and leads to low blood pressure. Therefore, treatment should be instituted immediately. Others types of VPCs may require treatment for underlying causes (e.g. improving ventilation, providing enriched oxygen, deepening anesthesia, or supplementing with additional analgesics).
- In the cases of multiple VPCs (ventricular tachycardia, **Fig. 22.10**) or multifocal VPCs, 2 mg/kg of lidocaine (containing no epinephrine in the solution) should be given as an IV bolus of up to 8 mg/kg with 2–3 minutes in between each treatment.
- Idioventricular rhythm (**Fig. 22.11**) may be seen in some critically ill or trauma cases under general anesthesia. It may be due to a heart reaction to myocarditis, electrolyte imbalance, hypoxia, or drugs. Idioventricular rhythm is usually benign and does not require immediate treatment. However, it should be closely monitored, especially blood pressure and hemodynamic stability, before it becomes ventricular tachycardia or ventricular fibrillation.

CARDIAC ARRHYTHMIAS ASSOCIATED WITH CARDIAC EMERGENCY AND ARREST

- Cardiac arrest and resuscitation are described in detail in Chapter 21.
- Cardiac arrest may be associated with three types of electrical activity of the heart, namely ventricular fibrillation, asystole, and electrical mechanical dissociation.
  - Ventricular fibrillation is when there is a rapid and totally erratic ventricular heart waveform with no rhythm. A general description for

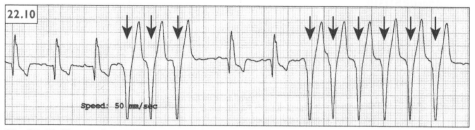

Fig. 22.10 Ventricular tachycardia as indicated by the blue arrows. These are VPCs in a run and severely affect cardiac output.

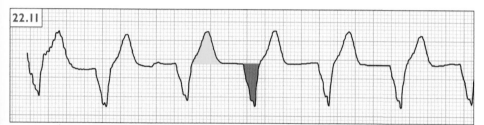

Fig. 22.11 Idioventricular rhythm in a dog. Note the distinct discordant (heading in different direction) of the QRS (yellow area) and ST-T (purple area) segments.

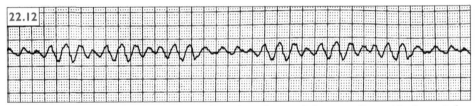

Fig. 22.12 Ventricular fibrillation is one of the three forms of electrocardiographic diagnosis for cardiac arrest. A coarse form of ventricular fibrillation is shown here.

the myocardial movement is 'a bag of worms'. This type of uncoordinated electrical activity generates no blood flow in or out of the heart.

- Coarse ventricular fibrillation (**Fig. 22.12**) is usually the early stage of ventricular fibrillation. It is characterized by bigger erratic waveforms and appears on the ECG screen to be random looking. Coarse ventricular fibrillation is usually followed by fine ventricular fibrillation with smaller erratic waveforms. As the cardiac arrest continues, it eventually goes into asystole.

- Asystole is a total cardiac standstill with no detectable cardiac activity. It is frequently called 'flat line' because there is no electrical activity with the heart.

- Electrical mechanical dissociation is when there is no mechanical activity of the heart but there is a near normal electrical wave form of heart activity.

Further reading

Chang HK, Seong-Hyop K (2017) Intraoperative management of critical arrhythmia. *Korean J Anesthesiol* **70(2)**:120–6.

Dua N, Kumra VP (2007) Management of perioperative arrhythmias. *Indian J Anaesth* **51**:310.

Dubin D (2000) *Rapid Interpretation of EKGs*, 6th edn. Cover Publishing Company, Tampa.

Lorentz MN, Vianna BSB (2011) Cardiac dysrhythmias and anesthesia. *Rev Bras Anestesiol* **61(6)**:798–813.

Local anesthetic agents and anesthetic techniques

Jeff C Ko and Tomohito Inoue

Introduction

Appropriately applied local anesthetic techniques offer additional perioperative analgesia, muscle relaxation, and anesthetic-sparing effects. Local anesthetic techniques, in general, are still underutilized in small animals when compared with large animal practice. Local anesthetic agents not only provide local and regional anesthesia and muscle relaxation but, when used parenterally as part of a CRI, also have profound systemic effects. This chapter describes the pharmacology of local anesthetic agents and the different injection techniques for local anesthesia.

Pharmacodynamics

TYPES OF LOCAL ANESTHETIC AGENT
- Local anesthetic agents can be divided into two groups, esters or amides, based on their chemical structure:
  - Esters include cocaine, procaine, tetracaine, and benzocaine.

They undergo hydrolysis by pseudocholinesterase in the blood and require minimal liver metabolism.
- Amides include lidocaine, mepivacaine, bupivacaine, prilocaine, ropivacaine, and etidocaine. They undergo

Table 23.1 Duration of action of the three most commonly used local anesthetic agents in small animal practice

Local anesthetic agent	Onset of action (minutes after injection)	Duration of action (min)
Lidocaine	2–4	60–90
Mepivacaine	3–5	120–180
Bupivacaine	5–10	240–360

extensive oxidative metabolism in the liver via cytochrome P450. Hepatic blood flow and hepatic function determine the clearance of amide local anesthetics. Patients with heart failure or liver disease are at increased risk for amide local anesthetic toxicity.

- In veterinary medicine the most commonly used agents are lidocaine, mepivacaine, and bupivacaine. This chapter focuses on the use of these three agents. Their duration of action is listed in *Table 23.1*.

MECHANISM OF ACTION

- Local anesthetics induce local anesthesia by blocking the voltage-gated sodium channels on the neuron cell membranes, inhibiting sodium permeability and resulting in low-acting potentials blocking transmission of signals between neurons.

SPECIFIC ACTIONS

- In addition to their local anesthetic effects, systemic administration of local anesthetic agents can have antiarrhythmic, anti-inflammatory, microcirculatory, postoperative gastrointestinal, and systemic analgesic effects. (See Chapter 24 for a description of the use of lidocaine as a systemic CRI for acute intra- and postoperative pain management.)
- In order to achieve local anesthesia, the local anesthetic agent must cover a sufficient length of nerve (or Ranvier nodes in the neurons) in order to block nerve conduction. This can usually be accomplished by administering an appropriate injection volume, concentration, and mass of local

anesthetic drug. It is still unclear which of volume, concentration, or mass is the most important factor in determining the success of a local anesthetic technique.

- DepoFoam (a recently developed extended-release formulation) has been combined with bupivacaine to induce a sustained action. DepoFoam is a biocompatible, biodegradable lipid-based suspension of spherical small particles (10–30 μm) that encapsulate the bupivacaine and allow diffusion over an extended duration. The veterinary product is called Nocita® (see **Fig. 19.1**) and the human product Exparel®. If 5.3 mg/kg of liposome bupivacaine injection suspension is infiltrated into the surgical site once, it induces analgesia lasting up to 72 hours. The suspension can be administered directly or diluted in a 1:1 ratio with sterile physiologic saline or lactated Ringer's solution for volume expansion.
- It is important to note that the liposome bupivacaine injection is for infiltration of the surgical site. It is not intended for regional nerve block, epidural, or injection into any of the dental nerve foramens. Nocita® is also approved for use in cats as a peripheral nerve block for postoperative analgesia following onychectomy.
- The economic downside of liposome bupivacaine injection suspension is that it does not contain preservative and, as a result the manufacturer recommends that the solution is kept for only 4 hours once the vial is broached. Practitioners are advised to plan ahead so that an opened vial can be used on several patients within a 4-hour period.

FACTORS THAT DETERMINE THE POTENCY, ONSET, DURATION, AND TOXICITY OF A LOCAL ANESTHETIC AGENT

- The onset and duration of action and toxic dose varies between the different agents and these factors should be taken into consideration when selecting the most appropriate one for a particular case.
- The maximum dose that can be administered is based on several factors. These include previously documented

doses associated with neurologic or cardiologic toxicity, anatomic site of injection, the patient's overall health, body weight and age, the desired duration of effect, and the coadministration of other drugs.

- Local anesthetic agents have different potencies. Those with larger molecular weights, greater lipid solubility, and higher protein binding (e.g. bupivacaine) have greater affinity for the sodium ion channel and, consequently, a longer duration of action. The more potent a local anesthetic agent, the higher the risk of cardiac toxicity. Bupivacaine is more cardiotoxic than lidocaine when compared on a mg/kg basis in dogs and cats.
- The onset of action is related to the lipid solubility of the agent.
- The rate at which a local anesthetic agent diffuses into a nerve is determined by its concentration. The higher the concentration, the more rapid the onset of the block.

ADDITIVES

- Drugs such as epinephrine, alpha-2 agonists, opioids, sodium bicarbonate, and midazolam have been used as additives to local anesthetic agents to increase the quality, intensity, duration, and safety of local anesthesia.
- Epinephrine is added to produce local vasoconstriction and prevent blood loss and to delay the absorption of the local anesthetic, thereby prolonging the duration of action. However, excessive epinephrine may lead to tachycardia and arrhythmias.
- In addition to their vasoconstrictive effects, alpha-2 agonists also have local anesthetic properties. Adding an alpha-2 agonist to a local anesthetic agent may also induce systemic sedation depending on the dose.
- Opioids enhance analgesia when administered together with a local anesthetic agent into the epidural or intrathecal (subarachnoid) space. They may also provide additional systemic sedation and analgesia.
- A recent study has shown that bupivacaine block induces a lower nerve blood flow.

However, this low blood flow does not induce relevant nerve ischemia. In the same study, coadministering clonidine (an alpha-2 agonist similar to xylazine) or epinephrine as an adjuvant to bupivacaine block for extending the local anesthetic effect, had no impact on nerve tissue oxygenation (as measured by tissue oximetry).

- Sodium bicarbonate is added (1 mmol (mEq) of $NaHCO_3$ per 10 ml of lidocaine or mepivacaine) to decrease the pain associated with injection of the agent and to facilitate the onset of action of some nerve blocks.
- Midazolam mainly acts on γ-aminobutyric acid type A (GABA-A) receptors for its sedative action. Despite the lack of presence of GABA-A receptors along peripheral nerve axons, midazolam has been shown to hasten the onset as well as prolong local anesthetic effects when used with a local anesthetic agent. Furthermore, when midazolam is combined with a local anesthetic agent, it also reduces the risk of neurotoxcity and motor blockade than when using the local anesthetic alone. A recent study found that midazolam may act on the 18 kDa translocator protein (TSPO), previously named peripheral benzodiazepine receptor. The TSPO is a nuclear-encoded mitochondrial protein. This author has successfully used 0.1–0.2 mg/kg of midazolam with either bupivacaine (2 mg/kg) or lidocaine (up to 6 mg/kg) for local infiltration, or with 0.5 mg/kg of bupivacaine and physiologic saline (to make up 1 ml/4.5 kg in total injection volume) for epidural injection in dogs and cats for regional anesthesia. Anecdotally, midazolam greatly enhances the analgesic intensity and duration of the treated animals.

TOXICITY OF LOCAL ANESTHETICS AND TREATMENTS

- Potential toxic doses of lidocaine, mepivacaine, and bupivacaine are listed in *Table 23.2*.
- An overdose is usually characterized by CNS symptoms including muscle tremors and seizures. Marked overdose results

Table 23.2 Potential toxic and clinical upper limit doses of lidocaine, mepivacaine, and bupivacaine

Agent	Dogs	Cats
Lidocaine	Convulsive IV bolus dose: 11–20 mg/kg Lethal IV bolus dose: 16–28 mg/kg Cumulative IV dose to collapse: 127 mg/kg Upper limit dose: 8–9 mg/kg by any route	Convulsive IV bolus dose: 8–22 mg/kg Lethal IV bolus dose: unknown, but likely similar to dogs Upper limit dose: 6–8 mg/kg by any route
Mepivacaine	Convulsive IV bolus dose: 9–20 mg/kg Upper limit dose: 3–4 mg/kg by any route	Convulsive IV bolus dose: 22 mg/kg Upper limit dose: 3–4 mg/kg by any route
Bupivacaine	Convulsive IV bolus dose: 2–8 mg/kg Lethal IV bolus dose: 10 mg/kg Cumulative IV dose to collapse: 22 mg/kg Upper limit dose: 2–3 mg/kg by any route	Convulsive IV bolus dose: 3–6 mg/kg Lethal IV bolus dose: similar to dogs Upper limit dose: 2–3 mg/kg by any route

in severe hypotension and ultimately cardiorespiratory arrest.

- Bupivacaine is more arrhythmogenic and a greater myocardial depressant than lidocaine in dogs and cats. Mepivacaine has intermediate toxicity (between bupivacaine and lidocaine).
- Muscle tremors and seizures induced by an overdose can be managed with diazepam or midazolam (0.2–0.4 mg/kg IV). Alternatively,

propofol (3–4 mg/kg IV) or alfaxalone (1–2 mg/kg IV) can be given.

- Hypotension induced by local anesthetic agents can be treated with a combination of IV fluids and vasopressors (phenylephrine [5–10 µg/kg/min] or norepinephrine [2–5 µg/kg/min]).
- If cardiac arrest occurs, epinephrine (10–100 µg/kg) should be administered IV and cardiopulmonary resuscitation performed.

Dental blocks

- Traditionally, dental blocks have involved blocking the infraorbital, mental, and mandibular foramens (**Fig. 23.1**). Recent work suggests that blocking the infraorbital and

mental foramen is sufficient to provide analgesia extending from the canines to the molars in both the maxilla and the mandible.

- The use of bupivacaine liposome injection suspension (Nocita®) around the tooth extraction site will provide analgesia in addition to the following tooth never blocks. The suspension can be injected, in a similar away to infiltration, above and below the gingival margin and into the periodontal ligament and fibers. The analgesic effect lasts approximately 72 hours and greatly enhances the comfort of the dogs and cats. Some anesthesiologists have used Nocita® for dental foramen blocks (see the following). However, the pros and cons for such prolonged (72 hours) blocks via these foramens have not been studied in detail. It is therefore not currently recommended to use Nocita for foramen blocks.

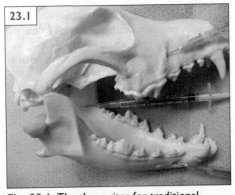

23.1

Fig. 23.1 The three sites for traditional dental blocks are the infraorbital (top syringe), mandibular foramen (middle syringe), and mental foramen (bottom syringe).

INFRAORBITAL BLOCK

INDICATIONS
- To provide intra- and postoperative analgesia for maxillary canine, molar, and premolar extractions.
- The same technique also provides analgesia to the area around the upper lips and nares.

AREA AND NERVES BLOCKED
- The infraorbital nerves supply the caudal, medial, and rostral superior alveolar nerves with multiple nerve branches innervating the upper lip, buccal, and nasal areas (**Fig. 23.2**).

LANDMARKS
- The infraorbital foramen ipsilateral to the tooth to be extracted is located just below the zygomatic arch. The lateral bone margin of the infraorbital foramen is easily palpated immediately dorsal to the root of the maxillary third premolar (**Fig. 23.3**). The foramen is triangular and easily palpated in medium- and large-sized dogs both intraorally (**Fig. 23.4**) and extraorally (**Fig. 23.5**).

DRUGS AND EQUIPMENT
- A combination of 0.5 ml 2% lidocaine and 0.5 ml 0.5% bupivacaine, dosed at 0.15 ml/4.5 kg (10 lb), is administered.

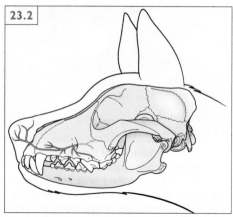

Fig. 23.2 Schematic drawing of the innervation of the upper lips, nares, canines, and molars.

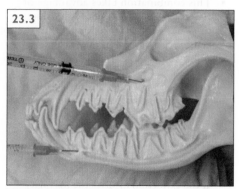

Fig. 23.3 The infraorbital foramen (upper syringe) and mental foramen (lower syringe).

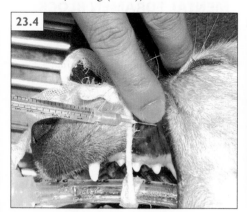

Fig. 23.4 Intraoral approach for the administration of a lidocaine–bupivacaine mixture to block nerves that innervate the infraorbital foramen.

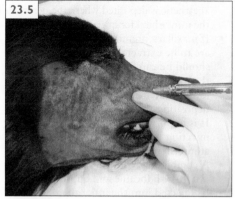

Fig. 23.5 Extraoral approach for an infraorbital nerve block. The infraorbital foramen can be easily palpated in a medium- to large-sized dog.

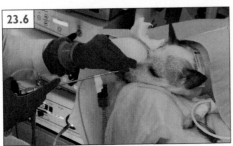

Fig. 23.6 An infraorbital block was performed on this dog prior to rhinoscopy. The area of the maxillary sinus region (the red lighted area) was desensitized to reduce the potential reaction of the dog during the biopsy and scoping procedures.

- This combination takes advantage of the fast onset of action of lidocaine (3–5 minutes) and the longer duration of action (6–8 hours) of bupivacaine.
- A 22–25 gauge, 1–1.5 inch needle should be used.
- Lidocaine with epinephrine (1:100,000) may be used to prolong the duration of the effect.

APPROACH
- The infraorbital foramen is palpated intra- or extraorally (**Figs. 23.4, 23.5**).
- If the extraction involves the maxillary canine tooth and incisor, the needle is inserted through the gingiva of the oral cavity just above the premolar. The local anesthetic is deposited where the nerves exit the infraorbital foramen.
- If maxillary premolars and molar are to be extracted, the needle should be carefully advanced into the infraorbital foramen to the level of the medial canthus prior to depositing the local anesthetic agent. It is important to aspirate prior to injecting to ensure that the agent is not administered IV.
- A combined volume of 0.15 ml/4.5 kg (10 lb) of lidocaine and bupivacaine can be injected into the infraorbital foramen for this block.
- The effectiveness of the block can be confirmed by lowering the maintenance concentrations of the inhalant anesthetic agent. This is because the local anesthetic, through

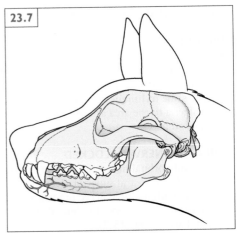

Fig. 23.7 Schematic drawing of the innervation of the lower lips and the canine, premolar, and molar teeth of the mandible.

the effectiveness of the block, has an inhalant anesthetic-sparing effect.
- The infraorbital foramen block is also useful to alleviate the nociceptive reactions from rhinoscopy and nasal biopsy (**Fig. 23.6**). Studies have shown that cardiorespiratory reactions (drastically increased heart rate, respiratory rate, and/or blood pressure) of the animals were much less with this foramen blocks than of the animals without the block during the rhinoscopic procedures.

MENTAL FORAMEN BLOCK

INDICATIONS
- To provide intra- and postoperative analgesia for mandibular canine, molar, and premolar tooth extractions. Analgesia also extends to the lower lip.

AREA AND NERVES BLOCKED
- The nerves that innervate and exit the mental foramen (**Fig. 23.7**) include the rostral alveolar branch of the inferior alveolar nerve.

LANDMARKS
- The mental foramen ipsilateral to the tooth to be extracted.
- The mental foramen can be palpated through the gingiva of the mandible below the premolar immediately caudal to the canine tooth (**Fig. 23.8**).

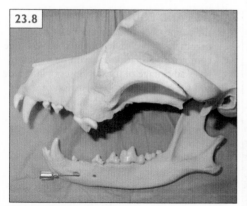

Fig. 23.8 The mental foramen is located just below the first premolar.

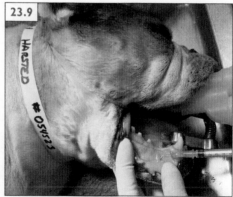

Fig. 23.9 Injection of local anesthetic into the mental foramen canal for desensitizing the canine, premolars, and molars of the mandible.

DRUGS AND EQUIPMENT
- As for maxillary tooth extractions.

APPROACH
- The mental foramen is approached intraorally (**Fig. 23.9**).

Brachial plexus block

INDICATIONS
- To provide analgesia and muscle relaxation for the forelimb, from the shoulder to the toes, to facilitate orthopedic or soft tissue surgeries.
- If an amputation is to be performed, injecting local anesthetic around the brachial plexus nerves is thought to prevent phantom limb pain (neuropathic).

AREA AND NERVES BLOCKED
- Brachial plexus nerves derived from the ventral branch of spinal nerves exiting from C6–T1, branches into the suprascapular nerve, musculocutaneous nerve, axillary nerve, radial nerve, median nerve, ulnar nerve, and thoracodorsal nerve, which innervate the forelimb.

LANDMARKS
- Tip of the greater tubercle of humerus (**Fig. 23.10**).

- In cats, palpating the mental foramen is difficult as the labial frenulum lies over the canal. The easiest way to administer the drug appropriately is to 'walk' the needle along the bony mandible until the mental foramen is encountered.

- During forelimb amputation, the nerves of the brachial plexus are directly exposed (**Fig. 23.11**).

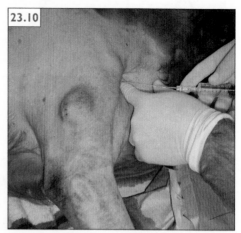

Fig. 23.10 Brachial plexus block. The left index finger is firmly palpating the first rib and preventing the needle accidentally entering the thorax. Note the tumor nodule in the center of the scapula.

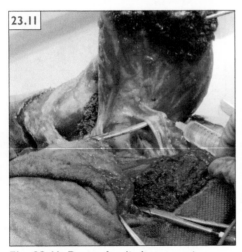

Fig. 23.11 During forelimb amputation, the brachial plexus nerves are directly exposed, allowing for the administration of lidocaine–bupivacaine in and around the nerves.

DRUGS AND EQUIPMENT

- ·Lidocaine or bupivacaine alone or mixed together. Mepivacaine can also be used. The combination of lidocaine with bupivacaine takes advantage of the fast onset of lidocaine and the longer duration of action of bupivacaine, as discussed previously.
- Dose: 1–2 mg/kg of 0.5% bupivacaine. For smaller-sized dogs, if the volume of local anesthetic is too small, it can be diluted with sterile saline to a volume of 5–12 ml for administration.
- A 22 gauge, 1.5–2.5 inch spinal needle is suitable for most dogs and cats.
- An insulated catheter needle (**Fig. 23.12**) can also be used, together with a low-current nerve stimulator (different to that used for neuromuscular blocks) (**Fig. 23.13**), to locate the nerves.

APPROACH

- The hair is clipped and the area surgically prepared. Sterile technique must be used

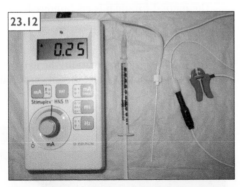

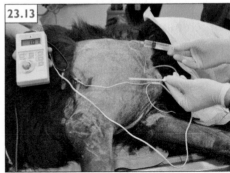

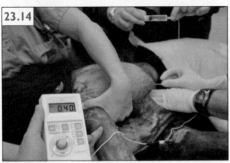

Figs. 23.12–23.14 (**23.12**) An insulated needle with an injection catheter, which may be used with a low-current nerve stimulator to locate the nerves of the brachial plexus. (**23.13**) The dog is placed in lateral recumbency with the area aseptically prepared. The positive lead (red color) is attached to the skin and the negative lead is connected to the needle. The catheter is filled with local anesthetic. The needle shows the direction of insertion. (**23.14**) Once the needle is in place, the current of the nerve stimulator is turned up and the needle inserted further to search for the brachial plexus nerves. On approaching the nerves, the muscle twitches becomes obvious and at this time the current of the stimulation is reduced (down to 0.4 volts or less). If the muscle twitching remains, the local anesthetic (either lidocaine or bupivacaine) is injected. On injection, the muscle twitches stop and the nerve is considered blocked.

in order to perform the block aseptically. The patient must be anesthetized or profoundly sedated.

- The patient is placed in lateral recumbency with the affected limb dorsal and parallel to the body wall (**Fig. 23.14**).
- The person performing the block should wear sterile gloves and place his or her index finger between the medial aspect of the scapula and the first rib (**Fig. 23.15**). This prevents accidental insertion of the spinal needle into the thoracic cavity.
- The spinal needle is placed parallel to the spinal column and enters the space between the medial aspect of the scapula and the first rib at a level slightly above the greater tubercle of the humerus. The needle is then directed caudally (for approximately 1.25–1.9 cm [0.5–0.75 in]) to the level of the second or third rib.
- The needle is aspirated to ensure that there is no blood or air and the local anesthetic is slowly injected as the needle is withdrawn.
- This procedure is repeated so as to create a fan-shaped area covering the brachial plexus nerves.

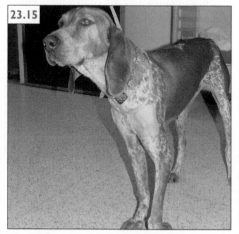

Fig. 23.15 This dog has recovered from general anesthesia immediately following a brachial plexus block to assess the success of the motor (muscle relaxation) and the sensory (analgesia) block. Note the dropped shoulder and forelimb knuckling, which indicate a successful brachial plexus blockage.

- If a low-current nerve stimulator is used to locate the nerves, an insulated needle is used for the brachial plexus nerve block instead of a spinal needle.
- An insulated needle will not penetrate the skin, therefore a small incision must be made to facilitate insertion of the needle. The nerve stimulator is switched on as the insulated needle is advanced. A higher current should be used initially (**Fig. 23.13**) until twitching is observed, at which point the current is reduced to the lowest possible setting to allow for detection of the point of maximal muscle twitching. This signifies that the needle tip is close to the nerve. Local anesthetic is then injected through the needle catheter onto the branches of the brachial plexus nerves. This method allows the local anesthetic to be deposited in close proximity to the nerves. As the local anesthetic reaches the nerve it pushes the nerve away, the twitching stops (Raj Test – see Chapter 18) despite the electrical current.
- If an animal is recovered from general anesthesia shortly after completion of a successful block, shoulder paresis will be evident (**Fig. 23.15**). The sensory and motor nerves recover gradually over time, with the animal regaining full use of the limb.
- Occasionally, Horner's syndrome (**Fig. 23.16**), which is characterized by a drooping eye, small size pupil,

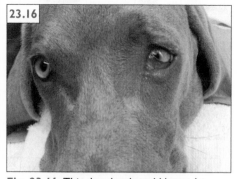

Fig. 23.16 This dog developed Horner's syndrome, which is characterized by a drooping eye, small size pupil, sunken-in eye, and a prominent third eyelid following a brachial plexus block.

sunken-in eye, and a prominent third eyelid, may develop after brachial plexus block. The symptoms are similar to the development of brachial plexus avulsion; however, the main reason is due to sympathetic blockage by the local anesthetic agent, which affects the normal function of the cervical 6th–8th to thoracic 1 and 2 sympathetic neurons. Horner's syndrome usually spontaneously resolves within 12 hours of its development.

Ring and three-point blocks

INDICATIONS
- Provision of intra- and postoperative analgesia when performing a feline forelimb declaw or removal of any interdigital growth (tumors). This technique can also be applied to hindlimb declaws or similar growth removal. (**Note:** The declawing of cats is prohibited in a number of US states and in certain countries.)

AREA AND NERVES BLOCKED
- Forelimbs: the radial nerve, palmar and dorsal branches of the ulnar nerve, and the palmer median nerve are blocked at the level of the carpus (**Fig. 23.17**).

- Hindlimbs: the superficial peroneal nerve on the dorsal side of the limb and the tibial nerve on the plantar side at the level of tarsus are blocked (**Fig. 23.18**).
- If using a ring block, these nerves are blocked at the level of the carpus.

LANDMARKS
- Ring block: a circular block is performed immediately above the metacarpal pad of the fore- or hindlimb (**Figs. 23.17, 23.18**).
- Three-point block: the anatomic landmarks on the dorsal and ventral portion of the forelimb are illustrated in **Fig. 23.17**.

DRUGS AND EQUIPMENT
- 2% lidocaine and 0.5% of bupivacaine combined without epinephrine.
- 0.6 ml of 2% lidocaine and 0.6 ml of 0.5% bupivacaine are drawn up in the same syringe and administered at 0.2 ml per site.

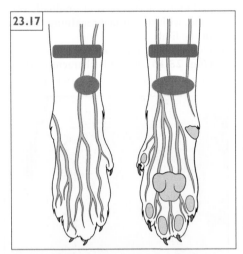

Fig. 23.17 Schematic drawing of the distal forelimb innervation in a cat. Note the anatomy of the nerve distribution. A three-point block may be used to selectively block the nerve conduction of the dorsal and ventral branches of the radial and ulna nerves.

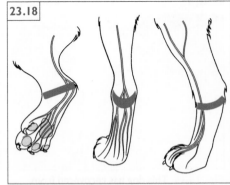

Fig. 23.18 Schematic drawing of the distal hindlimb innervation in a cat. Note the anatomy of the nerve distribution. A three-point block may be used to selectively block the nerve conduction of the superficial peroneal nerve on the dorsal side of the limb and the tibial nerve on the plantar side at the level of tarsus.

- Recently, Nocita® has been approved for use in cats as a peripheral nerve block to provide regional postoperative analgesia following onychectomy. Nocita can be used instead of lidocaine or regular bupivacaine for these ring block or three-point blocks to induce a 72-hour duration of analgesia.
- A 22 gauge needle with a 1 ml tuberculin syringe is used to administer the block.
- A tourniquet is applied distal to the elbow to prevent bleeding. Epinephrine can potentiate an ischemic response by constricting blood vessels. This could result in tissue necrosis and sloughing of the paw. As a consequence, use of a local anesthetic without epinephrine is preferred.

APPROACH

- Two approaches can be used: a ring block or a three-point block.
- The block is usually performed immediately prior to surgery (i.e. soon after the animal has been anesthetized). The injection site is prepared as for a sterile procedure.
- A ring block is performed by inserting a 22 gauge needle subcutaneously (**Fig. 23.19**) at the level above the

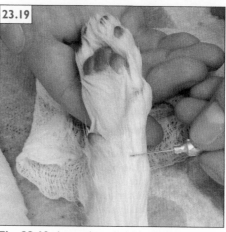

Fig. 23.19 A ring (circular) block in a cat. This can be used for removal of a front declaw or an interdigital growth.

metacarpal pad and injecting in a circular pattern. The area is seen to bulge post injection as the local anesthetic infiltrates the tissues around the limb.
- A three-point injection involves infiltration of 0.2–0.3 ml of local anesthetic at both the radial and ulna branches.

Nerve blocks for thoracic surgeries

INTERCOSTAL NERVE BLOCK

INDICATIONS

- To provide intra- and postoperative analgesia for lateral thoracotomy in dogs and cats.
- This technique also provides analgesia to the surgical area in the thoracic wall surrounding the incision and allows for improved ventilation, thus minimizing pain during respiration as the animal recovers.

AREA AND NERVES BLOCKED

- The internal surface of the thoracic wall is covered by costal parietal pleura. The internal intercostal muscle fascicles run between the ribs together with the intercostal nerve. The artery and vein run along the caudal border of each rib. The intercostal nerve block desensitizes the intercostal nerves innervating the intercostal spaces on the same (ipsilateral) side of the thorax as the surgical site.
- The nerves are blocked where they exit the spinal column and innervate the intercostal space (**Fig. 23.20**).

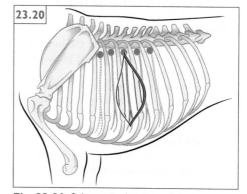

Fig. 23.20 Schematic drawing of the nerves innervating the intercostal nerve space in a dog undergoing lateral thoracotomy.

LANDMARKS

- Depending on the size of the animal, the injection should be made approximately 5–10 cm (2–4 in) from the ventral portion of the paravertebral area of the pleura.

DRUGS AND EQUIPMENT

- Bupivacaine 0.5% with or without epinephrine (0.3–0.5 ml per site).
- Alternatively, 0.25 ml of lidocaine 2% in combination with 0.25 ml of 0.5% bupivacaine can be used (administer 0.5 ml per site).
- A tuberculin syringe with a 22 gauge needle is usually used.

APPROACH

- The procedure is performed aseptically either at the beginning of the thoracotomy or at the conclusion prior to closure of the pleural layer of the thorax.
- Three injections are administered (**Fig. 23.20**): (1) dorsal to the surgical incision site in the ventral portion of the pleura; (2) intercostal cranial nerve; and (3) intercostal nerve caudal to the incision site.

INTRAPLEURAL INFUSION NERVE BLOCK

INDICATIONS

- To provide intra- and postoperative analgesia for sternal or lateral thoracotomy in dogs and cats.
- Can be used for multiple rib fractures or painful conditions in the thorax.

AREA AND NERVES BLOCKED

- The nerves that innervate the intercostal spaces on the ipsilateral side of the thorax involved in surgery.
- This technique provides regional analgesia by desensitizing the nerves that innervate the thorax.

LANDMARKS

- Depending on the size of the animal, the block is administered through a preplaced

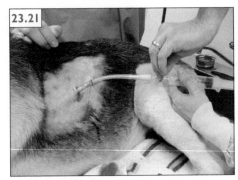

Fig. 23.21 Intrapleural infusion nerve block. Local anesthetic diluted with sterile saline is infused into the pleural space via a chest tube. A three-way stopcock is required for repeated injection to seal the chest and prevent iatrogenic pneumothorax.

chest tube or catheter tunneled into the thorax through the fifth or sixth rib interspace.

DRUGS AND EQUIPMENT

- Bupivacaine 0.5% without epinephrine (0.3–0.5 ml/kg diluted with 5–20 ml of sterile saline depending on the size of the animal).
- A chest tube or a catheter.
- A three-way stopcock is required to enable repeated injections and to seal the chest to prevent pneumothorax (**Fig. 23.21**).

APPROACH

- The block is administered under sterile conditions post thoracotomy prior to recovery from anesthesia.
- After placement of the chest tube, the diluted local anesthetic is slowly infused into the thorax. The chest tube should then be flushed with 3–5 ml of saline.
- The animal is positioned with the surgical or fracture site ventral to allow the local anesthetic to gravitate to the affected region. The animal should be maintained in that position for approximately 10 minutes.

Lumbosacral epidural block

INDICATIONS
- Intra- and postoperative analgesia for hindquarter surgeries in dogs and cats (e.g. tail amputation, anal–rectal surgeries, tibial–femoral fractures, total hip replacement, cruciate ligament repair), exploratory laparotomy, cesarean section, and surgical procedures in the region of the twelfth or thirteenth ribs.

AREA AND NERVES BLOCKED
- Pelvic plexus nerves.

LANDMARKS
- Lumbosacral junction (**Figs. 23.22, 23.23**).
- When performing an epidural, the acronym ED-SAS-PS ('Ed says PS') can help recognize the regional anatomy: Epidural space (the first anatomic space encountered by the needle), Dura mater, Subdura, Arachnoid, Subarachnoid space (where the CSF is located), Pia mater, Spinal cord.
- The spinal (also called epidural) needle should be angled toward the ventral aspect of the spinal column, passing through the skin, the interspinous muscles and ligaments, and the ligmentum flavum (where a 'pop' will be felt on penetration).
- Before entering the epidural space, the anatomic structures passed through are the skin, the interspinous muscles, the spinal muscles, and the ligmentum flavum.

DRUGS AND EQUIPMENT
- Various drugs may be used (e.g. opioids, opioids with local anesthetics, alpha-2 agonists, local anesthetics with alpha-2 agonists, opioids with alpha-2s)
- The *Further reading* list contains an excellent review of epidural analgesic drugs and techniques. The key features of some of the drugs used are described below.

Morphine
- Can be given with or without a preservative (preferred).
- Dose is 0.1 mg/kg.
- Onset of action is 20–60 minutes.
- Duration of action is 6–8 hours.

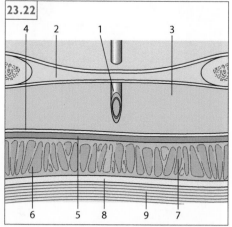

Fig. 23.22 Diagram showing the regional anatomy for an epidural injection in cats. Note that the subarachnoid space extends into the first sacrum. 1, spinal needle; 2, ligamentum flavum; 3, epidural space; 4, dura mater; 5, arachnoic membrane; 6, subarachnoid space (where the cerebrospinal fluid is located); 7, cerebral spinal fluid; 8, pia mater; 9, spinal cord.

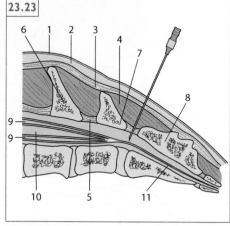

Fig. 23.23 Schematic drawing of the anatomic structures of the lumbosacral region in dogs. 1, skin; 2, subcutaneous tissue; 3, supraspinous ligament; 4, interspinous ligament and muscles; 5, ligamentum flavum; 6, 6th lumbar vertebra; 7, 7th lumbar vertebra; 8, 1st sacrum; 9, subarachnoid space; 10, spinal cord; 11, cauda equina. (Note: The spinal cord of the dog, unlike that in cats, ends between the 6th and 7th lumbar vertebrae.)

Oxymorphone or hydromorphone
- Dose of 0.1 mg/kg.
- Duration of action is 2–3 hours in dogs.

Fentanyl
- Dose is 5–10 µg/kg.
- Short duration of action (less than 1 hour) due to high lipid solubility makes it of minimal benefit when administered epidurally.

Butorphanol
- Dose is 0.25 mg/kg.
- Reduces isoflurane MAC by 31%.
- Duration of action is 2–3 hours.

Medetomidine (and dexmedetomidine)
- Dose is 15 µg/kg (10 µg/kg for dexmedetomidine) for dogs and 10 µg/kg (7–10 µg/kg for dexmedetomidine) for cats.
- Duration of action is 4–8 hours in dogs and 20 minutes to 4 hours in cats.

Bupivacaine and morphine combinations
- The most common combination is bupivacaine at 0.2 mg/kg with preservative-free morphine at 0.1 mg/kg (final injection volume dosed at 1 ml/4.5 kg [10 lb] in dogs and cats).
- Duration of analgesia is approximately 8 hours.

APPROACH
- This procedure is performed aseptically under general anesthesia or profound sedation.
- The animal can be in lateral (**Figs. 23.24, 23.25**) or sternal (**Fig. 23.26**) recumbency.
- Sternal recumbency is easier than lateral recumbency given that the landmarks are easily identifiable (**Figs. 23.27, 23.28**). The hanging drop technique can be applied to animals in sternal recumbency.
- With the hanging drop technique (**Fig. 23.29**), a few drops of sterile saline are used to fill the hub of the spinal needle so that a bleb of saline is formed in the spinal needle hub. As the spinal needle is advanced ventrally into the epidural space (in a sternally recumbent

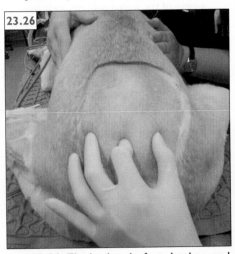

Fig. 23.26 The landmarks for a lumbosacral epidural injection are easier to identify when the dog is in sternal recumbency. The index finger is pointed at the lumbosacral junction and the thumb and middle finger rest on top of the wing of the right and left ileum, respectively. The limbs are pulled forward and the body is stabilized in a central position to facilitate palpation of the landmarks.

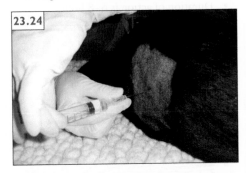

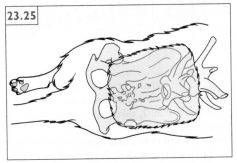

Figs. 23.24, 23.25 A lumbosacral epidural injection (see highlighted area **Fig. 23.25**) being performed in a dog in lateral recumbency (**Fig. 23.24**).

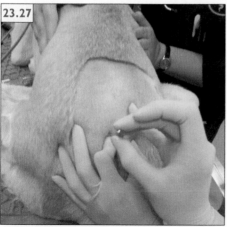

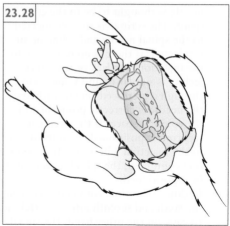

Figs. 23.27, 23.28 Placement of the epidural needle with an index finger identifying the lumbosacral junction (**Fig. 23.27**) while inserting the epidural needle ventrally into the lumbosacral junction (highlighted area, **Fig. 23.28**).

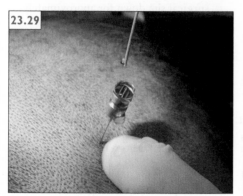

Fig. 23.29 The hanging drop technique for epidural needle placement. The stylet is removed and a few drops of sterile saline are used to fill the hub of the epidural (also called spinal) needle. The saline is left to 'hang' onto the needle hub. The needle is advanced ventrally and on entering the epidural space, the negative pressure will aspirate the saline into the epidural space, providing clear evidence of proper placement of the needle.

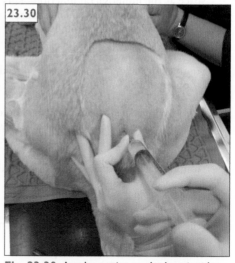

Fig. 23.30 An alternative to the hanging drop technique is to detect a lack of resistance on injection. The lack of resistance during the epidural injection is similar to that of giving an intravenous injection.

animal, see **Figs. 23.26, 23.27**), the saline in the hub is aspirated into the epidural space as a result of the negative pressure within this space. This technique is less likely to work in animals in lateral recumbency.

- The technique is not always successful even when performed in animals in sternal recumbency, and seems to occur more readily in larger (>15 kg) dogs.
- An alternative (concurrent) technique is 'the lack of resistance method' of epidural placement (**Fig. 23.30**). This method uses a syringe filled with 3 ml of sterile saline or air. The spinal needle is positioned to a point where the

needle is thought to be in the epidural space. The syringe is then connected to the spinal needle and saline or air is injected. If there is no resistance to the injection (the lack of resistance feeling is similar to an IV injection through a preplaced venous catheter), the needle is correctly positioned in the epidural space. If the needle is incorrectly positioned, high resistance to the injection will occur. If resistance is encountered, the spinal needle must be repositioned.

- In dogs, the spinal cord ends between the sixth and seventh lumbar vertebrae. In cats, on the other hand, the spinal cord ends at the level of first sacrum. When performing an epidural injection in cats, CSF may be encountered if the spinal needle enters the subarachnoid space at the lumbosacral junction. This does not occur in dogs when epidural needle is placed in the lumbosacral junction.
- If CSF is encountered in cats, the drug volume administered should be reduced by one-half to avoid an anesthetic overdose. The analgesic agent(s) is deposited directly into the subarachnoid space, contacting neural tissues directly, with less filtering by the meninges (dura and arachnoid).
- Administration of drugs into the epidural or spinal space should be performed slowly over 60–90 seconds and not as a rapid bolus.
- The correct position of the animal after an epidural injection is important to ensure full action of the analgesic drug.
- For a unilateral effect, the animal should preferably be positioned

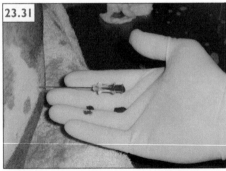

Fig. 23.31 Occasionally, blood will be encountered during epidural needle placement. If this occurs, the needle should be removed and flushed with saline or replaced. The procedure can then be repeated.

surgical site down for approximately 10–15 minutes.
- For a bilateral effect, the animal is placed in dorsal recumbency.
- If blood is encountered during an epidural injection (**Fig. 23.31**), the procedure should be abandoned with the needle being withdrawn and flushed with the saline to clear the blood or replaced altogether. The procedure can then be attempted again.
- Complications that have been reported with epidural/spinal injections include lack of efficacy, hypotension, urinary retention, CNS toxicity, pruritus post-morphine epidural, self-mutilation following the use of an opioid containing preservative, and failure of hair regrowth at the injection site.

Epidural catheter placement

- Same approach as for performing an epidural injection at the lumbosacral junction.
- Using a Touhy needle (**Figs. 23.32, 23.33**) instead of a regular epidural needle allows an epidural catheter to be placed into the epidural space for repeated administration of local anesthetic. An appropriately-sized

epidural catheter is required in order for it to be thread through the lumen of the epidural needle. Failure to use the correctly sized epidural catheter, and therefore an inability to thread the catheter through the epidural needle, should be differentiated from inappropriate placement of the epidural needle and

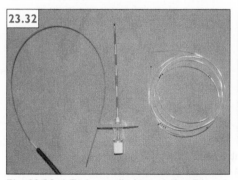

Fig. 23.32 A Touhy needle (named after Edward Boyce Tuohy) with two different sizes of epidural catheters. Note the 1 cm markings (called Lee markings after John Alfred Lee, who added these marks so that anesthetists would know accurately the depth of the Touhy needle tip) on the needle shaft. The Touhy needle has a curved tip (called the Huber point after its designer Ralph L. Huber), which allows an epidural catheter to be introduced into the epidural space.

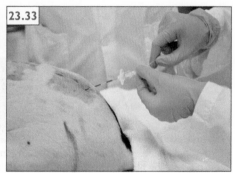

Fig. 23.33 A Touhy needle being inserted at the lumbosacral junction, with an epidural catheter being fed into the epidural space.

resulting failure to insert the catheter into the desired place.
- The use of an epidural catheter also allows the catheter to be placed in different regions (thoracic versus lumbar) of the epidural space for drug administration.

Specific nerve blocks

- In addition to regional blocks of the brachial or pelvic plexus, techniques are available to apply local anesthetic agents directly aimed at specific nerves. Femoral and sciatic nerve blocks (see Chapter 18) are examples of using a low-current nerve stimulator with an insulated needle to find the specific nerve with or without ultrasound visual aid.
  - The advantages of a specific nerve block are that it is less invasive, blocks only the specific region that is needed for surgery, and has fewer complications (e.g. urinary retention, constipation induced by pelvic plexus epidural administration).
  - The disadvantage is that this technique also takes time to master and is considered slightly more difficult than epidural administration. Furthermore, the use of a low-current nerve stimulator with insulated needles is necessary to ensure a high successful block rate.

Intravenous regional blocks (Bier block and hindlimb blocks)

INDICATIONS
- To provide intra- and postoperative analgesia for fore- or hindlimb soft tissue surgeries.

AREA AND NERVES BLOCKED
- The nerves that innervate the distal portion of the limb below the elbow or stifle.

LANDMARKS
- The cephalic vein of the forelimb or the saphenous vein of the hindlimb.

DRUGS AND EQUIPMENT
- 2% lidocaine without epinephrine is administered IV at 5 mg/kg. A lidocaine (3 mg/kg) and bupivacaine mixture (1 mg/kg) may also be used.
- Rubber tubing is used as a tourniquet.
- A blood pressure cuff can also be used to block local circulation.

APPROACH
- The limb must be exsanguinated prior to application/inflation of the tourniquet.

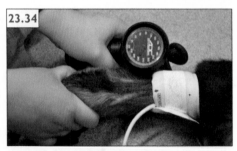

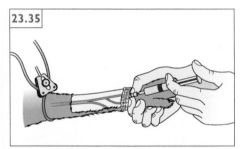

Figs. 23.34, 23.35 A Bier block of the forelimb is used to desensitize the area distal to the tourniquet. The blood pressure cuff is used as a tourniquet in this case and the cuff pressure is inflated to exceed systolic pressure in order to retain local anesthetic regionally. The local anesthetic agent is administered through the cephalic vein, as shown here.

This is accomplished by wrapping a bandage tightly around the limb proximal to the needle placement site.

- Alternatively, the limb can be elevated for 30 seconds prior to application of the tourniquet.
- If using a blood pressure cuff for a tourniquet, the cuff is inflated to a pressure 50 mmHg higher than the animal's systolic blood pressure (**Figs. 23.34, 23.35**).
- Adequate inflation has been achieved when the distal pulse disappears.
- Surgery should last no more than 60 minutes to prevent ischemia of the extremity with the tourniquet.

Local anesthetic as an adjunct to general anesthesia for eye surgery

INDICATIONS
- Enucleation and eyelid surgery (e.g. entropion, ectropion, wedge resection, canthoplasty).
- To provide additional intraoperative and postoperative analgesia for eye surgery.
- Anesthetize the palpebral nerve and all the eyelid muscles except the levator palpebrea.

AREAS AND NERVES BLOCKED
- Retrobulbar block: trigeminal nerve, oculomotor (cranial nerve III), trochlear (cranial nerve IV), and abducens (cranial nerve VI) nerves.
- Local eyelid block: palpebral nerve. The palpebral nerve is a branch of the auriculopalpebral nerve, which in turn is a branch of the facial nerve.

LANDMARKS
- Retrobulbar block. A retrobulbar block is performed by stabilizing the sclera with an ophthalmic forceps and pushing the eyeball upward and medially. A 22 gauge needle (a spinal needle can be used instead) of sufficient length (1–1.5 in) is then introduced through the inferior rectus muscle and there should be a feeling of a 'pop' as soon as the muscle is penetrated. The needle is then tangentially moved towards the maxillary bony floor. On striking the floor, the needle is directed slightly upwards towards the back of the globe until it reaches the retrobulbar space (**Figs. 23.36, 23.37**). The correct placement is confirmed by free motion of the needle tip and protrusion–rotation of the eyeball on injection of 1 ml of anesthetic agent (**Figs. 23.38–23.40**).
- Palpebral nerve block. The palpebral nerve can be anesthetized by SC injection of 1 ml of local anesthetic approximately 1 cm dorsal to the zygomatic arch at its most lateral projection.

DRUGS
- One to 3 ml of 2% lidocaine or bupivacaine without epinephrine.

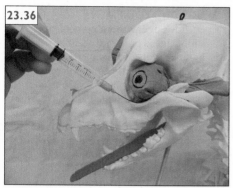

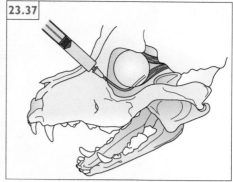

Figs. 23.36, 23.37 A 22 gauge needle of sufficient length is introduced through the inferior rectus muscle in this canine skeletal model. The needle is then tangentially moved towards the maxillary bony floor. On striking the bony floor, the needle is then directed slightly upwards towards the back of the globe and reaches the retrobulbar space.

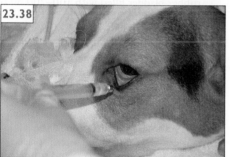

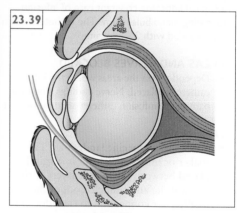

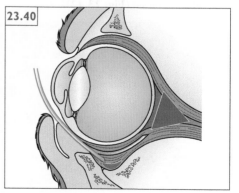

Figs. 23.38–23.40 (**23.38**) This photograph shows a 22-gauge spinal needle being introduced through the inferior rectus muscle of a dog, with the needle being repositioned toward the retrobulbar space. (**23.39**) The needle (shown in green) is moved tangentially towards the bony floor of the maxilla (red colored area). On striking the bony floor, the needle is directed slightly upward towards the back of the globe until it reaches the retrobulbar space (blue colored area). (**23.40**) The sequence of needle movements from the rectus muscles toward the retrobulbar space is shown in this drawing. The correct placement of the needle in the retrobulbar space is confirmed by free motion of the needle tip and protrusion–rotation of the eyeball on injection of 1 ml of anesthetic agent.

Lidocaine regional constant rate infusion

INDICATIONS
- To provide additional postoperative analgesia for up to 3–5 days whenever a fenestrated infusion catheter can be placed.

- This technique is useful in procedures such as mastectomies, mandibulectomies (**Fig. 23.41**), amputations, and ear canal ablations.

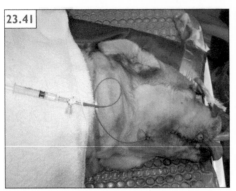

Fig. 23.41 A home-made fenestrated catheter (in this case a sterile catheter normally used in the urinary tract) has been placed between the muscle layers to allow for a topical lidocaine constant rate of infusion following mandibulectomy. The catheter lumen is preloaded with 2% lidocaine.

AREAS AND NERVES BLOCKED

- Dependent on the areas where the infusion catheter is placed. Nerve endings along the path of the infusion catheter are desensitized.

LANDMARKS

- There are no specific landmarks. The soaker or infusion catheter is surgically placed between the muscle layers at the surgical site and tunneled out of the skin to allow for connection to the lidocaine infusion pump (**Fig. 23.42**).

DRUGS AND EQUIPMENT

- 2% lidocaine without epinephrine. Lidocaine is preferred to bupivacaine because of its less toxic effect. In addition, if lidocaine is given by CRI, there is no need to use a long-acting anesthetic (such as bupivacaine). Furthermore, if there is a suspicion of toxicity, the lidocaine infusion can be stopped immediately and, because of its short duration of action, its effects will wean off relatively quickly.
- An infusion pump and a fenestrated catheter (15–20 fenestrations).
- Infusion pumps that do not require battery power or electricity are available. They are powered via inflation of a rubber bladder filled with 100–200 ml of lidocaine (**Fig. 23.43**).
- Fenestrated catheters are available commercially or they can be manufactured using a sterile urinary catheter with the tip flamed shut and fenestrated (15–20 holes) with a needle.

APPROACH

- Just prior to the conclusion of the surgery, the infusion catheter is placed between the muscle layers and tunneled outside the skin (**Figs. 23.44, 23.45**). The catheter is secured to the skin with sutures and connected to an infusion pump.

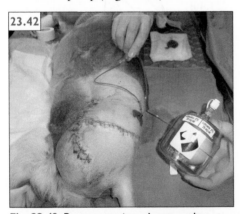

Fig. 23.42 Post amputation, a home-made fenestrated catheter is surgically placed between the muscle layers at the amputation site. The regional topical lidocaine infusion technique is used to provide additional analgesia in combination with systemic opioid pain management.

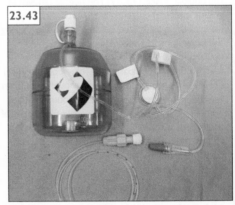

Fig. 23.43 An infusion pump that does not require any external power source. The rubber bladder within the plastic casing accommodates 100 ml in volume. Note the bacteria filter located mid-way in the infusion line.

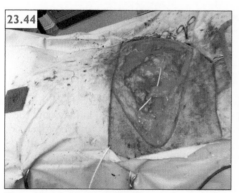

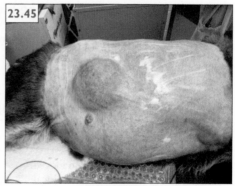

Figs. 23.44, 23.45 (**23.44**) A commercial fenestrated catheter being inserted between the muscle layers to provide topical local anesthesia post tumor removal. (**23.45**) A large tumor before surgery is shown.

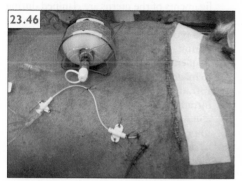

Fig. 23.46 An infusion pump connected to a fenestrated catheter. Several lidocaine patches (white colored patches) are also usable on the surgical site for additional topical analgesia.

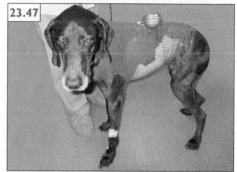

Fig. 23.47 The lidocaine infusion pump is secured with a surgical dressing and a stockinet (red color) on the back of the dog. The pump is attached to the dog and provides mobility without any power source or electrical attachment, while still providing lidocaine infusion.

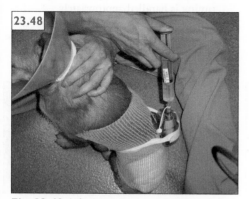

Fig. 23.48 Infusion pumps can be reloaded with additional lidocaine (up to 100 ml). The pump and catheter can be left in place for 3–7 days.

- The infusion pump is secured to the surgical dressing (**Figs. 23.46, 23.47**). The pump can operate for 48 hours without requiring reloading with lidocaine. If needed, an additional 100 ml of lidocaine can be reloaded (**Fig. 23.48**) every 48 hours.
- The infusion pump can be turned off if there is any suspicion of lidocaine toxicity.
- A soaker catheter can be removed by simply pulling it out of the skin.

Intratesticular and intrauterine blocks using a local anesthetic

- Intratesticular and intrauterine blocks can be performed relatively easily using 2% lidocaine without epinephrine.
- This technique allows 2% lidocaine to be deposited in the testicular parenchyma (**Fig. 23.49**) or uterine lumen (**Fig. 23.50**) as a depot and allows it to be absorbed through the local blood circulation into the nerve tissues before the testicles/uterine horns are surgically removed.
- Lidocaine is the most suitable local anesthetic agent for intratesticular and intrauterine blocks due to its relatively fast onset of action and is of lower toxicity than other local anesthetic agents. The drawback is that its duration is relatively short when compared with other local anesthetics.
- The timing of the intratesticular/intra-uterine block is important because it has to be a balance between leaving the local anesthetic long enough to take effect while taking into account that leaving it in the tissue for too long might cause systemic absorption and result in potential systemic toxicity.
- The best time to perform an intratesticular block is soon after anesthetic induction and prior to sterile surgical preparation. The hair on the caudal epididymis should be clipped and a quick prep performed. A 22 gauge needle is then inserted into each testicular parenchyma (**Fig. 23.49**), after a withdraw to ensure that the tip of the needle is not in a blood vessel, then 0.5–1.0 ml of 2% lidocaine can be deposited into the tissue and the needle is withdrawn. The same can be repeated

for the second testicle. Therefore, a total of 2 ml maximum (40 mg per animal) is used. The testicles will appear to be distended with the lidocaine. The dog is then prepared for surgery. The testicles are removed within 10–20 minutes and the depot of the lidocaine removed together with the testicle. However, by this time, the lidocaine is already taking its action along the absorption site.

- The most noticeable analgesic effect of such testicular/uterine blocks is the animal is not suddenly awaking from general anesthesia when the spermatid cords or the board ligaments of the uterus are clamped during the surgical removal procedures. These two procedures are the most painful part during reproductive surgeries and animals frequently have premature awakening due to inadequate anesthesia/analgesia.
- Intrauterine block is not as effective as intratesticular block and therefore not as commonly practiced, because the timing to perform such technique is difficult to determine. Unlike an intratesticular block, an intrauterine block cannot be performed until the uterine horns are exteriorized. The time needed to allow the lidocaine to be absorbed into the uterine blood flow may not be long enough before the uterus is removed.
- Nevertheless, an intrauterine block can be applied to effectively alleviate pain if timing is handled appropriately.
- When performing an intrauterine block, 1–3 ml of 2% lidocaine without epinephrine is injected into the lumen of the uterine horns. A slight distension of the horns can

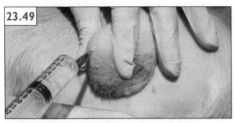

Fig. 23.49 An intratesticular block is performed by inserting the needle into the testicular parenchyma and depositing 0.5–1 ml of 2% lidocaine. The same procedure is repeated on the other testicle.

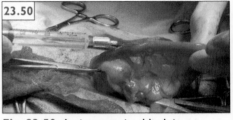

Fig. 23.50 An intrauterine block is performed by inserting the needle into the uterine lumen and filling the uterine lumen with 1–3 ml of 2% lidocaine, depending on the size of the uterus.

be seen as the local anesthetic liquid fills the uterine lumens. Once injected, the local anesthetic and the horns are left alone and the surgical work is directed to ligate the uterine broad ligament or uterine body. At least 7–8 minutes should be allowed for the local anesthetic to be absorbed into the blood stream and become effective.

Intra-articular injection of a local anesthetic or other medication

- Intra-articular administration of a local anesthetic is an effective method for providing perioperative analgesia in dogs. However, many studies have shown that local anesthetics are chondrotoxic and impair chondrocyte metabolism. Among local anesthetics, lidocaine and bupivacaine are found to be more chondrotoxic than mepivacaine and ropivacaine.

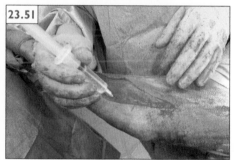

Fig. 23.51 Intra-articular administration of bupivacaine has been used routinely as part of a multimodal perioperative approach after arthrotomy or arthroscopy in dogs. The needle is placed into the knee joint aseptically and approximately 5–8 ml of bupivacaine is administered in this 45 kg (100 lb) dog.

- The chondrotoxicity is characterized by damage to membrane integrity and mitochondrial DNA, and nuclear changes in the superficial layer of the chondrocytes. Therefore, the use of local anesthetic agents for intra-articular injection should be avoided.
- Dexmedetomidine (2.5–5.0 μg/kg) and preservative-free morphine (0.1 mg/kg) diluted with saline up to 0.15 ml/kg body weight can be used for intra-articular injection. This single injection induces a median analgesic duration of 10 hours (range 6–14 hours in dogs). The technique has been used routinely as part of a multimodal perioperative approach after arthrotomy or arthroscopy (**Fig. 23.51**).
- A 22 gauge or large needle is placed into the knee or elbow joint aseptically (usually during the arthrotomic or arthroscopic surgery) and the anesthetic agent administered slowly for perioperative analgesia.
- An alternative to intra-articular injection is to perform local infiltration of the muscle layers around the surgical site using liposomal bupivacaine; this will give 72 hours analgesia.

Further reading

Bailard NS, Ortiz J, Flores RA (2014) Additives to local anesthetics for peripheral nerve blocks: Evidence, limitations, and recommendations. *Am J Health Syst Pharm* 71(5):37–85.

Fizzano KM, Claude AK, Kuo LH et al. (2017) Evaluation of a modified infraorbital approach for a maxillary nerve block for rhinoscopy with nasal biopsy of dogs. *Am J Vet Res* 78(9):1025–35.

Groban L, Deal DD, Vernon JC et al. (2001) Cardiac resuscitation after incremental overdosage with lidocaine, bupivacaine, levobupivacaine, and ropivacaine in anesthetized dogs. *Anesth Analg* 92:37–43.

Gulihar A, Robati S, Twaij H et al. (2015) Articular cartilage and local anaesthetic: a systematic review of the current literature. *J Orthop* 12(Suppl 2):S200–10.

Hennig GS, Hosgood G, Bubenik-Angapen LJ et al. (2010) Evaluation of chondrocyte death in canine osteochondral explants exposed to a 0.5% solution of bupivacaine. *Am J Vet Res* 71:875–83.

Jones RS (2001) Epidural analgesia in the dog and cats. *Vet J* 161:123–31.

Lantz GC (2003) Regional anesthesia for dentistry and oral surgery. *J Vet Dent* **20**:181–6.

Soto N, Fauber AE, Ko JC *et al.* (2014) Analgesic effect of intra-articularly administered morphine, dexmedetomidine, or a morphine-dexmedetomidine combination immediately following stifle joint surgery in dogs. *J Am Vet Med Assoc* **244(11)**:1291–7.

Yilmaz E, Hough KA, Gebhart GF (2014) Mechanisms underlying midazolam-induced peripheral nerve block and neurotoxicity. *Reg Anesth Pain Med* **39(6)**:525–33.

Acute pain management

Jeff C Ko

Introduction

Pain management in veterinary medicine has advanced rapidly in recent years and can largely be classified into acute, chronic, and cancerous pain management. This chapter reviews acute pain management.

Principles of acute pain management

- Management of acute pain includes managing pain immediately after trauma and surgical pain prior to, during, and after surgery. In addition, some patients require continued pain medications at home. Therefore, managing acute pain cases can encompass perioperative pain management up to, and including, take-home pain medication.
- In contrast to acute pain, chronic pain is pain that persists beyond 6 months and chronic pain management requires not only alleviating the pain, but also improving function. Therefore, management of chronic pain is different to acute pain. Details of managing chronic pain, including osteoarthritic pain, are discussed in Chapter 28 and managing cancerous pain, a form of chronic pain, in Chapter 27.

- It is important to treat acute pain (adaptive pain) aggressively with multimodal analgesia. If acute pain is not treated appropriately, a condition called chronic acute pain (maladaptive pain) may result. Chronic acute pain describes acute pain that persists beyond the regular time frame and becomes chronic pain. Chronic acute pain is likely due to both peripheral and central sensitization (a 'wind-up' response) from the initial injury, which results in increased sensation over time.
- The term *adaptive pain* is defined as pain that triggers the initiation of responses and behaviors that contribute to animal survival and promote wound healing or prevent further injury.
- *Maladaptive pain* is defined as pain that is persistent or recurrent after healing and

acts as a disease with abnormal sensory processing.

- *Multimodal analgesia*, similar to multimodal anesthesia, is the use of more than one class of analgesic agent or analgesic technique to treat pain. It is also called balanced analgesia.
- *Peripheral sensitization* is defined as an increase in sensitivity or decrease in the threshold of peripheral nociceptive neurons produced by various inflammatory mediators such as histamine, serotonin, prostaglandins, and bradykinin. Central sensitization is defined as an increased response of spinal dorsal horn neurons, especially to NMDA receptors, to afferent inputs.
- Patients suffering from acute trauma (e.g. hit by a car, fractures, bite wounds) should receive rescue analgesic therapy, in addition to medical stabilization, as soon as possible in order to minimize and prevent a further wind-up pain response (through peripheral and central sensitizations) stimulating more pain and inflammatory responses.
- Dogs and cats undergoing elective surgical procedures benefit the most from pre-emptive analgesic premedication prior to initiation of surgical trauma. This is called *pre-emptive analgesia* and helps to prevent a wind-up response.
- The degree of pain associated with elective or therapeutic surgeries (both orthopedic and soft tissue) should be anticipated and the appropriate pain management provided. Following surgery, analgesic therapy should be continued until the patient returns to a normal or comfortable condition. Continuous evaluation for pain during the postoperative period provides vital feedback for pain management and adjustment of pain medication (see Chapter 6). The type of analgesic drug and dosages should be tailored to each patient's specific needs according to the degree of pain and the recovery stage.
- Take-home pain medications should be relatively safe and easy to administer by the owner. Owners should be educated about risk factors they may not immediately recognize as serious side-effects. Follow-up for feedback is necessary to ensure the patient's comfort and safety even after discharge from the hospital.

Mechanisms of pain and mechanism-based pain management

The mechanisms of pain and mechanism-based pain management can be presented as follows:

- Pain, such as inflammatory or neuropathic pain, resulting from surgery, trauma, or disease can be classified as somatic (which includes orthopedic pain) pain or visceral pain. Some authors also refer to articular and musculotendinous pain. For the purposes of this chapter these are considered to be somatic pain.
- Mechanism-based analgesic therapy is based on understanding the pain pathway and anatomic origin of pain in order to select the most effective analgesic agents for interventional action (*Table 24.1* and **Fig. 24.1**).

ORIGINS OF SOMATIC AND VISCERAL PAIN AND PAIN MANAGEMENT
Somatic pain

- Somatic pain (see **Fig. 24.1**) arises from skin, connective tissues, muscles (musculotendinous tissues), joints, and bones (articular tissues).
- Somatic pain sensations are usually described as localized, sharp, aching, throbbing, or pressure-like.
- The nociceptors in somatic, articular, and musculotendinous tissues, such as muscles, tendons, and fascia, are well innervated with A-delta fibers and C-fibers.
- Activation of the A-delta fibers typically produces 'fast' pain characterized by localized stinging with rapid onset

Table 24.1 Mechanism-based pain management using pharmacologic interventions aimed towards the pain pathway of nociception that includes transduction, transmission, modulation, and perception

Pain pathway	Transduction	Transmission and projection	Modulation	Perception
Noxious stimuli (mechanical, thermal, chemical, and electrical)-induced tissue damage and inflammation	Afferent nerve endings (nociceptors) detecting damaged tissue release chemical mediators that include prostaglandins, bradykinin, leukotrienes, and histamine. The nociceptors then participate in converting these factor-mediated painful stimuli into pain-related nerve impulses	Pain-related nerve impulses are sent from peripheral site to the dorsal spinal horn cells regions in the spinal cord as well as brainstem	Minimize the pain-related signal and contained in the spine, or amplify pain signals and continue on to the brainstem and thalamus	Conscious awareness (mainly cerebral cortex) of pain-related signals from transduction, transmission, and modulations pain pathway
Afferent nerves and tissues	Peripheral nociceptive receptors	A-beta, A-delta, C-fibers	Spinal neurons in the dorsal horn cells contain all the receptors for alpha-2 adrenergic, NMDA, and serotonin for response to pain signals	Alter the consciousness of the animal, reducing the perception of the pain-related signals
Pharmacologic agents act on the pain pathway	Prevention of peripheral sensitization: NSAIDs, local anesthetic agents, steroidal drugs	Prevention of peripheral sensitization: local anesthetics	Prevention of central sensitization: opioids, alpha-2 agonists, ketamine or other NMDA antagonists, gabapentin, tramadol	Sedatives (acepromazine, diazepam, midazolam, alpha-2 agonists)

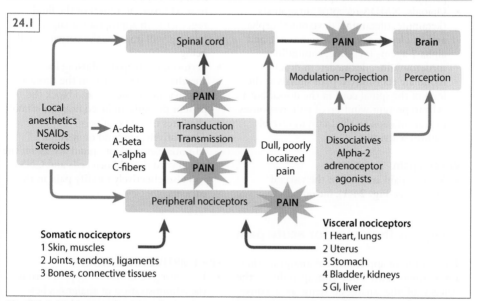

24.1

Fig. 24.1 Mechanism-based analgesic therapy (green arrows) is based on understanding the pain pathway and anatomic origin of pain. This will allow selection of the most effective analgesic agents to block specific pain along its pathway. GI, gastrointestinal; NSAID, non-steroidal anti-inflammatory drug.

of sharp pain. Activation of C-fibers produces 'slow' pain, characterized by a slower onset, burning, intense, but non-localized pain.

- Both A-delta fibers and C-fibers are activated by noxious stimuli, such as chemical irritants, intense heat (e.g. noxious stimuli from cautery, bone sawing, and LASER), strong chemical contractions, pressure, and stretching during surgery or trauma. The pain signals are converted through the nociceptors and transmitted via the pain pathway in order to produce pain responses and sensations.
- A-delta fibers and C-fibers are also well innervated with free nerve endings in the joint capsules, adipose tissue, and ligaments. These tissues show a marked response to noxious stimuli, and the nociceptive reactions are enhanced by prostaglandins, as well as other pain mediators.
- Analgesics, including NSAIDs and local anesthetics, act on these peripheral pain mediators to effectively block their transduction into painful signals and prevent transmission of pain signals from peripheral sites to the spinal cord.
- Opioids, NMDA-receptor antagonists (ketamine, tiletamine, dextromethorphan, and to a lesser degree methandone), and alpha-2 agents (xylazine, romifidine, medetomidine, dexmedetomidine) modulate transmitted pain signals at the level of the spinal cord in the dorsal horn cells to prevent wind-up of pain responses or transmission to the brain in severely painful reactions.

Visceral pain
- Visceral pain arises from the visceral organs (see **Fig. 24.1**), including the heart, lungs, kidneys, liver, gastrointestinal tract, uterus, and bladder. Visceral pain is usually dull and poorly defined. Visceral pain is transmitted exclusively by C-fibers. Since it is in close proximity with the autonomic nervous system, when C-fibers are activated, visceral pain also causes autonomic responses such as an increase in heart rate, respiration, and blood pressure.
- Tumors or obstructions can be associated with marked visceral pain. The obstruction of hollow organs is associated with intermittent cramping or poorly localized pain. Constipation, pyometra, pancreatitis, ascites, or urethral blockage are examples of visceral pain.
- Interestingly, many noxious stimuli (clamping, cutting, or burning) when applied to visceral structures appear to produce less severe pain than the same noxious stimuli applied to peripheral tissues. In contrast, dilation or spasm of hollow viscera or organs, together with inflammation, ischemia, or stretching of the mesentery, produces severe visceral pain.
- Dogs and cats with a fluid-filled thoracic or abdominal cavity (pyo-, chylo- or hemothorax and ascites) are in moderate to severe pain. Removal of the fluid, together with appropriate analgesic therapy, will improve the patient's well being.
- Performing an epidural using local anesthetic drugs to act on the thoracic or pelvic plexus nerves and block the pain or pressure-induced noxious stimuli alleviates this type of pain.
- Alternatively, epidural or systemic administration of an opioid acting on the spinal cord dorsal horn cells and CNS will also effectively modify pain in these patients.

Analgesic therapies for acute pain

The timing of application of analgesic therapy is important. Poor timing reduces the efficacy of the analgesic drug as a consequence of peripheral/central sensitization. The timing of analgesic therapy, types of analgesics, and benefits are listed in *Table 24.2*.

PRE-EMPTIVE ANALGESIA
- Preventing or minimizing pain through the administration of analgesics before a surgical or painful procedure is called pre-emptive analgesia.
- The goal of pre-emptive analgesia is to provide therapeutic intervention prior

Table 24.2 Timing of analgesic therapy, analgesics used, and their benefits

Preoperative (including prior to visit the clinic)	Intraoperative	Postoperative (including take-home medication)
Pre-emptive analgesia and prevention of wind-up response both peripherally and centrally Reduction of IV induction and inhalant anesthetic requirement; NSAIDs may provide immediate anti-inflmmatory action Provide both intra- and postoperative pain relief	Provide intraoperative pain relief Reduction of inhalant anesthetic requirement during the surgery Provide immediate postoperative pain relief Smooth recovery	Provide postoperative pain relief Reduce inflammation Provide patient comfort and facilitate long-term recovery
Alpha-2 agonists, dissociatives, opioids, local anesthetic agents, sedatives, NSAIDs, tramadol	Alpha-2 agonists, dissociatives, opioids, local anesthetic agents	Alpha-2 agonists, dissociatives, opioids, NSAIDs, sedatives, tramadol

to a painful experience in order to prevent or minimize both peripheral and CNS sensitization to the noxious stimulus.

- If an analgesic is provided to the animal before surgical stimulation, then the effect of the analgesia is more profound than analgesia provided following surgical trauma.
- Pre-emptive analgesia can be provided by opioids, NSAIDs, or other analgesic agents as part of the premedication protocol prior to anesthetic induction.
- Analgesic agents can also be administered intraoperatively and postoperatively, and continued as take-home medication.

INTRAOPERATIVE ANALGESIA

- The goals of providing analgesic drugs intraoperatively are to reduce inhalant anesthetic requirement, provide additional analgesia throughout the surgical procedure, and smooth the transition from anesthetic maintenance into recovery.
- All inhalant anesthetic agents (isoflurane and sevoflurane) induce a degree of dose-dependent cardiorespiratory depression with a reduction of cardiac output and potent vasodilation, while most analgesic agents are much less cardiorespiratory depressant than inhalants, with minimal effect on the cardiovasculature. Reducing the total inhalant requirement through the use of appropriate analgesic agents will lesson a patient's cardiorespiratory depression.

POSTOPERATIVE ANALGESIA

- The goals of postoperative analgesia are to ensure a smooth recovery, minimize

postoperative pain, increase patient comfort, and facilitate wound healing.

DRUGS USED IN ANALGESIC THERAPIES FOR ACUTE PAIN

- Anesthetics–analgesics that can be used for pre-emptive, intraoperative, and postoperative pain management include opioids, alpha-2 adrenoceptor agonists (xylazine, romifidine, medetomidine, dexmedetomidine), and local anesthetic agents. Other analgesic agents include dissociatives (ketamine and, likely, tiletamine), tramadol, steroids, and NSAIDs.
- Opioids (e.g. morphine, fentanyl, hydromorphone, oxymorphone, buprenorphine, butorphanol) are among the most effective analgesics for acute pain. Opioids, when administered in intermittent bolus doses or as a CRI perioperatively, activate opioid receptors in the CNS, producing good to excellent analgesia with mild to moderate sedation.
- Preoperative administration of opioids, with or without a local anesthetic (usually lidocaine or bupivacaine) administered via an epidural or spinal route (see Chapter 23) provides another alternative for acute pain management in the intraoperative to postoperative stages.
- A fentanyl patch (**Fig. 24.2**) applied to a shaved area (**Fig. 24.3**) 12–24 hours prior to surgery is another systemic route for opioid administration. A fentanyl patch applied post surgery will treat pain from 12–24 hours to up to 3 days after application.
- Dexmedetomidine, medetomidine, romifidine, and xylazine are

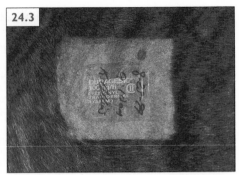

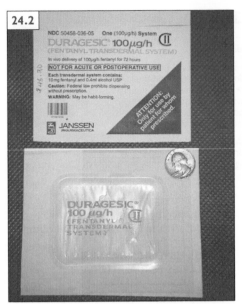

Fig. 24.2 Fentanyl patches come in different concentrations. A 100 μg/hour patch is illustrated. The patch is contrasted in size with a small coin. In the upper picture the patch label indicates 'not for acute or postoperative use' – this means that the patch will not be effective in treating pain until 12–24 hours after its application and it is therefore not for treating immediate pain.

sedative–analgesics that induce muscle relaxation and analgesia by stimulating presynaptic alpha-2 receptors in the CNS. These agents can be used for premedication, intraoperative CRI, or postoperative pain management in conjunction with other analgesic agents.

Fig. 24.3 A fentanyl patch applied to an area of shaved skin on a dog. A fentanyl patch can also be applied to a cat.

- The use of a microdose of medetomidine or dexmedetomidine as an adjunct analgesic is popular in many perioperative and intensive care unit settings. This is especially true in cases of opioid-associated dysphoria. A sedative may significantly comfort and quieten the patient by altering the patient's perception of pain.
- In cases of trauma, pre-emptive administration of analgesics is not possible as the pain is already induced by the injury. In this situation, the pain is best managed by providing rescue analgesics as soon as possible after the initial trauma to reduce further wind-up (allodynia and hyperalgesia) from the injured tissue or to prevent the development of chronic pain.
- Allodynia is defined as pain caused by a stimulus that normally does not induce pain. Hyperalgesia is defined as increased painful response to a normally painful stimulus.

Pre-emptive/preoperative pain management

OPIOIDS
- See also Chapter 3.
- Preoperative administration of opioids not only provides some sedation, but it also provides pre-emptive analgesia and reduces the amount of IV induction agent and inhalant maintenance anesthetic (sevoflurane or isoflurane) required intraoperatively. A fentanyl patch may be applied before or after surgery as an alternative to pre-emptive or postoperative pain management.
- Doses and routes (dogs and cats) are listed in *Table 24.3*.
- Opioids are commonly combined with sedatives/tranquilizers (neuroleptic–analgesic combinations), including diazepam, midazolam, acepromazine, xylazine, romifidine, medetomidine, or dexmedetomidine, as part of premedication. Details of neuroleptic–analgesic combinations can be found in Chapters 3 and 9.

Table 24.3 Doses and routes of administration of opioids for pre-emptive/preoperative pain management in dogs and cats

Opioid	Dosage	Route
Morphine	0.25–1.0 mg/kg	IV, IM, or SC
Hydromorphone, oxymorphone	0.05–0.1 mg/kg	IV, IM, or SC
Fentanyl	3–5 µg/kg	IV
Butorphanol	0.2–0.6 mg/kg	IV, IM, or SC
Buprenorphine	40–120 µg/kg	IV, IM, or SC
Buprenorphine	40–180 µg/kg	Sublingual or OTM, with the larger the dose, the longer the duration of effect up to 0.12 mg/kg in dogs and up to 0.18 mg/kg in cats

ALPHA-2 AGONISTS

- Alpha-2 agonists can be used as sedatives, but they also provide pre-emptive and perioperative analgesia. Studies have shown that premedication with medetomidine or dexmedetomidine is capable of providing analgesia into the early hours (1st to 2nd hour) of recovery.
- The doses and routes of administration are listed in *Table 24.4*. The doses and routes of administration for alpha-2 agonist combinations with opioids for premedication are outlined in Chapter 3.
- Dexmedetomidine (or medetomidine), together with an injectable NSAID such as carprofen (4.4 mg/kg SC) or meloxicam (0.2 mg/kg SC), provides an attractive pre-emptive analgesic combination in dogs and cats that is likely to provide longer postoperative analgesia than either drug used alone.

NON-STEROIDAL ANTI-INFLAMMATORY DRUGS

- For premedication, oral formulations of NSAIDs can be administered 1–2 hours prior to anesthetic induction or injectable NSAIDs can be given as a preanesthetic medication or after anesthetic induction and just prior to surgery for both intraoperative and postoperative analgesia as well as anti-inflammatory effects.
- Doses and routes (dogs and cats) are listed in *Table 24.5*.

Table 24.4 Doses and routes of administration of alpha-2 agonists for pre-emptive/preoperative pain management in dogs and cats

Alpha-2 agonist	Dogs	Cats
Dexmedetomidine	5–10 µg/kg IV, IM	10–30 µg/kg IV or IM
Medetomidine	10–20 µg/kg IV, IM	20–60 µg/kg IV or IM
Romifidine	5–10 µg/kg IV, IM	20–40 µg/kg IV or IM
Xylazine	0.15–0.25 mg/kg IV, IM	0.5–1 mg/kg IV or IM

Table 24.5 Doses and routes of administration of NSAIDs for pre-emptive/preoperative pain management in dogs and cats

NSAID	Dosage	Route
Carprofen	2.2–4.4 mg/kg	SC or PO
Meloxicam	0.2 mg/kg	SC or PO
Firocoxib	5 mg/kg (dogs only)	PO, once daily
Deracoxib	3–4 mg/kg (dogs only)	PO, once daily
Ketoprofen	1–2 mg/kg	SC, IM
Robenacoxib	1–2 mg/kg	SC or PO, 45 minutes prior to surgery and then for an additional 2 days after the surgery

- Minimal renal or hematologic side-effects are noticed in normal, non-dehydrated dogs and cats when these agents are administered preoperatively. Some studies caution against the use of ketoprofen pre-emptively because of its enhanced potential for anti-platelet effects.
- A significant disadvantage of using oral NSAIDs preoperatively is their potential loss through vomiting following premedication. Opioids, such as morphine and occasionally hydromorphone, may induce vomiting, with the result that orally-administered NSAIDs may be lost before they are fully absorbed.

LOCAL ANESTHETIC AGENTS

- Local or regional blocks (epidural and brachial plexus blocks) with local anesthetic agents (e.g. lidocaine, mepivacaine, or bupivacaine) provide excellent pre-emptive analgesia. Techniques and dosages for local anesthetic agents are described in Chapter 23.
- A slow-release liposome bupivacaine injectable suspension (Nocita®, see Chapter 19) is commercially available. It can be infiltrated into various layers of skin, muscle, and tendon tissues and induces an analgesic duration of up to 72 hours after a single infiltration. However, it is not currently recommended for any of the regional blocks or epidural, because it may produce prolonged motor blockage of the animal. The use of Nocita in cats has recently being approved for use as a peripheral nerve block anesthetic. The label cautions the use of such a product

in dogs and cats younger than 5 months of age, that are pregnant, lactating, or intended for breeding. Nocita also should not be administered intravenously or intra-arterially. The adverse reactions of Nocita in cats may include elevated body temperature, infection, or chewing/licking at the surgical site. Concurrent use of Nocita with other amide local anesthetic such as bupivacaine or lidocaine is not recommended in cases with concerns of systemic toxicity.
- Doses and routes:
  - Lidocaine: 4–6 mg/kg via infiltration.
  - Mepivacaine: 3–5 mg/kg via infiltration.
  - Bupivacaine: 2–3 mg/kg via infiltration.
  - Nocita (slow-release liposome bupivacaine): 5.3 mg/kg (0.4 ml/kg).
- Local anesthetic infiltration can be used to provide pre-emptive, intraoperative, as well as immediate postoperative pain management using the following techniques:
  - Ring (or three-point) block for cat claw removal or digital growth removal.
  - Incisional infiltration block along the surgical site into the skin and muscles.
  - Intratesticular and intrauterine infiltration blocks.
  - Infraorbital and mental foramen blocks for dental analgesia.
  - Retrobulbar block for enucleation.
  - Regional blocks, such as brachial plexus, epidural, and Bier blocks, can also be used effectively for perioperative pain management.

Intraoperative pain management

OPIOIDS

- Opioids can be administered as an IV bolus or CRI (e.g. fentanyl) to reduce intraoperative pain and, subsequently, reduce the total amount of sevoflurane or isoflurane required for surgery, thus minimizing the cardiovascular depression associated with the inhalant.
- The opioids themselves, given intraoperatively, may induce or increase respiratory depression, characterized

by hypoventilation or even apnea, and the use of positive-pressure ventilation to assist or control ventilation may be necessary to maintain normal respiratory function.
- Doses and routes are listed in *Table 24.6*.

ALPHA-2 AGONISTS

- Intermittent IV boluses of microdoses of alpha-2 agonists may be given to alleviate pain. At the doses shown below, minimal

Table 24.6 Doses and routes of administration of opioids for intraoperative pain management in dogs and cats

Opioids	Dosage and route
Morphine	0.25–0.5 mg/kg IV bolus 240 µg/kg/h CRI
Hydromorphone	0.05–0.1 mg/kg IV bolus, 10 µg/kg/h CRI
Oxymorphone	0.05–0.1 mg/kg IV bolus
Fentanyl	5–10 µg/kg IV bolus 2–10 µg/kg/h CRI
Methadone	0.4–1.0 mg/kg IV bolus
Butorphanol	0.2–0.4 mg/kg IV bolus 40–50 µg/kg/h CRI
Buprenorphine	20–120 µg/kg IV bolus

cardiorespiratory side-effects will be induced, but analgesia will be provided by direct mediation of the drug's analgesic action and/or via its sedative–hypnotic action.

- Doses and routes:
  - Xylazine: 0.05 mg/kg IV.
  - Medetomidine: 1–2 µg/kg IV.
  - Dexmedetomidine: 0.5–1.0 µg/kg IV.
- Alternatively, medetomidine or dexmedetomidine can be given by CRI intraoperatively.
  - A CRI can be set up with 1–2 µg/kg/hour of medetomidine or 0.5–1.0 µg/kg/hour of dexmedetomidine. This is added to 6–12 ml of sterile water or saline and delivered over a course of 1 hour using syringe pump.
  - A CRI is made up by adding 0.1 mg (100 µg or 0.1 ml) of medetomidine or 0.05 mg (50 µg or 0.1 ml) dexmedetomidine into a 1 liter bag of balanced electrolytes. This results in 0.1 µg/ml medetomidine (0.05 µg/ml dexmedetomidine) for a nanodose medetomidine or dexmedetomidine infusion.
  - The resulting electrolyte-alpha-2 mixture is administered at a rate of 10 ml/kg/hour, which yields approximately 1 µg/kg/hour CRI of medetomidine or 0.5 µg/kg/hour dexmedetomidine.
  - This takes advantage of the sedative–hypnotic activity of the alpha-2 agonist

to enhance the analgesic and anesthetic properties of the inhalant or opioids administered previously, and spares about 20–40% of the inhalant during anesthetic maintenance.
- Potential side-effects with medetomidine or dexmedetomidine CRIs are second-degree heart block and/or bradycardia developing over time. However, blood pressure remains within the normal range when used with isoflurane or sevoflurane.
- The nanodose of medetomidine or dexmedetomidine can be combined with ketamine in a CRI. This is achieved by adding 0.1 mg (100 µg) of medetomidine or 0.05 mg (50 µg) dexmedetomidine and 60 mg ketamine into a 1 liter bag of balanced electrolyte crystalloid solution. The rate of administration is identical (i.e. 10 ml/kg/hour).

OTHER CONSTANT RATE INFUSION ALTERNATIVES

- Morphine, ketamine, and lidocaine can be either used alone or in combination for CRI intraoperative and postoperative pain management in dogs and cats.
- Side-effects occur if too much morphine or ketamine is infused during the intraoperative or postoperative period. Intraoperative side-effects include tachycardia and hypotension. Postoperative side-effects include dysphoria, vocalization, and restless behavior without pain. If these side-effects develop, the infusion should be discontinued. A microdose of medetomidine (2 µg/kg IV) or dexmedetomidine (1–2 µg/kg IV), diazepam (0.4 mg/kg IV), or a low dose of acepromazine (0.02 mg/kg IV) can be administered to induce sedation (alter perception) and reduce dysphoria.

Traditional morphine–lidocaine–ketamine constant rate infusion

- The morphine–lidocaine–ketamine (MLK) combination utilizes the analgesic and maintenance inhalant sparing effects of morphine, the local anesthetic, antiarrhythmic, systemic anti-inflammatory, and inhalant-sparing effects of lidocaine, and ketamine as an NMDA receptor antagonist to prevent wind-up.

- *Table 24.7* describes how to create a traditional MLK infusion bag. The solution is administered at a CRI of 10 ml/kg/hour. It reduces the inhalant anesthetic agent by 25–30%. Once made up, the MLK solution lasts approximately 1 week.

Alternative morphine–lidocaine–ketamine constant rate infusions

- An alternative MLK combination for CRI is shown in *Table 24.8*. 60 mg of morphine, 300 mg of lidocaine, and 60 mg of ketamine are added to a 1 liter bag of balanced electrolyte fluid.
- This modified MLK is given at a CRI of 1 up to 8 ml/kg/hour or through a 60 drop IV drip set at a rate equal to the animal's body weight in kg as drops per minute.
- For example, a 20 kg dog receives 20 drops/minute of this modified MLK combination, giving the dog 1 µg/kg/minute of morphine, 5 µg/kg/minute of lidocaine, and 1 µg/kg/minute of ketamine.

Table 24.7 Morphine–lidocaine–ketamine CRI at 10 ml/kg/hour

Drug (concentration)	ml (mg) to add to 1 liter of fluid	Individual dose rate
Morphine (15 mg/ml)	1.33 ml (20 mg)	3.3 µg/kg/min
Lidocaine (20 mg/ml)	15 ml (300 mg)	50 µg/kg/min
Ketamine (100 mg/ml)	0.6 ml (60 mg)	10 µg/kg/min

Table 24.8 Alternative morphine–lidocaine–ketamine CRI at 1–8 ml/kg/hour

Drug (concentration)	ml (mg) to add to 1 liter of fluid	Individual dose rate
Morphine (15 mg/ml)	4 ml (60 mg)	1–8 µg/kg/minute
Lidocaine (20 mg/ml)	15 ml (300 mg)	5–40 µg/kg/minute
Ketamine (100 mg/ml)	0.6 ml (60 mg)	1–8 µg/kg/minute

- The amount of the MLK combination with balanced electrolyte (1 ml/kg/hour) fluid is deducted from the total intraoperative fluid administration (10 ml/kg/hour).
- The alternative MLK, administered at a CRI of 10 ml/kg/hour, yields 10 µg/kg/minute of morphine, 50 µg/kg/minute of lidocaine, and 10 µg/kg/minute of ketamine.

Lidocaine constant rate infusion in dogs

- A recent study demonstrated that lidocaine CRI reduces the MAC of sevoflurane in dogs.
- Lidocaine (2 mg/kg IV) can be administered as a bolus loading dose followed by CRI at one of the following rates:
  - 50 µg/kg/minute (reduces sevoflurane by 22.6%).
  - 100 µg/kg/ minute (reduces sevoflurane by 29%).
  - 200 µg/kg/ minute (reduces sevoflurane by 39.6%).

Ketamine constant rate of infusion in dogs

- Ketamine as a CRI reduces the MAC of sevoflurane in dogs.
- Ketamine (3 mg/kg IV) can be administered as a bolus loading dose followed by a CRI at one of the following rates:
  - 50 µg/kg/minute (reduces sevoflurane by 40%).
  - 100 µg/kg/minute (reduces sevoflurane by 44.7%).

Lidocaine and ketamine constant rate of infusion in dogs

- Lidocaine (2 mg/kg) and ketamine (3 mg/kg) administered IV as a bolus loading dose.
- A CRI at 100 µg/kg/minute of both lidocaine and ketamine reduces sevoflurane by 62.8%.

LOCAL ANESTHETIC BLOCKS DURING SURGERY

- Local anesthetics can be used either by infiltration or by direct injection around and onto the nerves (see Chapter 23).

- Local anesthetics are injected into the joint when performing arthroscopy or arthrotomy, into the eye socket for enucleation, or intrapleurally into the intercostal nerves during thoracotomy.

- Local anesthetics can also be used as 'splash blocks' directly onto the nerve during an amputation or ear canal ablation.
- All of these techniques can alleviate pain intraoperatively and postoperatively.

Postoperative pain management

OPIOIDS
- Opioids (e.g. fentanyl, morphine, hydromorphone, oxymorphone, butorphanol, and buprenorphine) administered IV or IM 5–10 minutes prior to termination of the inhalant anesthesia or soon after extubation reduce postoperative pain.
- If the dog or cat received an opioid preoperatively or intraoperatively, the dose should be reduced by one-third to one-half of the original opioid dose for postoperative analgesia.

ALPHA-2 AGONISTS
- Microdoses of medetomidine (1–2 µg/kg), dexmedetomidine (0.5–1.0 µg/kg), or xylazine (0.05 mg/kg) may be administered IV for a smoother recovery. At these doses,

minimal cardiorespiratory effects are induced, but the pain and delirium immediately following recovery are reduced.

NON-STEROIDAL ANTI-INFLAMMATORY DRUGS
- Oral formulations of carprofen, etodolac, deracoxib, firocoxib, or meloxicam can be used for postoperative pain management.
- If not provided pre-emptively, tablets can be administered as soon as the animal regains consciousness and continued once daily for 2 or 3 days to alleviate postoperative surgical pain in dogs.
- For managing moderate to severe postoperative pain, NSAIDs can be combined with an oral opioid (butorphanol, buprenorphine, or tramadol) for several days postoperatively.

Take-home pain medication

Several analgesics are attractive for take-home pain management for patients discharged from hospital but requiring ongoing analgesia to keep them comfortable. These analgesics include buprenorphine, tramadol, fentanyl patches, lidocaine patches, and NSAIDs.

BUPRENORPHINE
- In addition to premedication and postoperative analgesia, buprenorphine is a good choice for take-home medication.
- When administered orally, buprenorphine, like other opioids, has a poor bioavailability (3–15%); however, when administered oral transmucosally (OTM), buprenorphine has approximately 38–47% bioavailability in dogs and cats. Recent studies have shown that dogs and cats have similar bioavailability following OTM dosing of injectable buprenorphine.

- Buprenorphine has a long duration of analgesic action, providing up to 12–24 hours of analgesia following a single dose administered IV or OTM. The duration of analgesic action appears to be dose dependent. The larger the dose, up to 120 µg/kg, the longer the duration.
- A commercially available buprenorphine (Simbadol™) has been approved for use in cats with a single SC injection providing 24 hours analgesia for postoperative pain. This buprenorphine preparation is no different from a regular human version of buprenorphine. It is not an extended-release form. The main difference is that when using the higher dosage, buprenorphine provides a longer-lasting analgesic effect than lower doses

(10–40 µg/kg) that were previously recommended.

- Although Simbadol is approved for use in cats, it can also be used off-label for dogs. Dogs are more sensitive to buprenorphine than cats. More profound sedation may occur in dogs. A dose of up to 120 µg/kg, IV, IM, SC, or OTM should be used in dogs, instead of 240 µg/kg as labeled for cats. Simbadol can be used by the OTM route for both dogs and cats. This high concentration of buprenorphine (Simabdol 1.8 mg/ml versus human label of buprenorphine at 0.3 mg/ml) provides a significant advantage in terms of smaller volume for OTM administration. This resolves the use of OTM buprenorphine in large-sized dogs and cats. An OTM dose of 120 µg/kg can be given to dogs and 120–180 µg/kg to cats, providing a duration of analgesia of 20–24 hours.
- Salivary pH plays a role in OTM absorption of buprenorphine, which is a weak base with a pKa of 8.24. The saliva of dogs and cats is approximately pH 9–10. In alkaline saliva, buprenorphine is primarily non-ionized, enhancing its lipophilicity, thus facilitating absorption across the oral–cheek–lingual mucosa into the blood stream.
- Studies have shown that when administered OTM buprenorphine absorption can be successfully achieved through the non-specific placement of buprenorphine either on or beneath the tongue or into the cheek pouch of dogs (**Fig. 24.4**) and cats. This makes administration easy and convenient for owners.
- Studies indicate that buprenorphine administered via the OTM route induces a dose-dependent duration of quantifiable plasma concentrations in dogs and cats. The higher the dose, the longer the duration of analgesic action and the more consistent the response among dogs.
- Buprenorphine doses between 20 and 180 µg/kg IV or OTM do not induce apnea, bradycardia, or excitement in dogs and cats. It appears that there is a ceiling effect of these side-effects.
- The only side-effects are salivation and moderate sedation at the higher doses in dogs (**Fig. 24.5**). Minimal to mild sedation and salivation are observed in cats.
- A dose of 120 µg/kg OTM will produce a plasma concentration similar to that produced by giving 20 µg/kg IV, with a duration of quantifiable plasma concentration of up to 20 hours in dogs.
- The dose for take-home pain management via OTM in dogs and cats is 40–180 µg/kg. For example, 1 ml (i.e. 300 µg if using a 300 µg/ml solution) of buprenorphine given OTM to a 4.5–6.8 kg (10–15 lb) dog or cat provides a satisfactory analgesia

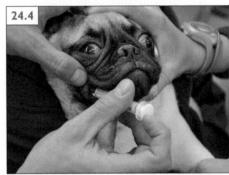

Fig. 24.4 The injectable formulation of buprenorphine is shown being administered OTM to a dog by placing a syringe into its cheek pouch. The bioavailability of this route of administration has proved to be 38–47% in dogs.

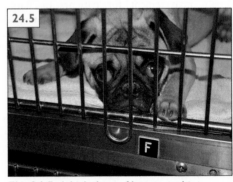

Fig. 24.5 A high dose of buprenorphine (0.12 mg/kg) administered OTM has induced moderate sedation and salivation in this dog. However, the dog is responsive to his name being called despite the moderate degree of sedation.

of 12–16 hours duration. This dose is equivalent to 66.6 µg/kg for a 4.5 kg (10 lb) animal and 44.1 µg/kg for a 6.8 kg (15 lb) animal.

TRAMADOL

- Tramadol is a synthetic product similar to codeine. It undergoes extensive liver metabolism to an 'M1' (O-desmethyltramadol) metabolite with a higher affinity for opioid receptors than the parent compound. However, the M1 metabolite is not as potent as morphine.
- Tramadol is a centrally-acting analgesic with proposed dual mechanisms of action: as an opioid and as a non-opioid.
- The proposed opioid mechanism suggests that tramadol selectively interacts with mu receptors and induces analgesia. The proposed non-opioid mechanism suggests that tramadol inhibits central norepinephrine and serotonin reuptake, as well as reducing the 5-HT turnover. These actions block nociceptive impulses at the spinal level and may contribute to the analgesic effects of tramadol.
- Tramadol is available in both injectable and oral formulations in some countries. In the US, tramadol is only available as 50 mg tablets.
- Tramadol has a relatively high bioavailability (60–80%) in humans, dogs, and cats, with similar patterns after oral administration.
- The use of tramadol in managing acute and chronic has become popular both in dogs and cats because of the low incidence of ileus and cardiorespiratory depression. As more studies evaluate the pharmacokinetic/dynamic (PK/PD) effect of tramadol, questions regarding its efficacy and appropriate dosing interval have arisen.
- It has been found that in dogs, the major metabolite M1 is not as high as previously thought and the duration of action is also short. Furthermore, multiple dosing of tramadol in dogs seems to decrease its bioavailability. These may account for the weak analgesic effect of using tramadol in dogs over time. Current recommendation based on the PK/PD study suggests a dose of 4–5 mg/kg q8 h.

- In contrast to dogs, cats have high plasma concentrations of M1 after oral tramadol administration, which suggests a more opioid-like response to tramadol than in dogs. The recommended dose of tramadol in cats is 5–10 mg/kg q12 h. Because of its unpleasant taste, the principle side-effect observed with oral administration of tramadol in cats is vomiting. Many cats will not tolerate the bitter taste of oral tramadol tablets. The use of a piller is an alternative for drug administration. Some pharmacies may be able to compound a better tasting syrup form of tramadol for easy administration in dogs and cats.
- Combinations of tramadol and NSAIDs seem to be better than either drug used alone. These two drugs act on different mechanisms to treat pain and appear to be complementary. In some cases where an NSAID is not working well, tramadol can be used as an adjunct treatment.
- In one study, using tramadol at 2 mg/kg IV immediately following induction produced a minimal inhalant-sparing effect when compared with morphine in dogs. Studies in dogs and cats using tramadol as an anesthetic adjunct suggest that tramadol minimally affects cardiorespiratory function in these animals.
- In humans, the incidence of side-effects, such as constipation and respiratory depression, following tramadol is lower than with other opioids. In animals there is concern about using tramadol in patients with elevated intracranial pressure, head trauma, or seizures.
- Studies in dogs as a model for humans suggest that the seizure-like activity in dogs is due to monoamine reuptake inhibition, with an increase in transmission triggering excitatory phenomena in the CNS. Such excitatory effects, however, may only be seen when tramadol is used in doses exceeding the therapeutic range (5–10 mg/kg IV).
- Some authors suggest that companion animals with liver or kidney disease tend to have slower metabolism and elimination of tramadol and that the dose should be adjusted accordingly.
- Studies in humans suggest tramadol is comparable to buprenorphine in

treating advanced tumor pain. Similar comparisons between these two analgesics have not been performed in companion animals.

- Clinical impressions are that tramadol is a weak opioid analgesic; however, it is a convenient medication that can be dispensed at dose of 4–5 mg/kg PO q24 h with an NSAID for at-home administration following surgery in dogs and cats. Higher doses of tramadol (up to 10 mg/kg PO) have been used. Sedation has been reported to be the main side-effect when using this higher dose.
- One study found that 10 mg/kg PO of tramadol prior to anesthetic induction reduced the sevoflurane MAC in a similar fashion to opioids (butorphanol and hydromorphone) in dogs and cats.
- In cats, there is no significant advantage of using oral tramadol in combination with an IV opioid to further reduce the sevoflurane concentration, while in dogs, combining tramadol with butorphanol or hydromorphone has an additive effect in further reducing the sevoflurane required for anesthetic maintenance.

FENTANYL PATCH

- Studies show that a fentanyl patch (**Fig. 24.2**) is an effective alternative method to alleviate pain in dogs and cats postoperatively and for ongoing pain management postoperatively.
- The main advantage of the fentanyl patch is that it provides a more convenient route for fentanyl administration than a CRI.
- The disadvantages of using a fentanyl patch are that transdermal absorption is irregular and unpredictable, such that therapeutic plasma concentrations are not always reached. The patch takes 12 hours in cats and 24 hours in dogs to reach therapeutic plasma concentrations, therefore the patch is not suitable for treating immediate pain.
- Fentanyl is a controlled substance and carries some risk of abuse as a take-home medication.
- It is also relatively expensive compared with a lidocaine patch.
- The size of the patch may not fit all sizes of animal and titration of the patch is

difficult in terms of balancing the need to alleviate pain and preventing side-effects.
- Oral ingestion of the fentanyl patch by the animal is also possible This could potentially cause significant sedation, bradycardia, and respiratory depression or apnea because of the systemic absorption of the fentanyl.
- Fentanyl patches come in 25, 50, 75, and 100 μg/hour sizes.
- The recommended doses of fentanyl patches in dogs and cats are as follows:
  - Use the 25 μg/hour patch for cats and small dogs.
  - Use the 50 μg/hour patch for 10–20 kg (22–44 lb) dogs.
  - Use the 75 μg/hour patch for 20–27 kg (44–59.4 lb) dogs.
  - Use the 100 μg/hour patch for 27–34 kg (59.4–74.8 lb) dogs.
  - A combination of different sizes of patches can be used for larger-sized dogs.

LIDOCAINE PATCH

- The use of lidocaine topical patches (**Fig. 24.6**) to treat pain in animals is increasing. The patch used is an analgesic patch (not a transdermal patch) approved in 1999 for treating human neuropathic pain induced by herpes zoster (shingles).
- Patches containing 5% lidocaine have been shown to treat three types of pain induced by shingles-related neuropathic pain, namely: (1) constant deep aching

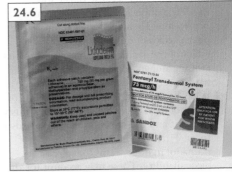

Fig. 24.6 Five percent lidocaine patches are currently available. In contrast to fentanyl, lidocaine is not a controlled substance, therefore no record keeping of its use is required.

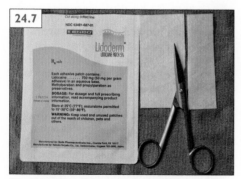

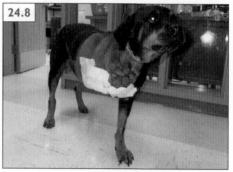

Fig. 24.7 This lidocaine patch is 10 × 14 cm in size and contains 700 mg of lidocaine at a concentration of 50 mg of lidocaine/g of adhesive. Unlike fentanyl patch, the lidocaine patch can be trimmed or cut into pieces without disrupting its delivery mechanism.

Fig. 24.8 This dog has had a forelimb amputation. Perioperatively, the dog received a morphine–lidocaine–ketamine CRI with an intraoperative bupivicaine brachial plexus block. Lidocaine patches were applied to the surgical site for topical analgesia and the dog was resting well. A lidocaine patch (white color tapes) has now been applied to the surgical site and secured with adhesive tape. The dog is able to walk and is feeling comfortable during its postoperative recovery. The patch will provide additional analgesic postoperative pain management for up to 5–7 days. The total amount of local anesthetic (lidocaine and bupivacaine) this dog has received has been carefully calculated so as not to exceed the toxic dose.

or burning pain; (2) intermittent sharp, lancinating or jabbing pain; and (3) dysesthetic pain provoked by normally innocuous stimuli such as light touch, heat, or cold (allodynia), which lasts well beyond the duration of the stimulus (hyperpathia).

- The current brand name of the lidocaine patch is Lidoderm, and it comes as an adhesive material containing 5% lidocaine.
- The current formulation is applied to a non-woven polyester felt backing and covered with a polyethylene terephthalate film release liner. The release liner must be removed prior to being applied to the skin. The patch is 10 cm by 14 cm in size (**Fig. 24.7**) and is supplied as a carton of 30 patches. Each adhesive patch contains 700 mg of lidocaine (i.e. 50 mg of lidocaine/g of adhesive) in an aqueous base with other inactive ingredients.
- The proposed mechanism of action is that the lidocaine binds to neuronal membrane receptors, stabilizing the Na^+ channel and reducing the pain signal initiation and transmission from peripheral nerves and tissues. In humans, the lidocaine patch is sufficient to produce an analgesic but not an anesthetic effect (i.e. lack of complete sensory blockade).
- A lidocaine patch can be applied to both intact skin and skin over a surgical incision in dogs and cats without complications (**Fig. 24.8**).

- Recent studies indicate that the use of the lidocaine patch is relatively safe in dogs and cats. The plasma concentration of lidocaine increases rapidly after initial application and reaches a constant rate of absorption 12–72 hours after patch application. Patches can be left in place for 3–5 days. Approximately 45% of the lidocaine remains in the patch after 3 consecutive days of application, with minimal side-effects observed in dogs and cats.
- Clinically, lidocaine is used as an analgesic adjunct to other analgesic agents for managing cases ranging from ovariohysterectomy to limb amputation and thoracotomy in dogs and cats.
- The advantages of using a lidocaine patch include:
  - Peripheral action with minimal systemic side-effects.
  - Incomplete sensory block in the area of application.

- A physical barrier against mechanical stimulation.
- It is not a controlled drug.
- The patch can be cut to fit any application area without affecting the drug delivery system.
- To use the patch in dogs and cats, it is cut to the length of the surgical incision and applied either directly on top of the incision or on each side of the incision after skin closure to alleviate skin and muscle pain following laparotomy or similar surgeries. It is left in place for up to 3–7 days.

SIMILARITIES AND DIFFERENCES BETWEEN LIDOCAINE PATCHES AND FENTANYL PATCHES

- Because systemic absorption of lidocaine from the patch is low and the mechanism of action is different, lidocaine patches have fewer systemic side-effects than fentanyl patches.
- Lidocaine patches act locally through topical absorption with low systemic concentrations of lidocaine. Fentanyl patches require transdermal delivery and systemic absorption.
- The greater the systemic absorption of fentanyl from the patch, the more the systemic side-effects and potential interactions with other drugs. Large lidocaine overdoses can be lethal, while fentanyl is reversible and toxicosis is treatable, if detected early.
- Lidocaine patches have a shorter onset of action in humans than fentanyl patches (30 minutes versus 12–24 hours). In dogs and cats, however, peak plasma lidocaine concentrations are reportedly reached in 10–24 hours after lidocaine patch application.
- The lidocaine patch must be applied directly on or close to the site of pain to function, while fentanyl patches can be applied anywhere for systemic uptake.
- Lidocaine patches can be cut to fit without affecting the drug delivery system. The delivery of lidocaine from a patch is through passive skin absorption with no reservoir or other delivery mechanism involved. In contrast, cutting a fentanyl patch disrupts the

delivery system, resulting in increased and uncontrolled delivery of the drug. Clinicians are advised to fold back the adhesive of the fentanyl patch for partial exposure when using the patch on cats and small dogs.

- As it is applied directly on top of an injury site, the lidocaine patch provides a physical barrier to prevent external mechanical stimulation of the painful site.
- Oral ingestion of a lidocaine patch is possible. The toxicity of oral ingestion is unknown, but it is not likely to be significant since the acidity of the stomach should destroy the lidocaine or inactivate it.
- Lidocaine is not a controlled substance; fentanyl is.
- Lidocaine patches are less expensive than fentanyl patches.
- Unused, cut portions of lidocaine patches can be stored and used on other animals without a problem.
- The duration of effect of lidocaine patches exceeds 3 days and may last up to 1 week.
- A lidocaine patch dosing guideline for dogs and cats is outlined in *Table 24.9*.

NSAIDs

- NSAIDs are very useful for providing take-home medication. They act in three ways to alleviate pain including analgesic, anti-inflammatory, and antipyretic actions.
- NSAIDs are versatile since they can be used for both soft tissue and orthopedic acute or chronic pain.
- They are flexible and convenient for administration. They can be administered as an injection or orally and the route

Table 24.9 Dosing guidelines for dogs and cats for using 5% lidocaine patches. The patch/s can be left in place for up to 7 days

Body weight in kg (lb)	Patch(es)
2.3 (5)	0.25
4.5 (10)	0.5
9.1 (20)	1.0
18.2 (40)	2.0
27.3 (60)	2.5
36.4 (80)	3.0

of administration can be interchanged between doses.
- NSAIDs have a long duration of analgesic and anti-inflammatory action following a single administration in dogs and cats.
- NSAIDs are relatively economical and they are not controlled substances.
- They do not cause sedation or other immunosuppressive side-effects.
- Precautions or contraindications for using NSAIDs for acute pain management or take-home pain medication include:
  - Should not be used in severely dehydrated dogs and cats or in animals with acute blood loss or homeostatic problems.
  - Should not be used in dogs and cats with gastrointestinal, renal, hepatic, or coagulation dysfunctions.
  - Should not be used together with steroidal analgesics.

- Patients must be closely monitored for signs of vomiting, diarrhea, abnormal bleeding, and lethargy as adverse reactions to NSAIDs.
- Approved indications for NSAIDs vary from country to country and practitioners should ascertain which NSAIDs are approved for postoperative acute pain management in their country.
- The dosages for NSAIDs are as follows:
  - Carprofen: 4.0–4.4 mg/kg PO q24 h or 2.0–2.2 mg/kg q12 h (dogs and cats).
  - Meloxicam: 0.2 mg/kg PO on day 1, followed by 0.1 mg/kg PO q24 h (dogs and cats).
  - Firocoxib: 5 mg/kg PO q24 h (dogs only).
  - Deracoxib: 3–4 mg/kg PO q24 h (dogs only).

Further reading

Abbo LA, Ko JC, Maxwell LK *et al.* (2008) Pharmacokinetics of buprenorphine following intravenous and oral transmucosal administration in dogs. *Vet Ther* **9**:83–93.

Benitez ME, Roush JK, McMurphy R *et al.* (2015) Clinical efficacy of hydrocodone-acetaminophen and tramadol for control of postoperative pain in dogs following tibial plateau leveling osteotomy. *Am J Vet Res* **76(9)**:755–62.

Ebner LS, Lerche P, Bednarski RM (2013) Effect of dexmedetomidine, morphine-lidocaine-ketamine, and dexmedetomidine-morphine-lidocaine-ketamine constant rate infusions on the minimum alveolar concentration of isoflurane and bispectral index in dogs. *Am J Vet Res* **74(7)**:963–70.

Evangelista MC, Silva RA, Cardozo LB *et al.* (2014) Comparison of preoperative tramadol and pethidine on postoperative pain in cats undergoing variohysterectomy. *BMC Vet Res* **10**:252–60.

Ko JC, Abbo LA, Weil AB *et al.* (2008) The effect of oral tramadol alone or concurrent with opioid administration on sevoflurane minimum alveolar concentration in cats. *J Am Vet Med Assoc* **232**:1834–40.

Ko JC, Freeman LJ, Barletta M *et al.* (2011) Efficacy of oral transmucosal and intravenous administration of buprenorphine before surgery for postoperative analgesia in dogs undergoing ovariohysterectomy. *J Am Vet Med Assoc* **238**:318–28.

Ko JC, Lange DG, Mandsager RE *et al.* (2000) Effects of butorphanol and carprofen on the minimal alveolar concentration of isoflurane in dogs. *J Am Vet Med Assoc* **217**:1025–28.

Ko JC, Maxwell LK, Abbo AL *et al.* (2008) Pharmacokinetics of lidocaine following the application of 5% lidocaine patches to cat. *J Vet Pharmacol Ther* **31**:359–67.

Ko JC, Weil AB, Maxell LK *et al.* (2007) Plasma concentration of lidocaine in dogs following 5% lidocaine patch application. *J Am Anim Hosp Assoc* **43**:280–3.

Lascelles BDX, McFarland JM, Swann H (2005) Guidelines for safe and effective use of NSAIDs in dogs. *Vet Ther* **6**:237–51.

Liu PL, Feldman HS, Giasi R *et al.*
(1983) Comparative CNS toxicity of
lidocaine, etidocaine, bupivacaine, and
tetracaine in awake dogs following rapid
intravenous administration. *Anesth
Analg* **62**:375–9.

Muir WW 3rd, Wiese AJ, March PA (2003)
Effects of morphine, lidocaine, ketamine,
and morphine-lidocaine-ketamine drug
combination on minimum alveolar
concentration in dogs anesthetized with
isoflurane. *Am J Vet Res* **64**:1155–60.

Muir WW, Woolf CJ (2001) Mechanisms of
pain and their therapeutic implications.
J Am Vet Med Assoc **219**:1346–56.

Uilenreef JJ, Murrell JC, McKusick BC *et al.*
(2008) Dexmedetomidine continuous
rate infusion during isoflurane anaesthesia
in canine surgical patients. *Vet Anaesth
Analg* **35**:1–12.

Weil AB, Ko JC, Inoue T (2007) Use of
lidocaine patches in dogs and cats. *Comp
Contin Educ Pract Vet* **29**:208–10, 212,
214–16.

CHAPTER 25

Photobiomodulation therapy in pain management

Andrea L Looney

Introduction

Utilizing (light-emitting diodes) (LEDs) and photobiomodulation (PBM; previously known as low-level light therapy [LLLT]) for analgesia and healing has become a routine procedure within small and large animal practices in the last half decade. The recognition and application of light energy for healing are not new. Light energy has had numerous applications in health care throughout history; to date over 500 randomized double-blinded placebo-controlled studies have been published concerning PBM's medical applications. Lasers are the most refined form of light energy. Low-level lasers have been used extensively in physical medicine throughout Europe and Canada for many years prior to FDA approval for clinical application in the setting of musculoskeletal pain in the USA.

MECHANISM OF ACTION IN DEVICE AND *IN VIVO*

- A laser is a device that generates light through the process of optical amplication; low energy level atoms absorbing light become excited to a higher energy level. As a photon strikes another excited atom, it stimulates the release of an additional photon as the electron returns to its resting orbit.

Thus, as more and more photons are generated, increasing amounts of light energy are produced (amplification). This excitation is exponential in that emitted photons are created in the excitation, and suddenly a wavelength of light is produced that is coherent (organized) and collimated (concentrated); this stimulated and sustained emission of photons by atoms of a certain medium creates the actual laser beam capable of healing.

In contrast to the LEDs that produce a narrow band of electromagnetic wavelengths, laser light is very wavelength and energy specific.

- Light of a wavelength of red (visible) to near infrared (NIR, invisible) is normally utilized for medical laser or light therapy because these wavelengths have the ability to penetrate skin and soft and boney tissue. When doing so, they have been proven to provide beneficial anti-inflammatory, analgesic, and healing effects.

- There are four categories of lasers that produce this light and these include gas (helium-non), solid (ruby), liquid (dye), and semiconductor (diode). The lasing medium or power source contains specific elements that will discharge photons of a specific wavelength and, therefore, energy. The resonating chamber contains the amplification and is normally a channel or rod that further concentrates the production of the photons by the use of mirrors.

- The effect of PBM is physiochemical, versus thermal, and the biochemical changes are comparable to photosynthesis, where photons or energy from the sun trigger chemical reactions. In order for light to have an effect on living tissues, photons of light must be absorbed by a chromophore or by a molecule that imparts color to a compound. Since mitochondria are the cellular power plants in our cells, it has been proposed that the mixed valence copper components of cytochrome c oxidase (Cytocox) are the primary photo-acceptor for the red-NIR wavelength range in mammalian cells. Nitric oxide (NO) binds to Cytocox and displaces oxygen, especially in injured or hypoxic cells.

- PBM is capable of reversing the mitochondrial inhibition of respiration by NO by increasing reactive oxygen species (ROS) and decreasing reactive nitrogen species. The long-term effects of PBM are thought to be due to the activation of various transcription factors by the immediate chemical signaling molecules produced via mitochondrial stimulation, namely adenosine triphosphate (ATP), cyclic adenosine monophosphate (cAMP), NO, and ROS.

- A long series of discoveries has demonstrated that ATP is not only an energy currency inside cells, but is a critical signaling molecule for neurons. When bound by ATP, ATP P2X receptors form a channel that allows sodium and calcium ions to enter cells; this influx further results in intracellular calcium stores being released. This intracellular calcium has been likened to a trigger for protective connective tissue building and cellular proliferation. The increased ATP synthesis and increased proton gradient leads to an increasing activity of the antiporter and Ca pumps. The resultant neovascularization via angiogenesis and increased collagen synthesis has been implicated in enhanced cell proliferation of fibroblasts, keratinocytes, endothelial cells, and lymphocytes.

- PBM has been said to exhibit a biphasic dose response curve wherein lower doses of light are more effective at healing and decreasing inflammation, and high doses/intensities seem to have an opposite effect inhibiting mitochondrial metabolism in C- and A-delta fibers and thereby reducing mitochondrial membrane potential, thus inducing a nerve blockade. This neural blockade occurs via temporary disruption of the cytoskeleton of axons. Dorsal root ganglia mitochondrial membrane potential decreases, and the proinflammatory mediators produced by attenuated second-order neural input are also lessened. Fast-acting pain relief occurs within minutes of application but the longer term decrease in edema and reduction in inflammation may indeed be due to a 'pile up' of mitochondrial upregulation that occurs at the nociceptors and tissue terminals largely aided by the initial vasodilation and neovascularization. The downregulated local mediator transduction and disrupted transmission of the nerve fibers are both thought to contribute greatly to reduced pain.

- Numerous other studies have shown that PBM is effective in reducing pain via production of endogenous opioids, NO, serotonin, and acetylcholine amongst other substances.

CLASSIFICATION OF DEVICES (*TABLE 25.1*)

- There are five levels of classification of laser energy: 1, 2, 3a, 3b, and 4. Categories 1–3a are considered safe, 3b requires precautions during use, and use of a Class 4 unit carries risk of injury to operator and patient.

- Laser manufacturers are required to certify and label their devices in the appropriate category. If we focus on true therapy lasers utilized in both veterinary and human medical application, Class 3 lasers are medium-power lasers, with Subclass 3a having a power output up to 5 mW, and Subclass 3b lasers an output of 5–500 mW.

- Class 4 lasers are high-power lasers that exceed 500 mW, which presents a hazard to both personnel, patient, and even

Table 25.1	Classification of laser energy and devices	
Category/class	*Energy*	*Risk to the patient and handler*
I, 2, and 3a	Low-power lasers, power output up to 5 mW	Safe
3b	Medium-power lasers, power output of 5–500 mW	Precautions
4	High-power laser, power output exceeds 500 mW	Chance of serious injuries

hospital if not used correctly; however, their reduced treatment times and increased penetration power often create the most immediate clinical responses.

- Class 3 lasers are still very useful, safer for in-clinic and at-home needs, and capable of eliciting an array of healing, anabolic, and analgesic outcomes in veterinary patients, especially for early acute pain and inflammation, superficial tissues, acupuncture point stimulation, and patients requiring longer treatment times.

PRECAUTIONS WITH PHOTOBIOMODULATION THERAPY

- Many of the potential hazards of PBM are ocular and thermal. It is important for the operator of the laser equipment to focus on appropriately-diagnosed conditions, know the laser strength, indication, and dangers involved, and become fully trained in its proper use prior to working on patients.
- A Class 4 laser poses the most danger given the combustibility of oxygen, the risk to unprotected eyes (staff, animals, and owners), and the thermal discomfort/tissue damage associated with non-moving application.
- The North American Association of Photobiomodulation Therapy (NAALT) makes the following recommendations regarding laser safety on its website:
  - Avoid inappropriate eye laser beam aiming and use safety glasses at all times.
  - Avoid treatment over any known primary neoplasia.
  - Avoid treatment over developing fetuses.
  - Beware that low frequency pulsed visible light may trigger photosensitization seizures.
  - Avoid use of higher power lasers over thyroid gland, active reproductive organs, and open growth plates.

LASER PARAMETER SELECTION AND TREATMENT TECHNIQUES

- Parameter selection is perhaps the most difficult aspect of understanding photobiomodulation since there are so many variables to consider. Many of these variables are centered around the patient, the type of condition, the acute or chronic nature of the condition, current medications, and even pigmentation, all of which can have an impact on outcomes.
- The laser parameters that must be considered in each treatment plan include:
  - Wavelength;
  - Output power;
  - Power density = intensity;
  - Energy density = dosage;
  - Time required;
  - Frequency of treatments; and
  - Application technique.
- Many of these parameters can be set by the operator or are included in preset programs with the units themselves (**Fig. 25.1**).

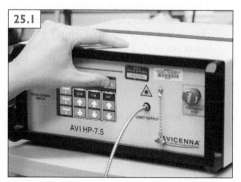

Fig. 25.1 Laser parameter selection is perhaps the most difficult aspect of understanding photobiomodulation. Many of these parameters can be set by the operator or are included in preset programs with the units themselves.

Wavelength

- The longer the wavelength (lower frequency), the greater the penetration. Wavelength is a function of the gas medium or semiconductor used, which includes combinations of gallium, aluminum, phosphide, arsenide, and indium, largely replacing the older HeNe lasers. Indium combinations usually emit wavelengths of 630–700 nm and, as such, penetrate to approximately a 1 cm depth, whereas gallium combinations often penetrate to deeper depths of 3–5 cm. Gallium combination lasers often are utilized for medium to deep tissue structures such as muscles, tendons, and joints.

Power = wattage

- Usually ranging from mW to W, this describes the rate at which the energy of the light is delivered, not the amount of energy. Keep in mind the formula watts = joules/second, which will become important when figuring out the dosage needed for treatment and the time required to treat a patient. Overall, the higher the power of the laser, the less time it takes to administer the correct therapeutic dosage, but more precautions must be taken to avoid combustion, inadvertent tissue injury, and discomfort during treatment.

Power density = intensity

- This is a variable that is normally programed into the lasers and is not changeable. It is reported simply as watts per cm^2. This parameter takes into consideration the actual beam diameter. Gas lasers have less divergence than semiconductor lasers.

Energy density = dosage = joules

- Treatment outcomes are dosage dependent, so this parameter must be consistently determined. If the wattage or power is known, then the number of joules is affected by the treatment time per irradiated area. Dose is calculated based on the laser power and the condition required to treat (*Table 25.2*).
  - Analgesic laser doses in the human literature are quoted as quite high

Table 25.2 Clinical condition versus dosage (joules, J)

Pain from	Dosage
Skin/wound/postoperative	3–4 J/cm^2
Otic/hot spot/abscess	3–4 J/cm^2
Tendon/ligament injury	4–6 J/cm^2
Osteoarthritis/degenerative joint disease	8–10 J/cm^2
Neck and back pain	4–8 J/cm^2
Trauma	3–6 J/cm^2
Neuropathy/neuritis	6–8 J/cm^2
Stomatitis	3–4 J/cm^2
Pancreatitis/cystitis	4–8 J/cm^2

(10–20 J/cm^2) compared with that in the veterinary literature, much of which is laser unit specific. In general, painful conditions are started low in dose and the owner is questioned as to adverse outcomes 3 days post treatment. If the animal has any adverse effects from the therapy, the dose can be decreased or treatment time/frequency increased. On the other hand, if there is no change in status of the patient, the dose is increased at the next treatment.

- If the animal is obese, consider an increase in the joules delivered. If the animal is thin, underweight, or frail, consider a decrease in the joules dosage. Fatigue has been reported after laser treatments, especially in animals with chronic conditions. Likewise, increased pain can be present in patients within 24 hours of a treatment given the activation of healing mechanisms that had become dormant over time in chronic conditions. Decreasing the dose +/– time of treatment +/– frequency can usually help reduce these immediate untoward responses.

Time

- The seconds or minutes used to treat a patient will depend on:
  - Size of the structure being treated.
  - Power/watts of the laser.
  - Acuteness or chronicity.
  - Depth of penetration needed.

- Application technique used (point versus grid versus scan).
- Pre-existing pain of the patient and the coat color/body: normally, smaller, darkly pigmented, acutely painful treatment areas are treated with shorter time periods. In addition, higher powered lasers require shorter time periods.

Treatment frequency

- A general recommendation is to use the least amount of energy that elicits the most benefit. Acute conditions should be treated more frequently (daily to every other day) than chronic conditions, but not more than once daily. Light energy has a cumulative effect, so smaller doses spaced farther apart have elicited more effective outcomes.

Application technique

- There are different methods of applying laser energy during the treatment. The laser should be maintained so that it is perpendicular to the treatment surface; however, it can be positioned directly on the skin for point treatment (as in acupuncture) or elevated off the skin and scanned back and forth near an area or in a grid fashion over the affected areas (**Fig. 25.2**).

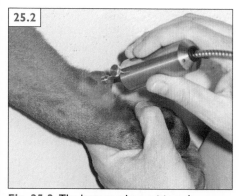

Fig. 25.2 The laser can be positioned directly on the skin for point treatment (as in acupuncture), or elevated off the skin and scanned back and forth near an area or in a grid fashion over the affected areas.

CONCLUSION

PBM is still under scrutiny using evidence-based research standards. It is making gains as research is more controlled and as multi-center studies and contemporary diagnostic measures/objective outcomes are utilized. Very few adverse effects have been reported in the literature, but additional research is required to obtain data concerning success rates in treating specific conditions, exact doses, frequency of treatment, depth of penetration required, as well as expected outcomes in both human and veterinary patients.

Treatment example

Using the chronic osteoarthritis-affected right elbow of a middle-aged, 27 kg (60 lb) dog as the target tissue, and an 8 W Class 4 therapy laser as our clinical tool:

- The area of treatment (bearing in a mind that a 3 × 5 card is approximately 100 cm^2) is roughly 75 cm^2 medial and 75 cm^2 caudolateral compartment. From *Table 25.1*, we can use a dosage of roughly 10 joules/cm^2 × 150 (75 + 75) cm^2 to get a total of 1,500 joules needed for treatment.
- Given that the laser unit is set at 8 watts and 1 watt =1 joule/second, the time required for treatment of this patient's elbow is 1,500 J divided by 8 watts = 187 seconds (or 3 minutes).
- The laser is moved with slow 'paintbrush' type strokes in a grid fashion over the medial epicondyle/joint compartment with the hand piece approximately 1 cm off the skin. Half of the total joules are delivered medially and the other half in the same manner over the caudolateral joint compartment.

Further reading

Chow RT, Armati PJ (2016) Photobiomodulation: implications for anesthesia and pain relief. *Photomed Laser Surg* **34(12)**:599–609.

Cotler HB, Chow RT, Hamblin MR *et al.* (2015) The use of low level laser therapy (LLLT) for musculoskeletal pain. *MOJ Orthop Rheumatol* 2 **(5)**:pii.

Denegar CR, Saliba E, Saliba S (2010) Low level laser therapy. In: *Therapeutic Modalities for Musculoskeletal Injuries*, 3rd edn. (ed CR Denegar) Human Kinetics Publishing, Champaign.

Draper WE, Schubert TA, Clemmons R *et al.* (2012) Low-level laser therapy reduces time to ambulation in dogs after hemilaminectomy: a preliminary study. *J Small Anim Pract* **53(8)**:465–9.

Hode L, Tuner J (2002) *Laser Phototherapy: Clinical Practice and Scientific Background.* Prima Books, Coeymans Hollow.

Kurach L, Stanley BJ, Gassola KM *et al.* (2015) The effect of low-level laser therapy on the healing of open wounds in dogs. *Vet Surg* **44(8)**:988–96.

McCauley L (2014) Lasers: more variables than power. *Clinicians Brief* **12(6)**:89–91.

Neibaum K (2013) Rehabilitation physical modalities. In: *Canine Sports Medicine and Rehabilitation.* (eds MC Zink, JB Van Dyke) Wiley Blackwell, Ames.

North American Association of Photobiomodulation Therapy. www.NAALT.org

Riegal RJ (2008) *Laser Therapy in the Companion Animal Practice.* Companion Therapy Laser/LiteCure LLC, Langeskov.

Riegel RJ, Godbold JC (eds) (2017) *Laser Therapy in Veterinary Medicine: Photobiomodulation.* J Wiley & Sons, Ames, Iowa.

Ritzman T, Griffin C, Kilgore A *et al.* (2015) Therapeutic laser treatment for exotic animal patients. *J Avian Med Surg* **29(1)**:69–73.

CHAPTER 26

Management of neuropathic pain in dogs and cats

Talisha M Moore and Stephanie A Thomovsky

Overview of pain

To understand neuropathic pain, it is important to have a basic understanding of the normal physiology of pain, as well as how pathologic or chronic pain develops.

Components of normal pain perception (see also Chapter 24)

- Transduction: conversion of noxious stimulus (mechanical, thermal, or chemical) received in the periphery at the level of the nociceptor into an electrical signal (action potential).
- Transmission: propagation of the action potential along the peripheral nerve into the spinal cord, and ultimately cerebrum. Peripheral nerve fibers: A-δ and C-fibers.
- Modulation: alteration of the nociceptive signal via inhibition or facilitation within the dorsal horn gray matter of the spinal cord; sensory information enters the spinal cord via the dorsal root of spinal nerves.

- Perception: somatosensory processing of noxious stimuli as painful. Occurs in the forebrain of the cerebral cortex.

ROLE OF THE PERIPHERAL NERVOUS SYSTEM IN PAIN PERCEPTION
- A-δ fibers:
  - Activated by noxious thermal or mechanical stimulus.
  - Localized receptive field.
  - Thin, myelinated fibers that produce rapid transduction and transmission of sensory information.
  - Responsible for the initial feeling of acute (e.g. pinprick) pain.

- Serve as a protective mechanism, warning the animal to remove the affected body part from the noxious stimulus.
- C-fibers:
  - Increased intensity of the stimulus, as may occur when tissue injury is present, results in recruitment of C-fibers.
  - Very thin, unmyelinated fibers with poorly localized receptive fields.
  - Slow transduction and transmission.
  - May be activated by mechanical, thermal, or chemical stimuli.
  - Perceived as burning, throbbing, or dull pain.
    - Source of 'chronic pain'.
  - No physiologic benefit; may be referred to as pathologic pain.
- A-β fibers:
  - Play a major role in proprioception.
  - Activated by low-intensity sensations (e.g. touch, vibrations).
  - Under normal circumstance, no role in pain pathway.

ROLE OF THE CENTRAL NERVOUS SYSTEM IN PAIN PERCEPTION

- Complex pathway in domestic animals, but the general concepts are:
  - After modulation occurs, afferent sensory information projects cranially through the spinal cord and brainstem, and synapses within the thalamus.
  - Axonal projections travel from the thalamus to the somatosensory cortex where the sensory information is further processed and is associated with an emotional response (pain).
- Development of chronic pain:
  - In the presence of tissue injury, C-fibers repetitively fire and are responsible for the ongoing or 'chronic pain' felt after the initial insult has occurred.
  - Repetitive firing of C-fibers is a result of inflammatory mediators, which are activated by the injured tissue.
  - As the injured tissue heals, transduction and transmission of sensory information via C-fibers ceases.

- Untreated or inadequately treated acute or chronic pain results in prolonged activation of pain pathways.
  - Results in augmented somatosensory transmission of pain:
    - Peripheral sensitization:
      - Lowered threshold of peripheral nociceptors via infiltration of inflammatory cells with subsequent release of chemical mediators: arachidonic acid (AA) cascade; eicosanoid production; substance-P (a pronociceptive chemical).
      - May lead to hyperalgesia.
    - Central sensitization ('wind-up') is considered multimodal:
      - Dysfunction of descending inhibitory pain pathways. Descending inhibitory system functions as an endogenous analgesic systems. Dorsal horn neurons are thought to play a major role in modulation of nociceptive transmission. Several substances are thought to be involved: GABA, glycine, norepinephrine, endogenous opioids (e.g. endorphins, enkephalins), and serotonin.
        - Recruitment of spinal neurons that release glutamate. Postsynaptic binding of glutamate to NMDA receptors causes a cascade of events that ultimately result in an amplified sensitivity of dorsal horn neurons. Enhanced transmitter release of spinal prostaglandin E_2 and amino acids.
      - Central sensitization may lead to allodynia.

Neuropathic pain

- A form of chronic pain.
- Proposed mechanisms for the development of neuropathic pain result from pathologic neuroplasticity:
  - Central sensitization.
  - Phenotypic change of mechanoreceptive A-β fibers.
- Occurs as a direct result of a primary lesion or disease within the peripheral or CNS.
  - Peripheral nervous system lesions:
    - Spinal nerves.
    - Spinal nerve root.
    - Damage to myelin sheath.
  - CNS lesions:
    - Meninges:
      - Well innervated by local nerves.
    - Spinal cord:
      - Nociceptive tracts (e.g. spinothalamic tract).
    - Intervertebral disc:
      - Comprised of annulus and nucleus pulpous.
      - The peripheral one-third of the annulus is innervated. Lesions (e.g. compression, tears within the annulus) may result in 'discogenic' pain.
    - Thalamus:
      - Thalamic pain syndrome. Spontaneous, poorly localized pain. Poorly understood mechanism. Most often associated with a thalamic neoplasm, but can occur with a vascular event.
- Any tissue or organ that possesses nerve endings can be the source of neuropathic pain.
  - Somatic nociceptors are those that originate from bone, joints, tendons, and skin.
  - Common veterinary neurologic diseases that result in neuropathic pain:
    - CNS:
      - Brain. Meningoencephalitis, intracranial neoplasia/tumor, diencephalic syndrome, head trauma/skull fracture.
      - Spinal cord. Intervertebral disc disease, spinal fracture/ luxation, lumbosacral disease, caudal cervical spondylomyelopathy, syringomyelia, meningomyelitis, spinal neoplasia/tumor, discospondylitis, spinal empyema, ascending/ descending myelomalacia.
    - Peripheral nervous system: Neuritis, myositis, brachial plexus avulsion, nerve root disease.
  - Referred pain:
    - Visceral (originating from organs) nociceptors share a common pathway with cutaneous (skin) nociceptors, and therefore lesions within organs may be poorly localized to cutaneous zones.

Common medications used for the treatment of neuropathic pain

With such a variety of etiologies, diagnosis and treatment of neuropathic pain is often challenging. When possible, it is always recommended to treat the primary disease. Strategies for treating neuropathic pain should focus on a multimodal drug approach. (Refer to *Table 26.1* for dosages and side-effects.)

- Anticonvulsants:
  - Gabapentin:
    - Structural analog of GABA.
    - Binds to calcium channels, in so doing reducing calcium influx.
    - Short half-life.
    - Binding of NMDA receptors by glutamate facilitates calcium conductance and upregulation of receptors, which may lead to amplified sensitivity of dorsal horn neurons.

Table 26.1 Common medications used for the treatment of neuropathic pain in dogs and cats

Medication	Dose (mg/kg) PO (unless otherwise specified)	Frequency (hours)	Common side-effects
Gabapentin	10–20 (dogs), 10-15 (cats)	q8–12	Ataxia, sedation
Pregabalin	3–4 (dogs), not evaluated in cats	q12	Ataxia, sedation
Tramadol	3–5 (dogs), 2–4 (cats)	q8	Ataxia, sedation, constipation
Fentanyl transdermal patch	25–100 µg/h (dogs) and 25 µg/h (cats)	n/a	Ataxia, sedation, constipation
Amantadine	3–5 (dogs), 2–5 (cats)	q12–24	Agitation, diarrhea
Amitriptyline	1.1–4 (dogs) 2.5–12.5 per cat	q12 (dogs) q24 (cats)	Sedation, constipation, urinary retention

- – GABA is thought to play a role in decreasing central sensitization (see previous discussion).
- Pregabalin:
  - – Structurally similar to gabapentin.
  - – Longer half-life with stronger binding affinity of receptors.
  - – Like gabapentin, it is thought to play a role in decreasing central sensitization.
  - – May be cost prohibitive.
- NMDA antagonists:
  - Amantadine HCl:
    - – Dopamine agonists and non-competitive NMDA antagonists.
    - – NMDA receptors have a major role in the development of central sensitization (see previous discussion) and therefore antagonism of these receptors may decrease central sensitization.
    - – Possible synergistic relationship with opioids, NSAIDs, and gabapentin.
- Tricyclic antidepressants:
  - Amitriptyline HCl:
    - – Antidepressant that may be used in small companion animals for behavioral problems, although

these effects are thought to be distinct from its pain-relieving effects.
- – Inhibits the reuptake of norepinephrine and serotonin, as well as antagonism of NMDA receptors.
- – Major role within the descending inhibitory pathway at the level of the dorsal horn neurons, decreases central sensitization.
- Opioids:
  - Tramadol HCl:
    - – Weak, synthetic opioid-like (mu receptor) agonist.
    - – Debate exists regarding the usefulness of this medication in the treatment of neuropathic pain, therefore it is not recommended that it is used as a monotherapy.
    - – Likely exerts its effects at the level of the spinal cord dorsal horn.
  - Fentanyl transdermal patch:
    - – Full mu receptor agonist.
    - – Variable absorption may limit its use in clinical setting.
    - – Similar to tramadol, exerts its effects at the level of the spinal cord dorsal horn.

Common medications used for the treatment of chronic pain

These medications may be used as adjunct therapy to neuropathic pain medications. Selection of adjunct therapy should be based on underlying disease. (Refer to *Table 26.2* for dosages and side-effects.)

- Non-steroidal anti-inflammatory drugs:
  - As a class, these medications function via inhibition of cyclooxygenase-1 (COX-1) and cyclooxygenase-2 (COX-2).

Table 26.2 Common medications used for the treatment of chronic pain in dogs and cats

Medication	Dose (mg/kg) PO (*unless otherwise specified)	Frequency (hours)	Common side-effects
NSAIDs			
Carprofen	2.2 or 4.4 (dogs)	q12 or q24	Gastrointestinal, renal, hepatic
Meloxicam	0.2 on the first day, then reduce to 0.1 (dogs)	q24	
Robenacoxib	1–2 (dogs); 1 tablet for 2.5–6 kg cat; 2 tablets for 6.1–12 kg cat	q24 (up to q3 days in cats)	Vomiting, diarrhea/soft stool
Grapiprant	2 (dogs); not evaluated in cats	q24	
Prednisolone/ prednisone	0.5–1 (dogs and cats)	q24	Polyuria, polydipsia, polyphagia, gastrointestinal ulceration, muscle atrophy (with high dose or chronic use)
Muscle relaxants			
Methocarbamol	15–20 (dogs and cats)	q8–12	Ataxia, sedation
Diazepam	0.25–0.5 (dogs); oral diazepam not recommended in cats	q8	Ataxia, sedation, increased appetite, CNS agitation or aggression

- Common therapy for the treatment of mild to moderate chronic pain.
- May be useful as an adjunct therapy, especially if an underlying inflammatory component to the disease exist.
- Carprofen and meloxicam are commonly chosen.
- Recent or upcoming medications to the market that should be considered:
  - Robenacoxib (Onsior®):
    - Coxib class NSAID.
    - Selective COX-2 inhibition.
    - FDA approved for use in cats (up to 3 days in the USA, longer in the UK).
  - Grapiprant (Galliprant®):
    - New piprant class of NSAID.
    - Mechanism of action via antagonism of prostaglandin receptors.
    - Specifically, the drug is a selective prostaglandin E_2 antagonist and exerts its effects via binding of EP4

  prostaglandin receptor with high affinity.
- Glucocorticoids (steroids):
  - As a class, has effects on many cell types throughout the body.
  - Pharmacokinetics varies based on the glucocorticoid chosen:
    - Prednisone/prednisolone is most commonly chosen.
  - May be useful as an adjunct therapy when inflammation and/or vasogenic edema are present.
- Muscle relaxants:
  - Methocarbamol (Robaxin®):
    - Skeletal muscle relaxant; exact mechanism of action is not well understood.
    - May be useful as an adjunct therapy when underlying disease causes muscle fasciculation or spasms.
    - Intervertebral disc disease (especially cervical), myositis.
  - Valium (Diazepam):
    - Benzodiazepine; functions at GABA receptors.
    - Used in a similar manner as methocarbamol.

Alternative therapies used for the treatment of neuropathic pain

- In human medicine, there exists a plethora of medications available for the treatment of neuropathic pain. However, for veterinary patients, some of these medications are cost prohibitive, have limited efficacy as a monomodal treatment, and can have severe side-effects.

- As a result, adjunct treatments, such as physical rehabilitation and massage, low-level laser therapy, and acupuncture are being recommended when traditional medications alone fail.
- Refer to Chapter 30 for additional readings on this topic.

Case examples

CASE 1
- Signalment: 7-year-old, female spayed Beagle.
- History: 1 month of cervical pain.
- Clinical signs: low head carriage, reluctance to go up and down stairs, reluctance to lateral flexion of the neck, cervical muscle spasms/fasciculation, and moderate/severe cervical hyperesthesia; no neurologic deficits noted.
- Diagnosis: Intervertebral disc disease at C3/4 and C4/5 causing spinal cord compression.
- Treatment:
  - Tier 1: medical management – cage rest and multimodality pain control. Use of an anti-inflammatory (steroids versus NSAID) and a medication targeting the pain pathway (gabapentin or tramadol). Consider a muscle relaxant such as methocarbamol for muscle fasciculations.
  - Tier 2: patient fails medical management, then surgery should be pursued:
    - Surgical decompression (ventral slot at C3/4 and C4/5) performed.
    - Patient remains painful postoperatively with muscle spasms/fasciculation.
  - Consider the addition of non-pharmaceutical therapy:
    - Acupuncture.
    - Transcutaneous electrical nerve stimulation (TENS).

CASE 2
- Signalment: 9-month-old, female spayed Golden Retriever.

- History: 1 month of thoracolumbar and pelvic limb pain, anorexia, and weight loss.
- Clinical signs: moderate kyphosis, marked atrophy of the caudal musculature of both pelvic limbs, narrow-based stance and crossing over in the pelvic limbs when walking, lowered tail carriage, and severe hyperesthesia noted on palpation of the cranial thoracic spine through the lumbar spine; no neurologic deficits noted.
- Diagnosis: discospondylitis at T10/11, T11/12, and L4/5.
- Treatment:
  - Tier 1: begin appropriate antibiotic therapy, as well as initiation of gabapentin and NSAID for pain management.
  - Tier 2: patient remains painful, consider the addition of an opioid.
  - Tier 3: no clinical improvement, consider the addition of amantadine or amitriptyline.

CASE 3
- Signalment: 9-year-old, female spayed Domestic Shorthair cat.
- History: 1 month of thoracolumbar pain and proprioceptive ataxia.
- Clinical signs: ambulatory paraparesis with moderate proprioceptive ataxia, hyperesthesia noted on cranial lumbar spinal palpation; no other neurologic deficits noted.
- Diagnosis: intradural-extramedullary mass at L3, suspect meningioma.
- Treatment:
  - Tier 1: surgery and/or radiation therapy declined, initiate conservative management with gabapentin and prednisolone.

- Tier 2: patient remains painful, consider the addition of an opioid (fentanyl patch or buprenorphine).

- Tier 3: no clinical improvement, consider the addition of amantadine.

Further reading

Cashmore RG, Harcourt-Brown TR, Freeman PM *et al.* (2009) Clinical diagnosis and treatment of suspected neuropathic pain in three dogs. *Aust Vet J* **87(1)**:45–50.

Corti L (2014) Nonpharmaceutical approaches to pain management. *Top Companion Anim Med* **29(1)**:24–8.

Greene SA (2010) Chronic pain: pathophysiology and treatment implications. *Top Companion Anim Med* **25(1)**:5–9.

Grubb T (2010) Chronic neuropathic pain in veterinary patients. *Top Companion Anim Med* **25(1)**:45–52.

Grubb T (2010) What do we really know about the drugs we use to treat chronic pain? *Top Companion Anim Med* **25(1)**:10–19.

Mathews KA (2008) Neuropathic pain in dogs and cats: if only they could tell us they hurt. *Vet Clin North Am Small Anim Pract* **38(6)**:1365–414.

Moore SA (2016) Managing neuropathic pain in dogs. *Front Vet Sci* **3**:12.

Rausch-Derra L, Huebner M, Wofford J *et al.* (2016). A prospective, randomized, masked, placebo-controlled multisite clinical study of grapiprant, an EP4 prostaglandin receptor antagonist (PRA), in dogs with osteoarthritis. *J Vet Intern Med* **30(3)**:756–63.

CHAPTER 27

Oncologic pain management and radiation therapy

Nicholas J Rancilio and Jeff C Ko

Overview of radiation therapy and its role in pain management

- Radiation therapy is a powerful tool for the treatment of cancer and the palliative management of painful conditions in cancer patients. Treatments (called fractions) are delivered under general anesthesia or heavy reversible sedation using protocols suggested elsewhere in this book. This chapter will focus on the palliative management of cancer pain, oncologic pain assessment, and commonly encountered painful conditions.

- In veterinary medicine the most common method of radiation delivery is using a device called a linear accelerator. Drugs that incorporate a radioactive isotope termed radiopharmaceuticals may also be used in certain cases. Other methods of delivery, such as the implantation of radioactive seeds into the tumor excision bed either temporarily or permanently, may also be attempted but are less commonly encountered in veterinary medicine.

- Delivery of radiation using a linear accelerator is termed external beam radiation therapy (EBRT). The beam of radiation is focused on the tumor outside of the patient using computer-controlled collimators and treatment plans. The radiation source in EBRT is mounted on a gantry that can aim the radiation beam 360 degrees around the patient to facilitate sparing of normal tissues by conformal avoidance. The net effect is that minimal volumes of normal tissues, such as the skin, small intestines, brain, or eyes, are included in the treated volume.

- Two different types of radiation therapy protocols may be used depending on the clinical situation encountered: definitive radiation therapy (DRT) and palliative radiation therapy (PRT). Radiation dose delivered to a patient is measured using a unit called the Gray (Gy) and is a representation of the energy deposited into the tissue irradiated.

- DRT protocols incorporate 16–20 daily fractions delivered over consecutive weekdays with breaks on the weekend. DRT uses small fractions sizes of between 2 and 3 Gy. DRT delivers the most dose of radiation possible and, depending on the anatomic location treated and treatment

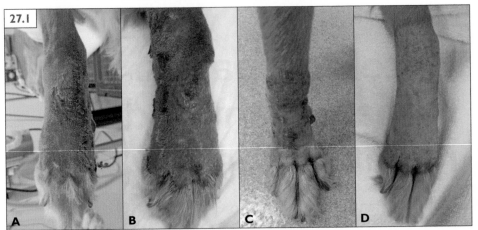

Fig. 27.1 (A) Moist desquamation after completing 19 fractions of definitive radiation therapy (DRT) for a soft tissue sarcoma, excised with dirty margins from the distal forelimb. The limb is swollen and there are several focal areas of redness, and edema. (B) 1 week after completion of DRT in the same patient, the reaction has become more severe with radiating redness, edema, crusting, and serum seepage. (C) 2 weeks after completion of DRT, note the near complete resolution of moist desquamation, the skin is pink and smooth with a few areas of crusts and redness. (D) 4 weeks after completion of DRT. Complete resolution of clinical signs.

technique, may result in reversible painful side-effects. Patients prescribed a course of DRT must have a favorable long-term prognosis with treatment. Definitive radiation therapy is used as a combined modality treatment with surgery in many cases. For example, the treatment of a scar on the carpus where a soft tissue sarcoma or mast cell tumor was removed with incomplete margins (Fig. 27.1).

- PRT is delivery of much smaller total doses of radiation over a shorter period of time. The dose delivered at each fraction of PRT is between 4 and 8 Gy. The overall goal of PRT is to alleviate pain and discomfort without inducing painful radiation side-effects in normal tissues. Measureable gross disease must be present in order for PRT to be effective.
  - PRT protocols may also play a role in the treatment of benign painful conditions such as osteoarthritis. PRT is a non-pharmacologic modulator of the pain response. Older patients are most suitable for this treatment option as their risk for a late side-effect is decreased relative to younger patients.
- Side-effects may result from radiation therapy. There are two categories of side effects:
  - Acute: occur in rapidly proliferating normal tissues such as the skin or mucous membranes. Acute side-effects are completely reversible but may be painful.
  - Late: occur in slowly proliferating normal tissues such as the nervous system or bones. Late side-effects are generally irreversible and the probability of their occurrence increases exponentially with fraction size and with time after exposure.

Head to tail approach to painful tumors and cancer (see *Table 27.1*)

BODY SYSTEMS COMMONLY AFFECTED BY ONCOLOGIC PAIN
Head and neck
- Invasion into oral cavity gingiva, dental nerves.
- Affect structures of the head/neck, such as the eyes, or afferent cranial nerves, which may cause pain or discomfort.
- Spinal nerve roots may be affected and cause particularly severe pain.
- Moderate to severe pain.

Table 27.1 Anatomic location and sensory nerve involvement of the commonly involved tumors

Anatomic location	Common tumor types	Sensory nerves	Tissue involvement	Degree of pain/functional interference
Head/neck	Oral malignant melanoma (dogs), squamous cell carcinoma (dogs/cats)	CNs V, VIII, IX	Invasive tumors that may involve the gingiva, soft tissues of the tongue/mouth, and invade bone	Diminished ability to prehend food. Tumors that invade into bone are exceptionally painful. May be infected and odiferous
Nasal	Nasal adenocarcinoma (60%), sarcomas (40%), lymphoma (cats)	CNs V, VIII, IX; CN I (olfactory nerve) involvement may affect ability of patient to detect food	Localized destruction of nasal turbinate bones. May invade into bones of the cribriform plate, frontal bone, orbit, or through the hard palate	Wide spectrum. Generally tumors that are small, rostral, and only involve the nasal turbinates have a mild degree of pain. Most clinical signs result from postnasal drip due to secretions from the tumor. The back of the oropharynx may be red and irritated on physical examination. Highly invasive masses involving the bones of the skull or orbit may cause severe pain
Skin/subcutis	Soft tissue sarcoma, mast cell tumor, vaccine-associated sarcoma (cats) (Fig. 27.2)	Variable, may occur anywhere on the body where there is skin. Pain is detected by sensory afferents and transmitted to the dorsal horn of the spinal cord	Soft tissue sarcomas as a rule tend to move along fascial planes but do not invade into them. Mast cell tumors may be very localized to the skin but can directly invade into deeper structures	Sarcomas tend to cause mechanical impingements of bones and joints. Mild–moderate pain may occur. If masses are allowed to grow to an advanced stage, there may be pressure from the mass causing severe pain. Sarcomas and mast cell tumors that are ulcerated can cause severe pain. Mast cell tumors as a group may secrete histamine and serotonin if irritated. These substances can directly cause pain and decrease the pain threshold in a given patient
Bone	Osteosarcoma, hemangiosarcoma, metastatic, other	Variable, may occur in any bone of the body (limbs are most common). Pain is detected by sensory afferents and transmitted to the dorsal horn of the spinal cord. Bone is richly innervated, especially on the periosteal and endosteal surfaces	Medullary cavity, periosteum, endosteum	Primary and metastatic tumors of bone may cause severe pain and inhibit mobility of the patient
Metastatic	Hemangiosarcoma, osteosarcoma, oral malignant melanoma	Variable, visceral sensory afferents, bone invasion	Body viscera such as lungs/pleura, liver/kidney/bone	Highly variable, little or no pain to severe unrelenting pain

CN, cranial nerve.

Fig. 27.2 (**A**) A cat after completing fraction 20/20 of definitive radiation therapy (DRT) for a vaccine-associated sarcoma on the left paralumbar-flank region. Dry, flaky skin is present with mild redness. (**B**) The same cat 1 week after finishing DRT; note the dry, flaky redness has progressed and there is more alopecia. No confluent moist desquamation is present as in the dog. (**C**) The same cat approximately 2 weeks after finishing DRT. Lesions have healed and the hair is beginning to grow back.

Central nervous system

- The brain itself paradoxically does not feel pain.
- Mass lesions in the brain may cause discomfort by stretching meninges.
- Mass lesions compressing spinal nerve roots may cause severe and debilitating pain.

Cardiorespiratory system

- Tumors of the heart base, pericardium, lungs, or pleura may cause irritation of visceral nociceptors.
- Irritation of pleural/pericardial surfaces or obstruction of venous return may cause plural or pericardial effusion if a mass lesion affects these structures.
- Clinically silent to severe pain.

Musculoskeletal system

- The musculoskeletal system is richly innervated, particularly on the periosteal or endosteal surfaces.
- Tumors of the bones and joints. Primary or metastatic tumors of bone may cause severe and debilitating pain.

Skin/subcutis

- Masses may present incidentally at annual examination and may be benign.
- Tumors such as soft tissue sarcoma or mast cell tumors have variable pain characteristics depending on the biology of the particular tumor and size of the mass.
- Mast cell tumors may degranulate, causing release of histamine, serotonin, and other substances that are painful and decrease the pain threshold.
- Sarcomas that are very advanced in the disease process may ulcerate the skin, causing severe pain.

Urogenital system

- Masses of the urethra or urinary bladder may cause dysuria and urinary blockage, which may cause stretching of visceral nociceptors and subsequent pain. Masses of the kidneys or ureter may be particularly painful as these structures are richly innervated.

Digestive system

- Masses of the rectum and anal sac are most commonly encountered. Mass effect causes stretching or blocking of excreta. Masses of the anal sac may ulcerate through the skin or rectal mucosa, causing severe pain. Variable levels of pain are encountered depending on the characteristics of the tumor.

Oncologic pain assessment and management

Systematic evaluation of oncologic pain is one of the best ways to approach treatment. This can be accomplished by using multiple recheck examinations. Pain score use by the owners and by the veterinarian can objectively track the progress of pain management. Two oncologic pain scoring systems have been developed by the authors: an owner pain scoring system (*Table 27.2*); and a veterinarian pain scoring system (*Table 27.3*).

PALLIATIVE PAIN MANAGEMENT
- Generally will be patients with tumors that are incurable.
- Pain management may be accomplished using medical management or by combining this with palliative radiation therapy, chemotherapy, and in some instances surgery.
- Palliative radiation therapy is highly effective for the management of pain in patients with gross bulky disease or bone tumors.

Table 27.2 The owner's pain brief inventory scoring system

Description of pain
Rate your pet's pain

Circle the one number that best describes the pain at its worst in the last 7 days

0	1	2	3	4	5	6	7	8	9	10
Not painful										Worst pain imaginable

Circle the one number that best describes the pain at its least in the last 7 days

| 0 | 1 | 2 | 3 | 4 | 5 | 6 | 7 | 8 | 9 | 10 |

Circle the one number that best describes the pain at its average in the last 7 days

| 0 | 1 | 2 | 3 | 4 | 5 | 6 | 7 | 8 | 9 | 10 |

Circle the one number that best describes the pain as it is right now

| 0 | 1 | 2 | 3 | 4 | 5 | 6 | 7 | 8 | 9 | 10 |

Description of function
Circle the one number that during the past 7 days pain has interfered with your pet's:

General activity

0	1	2	3	4	5	6	7	8	9	10
Does not interfere										Completely interferes

Enjoyment of life

| 0 | 1 | 2 | 3 | 4 | 5 | 6 | 7 | 8 | 9 | 10 |

Enjoying a peaceful night sleeping

| 0 | 1 | 2 | 3 | 4 | 5 | 6 | 7 | 8 | 9 | 10 |

Eating or drinking (appetite)

| 0 | 1 | 2 | 3 | 4 | 5 | 6 | 7 | 8 | 9 | 10 |

Interaction with people or other pets

| 0 | 1 | 2 | 3 | 4 | 5 | 6 | 7 | 8 | 9 | 10 |

Overall impression
Circle the one response that best describes your pet's overall quality of life over the last 7 days

| Poor | Fair | Good | Very good | Excellent |

Table 27.3 Pain scoring system for veterinary use in the hospitalized patient

Pain score	Behavioral signs
1 (minimum pain)	Relaxed, resting comfortably, not vocalizing, moving freely, calm or asleep, palpation of lesion elicits no reaction from patient
2 (faint pain)	Minimal agitation, resting calmly, barely noticeable alteration from signs of minimal pain, some position changes, palpation of lesion elicits minimal response
3 (mild pain)	Mild agitation, some position changes, responds to calm voice and stroking, some salivation, occasionally vocalizing, palpation of lesion may cause patient to turn their head, lick, and/or scratch the lesion
4 (moderate pain)	Moderate agitation, vocalizing, excessive salivation, muscle trembling, frequent position changes, some thrashing movements, palpation of the lesion may cause the patient to become aggressive or traumatize the lesion further
5 (severe pain)	Severe agitation, vomiting, vocalizing, excessive salivation, extremely depressed, inactive, palpation of the lesion increases the level of agitation

- Generally 4–5 treatments given on weekdays (4 Gy in 5 fractions or 8 Gy in 4 fractions) and with weekend rest.
- Low total doses are given such that there is an effect on the tumor but not enough radiation delivered to cause acute side-effects in normal tissues.
- Acute side-effects may occur as a result of radiation therapy delivered to rapidly dividing normal tissues. The acute side-effects have the following characteristics:
  - Commonly occur on skin, mucosal surfaces, and gastrointestinal tract.
  - Result from denudation of proliferating stem cells.
  - Side-effects are temporary, self-limiting, and reversible.
  - Clinically significant acute side-effects occur in less than 10% of veterinary patients undergoing palliative radiation therapy.
- Bone tumors:
  - Pain can be treated using 2 fractions of 8 Gy, 24 hours apart.
  - Can be effective for up to 80% of patients treated but there is variable durability in response of between 3 and 6 months.
  - Patients that have not developed a displaced or unstable fracture may be retreated with this protocol at any time.
  - May be an effective choice for large-breed dogs with forelimb masses that are not good candidates for amputation.

ONCOLOGIC TREATMENT-RELATED PAIN MANAGEMENT

- Surgical removal and definitive radiation therapy to reduce cancer bulk can also trigger pain and requires pain management.
- Surgical pain for oncologic conditions is treated similarly to other orthopedic and soft tissue surgeries discussed in this book.
- Patients undergoing definitive radiation therapy may develop acute side-effects depending on the location of their tumor and the technique used for radiation therapy.
  - Deep-seated masses may not develop any acute painful side-effects because the deposition of energy is sufficiently away from surfaces such as the skin or mucosa to induce significant pain.
  - New treatment techniques for nasal tumors allow sculpting of the radiation dose to avoid the skin, eyes, and oral mucosa. Dose sculpting can help reduce or eliminate side-effects from definitive treatment in nasal tumors and other locations.
- Acute side-effects' mechanism of action (skin):
  - Temporary and self-limiting condition.
  - Most commonly visible/encountered for treatment of scars on the skin in tumors such as soft tissue sarcoma/mast cell tumor. Especially on the distal limb.
- Results from denudation of stem cells:
  - Deposition of ionizing radiation into the skin.
  - Depopulation of keratinocyte stem cells.

- Differentiated keratinocytes go through their normal life cycle and shed.
- Diminished numbers of stem cells to replace differentiated keratinocytes results in a defect.
- Begins about 2 weeks into the course of therapy and results in a dry area or red scaling on the skin. This phase is called dry desquamation.
- As treatment progresses the lesion progresses to moist desquamation. An exudative and red lesion develops and is at peak pain severity about 1 week after finishing the course of DRT (or PRT should it occur).
- Pain is mediated by somatic sensory afferent C-fibers.
- Rapidly heals after it appears.
- Cats are less radiosensitive than dogs and will generally only develop dry desquamation, which is typically much less painful.

PHARMACOLOGIC THERAPY
- NSAIDs are first line and are generally started approximately 2 weeks into a course of definitive radiation therapy. For example: carprofen 4.4 mg/kg PO q24 h.
- As the lesion progresses over the course of therapy other drugs are added in:
  - Tramadol 5–10 mg/kg PO q6–12 h.
  - Gabapentin 5–10 mg/kg PO q6–12 h.
  - Amantadine 2–5 mg/kg PO q12 h.
- All the above drugs may be combined for maximum effect in addition to the following for patients that develop more severe clinical signs of pain:
  - Transdermal fentanyl patch 25, 50, 75, or 100 μg/hour.
  - Codeine 1–2 mg/kg PO q8–12 h.
  - Buprenorphine: dogs 80–120 μg/kg OTM q12–24 h; cats 80–180 μg/kg OTM q12–24 h. Highly concentrated formulations (Simbadol™) may be prescribed to help manage the volumes necessary for therapeutic administration.

Further reading

Fan TM (2014) Pain management in veterinary patients with cancer. *Vet Clin North Am Small Anim Pract* **44**(5): 989–1001.

Hall EJ, Giaccia AJ (2019) *Radiobiology for the Radiologist*, 8th edn. Walters Kluwer.

Henry CJ, Higginbotham ML (2010) *Cancer management in small animal practice.* Saunders/Elsevier, Maryland Heights.

Knapp-Hoch HM, Fidel JL, Sellon RK, Gavin PR (2009) An expedited palliative radiation protocol for lytic or proliferative lesions of appendicular bone in dogs. *J Am Anim Hosp Assoc* **45**(1):24–32.

Rancilio N, Ko J, Fulkerson CM (2016) Strategies for managing cancer pain in dogs and cats. Part II: Definitive and palliative management of cancer pain. *Today's Vet Prac* **6**(1):47.

Rancilio N, Poulson J, Ko J (2015) Strategies for managing cancer pain in dogs and cats. Part I: Pathophysiology and assessment of cancer pain. *Today's Vet Prac* **5**(3):60.

Rossi F *et al.* (2018) Megavoltage radiotherapy for the treatment of degenerative joint disease in dogs: Results of a preliminary experience in an Italian Radiotherapy Centre. *Front Vet Sci* **5**:74.

Chronic pain management for osteoarthritis in dogs and cats

Tamara L Grubb

Introduction

Osteoarthritis (OA) is a painful condition that limits the patient's quality of life. It is the most common cause of chronic pain in all species, including dogs and cats. It is believed to affect up to 40% of dogs over 1 year of age and, based on radiographic evidence, may affect a similar number of adult cats with up to 90% of geriatric cats affected.

Pathology of osteoarthritis

- Although age is a predisposing factor for OA development, OA is not a normal part of the aging process and pain from OA should not be tolerated just because a patient is 'old'.
- Secondary OA, the most common OA form in animals, is caused by factors that include previous trauma or surgery of the joint; joint instability due to injuries, tendon laxity, poor muscle tone or congenital abnormalities; and developmental conditions that directly affect the joint.
- OA is a progressive, degenerative, painful disease that can impact all structures of the joint, including articular cartilage, subchondral bone, synovial membrane, and soft tissue surrounding the joint.

Pain from osteoarthritis

- Protective pain, or physiologic pain, occurs with acute injury and it is initially useful because it causes the patient to limit movement, thereby protecting the injured tissue from further damage.
- Chronic pain, such as that caused by OA, is not protective but is pathologic, meaning that there is no reason for the pain to exist. 'Resting' an osteoarthritic joint will not improve healing nor prevent further tissue damage. Thus, the pain should be treated in the same way as any other disease process that limits quality of life would be treated.
- As with any chronic disease, the source of the problem (pain in this case) is likely to be complex and multifactorial, requiring that treatment be individually tailored to the patient. Advise the owner that treatment will be an ongoing and dynamic process that will include a drug/dosing trial to determine the initial effective therapy and changing therapy as the disease progresses.

SOURCES OF OSTEOARTHRITIS PAIN

- The sources of OA pain are multifactorial:
  - Pain of inflammation, which is a major component of OA pain.
  - Mechanical pain that results from reduced range of motion of joints, shortening of tendons/ligaments from disuse and muscle pain.
  - Central pain or central sensitization from activation of pain pathway components, such as the NMDA receptors in the spinal cord, that are not involved in the local OA pain. Once central sensitization (see Chapter 24) occurs, generalized pain may exist such that pain can be elucidated at sites remote from the original painful site. In addition, allodynia (pain elicited by non-painful stimuli) and hyperalgesia (exaggerated pain from normally low-pain stimuli) often occur.

Treatment of osteoarthritis pain

- Treatment should include weight loss:
  - Mild pain may decrease dramatically with weight loss, moderate pain will improve but will likely require analgesic therapy for adequate pain relief, and severe pain will definitely require analgesic therapy in addition to the weight loss.
  - Weight loss is often not possible without analgesia as pain is one of the most common causes of immobility.
- As with acute pain, moderate to severe chronic pain will require multimodal therapy, which could include both pharmacologic and non-pharmacologic options.

PHARMACOLOGIC AND NON-PHARMACOLOGIC THERAPY (SEE *TABLE 28.1*)

- The pharmacologic and non-pharmacologic therapy should address the following:

- **Inflammation**. A variety of NSAIDs are used in dogs and cats for chronic OA pain. A new anti-inflammatory drug, grapiprant, is now on the market in some countries for dogs and is being studied for cats.
- **Joint health**. Joint health may potentially be improved from the inside (e.g. administration of compounds that improve articular cartilage health, such as glucosamine chondroitin) and from the outside (e.g. exercising the patient to improve muscle strength, which improves joint stability). Weight loss, exercise, physical therapy, prescription joint diets, glucosamine, omega fatty acids, and polysulfated glycosaminoglycans (PSGAGs) (among others) potentially improve joint health. In some cases, such as stifle instability, surgery to improve joint stability may be used along with

Table 28.1 Drugs for use in the management of osteoarthritis pain in dogs and cats

Drug class/drug	Dose in dogs	Dose in cats	Adverse effects	Comments
NSAIDs: Pain of inflammation is a large component of OA pain and NSAIDs should be administered as a first-line therapy unless contraindicated				
Carprofen	2.2 mg/kg PO q12 h or 4.4 mg/kg once daily	Anecdotal: 2 mg/kg once every 3–5 days	All NSAIDs can cause GI (most common), renal, and hepatic adverse effects	NSAIDs that are FDA approved for dogs and cats will have specific dosing considerations on the label, which should be consulted before using that particular NSAID. **Not all of the NSAIDs listed here are actually FDA-approved for treatment of chronic pain in dogs and none are approved for treatment of chronic pain in cats in the USA.** However, unless otherwise indicated, the dosages listed here for both dogs and cats are commonly used to treat chronic pain
Firocoxib	5 mg/kg PO q24 h	Not known		
Deracoxib	1–2 mg/kg/day PO	Not known		
Piroxicam	0.3 mg/kg PO q24–48 h	0.3 mg/kg PO q 24–48 h		
Robenacoxib	1–2 mg/kg PO or SC q24 h	1 mg/kg PO or SC q24 h		
Meloxicam	0.2 mg/kg once followed by 0.1 mg/kg PO q24 h	0.1 mg/kg once followed by 0.01–0.05 mg/kg q24 h		
Piprant: Not a COX-inhibiting NSAID but is an anti-inflammatory drug				
Grapiprant (Galliprant®)	2 mg/kg PO q24 h for acute pain and commonly used at this dose for chronic pain	Currently in development	In safety studies at 15 times the dose for 9 months there was no effect on renal or hepatic systems. GI adverse effects were only mild and intermittent vomiting and soft stool. No ulceration. Slight reversible decrease in ionized calcium and albumin – likely no clinical impact	New and only drug in class. Piprant = prostaglandin receptor antagonist. Antagonizes receptor EP4, which is integral to inflammatory pain. No clinical studies on use for chronic pain but since the safety study was for 9 months, safety for chronic pain dosing has been extrapolated and the drugs is currently used in many clinics for treatment of chronic pain

(Continued)

Table 28.1 (Continued) Drugs for use in the management of osteoarthritis pain in dogs and cats

Drug class/drug	Dose in dogs	Dose in cats	Adverse effects	Comments
Anticonvulsants: Used to treat central pain, which is often a component of chronic pain				
Gabapentin	5–10 (anecdotally up to 50) mg/kg PO q6–12 h	5–10 (anecdotally up to 50) mg/kg PO q6–12 h	Sedation	Excellent adjunct for many drug protocols and effective for some patients when used alone. Inexpensive and wide safety margin. Analgesic dosages can be very individual so expect to work through several dosages to find the correct dose for each patient
Pregabalin (Lyrica®)	Maybe 2–4 mg/kg PO	Maybe 2–4 mg/kg PO	Sedation	More predictable dosing and rapid onset in humans but dog/cat pharmacokinetics and dose not known. More expensive than gabapentin. DEA Class V drug in USA
NMDA receptor antagonists: Used as adjunctive therapy to treat central pain since the NMDA receptor activation provides a major contribution to central pain				
Amantadine	1.25–4 mg/kg PO q12–24 h	3 mg/kg PO q24 h	RARE. No reports in veterinary patients. Sedation or agitation reported in humans. Maybe diarrhea	Technically called an 'antihyperalgesic' rather than a true analgesic. Use as a multimodal protocol with analgesic drugs (e.g. NSAIDs)
Ketamine	0.5 mg/kg loading dose followed by 2–4 µg/kg/ minute CRI for 2+ hours	0.5 mg/kg loading dose followed by 2–4 µg/ kg/min CRI for 2–4 hours	Maybe dysphoria but extremely unlikely at this dose	Ketamine infusions are used in human medicine to break the cycle of chronic pain. The patient receives an infusion and continues to receive other analgesic drugs, but the drugs are more effective. The duration of administration is unknown in both humans and animals. The best protocol would be to administer until pain is obviously decreased but set rates of anywhere from 0.5–24 hours have been used anecdotally

(Continued)

Table 28.1 (Continued) Drugs for use in the management of osteoarthritis pain in dogs and cats

Drug class/drug	Dose in dogs	Dose in cats	Adverse effects	Comments
Opioids: Other than tramadol in dogs and buprenorphine in cats, this class is rarely used for mild OA pain, but opioids may be added to the NSAID for moderate to severe pain or used with other drugs if NSAIDs are not appropriate for a particular patient				
Fentanyl patch	2–5 µg/kg/h	12.5 – 25 µg/kg/cat	Sedation, increased tone of certain sphincters (i.e. bile duct, urethra), respiratory depression, emesis, physical dependence, bradycardia, miosis, hypotension, constipation	Variable absorption and effectiveness
Morphine	0.5–2 mg/kg PO q6 h	0.2–0.5 mg/kg PO q6–8 h	Hypothermia or hyperthermia, respiratory depression, bronchoconstriction in dogs, GI; some dogs experience unacceptable constipation at doses exceeding 1 mg/kg	Can develop tolerance to pure mu agonists and need increasing dosages over time; most cats strongly dislike the taste. Low oral bioavailability but dose can be increased if no effect
Codeine +/– acetaminophen	0.5–2 mg/kg PO of the codeine portion q4–6 h	Same as dog but ensure that **codeine + acetaminophen is not administered to cats**	Sedation, constipation, high doses may cause respiratory depression	Analgesic activity probably due to its conversion to morphine. Weak analgesic with low oral bioavailability but dose can be increased if no effect. More consistent analgesia than tramadol
Buprenorphine	0.03–0.05 mg/kg OTM; 0.01–0.03 IM	0.03–0.05 mg/kg OTM; 0.01–0.03 IM	Rarely, may cause respiratory depression	Bioavailability from OTM administration is not as high as once thought, hence the new recommendation for higher OTM dosing
Tramadol	1–5 mg/kg PO q6–12 h	1–4 mg/kg PO q6–12 h	CNS effects (agitation, anxiety, tremor, dizziness) or GI (inappetence, vomiting, constipation to diarrhea)	Bioavailability is extremely variable and unpredictable in the dog, making tramadol best used as part of multimodal therapy. Do not use alone for treatment of moderate to severe pain. Bioavailability higher in cats but cats have a strong aversion to the taste of the drug. Mechanism of analgesia likely more due to serotonin/norepinephrine reuptake than to opioid effects

(Continued)

Table 28.1 (Continued) Drugs for use in the management of osteoarthritis pain in dogs and cats

Drug class/drug	Dose in dogs	Dose in cats	Adverse effects	Comments
Tricyclic antidepressants: Decrease pain through stimulation of the descending inhibitor pain pathway				
Amitriptyline	0.5–3 mg/kg PO q12–24 h	0.5–3 mg/kg PO q24 h	Sedation and anticholinergic effects	Provide only weak analgesia at best. Should be part of a multimodal protocol
Clomipramine	1–3 mg/kg PO q12 h for at least 4 weeks	0.5–1 mg/kg PO q24 h	Emesis, diarrhea, sedation, anticholinergic (dry mouth, tachycardia, etc.) effects; cats may be more sensitive than dogs	
Joint health modifiers: May not provide analgesia directly, but improving joint health may slow progression of the disease and may lead to pain relief				
Glucosamine and chondroitin sulfate	13–15 mg/kg chondroitin sulfate PO q24–48 h	15–20 mg/kg chondroitin sulfate PO q24–48 h	Maybe diarrhea	Not FDA approved and not regulated, so products should be investigated to ensure that they contain the amount of active ingredient that they advertise
Polysulfated glycosaminoglycan	5 mg/kg IM weekly	1.1–4.8 mg/kg IM every 4 days for six doses and then as needed	Dose-related inhibition of coagulation/hemostasis RARE	
Omega-6:omega-3 fatty acids	Ideal dietary ratio of omega-6:omega-3 fatty acids unknown; current recommendation is between 5:1 and 10:1	Ideal ratio unknown, probably similar to dogs	Maybe diarrhea	
Bisphosphonates: Inhibit osteoclasts, which cause breakdown of bone, which allows osteoblasts to build stronger bone, which decreases pain from instability				
Alendronate	10–20 mg/kg PO q24 h	3–5 mg/kg PO q24 h	Primarily GI, including nausea, vomiting, diarrhea and/or anorexia. May cause kidney toxicity. Pamidronate is reported to occasionally cause necrosis of the mandible	Used primarily for treatment of osteosarcoma but increasingly used in OA. Some patients will experience significant analgesia
Pamidronate	1–2 mg/kg diluted and administered over 2–4 hours IV or SC	1–2 mg/kg diluted and administered over 2–4 hours IV or SC		

CRI, constant rate infusion; FDA, Food and Drug Administration; GI, gastrointestinal; IM, intramuscular; IV, intravenous; NSAID, non-steroidal anti-inflammatory drug; OA, osteoarthritis; OTM, oral transmucosal; PO, oral; SC, subcutaneous.

medical management to decrease the progression of OA.

- **Central pain (central sensitization).** Drugs such as gabapentin (see below), amantadine, ketamine, serotonin/norepinephrine uptake inhibitors, and tricyclic antidepressants can be used to decrease central pain through direct impact on the receptor or neurotransmitters that contribute to central pain or through stimulation of the descending inhibitory pathway. Cannabinoids and non-pharmacologic techniques such as acupuncture (see Chapter 29) also effect this process. If pain is severe, a ketamine CRI may be beneficial in decreasing the severity of pain.

- **Pain from other sources such as sore muscles and trigger points from abnormal weight distribution caused by off-loading the painful limbs.** Many of the drugs already mentioned, along with acupuncture, massage, transcutaneous electrical nerve stimulation, and low-level laser therapy, may be useful. Although scientific evidence of efficacy is not available for all of these therapies, acupuncture does have robust scientific proof of efficacy and the other therapies have anecdotal clinical evidence.

Gabapentin for treating central pain

- Gabapentin is the most commonly used drug in this class. Although scientific studies are yet to be completed, anecdotally and clinically, gabapentin appears to be very successful in treating central pain.

- Dosing gabapentin can be difficult because of the wide range of dosages. Keep trying! Increase the dose, dosing frequency until pain relief, sedation (the major adverse effect), or ataxia (more common in older, large breed dogs) occurs. If sedation or significant ataxia occurs without pain relief, try a different treatment.

- Gabapentin does not have linear pharmacokinetics so increasing the dose will not increase the amount of drug absorbed by the same percentage as the dose increase.

OTHER ALTERNATIVE THERAPIES

- There are a number of emerging therapies that may be useful for treatment of OA pain:
  - Adult stem cells reportedly promote articular cartilage regeneration. Of the treatments listed here, this one has the most evidence of efficacy in veterinary patients. The therapy is currently expensive.
  - Platelet rich plasma supposedly contains compounds such as growth factors and cytokines that may stimulate soft tissue healing. There is no efficacy evidence in veterinary medicine.
  - Shock wave therapy produces acoustic waves that supposedly promote regeneration of bones, tendons, and soft tissues. The therapy causes moderate to profound discomfort and can only be done in sedated or anesthetized patients. There is no efficacy evidence in veterinary medicine.

Sample protocols for treating osteoarthritis pain

MILD PAIN

- Prescription 'joint' diet or addition of chondroprotective compounds to diet or administration of PSGAGs.
- NSAIDs as needed or regimen of several weeks of gabapentin.
- Consider addition of non-pharmacologic therapy such as acupuncture.

MODERATE PAIN

- As for mild pain but with consistent NSAID administration and non-pharmacologic therapy PLUS a regimen of gabapentin or amantadine.
- Consider addition of a mild opioid (e.g. buprenorphine), as needed.

- Consider addition of tricyclic antidepressant drug.

SEVERE PAIN
- As for moderate pain but with consistent opioid therapy; consider addition of more potent opioids.

- Consider ketamine CRI or treatment with bisphosphonates.
- Consider targeted therapy such as epidural injection of steroids for lumbosacral pain.

Further reading

Bennett D, Zainal Ariffin SM *et al.* (2012) Osteoarthritis in the cat: 2. how should it be managed and treated? *J Feline Med Surg* **14(1)**:76–84.

Comblain F, Serisier S, Barthelemy N *et al.* (2016) Review of dietary supplements for the management of osteoarthritis in dogs in studies from 2004 to 2014. *J Vet Pharmacol Ther* **39(1)**:1–15.

Godfrey DR (2005) Osteoarthritis in cats: a retrospective radiological study. *J Small Anim Pract* **46(9)**:425–49.

Hardie EM, Roe SC, Martin FR (2002) Radiographic evidence of degenerative joint disease in geriatric cats: 100 cases (1994–1997). *J Am Vet Med Assoc* **220(5)**:628–32.

Marshall W, Bockstahler B, Hulse D *et al.* (2009) A review of osteoarthritis and obesity: current understanding of the relationship and benefit of obesity treatment and prevention in the dog. *Vet Comp Orthop Traumatol* **22(5)**:339–45.

Rausch-Derra LC, Rhodes L (2016) Safety and toxicokinetic profiles associated with daily oral administration of grapiprant, a selective antagonist of the prostaglandin E2 EP4 receptor, to cats. *Am J Vet Res* **77(7)**:688–92.

Rychel JK (2010) Diagnosis and treatment of osteoarthritis. *Top Companion Anim Med* **25(1)**:20–5.

Sharkey M (2013) The challenges of assessing osteoarthritis and postoperative pain in dogs. *AAPS J* **15(2)**:598–607.

Acupuncture and Chinese medicine for pain management in dogs and cats

Patrick Roynard, Lauren R Frank, and Huisheng Xie

Introduction

Acupuncture is the most extensively researched modality under the umbrella of both Traditional Chinese Medicine (TCM) and Traditional Chinese Veterinary Medicine (TCVM) and has known local, segmental, central, and autonomic effects, many of which have the potential to strongly reduce nociceptive signals and pain perception. It has beneficial, studied effects for treating both acute and chronic pain, in addition to helping to prevent 'wind-up' or central sensitization that occurs in chronic pain states.

Other treatment modalities of TCM and TCVM include Chinese herbal formulations that are combinations of specific plants. Many of these formulations include specific chemical combinations that create a potent analgesic response, as well as containing many anti-inflammatory and immune-modulating effects. The wide variety of mechanisms targeted along the pain pathway using herbs and acupuncture – and the relative safety of these modalities – makes them a valuable option for a multimodal approach to pain management.

What is acupuncture?

- Acupuncture may be defined as the stimulation of specific point(s) on the surface of the body by insertion of a needle, resulting in a therapeutic or homeostatic effect.

- Recent research has indicated that most acupuncture points are located in the areas of decreased electrical resistance and/or increased electrical conductivity on the skin's surface.

- The morphologic basis of this bioelectrical phenomenon has been attributed to neural or vascular elements in the dermis or hypodermis.
- Recent histologic studies have revealed that acupuncture points are located in areas of dense innervation, neuroimmune modulation, high concentration of mast cells, lymphatics, and arteriovenous plexuses.
- Studies have indicated that many acupuncture points can have specific effects on the body, based on depth of stimulation. For example, acupuncture stimulation at Stomach 36 (ST-36) induced a decrease in sympathetic renal nerve activity (RNA) and mean arterial blood pressure (MAP) in rats under deep anesthesia. However, acupuncture stimulation at just the level of the skin of ST-36 did not induce any change of MAP and RNA. This suggests that the anatomic structures and physiologic effects of acupuncture points lie in the deeper tissues beneath the epidermis. Hence the inherent benefits in targeting deeper fascia using acupuncture over other superficial modalities such as transcutaneous electrical neuromuscular stimulation.

ACUPUNCTURE FOR TREATING PAIN

- Acupuncture targets all levels of the pain pathway including:
  - Transduction, transmission, modulation, and perception
- Response to acupuncture in pain states may be dependent on:
  - Training and skill level of practitioner.
  - Acupuncture method(s) and point(s) used.
  - Species and physiologic specificities of the patient.
  - Endogenous opioid capacities of the patient.
  - Type and pathophysiology of pain.
  - Accurate identification of the location of the pain.
  - Chronicity of the pain.

COMMON METHODS OF VETERINARY ACUPUNCTURE FOR PAIN

- Dry needle (**Fig. 29.1**):
  - Dry needle is the most commonly used technique.
  - Involves the insertion of fine, sterile needles into specific anatomic areas of the body ('acupoints').
  - Mechanical stimulation can be applied to the needles manually if electroacupuncture is not available and if the patient tolerates it.
- Electroacupuncture (**Fig. 29.2**):
  - Attaching electrodes and applying electric current to the needles.
  - Enables deeper penetration of electricity into the percutaneous tissue.
  - Promotes a more profound local and systemic analgesic response.

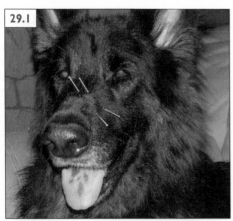

Fig. 29.1 Dry-needle technique. Four acupuncture needles are placed circling the area treated as shown in the picture ('Circle the Dragon' dry-needle technique for the local pain).

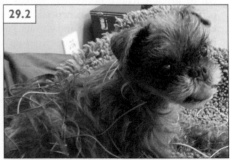

Fig. 29.2 Electroacupuncture technique. This dog is being treated for multifocal IVDD.

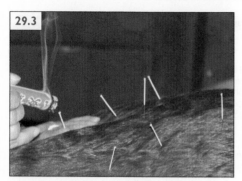
29.3

Fig. 29.3 Moxibustion technique. The stick of moxa is held close to the needles to provide warming *Qi*. Notice the hand of the practitioner positioned around the area treated to ensure the tolerability of the thermic stimulus provided.

- May be contraindicated in cases of seizures, neoplasia, pacemaker, or pregnancy.
- Aqua-acupuncture:
  - Injection of sterile liquids into acupuncture points in order to stimulate the point.
  - May stimulate a prolonged stimulus at the point.
  - Mildly caustic or autologous substances (i.e. blood) can be used.
  - Commonly used substances include:
    - Saline or water.
    - Polysulfated glycosaminoglycans.
    - Vitamin B complex.
    - Vitamin B12.
- Moxibustion (**Fig. 29.3**):
  - This involves the heating of either an acupuncture point or a needle inserted into an acupuncture point, with moxa, a type of bundled herb consisting primarily of *Artemesia* (mugwort).
  - Modern research indicates that the mechanisms of moxibustion mainly relate to the thermal, radiation, and pharmacologic effects of moxa and its combustion product.
- Low-level impulse light amplification by stimulated emission of radiation (LASER) stimulation of acupoints:
  - This is the stimulation of an acupuncture point using a low-level impulse LASER.

- A commonly utilized technique that may be better accepted than other acupuncture techniques in fractious animals.

EVIDENCE-BASED MECHANISMS OF ACUPUNCTURE

- Neuromodulation: targets multiple levels of the pain pathway:
  - Local (receptors in the skin and deeper tissues).
  - Segmental (peripheral nerves and dorsal root ganglion).
  - Central (spinal cord and brain):
    - Stimulates endogenous opioid pain pathways and others.
    - Many acupuncture meridians follow peripheral nerve pathways, for example: pericardium meridian and median nerve; gallbladder meridian and sciatic nerve.
- Autonomic effects:
  - Sympathetic nervous system (SNS):
    - Governing vessel point 26 (GV-26) and SNS:
      - Potent stimulator of endogenous catecholamines and dopamine.
      - Useful point in management of: shock, hypoventilation, bradycardia, hypotension, immediate postanesthetic period, neonates during cesarean section.
  - Parasympathetic nervous system.
- Other effects of acupuncture
  - Neuroparacrine.
  - Neurohumoral.
  - Neuroendocrine:
    - Modulates the hypothalamic–pituitary–adrenal axis.

ACUPUNCTURE CHANNELS/MERIDIANS

- These are pathways near the body's surface, where '*Qi*' is circulated.
- Each particular point along a pathway is a focal area of concentrated '*Qi*'.
- There are fourteen primary channels/meridians utilized in veterinary acupuncture:
  - Each acupuncture point is named by channel and number (*Table 29.1* and **Fig. 29.4**); for example, Liver 3 (LIV-3)

Table 29.1 Acupuncture points used for pain management in dogs and cats

Acupuncture point	Anatomic location	Common indications and uses in pain management and anesthesia
LI-4	Between the 2nd and 3rd metacarpal bones, at the midpoint of the 3rd metacarpal bone on the medial side. Around the level of the first phalanx (or where PI would insert). For cats: the alternative location is at the midpoint of the 2nd metacarpal bone on the medial side	Dental pain, facial pain, headaches
LI-11	At the lateral end of the cubital crease, one-half the distance between the biceps tendon and the lateral epicondyle of the humerus when the elbow is flexed	Elbow pain, inflammation
ST-36	Just off the lateral aspect of tibial tuberosity into the belly of the cranial tibialis muscle.	Gastrointestinal or abdominal pain, nausea, vomiting, gastric pain, gastric ulcers, food stasis
SP-6	3 cun* proximal to the tip of the medial malleolus in a small depression on the caudal border of the tibia	Uterine-associated pain
SI-3	Just proximal to the metacarpophalangeal joint on the caudolateral side of the 5th metacarpal bone	Cervical and spinal pain
SI-9	Caudal to the humerus, in a large depression along the caudal border of the deltoid muscle at its juncture with the triceps muscle (between the long and lateral heads of the triceps muscle, at the level of the shoulder joint). (Half the distance of the shoulder in dogs; in humans more caudal)	Otitis, shoulder pain, non-specific thoracic limb lameness
BL-23	1.5 cun* lateral to the caudal border of the spinous process of the 2nd lumbar vertebrae	Spinal pain, urinary tract-associated pain, pyelonephritis
BL-40	In the center of the popliteal crease. The point is found by directing the needle cranially towards the patella	Spinal and pelvic pain, pyelonephritis, urinary pain, coxofemoral joint pain
BL-60	In the thin fleshy tissue between the lateral malleolus and the calcaneus, level with the tip of the lateral malleolus. (The point is opposite but slightly distal to KID-3)	Pain during parturition, spinal pain, tarsal pain, headache, cervical pain, hypertension
PC-6	3 cun* proximal to the transverse crease of the carpus in the groove between the flexor carpi radialis and the superficial digital flexor muscles in the interosseous space. (Opposite TH-5 on the lateral side.) (Avoid tendons, needle medial aspect underneath tendons directing needle laterally)	Vomiting, anxiety, sedation, headache, chest pain, epilepsy
TH-5	3 cun* above the carpus on the craniolateral aspect of the forelimb in the interosseous space between the radius and ulna. (Directly opposite PC-6 on the medial aspect; finding TH-5 first is the best way to find PC-6)	Headache, febrile diseases, otitis, cervical pain, thoracic limb pain
GB-34	In the depression, just distal and cranial to the head of the fibula on the lateral side of the pelvic limb	Tendon and ligament pain, stifle pain
LIV-3	Between the 2nd and 3rd metatarsal bones, proximal to the metatarsophalangeal joint just prior to where the metatarsal bones fuse. (There is a large genetic variation of location of fusion in dogs so this point can have some anatomic variation between individuals)	Generalized pain, anxiety, pelvic limb lameness

(Continued)

Table 29.1 *(Continued)* Acupuncture points used for pain management in dogs and cats

Acupuncture point	Anatomic location	Common indications and uses in pain management and anesthesia
GV-26	In the philtrum (the vertical line on the upper lip and between the nostrils) at the level of the ventral limits of the nostrils in the non-haired skin	Shock, promotion of cardiovascular parameters during anesthesia and perianesthetic period, facial pain, spinal pain, IVDD
Hua-tuo-jia-ji	Between the vertebral bodies from TI to L7, 0.5 *cun** from the midline – just within the paraspinal musculature. Points are found inside the bladder meridian. (There are 19 acupoints on each side of the back)	IVDD, spinal pain
Bai-hui	Between the spinous processes of L7 and SI on dorsal midline. (Location of where lumbar–sacral epidurals are performed)	IVDD, pelvic limb pain
Jing-jia-ji	Immediately dorsal and ventral to the transverse processes at the level of the intervertebral spaces of CI/C2, C2/C3, C3/C4, C4/C5, C5/C6 (in humans also includes C6/C7 but these are not accessible in the veterinary patient)	Cervical pain, cervical myelopathies (including cervical IVDD, cervical vertebral instability/ligamentous hypertrophy, syringomyelia, Chiari and other craniocervical junction malformations)

* *cun*: A Chinese unit that is equal to the width of the individual's last rib. It is a unit of measure that approximates distances relative to the individual's own anatomy. This unit enables relative distances between individuals, breeds, and species. IVDD, intervertebral disc disease.

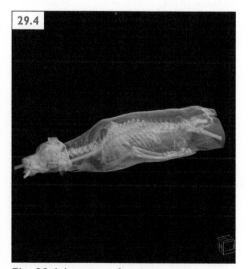

Fig. 29.4 Location of acupoints on 3-dimensional computed tomography reconstruction. Dorsal/lateral/oblique view of body with *Jing-jia-ji*.

is the third acupuncture point along the liver channel.

- Each particular point has a specific effect; for example, LIV-3 is commonly used in cases of general pain management.
- Classical points (*Table 29.1* and **Fig. 29.4**):
  - Points that are discrete or unique to channel pathways.
  - They are identified by their Chinese *Pin-yin* name; for example, *Hua-tuo-jia-ji* is located lateral to the dorsal midline of the body. It is a classical point because it is not directly associated with any of the fourteen channels.
  - There are approximately 173 major classical acupuncture points in horses and approximately 66 points in small animals.

Herbal medicine

There are classical herbal recipes that have been used for over 4,000 years in China to treat a variety of ailments. Most of these ancient Chinese herbal formulas have between 10 and 20 different herbs and plants. Modern day use has improved product quality, minimized heavy metal contamination, and substituted herbs when ethically questionable and/or endangered animal, fungi, or plant species were classically used. Most herbal formulations contain multiple active components with balancing effects, similar to the common use of multiple drugs in Western medicine to counterbalance the possible side-effects of the main drug used (e.g. gastroprotectant used concurrently with glucocorticoids).

Therefore, the different constituents of herbal formulations should not be analyzed for their effect individually, but rather synergistically as a whole formula. Many herbal formulations are used in Asia for the treatment of osteoarthritic and neuropathic pain syndromes.

TOP FIVE HERBS USED IN SMALL ANIMAL ANESTHESIA AND PAIN MANAGEMENT (*TABLE 29.2*)

- Shen Tong Zhu Yu Tang (Body Sore).
- Di Gu Pi.
- Da Huo Luo Dan (Double P II).
- Yunnan Bai Yao or Yunnan Pai Yao.
- Bu Gan Qiang Jin San (Tendon and Ligament Formula).

Table 29.2 Top five herbal formulas used for pain management in dogs and cats

Pinyin name	Brand names	Uses	Ingredients	Other
Shen Tong Zhu Yu Tang	Body Sore (JT)	Musculoskeletal pain, spinal pain, neuropathic pain	Ligusticum (*Chuan Xiong*), Notopterygium (*Qiang Huo*), Angelica sinensis (*Dang Gui*), Epimedium (*Yin Yang Huo*), Achyranthes (*Niu Xi*), Angelica pubescentis (*Du Huo*), Cuscuta (*Tu Su Zi*), Corydalis (*Yan Hu Suo*), Paeonia (*Chi Shao*), Eucommia (*Du Zhong*), Psoralea (*Bu Gu Zhi*), Myrrh (*Mo Yao*), Olibanum (*Ru Xiang*), Millettia (*Ji Xue Teng*), Persica (*Tao Ren*), Carthamus (*Hong Hua*)	One of the most widely used herbal formulations for any general pain management including osteoarthritis in dogs and cats
Di Gu Pi	Di Gu Pi	Osteoarthrosis, dysplastic joints (elbows, hips), degenerative joint disease, IVDD	Lycium (*Di Gu Pi*), Moutan (*Mu Dan Pi*), Rehmannia (*Shu Di Huang* and *Sheng Di Huang*), Gentiana (*Qin Jiao*), Psoralea (*Bu Gu Zhi*), Drynaria (*Gu Sui Bu*), Eucommia (*Du Zhong*), Alisma (*Ze Xie*), Salvia (*Dan Shen*), Angelica (*Du Huo and Dang Gui*), Phellodendron (*Huang Bai*)	Effectively for the treatment of osteoarthritis pain for Yin deficiency
Da Huo Luo Dan	Double P II (JT)	Paresis, paralysis, neuropathic pain, apparent excruciating pain, numbness, hyperesthesia, allodynia	Angelica (*Dang Gui*), Ligusticum (*Chuan Xiong*), Paeonia (*Chi Shao Yao*), Carthamus (*Hong Hua*), Myrrh (*Mo Yao*), Olibanum (*Ru Xiang*), Notoginseng (*Tian San Qi*), Draxonis (*Xue Jie*), Buthus (*Quan Xie*), Eucommia (*Du Zhong*), Dipsacus (*Xu Duan*), Drynaria (*Gu Sui Bu*), Morinda (*Ba Ji Tian*), Cibotium (*Guo Ji*), Achyranthes (*Niu Xi*), Psolarea (*Bu Gu Zhi*), Astragalus (*Huang Qi*), Strychnos (*Ma Qian Zi*), Aconite (*Fu Zi*), Lindera (*Wu Yao*), Licorice (*Gan Cao*)	Recommended usage is for short term (<2 months) at lowest effective dose, as risk of adverse gastrointestinal side-effects increases with duration of use

(Continued)

Pinyin name	Brand names	Uses	Ingredients	Other
Yunnan Bai Yao	Also known as 'Yunnan Pai Yao'	Potent antihemorrhagic, analgesia, antineoplastic, effective in: perioperative hemostatic control, ulcers (including gastric, colonic, and skin), hematuria, hematochezia, melena	Surmised main ingredients (others may not be listed): Notoginseng (*Tian San Qi*), Ajuga forrestii (*Li Zhi Hao*), Rhizoma dioscoreae (*Shan Yao*), Dioscorea hypoglauca and Dioscorea nipponica (*Chuan Shan Long*), Erodium stephanianum, (*Niu Er Miao*), Geranium thunbergii (*Lao Guan Cao*), Dioscorea parviflora (*Ku Liang Jiang*), Inulae cappae (*Bai Niu Dan*)	Actual formula is a 'secret recipe' owned by the Chinese Government
Bu Gan Qiang Jin San	Tendon and Ligament Formula	Tendinopathies, ligament injuries, IVDD	Lycium (*Gou Qi Zi*), Ligusticum (*Chuan Xiong*), Paeonia (*Bai Shao Yao*), Cornus (*Shan Zhu Yu*), Acanthopanax (*Wu Jia Pi*), Achyranthes (*Niu Xi*), Rehmannia (*Shu Di Huang*), Psolera (*Bu Gu Zhi*), Epimedium (*Yin Yang Huo*), Angelica (*Dang Gui*), Morus (*Sang Zhi*), Cinnamon (*Gui Zhi*)	

Table 29.2 *(Continued)* Top five herbal formulas used for pain management in dogs and cats

Clinical applications of acupuncture and herbs in pain management

NEUROLOGIC CONDITIONS
Intervertebral disc disease
- Commonly associated with nociceptive and earlier or later development of neuropathic pain.
- Acupuncture (specifically electroacupuncture) at local points surrounding the lesion (e.g. *Hua-tuo-jia¬ji, Bai hui*) and at distal points towards the limbs extremity (e.g. LIV-3, BL-60, SI-3). Suggested electroacupuncture protocol is 10–15 minutes of progressively increasing intensity at 20/40 Hz frequency (associated with endogenous opioid release), then 10–15 minutes of progressively increasing intensity at 80/120 Hz frequency (associated with non-opioid mediated endogenous pathways, such as serotoninergic and others), ending with 5–10 minutes of progressively increasing intensity at 200 Hz frequency (associated with nervous tissue modulation and regeneration).
- Electroacupuncture can be used both as an adjunct to medical/conservative management or during the postoperative recovery after surgical management (ideally starting from day 2, when the doses of IV opioids are progressively reduced).
- Clinically *Da Huo Luo Dan* can be used short term in appropriate patients, with severe myelopathies and/or neuropathic pain.
- *Bu Gan Qiang Jin San* can be utilized as a preventive to help reduce the incidence of IVDD in chondrodystrophic breeds of dogs.
- *Shen Tong Zhu Yu Tang* can be tried in cases of apparent neuropathic pain, such as in lumbosacral disease or lower motor neuron disorders.

Cervical pain and cervical myelopathies (Figs. 29.5–29.7)
- These conditions are very responsive to acupuncture (specifically electroacupuncture).
- Early and serial treatments are recommended for better outcomes (since neck pain can often relapse if treatment is discontinued too early/abruptly).
- Although the ideal recommendation remains with multiple treatments,

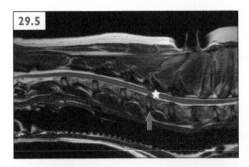

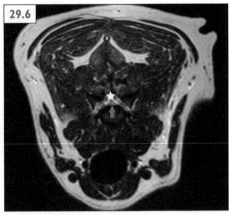

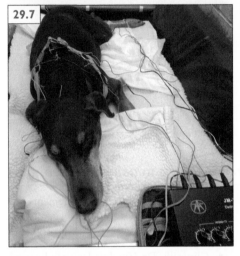

Figs. 29.5–29.7 Sagittal (**29.5**) and transverse (**29.6**) T2W MR images of a 9-year-old female spayed Doberman Pinscher with disc-associated cervical spondylomyelopathy or disc-associated wobbler syndrome. The spinal cord (star) is being displaced dorsally and compressed ventrodorsally by the intervertebral disc protrusion at C5/C6 (red arrow). The patient presented tetraplegic and recovered ambulatory status following surgical management with ventral slot at C5/C6, electroacupuncture, and herbs (including Double P II). (**29.7**) Patient receiving electroacupuncture in local (*Jing-jia-ji*, GV-14) and distal points (LI-11 and LI-4 in the thoracic limbs, LIV-3 in the pelvic limbs) during the postoperative recovery period. After any spinal neurosurgery, we consider the use of acupuncture in combination with standards analgesics (e.g. IV opioids) and other physical modalities (e.g. laser) to be standard of care.

cervical pain often has a pronounced response, as perceived by the caretakers, after just one electroacupuncture treatment.

- Many of the above mentioned IVDD herbal formulations can also be used in cases of cervical disorders.

'Nerve root signature,' radiculopathies, and neuropathic pain (Figs. 29.8–29.10)

- Signs of direct nerve involvement (sometimes called 'nerve root signature', such as in foraminal disc herniation) are an excellent candidate for acupuncture, specifically electroacupuncture.
- It is unclear if the sharp, acute pain encountered is a true example of neuropathic pain or a form of

nociceptive pain due to involvement of the local *nervi nervorum*.

- The role of the *nervi nervorum* in subsequent development of long-term neuropathic pain should not be underestimated, and electroacupuncture can help prevent this phenomenon.

Neuropathic pain

- Primary injuries of the peripheral nervous system including:
  - Nerve root signature (see above).
  - Sciatica.
  - Cases of self-mutilation or excoriation due to peripheral neuropathies (e.g. brachial plexus injury).
  - Obscure/nebulous pain syndromes (e.g. feline hyperesthesia disorder).

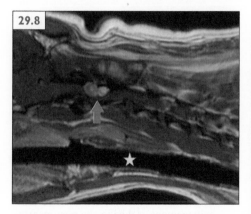

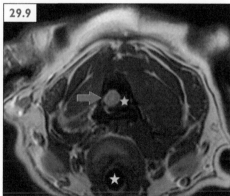

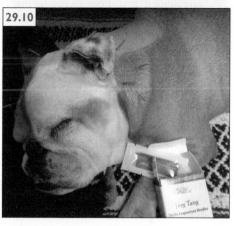

Figs. 29.8–29.10 Sagittal (**29.8**) and transverse (**29.9**) T1W postcontrast MR images of an 8-year-old female spayed English Bulldog with a peripheral nerve sheath tumor (PNST) of C2. The PNST is visible as a hyperintense lobulated mass (red arrow) invading the meninges and severely compressing the spinal cord (green star). The nearby trachea is identified (blue star). The tumor was surgically removed after dorsal laminectomy at C1/C2, durotomy, and rhizotomy, and the patient recovered ambulatory status post surgically. (**29.10**) Postoperative pain management of PNST and cases of rhizotomy can be challenging. The patient's level of pain was initially refractory to classical medical management with IV opioids. Judicious use of NMDA antagonists (here ketamine IV bolus at 5 mg/kg followed by a CRI) and acupuncture (here dry needle of Jing-jia-ji points, GB-20 and GB-21) can be of tremendous help in relieving pain due to acute insult to the nervous system, and prevent 'wind-up' and sensitization phenomenon.

- Given the refractory character of these cases to classical pain management methods, acupuncture (specifically electroacupuncture used early in the course of the disease) can be an effective modality for the management of neuropathic pain.
- Effects can be noted by the marked decrease in self-inflicted damage observed after treatment, as the translation in the veterinary medicine of the improvement of tingling, burning, or aching feeling reported in humans for various neuropathic pain condition (e.g. trigeminal neuralgia, diabetic neuropathy).
- In some types of neuropathic pain, such as tactile allodynia, non-nociceptive

nerve fibers such as A-β, faster than the C- and A-δ fibers traditionally associated with pain, become involved in the pain signal. The gate theory proposed in 1965, along with these changes in the function of nerve fibers, and with the ability of electroacupuncture to recruit A-α and A-β fibers prior to A-δ and C-fibers, might be an explanation to the ability of acupuncture to relieve neuropathic pain. For more chronic cases with central nervous system neuropathic pain, the lack of efficacy of acupuncture mentioned by some authors may be related to central sensitization but also remodeling of the dorsal horn and higher centers of pain processing.

'Nebulopathies' (e.g. feline hyperesthesia disorder/syndrome, Figs. 29.11, 29.12)

- When an actual physiologic explanation to the signs observed is unknown, but paresthesia/dysesthesia/pain are suspected, acupuncture, because of its relative safety, should be considered.
- In cases of regional allodynia, dysesthesia, or hyperpathia (i.e. in cases where the stimulus produced by the placement of the needle(s) is expected to be painful) the area affected might be 'surrounded' first, prior to narrowing the circle and getting in closer proximity during future treatments ('surround the dragon').
- Calming points located away from the lesion, and other techniques, can be used to render the animal more cooperative (**Figs. 29.11, 29.12**).

OSTEOARTHRITIS AND DEGENERATIVE JOINT DISEASE

- Acupuncture (specifically electroacupuncture if very painful or affected) is indicated for both acute and chronic pain from osteoarthritis and degenerative joint disease. Local points surrounding the lesion and distal points away from the joints (e.g. LIV-3, LI-4, SI-3) may be used.
- The amount of opioids received by the patient can alter the duration of treatment and frequencies applied. Endogenous opioid habituation and tolerance can develop if only low frequencies are used, therefore alternating the frequencies used in patients that are chronically treated can maximize response.
- Acupuncture can be used both as an adjunct to medical/conservative management or during the postoperative recovery after surgical management.

POSTOPERATIVE PAIN MANAGEMENT

- Acupuncture can be used to target local, segmental, and central components of the pain pathways.
- Acupuncture can help decrease wind-up or central sensitization, especially in surgeries that are expected to lead to chronic and/or excruciating pain (e.g. amputation, rhizotomy).
- Electroacupuncture can be used, but modified protocols and frequencies are advised for each patient, based on the concurrent use of synthetic opioids.

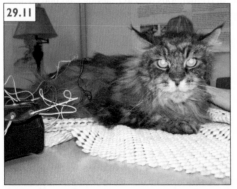 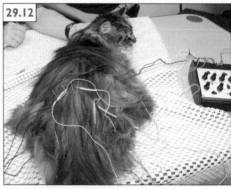

Figs. 29.11, 29.12 13-year-old spayed female Maine Coon receiving treatment for paroxysmal episodes of flank-biting, tail flicking, lumbar paraspinal allodynia, hyperesthesia, and hyperpathia. Diagnostics (CBC/chemistry, thoracic radiographs, MRI of the brain and lumbar area, CSF analysis) were unremarkable and feline hyperesthesia syndrome was suspected. Electroacupuncture treatment was applied to local area points, with the addition of dry needle at *Bai-hui* and GV-20. Acupuncture treatments, carried out every 3–4 weeks, resulted in marked reduction of the episodes' frequency and severity.

PALLIATIVE CARE AND ONCOLOGY

• The International Association for the Study of Pain (IASP) defined pain as "an unpleasant sensory and emotional experience associated with actual or potential tissue damage, or described in terms of such damage."

• This statement underlines the emotional/psychologic component of the perception of pain, difficult to assess with objective and repeatable criteria. Many suggest that acupuncture can be an invaluable asset to the patient's quality of life, especially in a busy and stressful environment such as a veterinary hospital; for example, acupuncture can help hospitalized patients relax and sleep.

• Acupuncture has been shown in numerous studies to help depression and anxiety and greatly improve quality of life in cancer patients. Its orexigenic and antiemetic benefits have been documented, such as the acupuncture point, PC-6 (*Nei Guan*). This point has a well-researched effect against postoperative and chemotherapy-related nausea and vomiting.

Conclusion

Acupuncture and herbs are relatively safe when practiced by skilled, accredited practitioners. They benefit the patient using numerous mechanisms that modulate different levels of the pain pathway. Acupuncture is valuable in the prevention of central sensitization, which can otherwise lead to chronic, excruciating pain if left untreated. Its multifaceted effects on the body make it an ideal therapy for analgesia, as an adjunct or sole therapy. It is now becoming increasingly understood that a multimodal approach to pain management (using both pharmaceutical and physical modalities such as acupuncture) is essential, as not all types of pain respond equally to the various therapeutic options available to the veterinary clinician. Acupuncture can also help ameliorate many of the side-effects of commonly used anesthetic drugs, as it can be a potent antiemetic and also stimulates the autonomic nervous system. Stringent training in veterinary acupuncture, with appropriate patient, herbal recipe, points, and acupuncture technique selection, are imperative for an optimum analgesic response. In addition, there can be varying species and individual sensitivities to acupuncture and herbs.

Further reading

Ashbury AK, Fields HL (1984) Pain due to peripheral nerve damage: a hypothesis. *Neurology* **34**:1587–90.

Barlas P, Lundeberg T (2006) Transcutaneous electrical nerve stimulation and acupuncture. In: *Wall and Melzack's Textbook of Pain*, 5th edn. (eds SB McMahon, M Koltzenburg) Elsevier Churchill Livingstone, Philadelphia, pp. 583–591.

Bove GM, Light AR (1997) The nervi nervorum: missing link for neuropathic pain? *Pain Forum* **6(3)**:181–90.

Campbell JN, Raja SN, Miyer RA *et al.* (1988) Myelinated afferents signal the hyperalgesia associated with nerve injury. *Pain* **32(1)**:89–94.

Campbell A (2016) History of medical acupuncture. In: *Medical Acupuncture: A Western Scientific Approach*, 2nd edn. (eds J Filshie, A White, M Cummings) Elsevier, Philadelphia, pp. 11–20.

Deng H, Shen X (2013) The mechanism of moxibustion: ancient theory and modern research. *Evid Based Complement Alternat Med* 2013:379291.

Hwang Y, Egerbacher M (2001) Anatomy and classification of acupoints. In: *Veterinary Acupuncture: Ancient Art to Modern Medicine*. (ed AM Schoen) Mosby, St. Louis, pp. 19–25.

Koltzenburg M, Torebjork H, Wahren L (1994) Nociceptor modulated central sensistization causes mechanical hyperalgesia in acute chemogenic and chronic neuropathic pain. *Brain* 117:579–91.

Li AH, Zhang JM, Xie WK (2004) Human acupuncture points mapped in rats are associated with excitable muscle/skin-nerve complexes with enriched nerve endings. *Brain Res* 1012:154–9.

Lindley S (2016) Acupuncture in veterinary medicine. In: *Medical Acupuncture: A Western Scientific Approach*, 2nd edn. (eds J Filshie, A White, M Cummings) Elsevier, Philadelphia, pp. 651–63.

Liu H, Li H, Xu M *et al.* (2010) A systematic review on acupuncture for trigeminal neuralgia. *Altern Ther Health Med* 16(6):30–5.

Melzack R, Wall PD (1965). Pain mechanisms: A new theory. *Science* 150(3699):971–9.

Ohsawa H, Okada K, Nishijo K *et al.* (1995) Neural mechanism of depressor responses of arterial pressure elicited by acupuncture like stimulation to a hindlimb in anesthetized rats. *J Auton Nerv Syst* 51(1):27–35.

Streitberger K (2016) Acupuncture for nausea and vomiting. In: *Medical Acupuncture: A Western Scientific Approach*, 2nd edn. (eds J Filshie, A White, M Cummings) Elsevier, Philadelphia, pp. 376–93.

Teixeira MJ, Almeida DB, Yeng LT (2016) Concept of acute neuropathic pain. The role of *nervi nervorum* in the distinction between acute nociceptive and neuropathic pain. *Rev Dor. Sao Paulo* 17(Suppl 1):S5–10.

Torebjork H, Lundberg L, LaMotte R (1992) Central changes in processing of mechanoreceptive input capsaicin-induced secondary hyperalgesia in humans. *J Physiol* 448:765–80.

Yang B, Xu ZQ, Zhang H *et al.* (2014) The efficacy of Yunnan Baiyao on haemostasis and antiulcer: a systematic review and meta-analysis of randomized controlled trials. *Int J Clin Exp Med* 7(3):461–82.

Yu C (1995) *Traditional Chinese Veterinary Acupuncture and Moxibustion* (in Chinese). China Agricultural Press, Beijing, pp. 66–226.

Rehabilitation and pain management for veterinary patients

Stephanie A Thomovsky

Introduction

The use of physical rehabilitation (therapy) for pain control has become increasingly more common in veterinary medicine. Today there are multiple commonly used manual and physical agent modalities for pain relief (*Tables 30.1* and *30.2*).

The decision as to which type of therapy to use, manual or physical rehabilitation, depends on the underlying disease being treated and the goals of therapy. For example, if muscle contracture is treated, the goals are to lengthen the muscle tissue and improve muscle flexibility and extensibility. Thus, agents that improve blood flow and tissue elasticity are desired. A combination of warm pack, massage, continuous therapeutic ultrasound, and therapeutic laser should be considered in this example.

The advantages and disadvantages of using manual rehabilitation are:
- Ease of use.
- Inexpensive, many manual therapies do not require equipment.
- Large storage space is not necessary for manual therapy modalities.
- There is a learning curve for appropriate and successful use of these techniques.

The advantages and disadvantages of using physical agents for rehabilitations are:
- These modalities can be utilized to heal tissue.
- These modalities can be utilized to improve muscle strength.
- Proper instruction is needed prior to using many of these modalities.
- There is an expense associated with the purchase of many of these modalities.
- A larger storage space is needed to house this equipment.

Table 30.1 Manual therapy modalities to provide analgesia in dogs and cats

Manual therapy modality	Goal of therapy	Use
Massage	Increase circulation; warm tissue; stretch, elongate, improve pliability of tissues; relax and reduce tension; improve circulation and lymphatic flow; reduce stress hormones; relieve pain; improve endorphin release	Improve mechanical function in cases of chronic musculoskeletal abnormalities; maintain mobility following surgical fixation/repair
Joint mobilization	Improve joint mobility; reduce pain and reduce stiffness; improve flexibility	For pain, grade 1 and 2 mobilizations are recommended: **Grade 1 mobilization:** small amplitude movements with 3–4 oscillations/second; **Grade 2 mobilization:** large amplitude movements with 3–4 oscillations/second. All grade 1 and 2 mobilizations are performed in the range of motion opposite to that which is causing the pain (e.g. if pain is on extension – oscillations are performed in flexion)
Stretching	Improve flexion and extension of joints, muscles and tendons; elongate muscle/tendon unit	Improve muscle, tendon and joint flexibility following neurologic injury, immobilization and/or surgery
Range of motion	Reduce the effects of disuse and immobilization; preserve normal joint function/synovial flow	**Passive range of motion:** improves muscle and joint mobility when a patient is unable to physically move his or her own limb **Assisted active range of motion:** when the therapist assists the patient in actively contracting his or her muscle or joint; the therapist guides the active motion of the joint **Active range of motion:** when the patient voluntarily contracts his or her muscles without any assistance – improving muscle mass and strength

Table 30.2 Physical agent modalities to provide analgesia in dogs and cats

Physical agent modality	Types	Goal of therapy	Use/settings
Warm pack	Hot pack; heating blanket	Superficial heating; increase circulation; vasodilation; improve tissue elasticity; muscle relaxation; pain relief	Heats from skin surface to 1.5 cm below the surface
Cold pack (**Fig. 30.1**)	Cold pack; compressive cooling; cold immersion; ice massage	Superficial cooling; decrease circulation; reduce edema; decrease histamine release; decrease nerve conduction velocity; decrease muscle contraction; pain relief	Cools from skin surface to 1.5 cm below the surface
Therapeutic ultrasound (**Fig. 30.2**)	Warming	Superficial and deep warming; improve circulation	A frequency setting of 3.3 MHz heats 1–3 cm below the skin surface A frequency setting of 1.0 MHz heats 2–5 cm below the skin surface

(Continued)

Table 30.2 (Continued) Physical agent modalities to provide analgesia in dogs and cats

Physical agent modality	Types	Goal of therapy	Use/settings (see also Chapter 25)
Therapeutic laser (**Fig. 30.3**)	Photobiomodulation – light interacts with cells to produce biochemical change	Slow nerve conduction velocity; suppress substance P; improve lymphatic drainage; decrease inflammation; improve wound healing; pain relief	**Acute pain setting:** $2-4$ J/cm^2 **Chronic pain setting:** $4-10$ J/cm^2
Electrical stimulation (**Fig. 30.4**)	Transcutaneous electrical nerve stimulation (TENS)	Increase blood flow; reduce muscle tone. Pain control: EITHER by activating A-β fibers $\rightarrow$ activates inhibitory neurons in spinal cord dorsal horn $\rightarrow$ blocks transmission of pain signals from the periphery to the brain (high frequency/short pulse duration/low intensity), OR by activating release of endogenous opiates $\rightarrow$ stimulates analgesia (low frequency/high pulse duration/high intensity)	**High frequency/short pulse duration/low intensity** $\rightarrow 50-150$ Hz, $2-50$ µsec pulse duration **Low frequency/high pulse duration/high intensity** (aka acupuncture-like TENS) $\rightarrow 1-10$ Hz, $100-400$ µsec pulse duration
Aquatic therapy (**Fig. 30.5**)	Swimming, underwater treadmill	Reduce joint concussive forces; improve soft tissue mobility; increase nerve conduction velocity; improve coordination and circulation; reduce edema; endorphin and enkephalin release, which improves mood, relaxation and provides pain relief	**Interval training:** shorter time intervals of activity interspersed with frequent, short, intermittent rest periods; best for immediate postoperative patients and patients in pain **Endurance training:** longer time intervals of activity, less total rest; best for patients whose end goal is improved cardiovascular fitness
Acupuncture (see Chapter 29)	Needle, electroacupuncture, acupressure	A-δ fibers $\rightarrow$ act on interneurons $\rightarrow$ inhibit C fibers $\rightarrow$ analgesia	Activation of various acupressure points results in analgesia

Types of patients who benefit from physical rehabilitation

Physical rehabilitation is commonly used to treat surgical patients, obese patients, and athletes. Surgical patients are treated both prior to and following surgical procedures with physical rehabilitation. Obese patients or patients who are unfit and need to improve cardiovascular fitness are also good candidates for physical rehabilitation. The opposite is also true; very active, healthy dogs are also perfect patients for physical therapy. High-level athletes that require endurance or sprint training or those that would benefit from improved athleticism in agility circles are also good candidates for a physical rehabilitation program.

ORTHOPEDIC PATIENTS THAT MAY HAVE ONE OR MORE OF THE FOLLOWING CONDITIONS

- Osteoarthritis.
- Postoperative orthopedic surgery.
- Most commonly following postoperative stifle surgery such as tibial plateau leveling osteotomy, lateral suture repair, fracture repair, hip surgery (include total hip or femoral head ostectomy), or arthroscopy.
- Muscle strain (such as the iliopsoas strain).
- Postoperative amputation patients.
- Patients with muscle atrophy.

NEUROLOGIC PATIENTS WITH ONE OR MORE OF THE FOLLOWING CONDITIONS

- Back or neck pain.
- Postoperative spinal cord surgery patients.
- Postoperative craniectomy patients.
- Patients with neuromuscular disease.
- Patients with muscle atrophy.
- Patients with cognitive decline.

OTHER TYPES OF PATIENTS

- Obese patients.
- Agility dogs.
- Endurance training (sled dogs).
- Sprint training (racing Greyhounds).
- Cardiovascularly unfit patients.

USE OF PHYSICAL REHABILITATION FOR PAIN CONTROL

- Physical rehabilitation techniques can be utilized as an adjunctive treatment of pain. Manual therapies, including massage and joint mobilizations, are techniques used to reduce pain and inflammation (*Table 30.1*). Physical agent modalities, including warm and cold therapy (**Fig. 30.1**), ultrasound (**Fig. 30.2**) therapeutic laser (**Fig. 30.3**), electrical stimulation (**Fig. 30.4**), aquatic therapy (**Fig. 30.5**), and acupuncture, also are potential therapies used to control pain (*Table 30.2*).

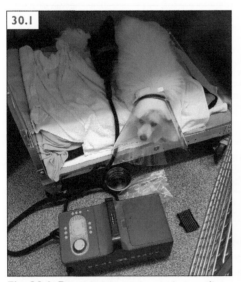

Fig. 30.1 Dog receiving compression cooling following stifle surgery.

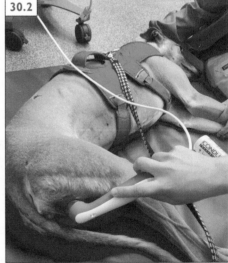

Fig. 30.2 Dog receiving therapeutic ultrasound for contracture of the hamstring muscles.

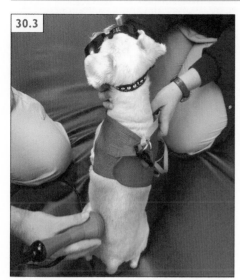

Fig. 30.3 Dog receiving therapeutic laser for hip osteoarthritis.

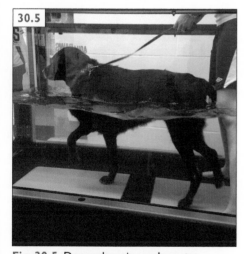

Fig. 30.5 Dog undergoing underwater treadmill therapy following surgical repair of the calcaneal tendon.

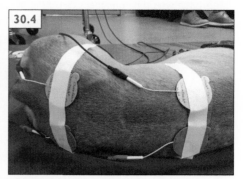

Fig. 30.4 Dog receiving transcutaneous electrical nerve stimulation (TENS) for lumbar spinal pain.

Further reading

Hanks J, Levine D, Bockstahler B (2015) Physical agent modalities in physical therapy. *Vet Clin North Amer Small Anim Prac* **45(1):**29–44.

Leem JW, Park EU, Paik KS (1995) Electrophysiological evidence for the antinociceptive effects of transcutaneous electrical stimulation on mechanically evoked responsiveness of the dorsal horn neurons in neuropathic rats. *Neurosci Letters* **192:**197–200.

Millard RP, Towle-Milard HA, Rankin DC et al. (2013) Effect of cold compress application on tissue temperature in healthy dogs. *Am J Vet Res* **74(3):**443–7.

Millard RP, Towle-Milard HA, Rankin DC et al. (2013) Effect of warm compress application on tissue temperature in healthy dogs. *Am J Vet Res* **74(3):**448–51.

Millis DL, Levine D (2014) (eds) *Canine Rehabilitation and Physical Therapy*, 2ⁿᵈ edn. Saunders, Philadelphia.

Anesthesia in shelter medicine and high-volume/high-quality spay and neuter programs

Jeff C Ko and Rebecca A Krimins

Introduction

Appropriate sedation and anesthesia is necessary for invasive and non-invasive procedures in shelter medicine, high-volume/high-quality spay and neuter clinics, and trap–neuter–release environments. Surgical procedures can range from spay and neuter to laparotomy and amputation. Other procedures such as tattooing and pre-euthanasia sedation all require proper selection of anesthetic and analgesic agents. Feral dogs and cats often require sedation or anesthesia prior to being handled. This chapter describes basic and advance anesthesia needs in these environments.

A typical high-volume spay and neuter program may require 9–10 minutes per surgery in order to achieve a goal of 30–40 surgical procedures daily per surgeon. This places a high demand on support personnel, speed of case turnover, surgical space, the availability of supplies, and monitoring equipment. In order to ensure successful anesthetic protocols capable of sustaining this high demand, three factors need to be considered: skilled personnel, effective and safe anesthetic drug combinations, and proper anesthetic monitoring.

Trained personnel are vital to support a successful program. Support personnel should be trained and familiar with anesthetic drug combinations, drug dosage calculation and record keeping, surgical preparation, instrument sterilization and packaging, anesthesia monitoring, and anesthetic and monitoring equipment and recovery care (**Figs. 31.1–31.3**). The required skills and areas of familiarity are listed in *Table 31.1*.

Other factors that need to be considered when dealing with shelters, high-volume/high-quality spay and neuter clinics, and trap–neuter–release environments are:

- **Environmental factors.** Crowded conditions, feral animals, budgetary constraints, animals with unknown history and vaccination status, minimal technical or personnel support.
- **Animal health status.** Neonates, estrus, pregnancy, pyometra, respiratory tract infections, parasitic infestations, heartworm disease, emaciation, animals suffering from cruelty/neglect.

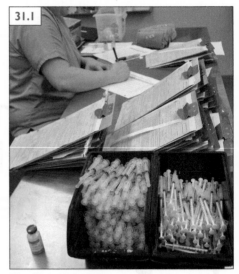

31.1

Fig. 31.1 Multiskills are needed for anesthetic dose calculation, proper drug withdrawal, record keeping, and surgical pack preparation in shelter and high-volume spay and neuter programs.

Table 31.1 Required skills and areas of familiarity for running a high-volume spay and neuter program

Area of familiarity	Familiarity of anesthesia and other drug protocols	Anesthesia and surgery preparation	Surgery and anesthesia maintenance	Anesthesia and postoperative recovery care
Skill and task requirements	Anesthetic drug combinations and their pharmacology Dose calculations for drug withdrawal of vaccines and antibiotics Record keeping for controlled substances Animal handling and drug administration	Endotracheal intubation and airway control Assembly of anesthesia machine, breathing circuit, and monitoring equipment Surgical field preparation for both animals and operational environment Set up and clean up of surgical instruments	Maintain proper surgical plane of anesthesia Recognize immediate anesthetic danger and be able to troubleshoot for both depth of anesthesia and equipment malfunction Provide surgical support for instrumentation and materials Safe animal transportation in and out of the operation room	Maintain body temperature and provide proper timing for extubation Recognize animal pain and provide proper treatment for delirium and pain Transport the animal from recovery to their cages, and ensuring smooth recovery Clean up and sterilize surgical instruments and recovery area Organize and provide anesthetic and surgical supplies

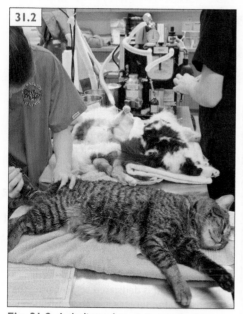

Fig. 31.2 A dedicated team is required to induce anesthesia and prepare animals for surgery. This approach facilitates the turnover of high-volume surgical case loads.

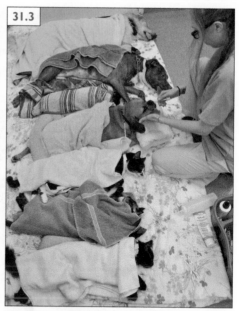

Fig. 31.3 High vigilance with properly trained/ skilled personnel is required to maintain a high quality of care when there are multiple animals at different stages of anesthesia recovery in a high-volume spay and neuter program.

Preimmobilization and anesthesia considerations

- Obtain or estimate the animal's age and body weight and assess its temperament prior to anesthesia.
- Physical examination should include auscultation of heart and lung sounds and an assessment of pulse quality and CRT. Body temperature should be obtained (if possible) for assessment of health status. Even with aggressive animals, a visual assessment is necessary.
- Fasting times prior to anesthesia are shown in *Table 31.2*.
- Factors to consider when using injectable anesthesia, inhalant anesthesia, or injectable followed with inhalant anesthesia for surgery include:
  - Injectable anesthesia may be used when an anesthesia machine and its related equipment is not available.
  - When using injectable anesthesia, if the animal becomes apneic, it will have to be intubated and ventilated and so an endotracheal tube and laryngoscope to

establish an airway plus an Ambu bag (see Chapter 1) to assist ventilation must be readily available. At best, a source of 100% oxygen should be available for either flow-by or insufflation during injectable anesthesia.
- Injectable anesthesia followed by inhalant anesthesia maintenance provides a time buffer for surgery turnover in multiple surgery cases in the operation room (**Fig. 31.4**).
- For inhalant anesthesia, the transportation of anesthetic equipment, oxygen source, and supply all play a role when performing trap–neuter–release. An integrated mobile unit equipped with both an anesthesia and a surgery suite is the ideal. It is critical to properly estimate the need of oxygen tanks, liquid anesthetic agents (isoflurane or sevoflurane) and CO_2 absorbent so that these materials are not depleted in the midst of a procedure.

Table 31.2 Fasting times prior to anesthesia for dogs and cats

Age of animal	6–16 weeks old	Older than 16 weeks
Food	Withhold for 2–4 hours before surgery, with 4 hours maximum	4–12 hours
Water	Free access	Free access

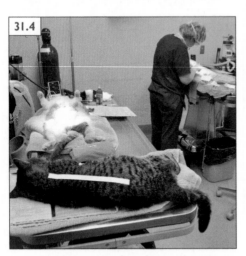

Fig. 31.4 Injectable anesthesia followed by inhalant anesthesia maintenance provides a time buffer for surgery turnover in multiple surgery cases in the operation room. In this photo, a surgeon is performing an ovariohysterectomy on an animal, while a second surgeon (not in the photo) is scrubbing and preparing for entering the surgery room. On the other operating table, a second animal is being maintained on inhalant anesthesia and a third animal is being maintained under injectable anesthesia. This enables a fast turnover of surgical cases. An anesthesia induction team is dedicated to preparing the next animal for surgery and an anesthesia recovery team is dedicated to recovering the animal waking up from surgery/anesthesia.

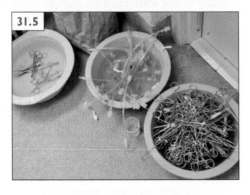

Fig. 31.5 A fast turnover of surgical instruments, surgical drapes, and endotracheal tubes, requiring a detailed cleaning and sterilization process, is essential for running a successful high-volume spay and neuter program.

- The efficiency of case turnover will rely on several factors:
  - The number of anesthesia machines (if using inhalant for anesthesia maintenance) and surgery tables available.
  - The number, and the skill, of the surgeons.
  - The number of support personnel to enable a rapid turnover of anesthetized animals and surgical instruments (**Fig. 31.5**).
  - The number of surgical packs and induction tables.
  - The induction, surgery, and recovery space.
- Some trap–neuter–release programs are conducted in the shelter environment, which is better than in the field because of controlled settings.

Anesthetic protocols

Ideally, anesthetic protocols for animals in shelter, high-volume spay and neuter programs, and feral environments should include some or all of the following properties:

- Wide margin of safety.
- Rapid induction of immobilization or unconsciousness.
- Excellent muscle relaxation.
- Provides intra- and postoperative analgesia.
- Effective and predictable for animals with a wide variety of ages, medical histories, and body sizes and conformations.
- Easy dose calculations and drug preparations for IV or IM administration.
- Small volume for rapid, smooth drug administration, especially for fearful or feral animals (**Fig. 31.6**).
- Being able to antagonize sedation or anesthesia will allow for faster recovery and improve efficiency of space utilization if necessary.
- Minimal cardiorespiratory side-effects.
- Versatility of dosage and capable of inducing a wide range of anesthetic depth ranging from mild sedation to a surgical plane of anesthesia in dogs and cats.
- Allow rapid and smooth recovery.
- Economical for drug cost.
- Minimal use of controlled substances.
- Commercially available and with a long shelf-life.

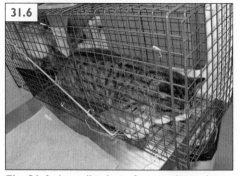

Fig. 31.6 A small volume for anesthetic drug administration, with a predictable sedative result, is important for the safety of both personnel and patients when handling feral animals.

TILETAMINE/ZOLAZEPAM (TELAZOL® OR ZOLETIL®), BUTORPHANOL (TORBUGESIC®), DEXMEDETOMIDINE (DEXDOMITOR®)

- The recommended anesthetic combination for shelter anesthesia is TTDex since it fits most of the aforementioned requirements. The dexmedetomidine may be substituted with medetomidine (TTD).
- Full details of the composition of TTDex and TTD can be found in Chapter 9.

Advantages of TTDex

- In the authors' clinical experience, TTDex can be stored at room temperature for up to 1–2 months following reconstitution, as it induces a constancy of anesthesia during this period. This assessment was based on the same anesthetic response of the patient when administered freshly made or as a 2-month-old mixture.
- Same drug combination can be used in dogs and cats using the same dose rate and induces a similar and consistent anesthetic response.
- Rapid onset of action (within 3–5 minutes following a single IM injection).
- Various depths of anesthesia (sedation to surgical plane) are attainable depending on the dosage used.
- Each drug of the TTDex combination contributes to analgesia.
- The TTDex combination can be antagonized for faster recovery.
- The combination is economical and provides both the safety and efficacy necessary for anesthetic procedures performed in a shelter and the feral (trap–neuter–release) environment.
- One of the most significant advantages of using TTDex is that it induces a rapid onset of action with a single IM administration. In situations where IV injection is preferred, one-half of the listed IM dose can be administered.

Mild to moderate sedation (premedication)

- The dose is 0.01–0.015 ml/kg IM.

- This is a premedication dosage and is ideal for non-invasive procedures such as IV catheterization or bandage changes. It is also a recommended dosage for premedication in geriatric animals or animals with systemic illness.
- If general anesthesia is desired, an induction agent such as propofol, or an inhalant delivered via face mask may be used. The general anesthesia should be maintained with an inhalant. Alternatively, in an overall healthy animal, an additional 0.01 ml/kg of TTDex can be administered IV to induce general anesthesia.

Moderate to profound sedation (immobilization)

- The dose is 0.015–0.025 ml/kg IM.
- This dosage is useful for diagnostic procedures (e.g. hip radiography) or moderately painful surgical procedures such as feline castration, laceration repair, simple dental procedures, suture removal, or deep ear cleaning. TTDex is also recommended at this dose for pre-euthanasia sedation (see Chapter 32 for details).
- If an animal appears to be too light with this dose, a low dose of an inhalant anesthetic agent can be delivered via face mask (e.g. isoflurane 0.5–1.0%) or propofol (0.5 mg/kg IV) titrated until the desirable degree of anesthesia is reached.

Profound sedation to surgical plane of anesthesia

- The dose is 0.03–0.04 ml/kg IM.
- A dose of ≥0.03 ml/kg IM is appropriate for procedures such as ovariohysterectomy, amputation, or other similarly painful surgical procedures.
- A dose of 0.03–0.04 ml/kg IM will provide a surgical plane of anesthesia for 30–45 minutes.
- If the anesthesia needs to be extended beyond this point, an inhalant agent or additional TTDex IV (one-half of the original volume) may be given.
- At this dosage, dogs and cats will assume lateral recumbency within 3–5 minutes after IM injection and respiratory depression may be seen.
- These patients should be intubated and placed on 100% oxygen if apnea occurs.

Other considerations when using TTDex

- In order to take advantage of the rapidity of onset of TTDex, it is recommended that all the anesthetic and surgical tools necessary for the procedure are prepared prior to administration.
- **Remember:** When using injectable anesthesia, the higher the dose used, or the more frequent the repeat dosing, the longer the recovery will be.

Variations of TTDex

- Several other opioids can be used in place of butorphanol in the TTDex protocol. Hydromorphone (2 mg/ml), morphine (15 mg/ml), and nalbuphine (20 mg/ml) can be used to replace the butorphanol using the identical volume (2.5 ml) in the TTDex combination. The same dose rate can be used for sedation, immobilization, and surgery.
- Detailed dose rates for practical use are provided in *Table 31.3*. The dose chart for each injection volume is identical regardless of the variation of TTDex used. This means that the same dose chart can be used to calculate the injection volume of TTDex, Telazol–morphine–Dexdomitor (TMDx), Telazol–hydromophone–Dexdomitor (THDex), or Telazol–nalbuphine–Dexdomitor (TNDex). The injection volume is the same regardless of whether TTDex, TMDx, THDex, or TNDex is used.
- Recently, the authors evaluated a combination that is similar to TTDex but with the butorphanol replaced with buprenorphine. In this combination, the 2.5 ml of the veterinary version of buprenorphine (Simbadol™, 1.8 mg/ml) is added to Telazol powder with 2.5 ml of dexmedetomidine, similar to TTDex; however, when dosing this combination using the same dosing chart, an additional dose of 88.5 µg/kg of buprenorphine is added to the 0.035 ml/kg of Telazol–Simbadol–Dexdomitor (TSDex) mixture. This amounts to a total of 120 µg/kg of buprenorphine being used in this combination. Adding 88.5 µg/kg of buprenorphine to the 31.5 µg/kg in the TSDex combination greatly increases the speed of onset of anesthesia and consistency of induction, and simultaneously provides a

Table 31.3 Dose rates for practical use of TTDex, TMDex, THDex, or TNDex. (Further dosing information can be found in *Table 9.17* in Chapter 9)

Body weight kg	lb	Premedication (0.01 ml/kg)*	Sedation (0.02 ml/kg)	Anesthesia (0.03 ml/kg)
0.45	1	0.005	0.01	0.02
0.91	2	0.01	0.02	0.03
1.36	3	0.01	0.03	0.04
1.82	4	0.02	0.04	0.05
2.27	5	0.02	0.05	0.07
2.73	6	0.03	0.06	0.08
3.18	7	0.03	0.06	0.09
3.64	8	0.04	0.07	0.10
4.09	9	0.04	0.08	0.12
4.55	10	0.05	0.09	0.14
5.00	11	0.05	0.10	0.15
5.45	12	0.06	0.11	0.16
5.91	13	0.06	0.12	0.17
6.36	14	0.07	0.13	0.19
6.82	15	0.07	0.14	0.20
7.27	16	0.08	0.15	0.22
7.73	17	0.08	0.16	0.23
8.18	18	0.08	0.17	0.25
8.64	19	0.09	0.17	0.26
9.09	20	0.09	0.18	0.28
9.55	21	0.10	0.19	0.29
10.00	22	0.10	0.20	0.30
10.45	23	0.11	0.21	0.31
10.91	24	0.12	0.22	0.33
11.36	25	0.12	0.23	0.34
11.82	26	0.12	0.24	0.35
12.27	27	0.13	0.25	0.37
12.73	28	0.13	0.26	0.38
13.18	29	0.13	0.27	0.40
13.64	30	0.14	0.27	0.41
14.09	31	0.14	0.28	0.42
14.55	32	0.15	0.29	0.44
15.00	33	0.15	0.30	0.45
15.45	34	0.15	0.31	0.46
15.91	35	0.16	0.32	0.48
16.36	36	0.16	0.33	0.49
16.82	37	0.17	0.34	0.51
17.27	38	0.17	0.35	0.52

Table 31.3 (Continued) Dose rates for practical use of TTDex, TMDex, THDex, or TNDex. (Further dosing information can be found in *Table 9.17* in Chapter 9)

Body weight kg	lb	Premedication (0.01 ml/kg)*	Sedation (0.02 ml/kg)	Anesthesia (0.03 ml/kg)
17.73	39	0.18	0.36	0.53
18.18	40	0.18	0.37	0.55
18.64	41	0.19	0.38	0.56
19.09	42	0.20	0.38	0.58
19.55	43	0.20	0.39	0.59
20.00	44	0.20	0.40	0.60
20.45	45	0.21	0.41	0.62
20.91	46	0.21	0.42	0.63
21.36	47	0.22	0.43	0.64
21.82	48	0.23	0.44	0.66
22.27	49	0.24	0.45	0.67
22.73	50	0.23	0.46	0.69
23.18	51	0.23	0.47	0.70
23.64	52	0.24	0.48	0.71
24.09	53	0.24	0.49	0.73
24.55	54	0.25	0.50	0.74
25.00	55	0.25	0.50	0.75
25.45	56	0.25	0.51	0.77
25.91	57	0.26	0.52	0.78
26.36	58	0.26	0.53	0.80
26.82	59	0.27	0.54	0.81
27.27	60	0.27	0.55	0.82
27.73	61	0.28	0.55	0.84
28.18	62	0.28	0.56	0.85
28.64	63	0.29	0.57	0.86
29.09	64	0.29	0.58	0.88
29.55	65	0.30	0.60	0.89
30.00	66	0.30	0.60	0.90
30.45	67	0.31	0.61	0.92
30.91	68	0.31	0.62	0.93
31.36	69	0.32	0.63	0.94
31.82	70	0.32	0.64	0.96
32.27	71	0.33	0.65	0.98
32.73	72	0.33	0.66	0.99
33.18	73	0.34	0.67	1.00
33.64	74	0.34	0.67	1.00
34.09	75	0.35	0.68	1.03
34.55	76	0.35	0.70	1.04

(Continued)

Table 31.3 *(Continued)* Dose rates for practical use of TTDex, TMDex, THDex, or TNDex. (Further dosing information can be found in *Table 9.17* in Chapter 9)

Body weight kg	lb	Premedication (0.01 ml/kg)*	Sedation (0.02 ml/kg)	Anesthesia (0.03 ml/kg)
35.00	77	0.35	0.70	1.05
35.45	78	0.36	0.71	1.06
35.91	79	0.36	0.72	1.08
36.36	80	0.37	0.73	1.09
36.82	81	0.37	0.74	1.10
37.27	82	0.38	0.75	1.12
37.73	83	0.38	0.76	1.13
38.18	84	0.38	0.77	1.15
38.64	85	0.39	0.77	1.16
39.09	86	0.40	0.78	1.17
39.55	87	0.40	0.80	1.19
40.00	88	0.40	0.80	1.20
40.45	89	0.41	0.81	1.22
40.91	90	0.42	0.82	1.23
41.36	91	0.42	0.83	1.24
41.82	92	0.42	0.84	1.26
42.27	93	0.43	0.85	1.27
42.73	94	0.43	0.86	1.28
43.18	95	0.43	0.87	1.30
43.64	96	0.44	0.87	1.31
44.09	97	0.45	0.88	1.33
44.55	98	0.45	0.89	1.34
45.00	99	0.45	0.90	1.35
45.45	100	0.46	0.91	1.36

* In general, a TTDex dose at 0.01 ml/kg is for premedication, 0.02 ml/kg is for profound sedation, and 0.03 ml/kg is for surgical plane of anesthesia. However, individual veterinarians and clinics will adopt their own approach to anesthetizing animals; for example, some will prefer to use TTDex as the preanesthetic medication, then follow with propofol induction and inhalant agent for maintenance, while others prefer to induce anesthesia with a single IM administration and finish surgery with only injectable anesthetic for maintenance. Therefore, the dosing rates listed in this Table should serve as a reference guideline. Each clinic is advised to factor in their own operational procedures and decide what is the best dosing rate to match up with their anticipated surgery turnover speed.

long duration of analgesia to the dogs and cats. The postoperative analgesic duration lasts for approximately 18–24 hours following a single premedication injection of buprenorphine.

- If TSDex is used without adding this additional dose (88.5 µg/kg) of buprenorphine, inconsistency of sedation and anesthesia are likely to occur. This is attributed to the fact that the low dose of buprenorphine (31.5 µg/kg) in this combination results in a slower onset of sedation and anesthesia. These lightly anesthetized animals need an isoflurane face mask to enable endotracheal intubation and maintenance for general anesthesia. The recovery, however, is relatively quick, but the analgesia is usually inadequate and requires additional supplementation with buprenorphine (up to 88.5 µg/kg).

Postoperative analgesia after TTDex anesthesia

- Depending on the type of surgical procedure being performed and the sensitivity of the animal to the painful stimulation, additional postoperative analgesia may be required. Opioids are frequently used for this purpose. The dose and type of opioid depends on the invasiveness of the surgery. Examples of postoperative analgesia are butorphanol (0.2–0.4 mg/kg IM or IV), hydromorphone (0.05–0.1 mg/kg IM or IV), morphine (0.25–0.5 mg/kg IM or IV), nalbuphine (0.4–0.6 mg/kg IM or IV), or buprenorphine (40–100 µg/kg SC or IV).
- **Note:** When TTDex (with butorphanol as part of the combination) is used, giving a different receptor type of opioid (i.e. mu receptor agonists such as morphine or hydromorphone) immediately after will allow these opioids to antagonize each other. Therefore, it is important to wait for at least 40 minutes to 1 hour from the initial injection before administering a different type of opioid as a postoperative analgesic. Ideally, the same receptor type of opioid should be used for postoperative pain management.
- A single dose of NSAID, such as carprofen (4.4 mg/kg SC), meloxicam

(0.2 mg/kg SC), or robenacoxib (1–2 mg/kg SC for dogs and cats), may be administered postoperatively. Alternatively, these NSAIDs may be given preoperatively or intraoperatively. Follow-up doses may be given orally for 3 days after surgery.

Reversal of TTDex

- Atipamezole is the most commonly used reversal agent for antagonizing the dexmedetomidine in TTDex.
- Use one-half the volume of the original TTDex dosage and administer IM.
- Cats can be reversed at any time after TTDex administration.
- In dogs, atipamezole should not be administered until at least 50 minutes after high doses of TTDex have been given. This will ensure that the tiletamine has been metabolized to a level that will not cause a rough recovery due to dissociative hangover. However, if a dose of TTDex <0.02 ml/kg IM has been used, the dog may be reversed earlier.

Side-effects of TTDex

- Hypoxia. Usually seen within 3–5 minutes of IM injection. The hypoxia is oxygen responsive and is resolved by providing 100% oxygen insufflation via a face mask, flow by, or endotracheal tube. The hypoxic response usually subsides with the start of surgical stimulation.
- Apnea may occasionally occur. If apnea does occur, the patient should be intubated and positive-pressure ventilation applied via an anesthetic breathing circuit or Ambu bag.
- Apneustic breathing pattern (inspiratory breath holding) may be observed. No treatment is necessary.
- Bradycardia is a baroreceptor reflex associated with hypertension, therefore no treatment is necessary. The concurrent use of an anticholinergic agent with TTDex is discouraged.
- Hypertension. No treatment necessary.
- In some patients, pain is seen on IM injection of TTDex.

Monitoring of anesthesia in shelters, high-volume/high-quality spay and neuter clinics, and trap–neuter–release environments

- In shelters, high-volume spay and neuter clinics, or trap–neuter–release programs, it is recommended that advanced anesthesia monitoring is carried out. If this is not feasible, then at least basic anesthesia monitoring should be performed.
- Basic anesthesia monitoring includes palpating pulses, observing mucous membrane color, monitoring respiratory rate/depth, assessing jaw tone, monitoring body temperature, and assessing eye position and general muscle tone.
- Advanced anesthesia monitoring includes all of the above plus the use of a regular or esophageal stethoscope, pulse oximeter, Doppler ultrasound and blood pressure monitor, ECG, and ETCO$_2$.
- Monitoring of postoperative pain is just as vital in the shelter animal as it is in private practice.
- Further details on monitoring anesthesia can be found in Chapter 6.

Further reading

Ko JC, Berman AG (2010) Anesthesia in shelter medicine. *Top Companion Anim Med* **25**:92–7.

Ko JC, Knesl O, Weil AB *et al.* (2009) FAQs – Analgesia, sedation, and anesthesia: making the switch from medetomidine to dexmedetomidine. *Compend Contin Educ Pract Vet* **31**:1–24.

Griffin B, Bushby PA, McCobb E (2016) The Association of Shelter Veterinarians' 2016 Veterinary Medical Care Guidelines for Spay-Neuter Programs. *J Am Vet Med Assoc* **249**(2):165–88.

Levy JK, Bard KM, Tucker SJ (2017) Perioperative mortality in cats and dogs undergoing spay or castration at a high-volume clinic. *Vet J* **224**:11–15.

Looney AL, Bohling MW, Bushby PA *et al.* (2008) The Association of Shelter Veterinarians veterinary medical care guidelines for spay neuter programs. *J Am Vet Med Assoc* **233**:74–86.

CHAPTER 32

Euthanasia

Jeff C Ko

Introduction

Euthanasia is derived from the Greek word meaning 'good death'. Veterinary professionals are often asked to perform euthanasia on research animals and pets for humane reasons. The American Veterinary Medical Association (AVMA) has published a detailed guideline for the appropriate euthanasia of animals, which should be consulted for further details.

This chapter primarily describes the situations in which the veterinarian is asked by the pet owner to perform euthanasia on an animal. Pet owners often request to be present during part of or for the entire euthanasia procedure. The euthanasia may take place in the veterinary hospital or in the owner's home or alternative place designated by the owner. The pet owner may also ask for a moment of grieving before their pet is euthanized. Veterinarians must structure the consultation to ensure that euthanasia is as painless and stress free for the pet as possible.

Principles of euthanasia

- The AVMA Guidelines indicate that the techniques used for euthanasia should rapidly produce a loss of consciousness followed by cardiac or respiratory arrest and, ultimately, loss of brain function (**Fig. 32.1**).
- Euthanasia techniques should be painless and minimize distress and anxiety prior to loss of consciousness. In addition, they should have a minimal negative impact on a person observing the euthanasia.
- The Guidelines also state that the choice of euthanasia agent or method is less critical if an animal is anesthetized or unconscious and does not regain consciousness prior to death.
- Euthanasia in general veterinary practice is largely classified into two categories: (1) euthanasia carried out by direct injection of euthanasia solution into a conscious dog or cat, or into animals under general anesthesia; (2) two-stage euthanasia where a sedative–anesthetic is injected into a conscious animal to induce profound sedation or general anesthesia prior to injection of the acceptable euthanasia solution (see below).

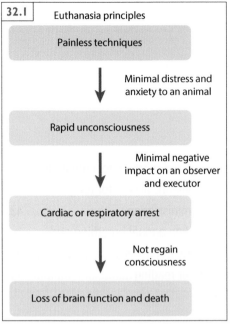

32.1 Euthanasia principles

Painless techniques

↓ Minimal distress and anxiety to an animal

Rapid unconsciousness

↓ Minimal negative impact on an observer and executor

Cardiac or respiratory arrest

↓ Not regain consciousness

Loss of brain function and death

Fig. 32.1 Key euthanasia principles should be followed to produce a rapid loss of consciousness followed by cardiac or respiratory arrest and, ultimately, loss of brain function.

- Oral administration has significant disadvantages when compared with parenteral administration, including lack of efficacy and predictability, lack of established drug dosages, difficulty of drug administration, and potential loss of euthanasia drug through vomiting or regurgitation. The oral route is generally unacceptable as the only means of administering a euthanasia drug. However, it is acceptable as a possible way to deliver a sedative prior to IV or IM administration of a euthanasia drug.

- Neuromuscular paralytic agents (e.g. succinylcholine, curare, atracurium, pancuroneum) or similar drugs that act as a neuromuscular blocking agent should not be used as part of the euthanasia protocol in an animal that is not properly anesthetized.

- IV injection is the preferred method of administering a euthanasia solution. If IV administration is not possible, an intraperitoneal or intracardiac injection may be used as an alternative. If either of these two alternative routes is required, the dog or cat should be profoundly sedated or anesthetized to minimize the pain and stress imposed on the animal.

- Some pet owners request oral administration of a sedative to their pets prior to euthanasia. In these cases, the dose and timing of administration of the sedative is very important (see *Table 32.1* for sedative drugs and doses).

Table 32.1 Anesthetic drugs used for sedation–anesthesia in dogs and cats prior to two-stage euthanasia

Sedative/anesthetic	Dosage (IM or SC)	Advantages	Disadvantages
Xylazine	Dogs: 2 mg/kg Cats: 3 mg/kg	Rapid onset sedation. Not a controlled substance	Vomiting, vasoconstriction, difficult IV drug administration
Medetomidine	Dogs: 50 µg/kg Cats: 100 µg/kg	Rapid and reliable onset of sedation. Not a controlled substance	Vomiting may occur in dogs and cats when administered SC. Severe vasoconstriction with associated difficult IV access
Dexmedetomidine	Dogs: 30 µg/kg Cats: 60 µg/kg	Rapid and reliable onset of sedation. Not a controlled substance	Vomiting may occur in dogs and cats when administered SC. Severe vasoconstriction with associated difficult IV access
Tiletamine/ zolazepam	Dogs: 10 mg/kg Cats: 20 mg/kg	Rapid and reliable onset of sedation. Facilitates IV injection due to minimal constriction of blood vessels	Controlled substance in most countries. Pain on injection
Acepromazine	Dogs: 0.5 mg/kg Cats: 1 mg/kg	Not a controlled substance	Slow onset of action. Sedation may not be as reliable. Hypotension makes venous access difficult

Euthanasia under general anesthesia

- Euthanasia under general anesthesia frequently occurs when a surgical repair is not possible following an exploratory procedure or when an animal suffers a severe injury prior to euthanasia.
- Sometimes, animals may be unconscious as a result of severe trauma or advanced disease or after an adverse surgical experience when the animal does not recover from general anesthesia and the owner elects euthanasia.
- Techniques to euthanize dogs and cats under general anesthesia are usually easily achieved as the animal is already unconscious or profoundly sedated, requiring minimal restraint.
- It is important to deepen the general anesthesia by turning up the inhalant vaporizer concentration or topping off with an IV anesthetic agent (e.g. propofol, alfaxalone, tiletamine/zolazepam, or ketamine) to prevent the animal from potentially suffering pain or regaining consciousness prior to euthanasia.
- Once the depth of anesthesia has been increased, the euthanasia solution

(e.g. sodium pentobarbital [**Fig. 32.2**] or saturated potassium chloride) is given as a rapid IV bolus. (**Note:** It is vital to ensure that if saturated potassium chloride is being used, the animal is under full general anesthesia [i.e. it is in an unconscious state] and not just under sedation. This is because it is inhumane to use saturated potassium chloride in a sedated animal as it is likely to cause pain prior to cardiac arrest.)

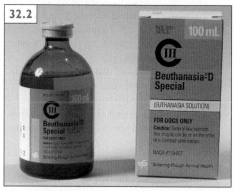

Fig. 32.2 Example of a commercially-available sodium pentobarbital solution for euthanasia.

Two-stage euthanasia: anesthesia–sedation prior to euthanasia

- Two-stage euthanasia reduces stress and anxiety for both the animal and the owner.
- It should be used when the pet owner wants to grieve with their pets for a few minutes prior to euthanasia. Grieving can take place while the animal is anesthetized and the euthanasia can be performed with minimal disruption.
- Frequently, 'at home' euthanasia requires a veterinarian to sedate the dog or cat prior to administration of the euthanasia solution.
- Some animals may be conscious but in pain, and two-stage euthanasia provides some relief to the pet, allowing the owner time to make the appropriate decision.

- Two-stage euthanasia allows preplacement of an IV catheter prior to euthanasia.
- There are times when venous access is difficult and IM administration of a sedative calms the animal, allowing for IV or an alternative route of euthanasia.
- Typically, two-stage euthanasia involves IM injection of an anesthetic agent followed by the IV administration of euthanasia solution.
- The anesthetic agents useful for IM injection in this procedure are xylazine, medetomidine, dexmedetomidine, tiletamine/zolazepam, and acepromazine.
- The dosages of drugs used for sedation–anesthesia in dogs and cats prior to two-stage euthanasia are listed in *Table 32.1*.

Drugs and solutions for euthanasia

BARBITURATE-BASED SOLUTIONS

- Several commercial barbiturate-based solutions are available. Most contain pentobarbital sodium (390 mg/ml) and phenytoin sodium (50 mg/ml) as the active ingredients. A dye is added to the formulation to distinguish it from other pentobarbital anesthetics intended for therapeutic use.
- The solutions cause death by inducing a barbiturate overdose, resulting in profound cerebral depression, respiratory arrest, and circulatory collapse. Cerebral death occurs prior to cessation of cardiac activity.
- The dose is 1 ml/4.5 kg (10 lb) IV or intraperitoneally.
- The advantages of using these solutions are that they are commercially available, effective, and easy to use. The main disadvantage is that they are controlled substances and strict recording keeping is required.

POTASSIUM CHLORIDE

- Potassium chloride (KCl) (10–20 mmol (mEq)/kg by IV bolus)

is an alternative euthanasia drug. A KCl overdose induces cardiac arrest by mimicking hyperkalemia, resulting in myocardial conduction blockage, cardiac arrhythmias (bradycardia, tall T-waves, prolonged Q-T interval, cardiac standstill), and eventually cardiac fibrillation.

- This method can only be used if an animal is adequately anesthetized (i.e. not just sedated), since sedation does not render the animal unconscious, and therefore the animal may still suffer KCl-induced pain (see above), as the cardiac arrest is painful.
- Chemical grade KCl dissolved in tap water until saturation can be administered at 1 ml/10 kg IV as a euthanasia solution for properly anesthetized dogs and cats.
- The advantage of using KCl is that it is not a controlled substance and it requires no record keeping. The disadvantage is that it is not a ready-to-use product and the animal must be properly anesthetized first to avoid any potential pain during the euthanasia procedure.

Intravenous access for drug administration

- All the proprietary euthanasia solutions are potentially irritating, which makes them difficult to be injected rapidly, so there is a greater opportunity for the venous access to be lost during the drug administration.
- Preplacing an IV catheter so that venous access is secured at a critical point will ensure an uneventful euthanasia.
- Two-stage euthanasia allows preplacement of an IV catheter in the sedated animal easily.

- The sedative used in two-stage euthanasia can affect vasoconstriction, causing increasing difficulty in placement of an IV catheter. Careful consideration is needed when choosing an appropriate sedative (see *Table 32.1*).
- It is important to have a trained nurse or technician available to assist in comforting the owner and, most important of all, to hold the animal correctly for injection of the euthanasia solution.

Avoiding agonal breathing and muscle spasms

- Agonal gasping is defined as spasmodic open-mouth breathing with contraction of the diaphragm and retraction of the hyoid apparatus that occurs at death.

- An agonal gasp occurs soon after the administration of any euthanasia solution in a percentage of dogs and cats.

- The use of two-stage euthanasia reduces the chance of an agonal gasp occurring. Administration of propofol, alfaxalone, or thiopentone immediately prior to giving the euthanasia solution reduces the frequency of agonal gasping, often abolishing it completely. Opened, left-over propofol from anesthetic induction can be saved and used for this purpose. Preplacement of an IV catheter will also facilitate propofol or alfaxalone administration.

- Propofol (4–8 mg/kg), alfaxalone (3–5 mg/kg), or thiopentone (10–15 mg/kg) can be used.

- Administering diazepam or midazolam (0.4 mg/kg IV) is an alternative method of minimizing the likelihood of agonal gasping.

Further reading

American Veterinary Medical Association (2001) Report of the AVMA Panel on Euthanasia. *J Am Vet Med Assoc* **218**:669–96.

American Veterinary Medical Association (2013) *AVMA Guidelines for the Euthanasia of the Animals: 2013 Edition.* American Veterinary Medical Association, Schaumburg.

British Veterinary Association (2016) *Euthanasia of Animals Guide*, 2nd edn. BVA.

Weng HY, Hart LA (2012) Impact of the economic recession on companion animal relinquishment, adoption, and euthanasia: a Chicago animal shelter's experience. *J Appl Anim Welf Sci* **15**(1):80–90.

Anesthetic dosage reference ranges

*	Authorized for veterinary use in the USA and UK
**	Authorized for veterinary use in the USA only
***	Authorized for veterinary use in the UK only
****	Authorized for human use in the USA and UK

Note: An indication that a product is authorized does not necessarily mean that it is authorized for all species listed in the monograph; users should check individual data sheets.

Acepromazine*	0.025–0.1 mg/kg IV, IM, SC. Max dose, 3 mg
Alfaxalone*	Dogs: 1–3 mg/kg IV; 0.1–0.15 mg/kg/min CRI Cats: 2–5 mg/kg IV; 0.1–0.18 mg/kg/min CRI
Amantadine****	Dogs: 3–5 mg/kg PO q24 h. NMDA receptor antagonist
Atipamezole*	Same volume as medetomidine or dexmedetomidine, IM
Atracurium	0.1–0.3 mg/kg IV; 2nd dose, 0.05–0.15 mg/kg IV, dose-dependent duration of action
Atropine*	0.02 mg/kg IV; 0.04 mg/kg IM
Bupivacaine	1–2 mg/kg for local anesthetic use in dogs and cats
Buprenorphine*	20–200 µg/kg IV, IM, SC; 40–200 µg/kg OTM. The larger the dose the longer the duration
Butorphanol***	0.1–0.4 mg/kg IV, IM, SC; 0.7–0.8 µg/kg/min CRI For butorphanol–lidocaine–ketamine CRI see Chapter 24
Carprofen*	Dogs: 4.4 mg/kg SC q24 h (UK: cats, 4 mg/kg SC or IV, one dose only); 2–4 mg/kg PO q24 h (dogs only)
Cisatracurium	0.2 mg/kg IV; 2nd dose, 0.1 mg/kg, IV
Deracoxib**	1–4 mg/kg q24 h (dogs only)
Dexmedetomidine*	Dogs: 2.5–20 µg/kg IV, IM; cats, 5–40 µg/kg IV, IM; 0.5–1.0 µg/kg/h CRI (cats and dogs)
Diazepam***	0.2–0.4 mg/kg IV; do not mix with any other anesthetic agent except ketamine. Precipitation will occur due to propylene glycol
Diphenhydramine****	2–4 mg/kg IV, IM
Dobutamine****	5–20 µg/kg/min CRI to effect
Dopamine****	5–20 µg/kg/min CRI to effect
Doxapram*	0.15–0.25 mg/kg IV, repeat dosing may be necessary
Endrophonium****	0.25–0.5 mg/kg IV
Ephedrine****	0.15–0.25mg/kg IV or 5–10 µg/kg/min CRI to effect
Epinephrine*	0.01–0.1 mg/kg IV
Etomidate****	0.5–2 mg/kg IV
Fentanyl***	2–40 µg/kg IV or 2–20 µg/kg/h CRI. For fentanyl–lidocaine–ketamine, see Chapter 24
Firocoxib**	Dogs and cats: 5 mg/kg PO q24 h
Flumazenil****	0.01–0.025 mg/kg IV, IM
Gabapentin****	Dogs: 3–5 mg/kg PO q24 h

Glycopyrrolate**	0.0075–0.01 mg/kg IM, SC; 0.005–0.0075 mg/kg IV
Grapiprant	Dogs: 2 mg/kg PO q24 h
Hydromorphone****	0.05–0.1 mg/kg IV, IM, SC
Ketamine*	3–6 mg/kg IM or IV when used with diazepam or other sedatives. For CRI see Chapter 24
Ketoprofen***	1–2 mg/kg IV, IM: dogs q12 h, cats one dose only
Lidocaine****	2 mg/kg for ventricular arrhythmias, up to 8 mg/kg IV. For CRI include morphine–lidocaine–ketamine, see Chapter 24
Liposome bupivicaine (Nocita)	Dogs and cats: 5.3 mg/kg (0.4 ml/kg) local infiltration
Medetomidine*	Dogs: 5–40 µg/kg IV, IM
	Cats: 10–80 µg/kg SC, one dose only
Meloxicam*	Dogs: 0.2 mg/kg SC or PO to start, then 0.1 mg/kg q24 h
	Cats: 0.1 mg/kg SC, one dose only
Meperidine****	1–4 mg/kg IV, IM
Methadone***	1.0–1.5 mg/kg IV, IM, SC
Midazolam****	0.1–0.4 mg/kg IM, IV, SC
Morphine****	0.25–1.0 mg/kg IM or SC in dogs and cats. For CRI see Chapter 24.
Morphine (Duramorph)	Preservative-free morphine for epidural use (0.1 mg/kg); give half the volume if performing spinal anesthesia. See Chapter 23
Nalbuphine	0.5–0.25 mg/kg IV, IM, SC
	For reversal of opioid mu agonists use 0.25–0.5 mg/kg IV, IM
Naloxone****	0.02 mg/kg IV, IM
Neostigmine****	0.01 mg/kg IV, IM
Oxymorphone****	0.05–0.2 mg/kg IV, IM
Pancuronium****	0.01–0.025 mg/kg IV
Phenylephrine****	5–10 µg/kg/min CRI to effect
Propofol*	Without premedication 6–8 mg/kg IV; with premedication 3–4 mg/kg IV. Giving 0.2–0.4 mg/kg of diazepam 45 seconds prior to propofol administration will reduce the induction dose of propofol by 33%; propofol CRI (loading dose: 1.5–2 mg/kg; CRI: 0.25–0.5 mg/kg/min)
Robenacoxib*	Cats only: 1–2 mg/kg PO q24 h for up to 3 days (in the USA) or 6 days (in the UK)
	Dogs and cats: 2 mg/kg SC 30 minutes before start of surgery (UK only)
Thiopentone	Without premedication 15 mg/kg IV; with premedication 10 mg/kg IV
Tiletamine–zolazepam*	For immobilization: 6–8 mg/kg IM (dogs); 10–12 mg/kg IM (cats) For induction: 2 mg/kg IV (dogs and cats)
Tolazoline**	1–2 mg/kg IV, IM
Tramadol****	2–10 mg/kg PO q12 h or q24 h
Vecuronium****	0.01–0.025 mg/kg IV
Xylazine*	Dogs: 0.25–0.5 mg/kg IM; 0.15 mg/kg IV
	Cats: 0.75–1 mg/kg IM; 0.5 mg/kg IV
Yohimbine**	0.05–0.2 mg/kg IM or IV

Index

Note: Page numbers in **bold** refer to figures in the text; those in *italic* refer to tables

Printed and bound by CPI Group (UK) Ltd, Croydon, CR0 4YY

18/10/2024

01776208-0015